Public Health Practice
in Australia

Public Health Practice in Australia
The organised effort

Second Edition

Vivian Lin, James Smith and Sally Fawkes
with Priscilla Robinson and Sandy Gifford

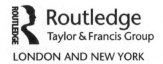

Routledge
Taylor & Francis Group

LONDON AND NEW YORK

First published 2014 by Allen & Unwin

Published 2020 by Routledge
2 Park Square, Milton Park, Abingdon, Oxon OX14 4RN
605 Third Avenue, New York, NY 10017

Routledge is an imprint of the Taylor & Francis Group, an informa business

Cataloguing-in-Publication details are available from the National Library of Australia
www.trove.nla.gov.au

Typeset in 11/13 pt Spectrum MT by Midland Typesetters, Australia
Printed and bound by CPI Group (UK) Ltd, Croydon, CR0 4YY

ISBN 13: 9781743314319 (pbk)

Contents

List of tables and figures

Tables

Figures

Abbreviations and acronyms

ABCD	Audit and Best Practice for Chronic Disease
ABS	Australian Bureau of Statistics
ACIR	Australian Childhood Immunisation Register
ACOSS	Australian Council of Social Services
ACSC	ambulatory care sensitive conditions
ACTU	Australian Council of Trade Unions
ADRAC	Adverse Drug Reaction Advisory Committee
AEA	Australian Epidemiology Association
AFL	Australian Football League
AHDG	Aboriginal Health Development Group
AHMAC	Australian Health Ministers' Advisory Council
AHMC	Australian Health Ministers' Conference
AHPA	Australian Health Promotion Association
AHPC	Australian Health Protection Committee
AHPRA	Australian Health Practitioner Regulation Agency
AHS	Area Health Service
AIEH	Australian Institute of Environmental Health
AIHW	Australian Institute of Health and Welfare
ALGA	Australian Local Government Association
AMA	Australian Medical Association
AML	Australian Medicare Local Alliance
AMS	Aboriginal Medical Service
ANAPH	Australian Network of Academic Public Health Institutions
ANCARD	Australian National Council on AIDS and Related Diseases
ANPHA	Australian National Preventive Health Agency
ANTA	Australian National Training Authority
ANZDATA	Australian and New Zealand Dialysis and Transplant Registry

ANZECC	Australian and New Zealand Environment and Conservation Council
ANZFA	Australia New Zealand Food Authority
ANZFSC	Australian New Zealand Food Standards Council
APHA	American Public Health Association
APHDPC	Australian Population Health Development Principal Committee
ARPANSA	Australian Radiation Protection and Nuclear Safety Agency
ARV	anti-retroviral therapies
ATSI	Aboriginal and Torres Strait Islander
ATSIC	Aboriginal and Torres Strait Islander Commission
AusAID	Australian Agency for International Development
BAT	British American Tobacco
BCG	Bacillus Calmette-Guerin
BF	Barmah Forest [virus]
BHOOC	Better Health Outcomes Overseeing Committee
BSE	bovine spongiform encephalopathy, commonly known as mad cow disease
CAPHIA	Council of Academic Public Health Institutions of Australia
CATI	computer-assisted telephone interview
CBA	cost-benefit analysis
CCNet	Cochrane Consumer Network
CDC	Centers for Disease Control and Prevention
CEA	cost-effectiveness analysis
CEDAW	Convention on the Elimination of All Forms of Discrimination Against Women
CEIPS	Centre of Excellence in Intervention and Prevention Science
CHF	Consumer Health Forum
CHINS	Community Housing and Infrastructure Needs Survey
CINDI	Countrywide Integrated Non-communicable Diseases Intervention
CIPHER	Centre for Informing Policy on Health with Evidence for Research
CJD	Creutzfeldt-Jakob disease
CLA	causal layered analysis
COAG	Council of Australian Governments
COPC	community-oriented primary care
COPD	chronic obstructive pulmonary disease
COSHG	Collective of Self-Help Groups
CQI	continuous quality improvement
CRC	cooperative research centre
CRCATSIH	Cooperative Research Centre for Aboriginal and Torres Strait Islander Health
CRIAH	Coalition for Research to Improve Aboriginal Health
CSDH	Commission on Social Determinants of Health
CUA	cost-utility analysis
DALY	disability-adjusted life year
DHC	District Health Council
DIAC	Department of Immigration and Citizenship
DIMIA	Department of Immigration and Multicultural and Indigenous Affairs

DoH	determinations of health
DoHA	Department of Health and Ageing
DOTS	directly observed treatment—short course
DPSEEA	Driving Forces, Pressure, State, Exposure, Effect, Action
EBM	evidence-based medicine
EFHIA	equity-focused health impact assessment
EHA	Environmental Health Australia
EIA	environmental impact assessment
EID	emerging infectious disease
EPA	Environment Protection Authority
ESD	ecologically sustainable development
FAO	Food and Agriculture Organization
FCGH	Framework Convention on Global Health
FCTC	Framework Convention on Tobacco Control
FOBT	faecal occult blood testing
FSANZ	Food Standards Australia New Zealand (successor to ANZFA)
GAVI	Global Alliance for Vaccines and Immunization
GM	genetically modified
GP	general practitioner
HACCP	hazard analysis critical control point
HBG	Health Benefit Group
HCV	hepatitis C virus
HIA	health impact assessment
HIC	Health Insurance Commission
HIPP	Health in Prisons Project
HIS	health impact statements
HIV/AIDS	human immunodeficiency virus/acquired immune deficiency syndrome
HPH	health-promoting hospital and health service
HPPC	health-promoting palliative care
HPV	human papilloma virus
HREOC	Human Rights and Equal Opportunity Commission
HRG	Health Resource Group
HWA	Health Workforce Australia
ICD	International Classification of Disease
IDD	iodine deficiency disorders
IEHW	Indigenous environmental health worker
ILO	International Labour Organization
IMR	infant mortality rate
IRISS	Institute for Research and Innovation in Social Services
ISCRR	Institute for Safety, Compensation and Recovery Research
IUHPE	International Union for Health Promotion and Education
JALI	Joint Action and Learning Initiative in National and Global Responsibilities for Health
LOAEL	lowest observed adverse effect level

MAE	Master of Applied Epidemiology
MCH	maternal and child health
MDGs	Millennium Development Goals
MMR	measles, mumps, rubella
MOsH	medical officers of health
MPH	Masters of Public Health
MSM	men who have sex with men
MTCT	mother-to-child transmission
MVE	Murray Valley encephalitis
NACCHO	National Aboriginal Community Controlled Health Organisation
NAGATSIHID	National Advisory Group on Aboriginal and Torres Strait Islander Health Information and Data
NAHS	National Aboriginal Health Strategy
NAHSWP	National Aboriginal Health Strategy Working Party
NAIHO	National Aboriginal and Islander Health Organisation
NCD	non-communicable disease
NDIS	National Disability Insurance Scheme
NEHS	National Environmental Health Strategy
NGO	non-government organisation
NHA	National Healthcare Agreement
NHIA	National Health Information Agreement
NHIPPC	National Health Information and Performance Principal Committee
NHISSC	National Health Information Standards and Statistics Committee
NHIMG	National Health Information Management Group
NHMRC	National Health and Medical Research Council
NHPA	national health priority area
NHS	National Health Survey
NIHIP	National Indigenous Health Information Plan
NOAEL	no observed adverse effect level
NOHSC	National Occupational Health and Safety Commission
NPCC	National Primary Care Collaboratives
NPHP	National Public Health Partnership
NPS	National Prescribing Service
NRT	nicotine replacement therapy
NWHP	National Women's Health Policy
OCS	Office of Chemical Safety
OECD	Organisation for Economic Co-operation and Development
OHP	Oregon Health Plan
OHS	occupational health and safety
OPAL	Obesity Prevention and Lifestyles
PBMA	program budgeting and marginal analysis
PBS	Pharmaceutical Benefits Scheme
PCM	prevention community model

PHAA	Public Health Association of Australia
PHC	primary health care
PHLI	Public Health Leadership Institute
PHOFA	Public Health Outcome Funding Agreement
PHRDC	Public Health Research and Development Committee
PIP	Poly Implant Prothese [breast implant]
PPP	public–private partnership
PSA	prostate-specific antigen
PYLL	potential years of lost life
QALY	quality-adjusted life year
QUM	Quality Use of Medicine
RACGP	Royal Australian College of General Practitioners
RCT	randomised controlled trial
RR	Ross River [virus]
SARS	severe acute respiratory syndrome
SMR	standard mortality rate
SOE	state of the environment
STI	sexually transmitted infection
SURE	Secure Unified Research Environment
TB	tuberculosis
TGA	Therapeutic Goods Administration
UN	United Nations
UNAIDS	Joint United Nations Programme on HIV/AIDS
UNEP	United Nations Environment Programme
UNFPA	United Nations Population Fund
UNGASS	United Nations General Assembly Special Session
UNHCR	United Nations High Commissioner for Refugees
UNICEF	United Nations International Children's Emergency Fund
WHO	World Health Organization

About the authors

Vivian Lin is Professor of Public Health at La Trobe University, Vice President for Scientific Affairs for the International Union for Health Promotion and Education and Senior Editor for Health Policy for *Social Science and Medicine*. She has been Chair of the Australian Network of Academic Public Health Institutions and served on the board of the Cooperative Research Centre for Aboriginal Health. She has held senior positions in a range of health authorities and non-government organisations across Australia, and is the co-author of *Health Planning* (2001) and co-editor of *Evidence-based Health Policy* (2003), *Health Policy in China* (2010) and *Intersectoral Governance for Health in All Policies* (2012). She consults on public health policy and system development for the World Bank, the World Health Organization and the UK Department for International Development, as well as Australian governments.

James Smith is an independent public health planning consultant and public health policy adviser to local government and its peak bodies. He is also a food safety risk-management consultant to the private sector in Australia. Jim is an Adjunct Associate Professor in the School of Public Health and Human Biosciences at La Trobe University and in the School of the Environment at Flinders University, where he teaches and researches environmental health policy and management. Jim's doctoral research was in reform and implementation of intergovernmental public health policy. He is a past President of Environmental Health Australia and former Editor-in-Chief of the journal *Environmental Health*.

Sally Fawkes is Senior Lecturer in Health Promotion and Leadership at La Trobe University where she teaches post-graduate subjects in public health policy, health promotion, and law and management in health. She has extensive national and international experience in health promotion policy development and practice. She has consulted for over a decade on leadership development and health system reform and capacity assessment projects for the World Health Organization, governments in Australia and Middle East and non-government health organisations. Her PhD was on the topic of health futures and the use of foresight methodologies in public health policy. She serves on the boards of Women's Health Victoria and the International Network of Health Promoting Hospitals and Health Services.

● About the authors

Priscilla Robinson is an epidemiologist and Senior Lecturer in the School of Public Health at La Trobe University. She has worked in surveillance and disease control in public health units in the west of England and in Victoria, Australia. She contributed updates to Chapter 12. Her expertise in these areas has led to increasing work in international health and disease control.

Sandy Gifford is Professor of Anthropology and Refugee Studies at the Swinburne Institute for Social Research, Swinburne University. She was the previous founding director of the La Trobe Refugee Research Centre at La Trobe University. Her background is in medical anthropology and her research has addressed ethnicity, migration, settlement and health in Australia.

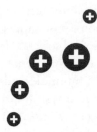

Introduction

Why our title?

Stories about health issues appear in the media almost every day, but each of us will read the information differently, putting our own slant on both the story and its evidence. Inevitably, any use we make of the story will be unique too.

A story about 'public health' in Australia is no different. For some people, public health means public hospitals or publicly funded health services. For others, it refers to the control of infectious diseases, or to the management of environmental health hazards, or to a set of programs aimed at disease prevention. The term may even provoke a sense of frustration in a person who has tried unsuccessfully to achieve a simple change that would have made their local community a healthier place in which to live.

We have chosen the title of this book, *Public Health Practice in Australia: The Organised Effort*, because we want to focus on what public health practitioners do, and to highlight some common threads that underlie all the seemingly disparate activities, ideas and entities included in the notion of public health. Our use of the term 'public health' refers to the social enterprise concerned with assuring the conditions in society that enable people to maintain and improve their health.

We are also focusing on the 'effort' involved in improving the health of the public. While others have written about and debated the concept of public health, and how to think about public health, we emphasise the 'doing' of public health. As we hope our book will demonstrate, the effort that is organised to achieve and sustain public health requires considerable knowledge, skill and wisdom. It is an effort that requires the contribution of many people, and it has been called both a science and an art form.

An evolving field of practice

As a field, public health has evolved over time, in terms of the priority issues that attract attention and the common practices adopted by its practitioners. It encompasses legislation and public policies, health services and community action that protect communities from a variety of health risks, prevent people from becoming ill from a range of diseases, and promote well-being. The practices are founded on the epidemiological, toxicological, behavioural and social knowledge bases that provide us with an understanding of the social and environmental determinants of health. Public health practice thus emphasises the impact of these factors on individuals, communities and populations, and aims to change these factors to bring about health outcomes.

The evolution of public health as a field has had a seemingly complex pathway. Along the way, there have been numerous debates—about the value of different scientific methods, the relative importance of particular health issues, the different approaches to intervening in the life of the community to improve health, whether interventions should be focused on individuals or the environment, the relative contribution of different disciplines and the range of philosophical positions that exist in relation to the roles of government, professionals, private industry and the community. Beneath these differences and arguments, however, are some principles that have provided a basic and constant frame of reference for public health practice. Upon this foundation, new methods, new understandings and new intervention strategies have been built.

Within the contemporary paradigm for public health practice, an emphasis on securing and maintaining basic conditions and resources for living (including housing, water, hygiene, food, sanitation, work, safety, nutrition and social stability) remains fundamental. A diverse range of practices are required to attain these conditions and resources, such as infrastructure development, building coalitions, policy advocacy and cooperation between different sectors, as well as the provision of information and the 'marketing' of health messages. These practices are now considered central to promoting health and well-being. Ensuring equitable access to health services also remains a cornerstone of public health practice. In terms of contemporary health service planning and delivery, the focus on equitable access to quality care is complemented by the recognition that services need to emphasise the prevention of problems as well as to provide continuity across the spectrum of prevention, treatment and rehabilitation, and community support.

The health of a population is not an incidental trait. It is central to economic and societal development, as well as being of major importance in the lives of individuals, families, communities and workplaces. How societies choose to invest, to prioritise and to act are core concerns of the organised effort called public health. Whether this organised effort leads to the best possible outcomes is also a key concern of the public health field. Yet there is no rule book for how to achieve the best outcomes. It is difficult to predict the extent to which science has universal application, in all communities, for all populations, under all socio-economic circumstances and in all health systems. It is also not easy to decide when societal norms demand a course of pragmatic action, rather than to adhere rigidly to the supposed scientific 'best practice'. Public health practitioners thus live with the everyday dilemma of making judgements about how and how much to interfere with individuals and families, communities, businesses and environments.

In reviewing contemporary practices in public health, this book recognises the importance, and inevitability, of history in shaping our current actions as well as our understanding. It also recognises that public health practices cannot be separated from the complex social and political systems within which they emerge and develop. The organised effort will always need to meet the challenges of changing systems and expectations. In updating this book for the second edition, we have found that these principles remain pertinent, while the specific issues, actors and contexts have evolved.

Why we wrote this book

This book arises from the collective experiences of the authors in teaching students from a mix of backgrounds, at both the undergraduate and postgraduate levels. We felt there was a need to introduce students (and practitioners who have moved into the field) to the breadth of concepts and practices that make up the field, particularly when people were asking for a book that would provide all the information they thought they needed on the discipline, and that would assist them to gain professional outcomes. We wanted to place the health issues that have received attention within the context of the structure of the health system. We wanted to discuss specific health issues and the range of possible intervention strategies within the context of changing population health needs. The aim was therefore to produce a book that would address the range of methods used in public health practice, their conceptual framework and the system components that underpin their delivery. As it is impossible to be comprehensive, given the continuous evolution of concepts and practices as well as their diversity, our aim was to focus on core concepts and activities, and offer illustrative examples through our choice of the health issues, situations and practices explored in this book.

Public health activities in Australia are delivered through a dynamic and mosaic-like system—by different professions, under different administrative arrangements, across different jurisdictions, and with different responsibilities and practices. The priority issues vary across geography and population groups, as well as over time. Many of the activities (such as control of communicable diseases, ensuring a supply of clean water and prevention of road accidents) are implicitly expected by members of the community as basic guarantees from government, yet these preventive efforts are virtually invisible to the public. Achievements are very much the result of organising resources and efforts across diverse segments of the community, as well as the contribution of public health practitioners.

The diversity of interests, professions and players has resulted in passionate debates, from time to time, about the field of public health—its definition, the priorities, the modes of practice, the essential skill base and the conceptual models. In this book, we do not argue for the hegemony of one approach over another. Indeed, we have seen students perplexed about the arguments within the field; we have also seen health professionals and decision-makers become frustrated with these recurring arguments. While we have seen the field move on from some of these interminable debates, we have yet to see a full embrace of the benefits of diversity.

We accept—indeed welcome—the simultaneous existence and legitimacy of different perspectives. We believe these perspectives are largely complementary, and therefore we believe the advancement of the public health effort will require better partnerships between different disciplines, professions, various government sectors and the public. These partnerships can be sustained by commitments to the values that are central to the public health enterprise: public interest, social justice and equity, and sustainable development.

Welcoming the reader to the field

While we respect the time-honoured tradition that books introducing a field should be written in as objective and balanced a fashion as possible, we want the subject of public health to come alive, as it has for us in our practice. To this end, we have included two sorts of case studies in the text. The first is a small 'challenge' that will appear at the beginning of each chapter to orient the reader to issues and concepts that are more broadly applicable in everyday life. The other kind of study is dotted throughout the chapters, either in a box or as a case study, and these will contain particular tellings of some of our fascinating public health stories. We hope that these stories will bring the colour and excitement of real public health practice into the book, and make the theories and concepts come alive.

The book is organised into five parts, each covering different dimensions of this organised effort. If the enterprise of public health depends on 'infrastructure', 'intelligence' and 'interventions', then Parts III and IV constitute the core of how public health in Australia is practised.

In *Part I*, the fundamentals of the field are covered. Chapter 1 introduces definitions and the debates, what public health practice involves, who makes up the body of professionals working in the field and what constitutes a public health system. Chapter 2 provides historical stories about where the field has come from, while Chapter 3 points to key health issues in Australia and the Australian health system today, including where public health sits in relation to the health sector.

Part II reviews the basic logic of public health practice by examining its basic toolkit. Chapter 4 reviews how our understanding of determinants of health has evolved, starting with a basic approach to understanding the distribution of health and illness in populations. Explanations for changing patterns of health and illness are offered in Chapter 5, based on the diverse disciplines that make up the public health knowledge base. Chapter 6 builds on 'discovery' and moves to 'delivery'. Approaches to acting on these health problems (that is, the fundamentals of public health practice) are discussed in this chapter, including what they are, how they continue to evolve, and how they are planned and evaluated. Chapter 7 moves to the system level and offers the tools for understanding why the system is so complex—that is, the political and economic underpinnings of decision-making.

Part III provides a guide to the basic intelligence required for public health action and the infrastructure needed to use the intelligence for public health program delivery. In other words, the foundation and the institutional arrangements in Australia are revealed. Starting with a contemporary history of the past 30 years in Australia, Chapter 8 reviews recent developments in Australia—from the renaissance of the 1980s through the neo-liberal threats of the 1990s to the more recent renewal of 'prevention'—and identifies the key players. Chapter 9 then sets out what authority is given for

public health activities in Australia, in particular how governmental and societal values come together into the legislative bases for public health action. Chapter 10 explains how public health intelligence—the informational and research base for action—is derived in Australia. Chapter 11 concludes the section by examining the basic human and financial resources that are necessary for public health program delivery, because public health action cannot happen without the right people and adequate funding.

Public health interventions are covered in *Part IV*. First, Chapter 12 begins with the fundamentals of surveillance as the basis for action, and explains how the concepts that developed with communicable diseases are applicable to other health issues. Chapters 13 to 16 discuss the main domains for public health action:

- health protection and its evolution from a focus on health hazards in the physical environment to a concern for ecological health
- preventive services and how public health programs are delivered through organised systems of personal health care
- health promotion and its shift from giving emphasis to changing individuals' lifestyles to securing socio-cultural and physical environments conducive to health
- how maintaining and restoring health and well-being for vulnerable populations shifts from a welfare orientation to an emphasis on empowerment.

Part V focuses on the contemporary decision points for public health policy and action. Insofar as public health policies reflect social values, political and community will and scientific evidence, they embody the judgement calls that are often made in the face of conflict and uncertainty. Chapter 17 considers how multiple interests must be balanced in making decisions, and implications for public health governance and priority-setting. Chapter 18 discusses emerging issues for Australia globally and contemplates an agenda for developing public health strategies and responses in the future. The formal and systematic use of foresight studies is suggested as a means of providing more rigour to policy-making that has long-term implications.

The book concludes with a brief endnote about ethical public health practice. The moral and ethical challenges in public health decision-making, which span the personal to the global, represent a recurring theme in public health work. In balancing science and societal interests, public health practitioners are faced constantly with ethical questions and dilemmas. This particular dimension is embedded throughout the various chapters in this book, as well as these final pointers.

This book is designed as an introduction to the principles and practice of public health. We hope that it captures the vast scope, endless complexities and ever-changing agenda in a form that can be understood by the uninitiated and enthuse the new practitioner. We also hope that it celebrates and reaffirms the work of established public health practitioners who may have arrived in the field through circuitous pathways.

The future challenges for the health of the public make it essential for the collective effort to remain organised. The initial local orientation of public health practice in the mid-nineteenth century broadened over the twentieth century to become national in scope. In the twenty-first century, public health practices and systems have global dimensions, as globalisation of trade and telecommunications and ecosystem changes become more important in influencing the health of communities. The specific problems will change, but the need for an organised effort will endure.

A note on institutions, names and terminology

A warning is necessary about the names and terms used in the field of public health in general, as well as the organisation of public health action in Australia in particular. As concepts and methods continue to evolve and are adapted to different national systems of public health practice and education, it is inevitable that there will be continuing debates about how words and terms are defined and used. New words and terms will also be introduced. We have provided a list of useful websites (see Useful resources)—various dictionaries, glossaries, encyclopaedias and handbooks—that provide an array of internationally recognised definitions. A search on the internet reveals that many public health organisations also develop and issue their own definitions.

Public health activities are typically funded, organised, coordinated or delivered by governments—albeit complemented by the resources and efforts of civil society and private-sector organisations. In Australia, as governments come and go, the names of government departments, statutory authorities and advisory committees change accordingly. In this book, we have tried to use the name of the body that existed at the time of the event under discussion, but when we discuss the generic roles or activities, we will adopt a generic term. So we variously refer to the national-level government either as 'the Commonwealth' or 'the federal government'. At the state/territory level, we have adopted the generic term of 'state health authority' to refer to the department with responsibility for health, unless we are referring to a specific event or policy during a specific time period.

It should also be noted that, just as government departments change names or become amalgamated or restructured over time, so do bodies created by government—be they statutory bodies or advisory committees. Organisational entities referred to in this book may well have changed or been replaced by the time it is in use. The more important point, in our view, is not the existence or the specific activities of any organisation, but the fact that particular issues were of concern, particular decisions were taken and a particular range of players were mobilised. These constitute the key characteristics of the organised public health effort in Australia and represent milestones in the field.

Acknowledgement—second edition

The authors wish to acknowledge the contributions made by a number of people to the first edition, namely Debra O'Connor, who was the instigator of this project, Gillian Sutton, who injected the element of 'art' into our thinking about the shape of the first edition, and Priscilla Robinson, Sue Chaplin and Sandy Gifford for their written materials. For the second edition, Priscilla again provided updates to the surveillance chapter while Bronwyn Carter worked tirelessly to support the authorship team in updating all chapters. We are grateful for the detailed feedback we received from users, which has contributed greatly to how we approached this second edition. We are also grateful to Lizzie Walton and everyone in the Allen & Unwin team for their assistance through all aspects of the process.

Vivian Lin, Jim Smith and Sally Fawkes

Part I

Background:
The basics

1

What is public health?
Definitions and applications

Challenge

Imagine your dearest friend or relative has fallen dangerously ill. A few hours later, someone else very close to you comes down with the same symptoms, and within just one day all of your neighbours are similarly affected. It becomes clear that you are the only person who will remain healthy in your area. What would your reaction be? Would you feel that your obligations had been fulfilled when you ensured that each of your ill friends was admitted to a hospital where they would receive the best possible care? Would you make sure that your neighbours received the same kind of care? Or would you also start to wonder what experience or environment these people had shared, and how it was that you were spared from illness? If so, you would have moved from thinking about your private concerns for particular people (and for yourself) to a broader concern for what has been called the public domain or the common good. These kind of concerns, and the activities that follow from them, shape an important area of effort in the public domain. It is called public health.

Introduction: Not just public hospitals or 'rats and drains'

Public health is not easy because different people hold strong opinions about what it is and is not. The meaning of 'public health' is very important to a wide range of people who work in the field (i.e. public health practitioners). In addition, the impact of public health actions is important to society as a whole.

Generally, what people think is meant by the term 'public health' depends on their awareness and level of engagement with the various elements that make up public health. Many are not aware of the scope of public health, and therefore the meanings and values ascribed to it are diverse. For example, some older people may think that public health is about past epidemics of flu or polio. A young mother may believe public health is all about child immunisation. A high school student may remember 'quit smoking' campaigns. A parent may conjure up an image from the 'Slip, Slop, Slap' campaign against skin cancer. A young person may recall a notice on an airport restroom door about condoms and safe sex. For others, public health means the public hospital system. Many also think of public health as the work of the historical health inspector—colloquially referred to as the 'rats and drains' part of local government's role of looking after 'rates, roads and rubbish'. Some health professionals might see public health as all those other health workers who 'do' public health work. In fact, all of these activities and messages are associated with modern public health practices; however, as you will see in the course of reading this book, the scope of public health is far greater than these important, but specific activities.

In the following chapters, we discuss some of the different ways in which the field of public health has been defined in the literature and how the practices of public health have been defined in different countries, along with the systematic underpinnings necessary for their delivery. Taking the perspective that what we do today is 'path dependent' (that is, historical decisions shape future choices) in relation to events over time and specific choices made by society, we will also provide a brief overview of the role of public health in history, and how the modern understanding of public health differs from the practices of our ancestors. Finally, we describe the health challenges facing Australia today, look at how well the Australian health system serves public health interests, and examine the place of public health in the Australian health system, including providing a sketch of its crucial relationship with other areas of public administration.

Society as the central feature: Not just the community or the country but also the world

> No man is an island, entire in itself; every man is a piece of the continent, and part of the main ... Any man's death diminishes me, because I am involved in mankind. (John Donne, in Carey 1990: 344)

As Donne observed in the seventeenth century, no person is truly isolated from others. This is particularly true of public health, which starts with a concern for many people, and is connected with almost everything important to people's lives, experiences and well-being. Historically, public health initiatives were concerned with the welfare of those people whom a particular community, city or nation-state considered worthy of care, and this might (or might not) have included all the people who lived in a particular place. One of the distinguishing features of public health as it is understood today is that it is concerned with the well-being of *all* people, largely (although by no means always) without regard to how important or valuable they are to society.

In 1958 the eminent medical historian George Rosen described the relevance of public health to communities, and then expanded the notion of public health to include nations and the international community. He noted that:

> Throughout human history, the major problems of health that men have faced have been concerned with community life, for instance the control of transmissible disease, the control and improvement of the physical environment (sanitation), the provision of water and food of good quality and in sufficient supply, the provision of medical care, and the relief of disability and destitution. The relative emphasis placed on each of these problems has varied from time to time, but they are all closely related, and from them has come public health as we know it today. (Rosen 1958: 25)

With regard to this wide range of problems, Rosen observed that:

> The manner in which these have been handled has always been connected with the way of life of the community and the scientific and technical knowledge available to it … In all countries, there are problems of community health that require social and political action guided by available knowledge … the horizon of health workers today can no longer be limited to the local or even the national community but must extend to the international community. Today, we are all members of one another; and so each in our own community, we must strive toward a goal of freedom from disease, want, and fear. (Rosen 1958: 495)

Rosen was guided by what he (and other public health experts of this period) described as 'humanism'—a general concern for the well-being of *all* people, regardless of their status in specific societies, or even the society from which they came. At the time he wrote his text, public health experts were beginning to explore the possibility of international health programs, delivered and coordinated through the emerging bureaucratic institutions,

the United Nations (UN) and the World Health Organization (WHO). Many people had long understood that epidemic disease, for example, was not confined to individual nations or communities and did not respect borders. However, prior to the latter half of the twentieth century, international health programs were restricted largely to the activities of colonial powers in their respective territories, and those of some charitable institutions, such as the Rockefeller Foundation. Subsequently, politicians and health experts around the world began to take important steps to approach public health from a global perspective, rather than being limited to the horizons of their own countries. Although this vision has not yet been achieved, a great deal of progress has been made in past decades to act upon this global perspective of public health. The international community is more interested in the health and well-being of people, regardless of which nation they come from. This is evident in international food-aid programs, war relief and coordinated efforts to control the spread of epidemic diseases from country to country. Events such as the 2003 Severe Acute Respiratory Syndrome (SARS) epidemic, the 2004 South-East Asia tsunami and 2009 H1N1 flu pandemic attest to the global nature of our health concerns and public health efforts.

The definitions

A science and an art

Given this breadth of concern and activity, what is a definition of public health? Rosen's statement about the focus of public health is similar to that provided by one of the early leaders of public health in the twentieth century, CEA Winslow (1877–1957). Winslow acknowledged that not all of the organised effort of public health could be achieved simply through the application of pure science. He saw public health as 'the science and the art of preventing disease, prolonging life, and promoting physical health and efficiency through organised community effort' (Winslow 1923).

The 'science' to which he referred was the research, biological, technical and medical knowledge used in the practice of public health, but the 'art' was more to do with the translation of that knowledge into practice. Like all arts, it relied on empathy and intuition rather than technique, depending on good (or fortuitous) timing, a sense of the subtleties of program implementation and comprehension of the relationship between parts of initiatives (for example, improved sanitation) to the whole (such as the improvement of general health).

Winslow catalogued a range of purposes that still occupy public health, including environmental sanitation, control of infections, education of individuals in personal hygiene, the organisation of health services for early diagnosis and preventive treatment, and the development of social machinery to ensure an adequate standard of living. His discussion of public health is important because it has been adopted, and subsequently updated, in many countries over the last century.

For example, the US Institute of Medicine, in its 1988 *The Future of Public Health* report, adopted a three-part definition for public health (Institute of Medicine 1988: 40–2). It expressed the profession's commitment to a healthy environment, the need to organise resources (human, financial, organisational and material) to achieve that end, and the importance of a framework that brings together all the different individuals, organisations and institutions that contribute to public health.

An Australian definition of public health

In Australia during the 1990s, senior representatives of Health Ministers from federal and state governments met regularly to participate in what was known as the National Public Health Partnership (NPHP). All Australian Health Ministers agreed on the following definition of public health in 1998 (NPHP 1998a):

> Public health is the organised response by society to protect and promote health and to prevent illness, injury and disability.

The definition confirms that public health is neither 'rats and drains' nor the public hospital system. Instead, it is a social enterprise that is concerned with the health of the public. Rather than listing all the issues that are addressed in public health measures, the definition recognises that the *organisation of effort* is key to public health, regardless of its specific goals. This 'effort' focuses on the population as a whole (or groups within it), and on the management of factors associated with health and illness.

The NPHP also defined three main components of public health work (NPHP 1998a). In doing so, it encapsulated the importance of knowing what is actually happening to the public's health, of organising interventions that make people healthier or less likely to suffer ill-health, and the key role of the infrastructural and legal framework within which such actions can take place.

According to these definitions, public health is a systematic approach to improve the health of, for and in the community. In that sense, it is a social enterprise—one that is concerned with the health

---

Box 1.1 Definition of public health

- The mission of public health is 'the fulfilment of society's interest in assuring the conditions in which people can be healthy'.
- The substance of public health is 'organised community efforts aimed at the prevention of disease and promotion of health'.
- The organisational framework of public health aims 'to encompass both activities undertaken within the formal structure of government and the associated efforts of private and voluntary organisations and individuals'.

Source: adapted from Institute of Medicine (1988).

> **Box 1.2 Main components of public health work**
>
> - **Public health intelligence:** Gathering and analysing information about the determinants of health, the causes of ill-health, and the patterns and trends of health and ill-health in populations.
> - **Public health interventions:** Developing policy; setting priorities for action; and implementing and coordinating services, strategies and interventions aimed at prevention, protection and promotion of the health of the community.
> - **Public health infrastructure:** Identifying infrastructure needs, such as workforce training and development, and information systems. This also involves ensuring that appropriate legislative and regulatory frameworks are in place.
>
> *Source:* NPHP (1998a).

of the *public*. The word 'public' is of particular significance in public health. Public health is an effort carried out *by* the public (community or collective effort) on behalf of or *for* the public (carried out in the public interest), making use *of* the public's actions (based on mobilisation of public resources, often using state investments and sanctions). But, as we describe in the next chapter, the definition of 'public' is also contested ground, and intimately connected with decisions made by specific societies (and/or their leaders) about who comprise their full and proper members. In contemporary Australia, for example, such debates have been evident in the consideration of whether asylum seekers, intravenous drug users and sex-industry workers are worthy recipients of government aid and attention.

Core public health function: What do public health practitioners 'do'?

Public health activities cover a broad spectrum of health issues (infectious diseases, chronic disease prevention), span a range of functions (epidemiology, health protection, health promotion) and include a range of interventions (policy, social marketing, community development, clinical service). Obviously, the scope of public health is diverse—public health is not concerned with a single issue and it has no single core activity. Therefore, just as the definition of public health can be very hard to pin down (even for people who practise it!), many people also find the question of what public health practitioners 'do' very difficult to answer.

Public health has always had close links with government, and in recent times changes in the organisation and ideology of governments around the world (and particularly in Western countries) have had a noticeable effect on resources for public health activities. Thus, there have been renewed attempts internationally to provide governments and communities with more specific definitions of what they should be able to expect from public health providers, what resources and capacities should exist in the community and what public health workers should do. This increased need for clear and unambiguous guidelines on the practice of public health has resulted in the emergence of the concepts of core public health functions and essential public health services in order to help define what services should be provided and what skills public health professionals should have.

Arising from the US Institute of Medicine's report *The Future of Public Health* (1988), a consensus approach was adopted by key professional organisations to elaborate on three major functions contained in that report: assessment, policy development and assurance. Box 1.3 presents the full statement.

Internationally, other countries were concerned about the impact of political changes on public health—for instance, the demise of the Soviet Union and the subsequent collapse of publicly planned infrastructure. The WHO surveyed public health leadership around the world in 1997 using a Delphi survey, which is a technique that encourages

Box 1.3 Essential public health services

Vision: Healthy people in healthy communities
Mission: Promote physical and mental health and prevent disease, injury and disability

Public health:
- prevents epidemics and the spread of disease
- protects against environmental hazards
- prevents injuries
- promotes and encourages healthy behaviours
- responds to disasters and assists with communities in recovery
- assures the quality and accessibility of health services

Essential public health services:
- monitor health status to identify community health problems
- diagnose and investigate health problems and health hazards in the community
- inform, educate and empower people about health issues
- mobilise community partnerships to identify and solve health problems
- develop policies and plans that support individual and community health efforts
- enforce laws and regulations that protect health and ensure safety
- link people to needed personal health services and assure the provision of health care when otherwise unavailable
- assure a competent public health and personal health-care workforce
- evaluate effectiveness, accessibility and quality of personal and population-based health services
- research for new insights and innovative solutions to health problems

Source: US Department of Health and Human Services (2001: 21).

comments by invited experts, stakeholders and other interested parties on forecasts of public health issues in order to develop consensus views through repeated rounds of questions and answers. The intent of the survey—in the face of reforms and cutbacks that have caused concern among people in the public sector in a number of countries—was to define the minimum functions required of an effective public health system. Box 1.4 lists the outcome of the survey. (Note that the WHO definitions combine the objectives and the services contained in the US definition.) Both statements attempt to encapsulate what public health practitioners do—today and into the future.

In Australia, a Delphi survey was also undertaken (NPHP 2000c) involving inputs from over 200 nominated public health leaders, including practitioners, researchers and policy-makers. Appendix A lists what Australians have defined as core public health functions. While the Australian definition mirrors that of the WHO in linking objectives with services (or functions), it differs

Box 1.4 Essential public health functions

- Prevention, surveillance and control of communicable and non-communicable diseases
- Monitoring of the health situation
- Health promotion
- Occupational health
- Protecting the environment
- Public health legislation and regulations
- Public health management
- Specific public health services (school health, emergency disaster management, public health laboratories)
- Personal health care for vulnerable and high-risk populations (maternal health and family planning, infant and child care)

Source: Bettcher, Sapirie and Goon (1998).

from previous efforts in identifying 'established' and 'evolving' practices. This approach recognises that health and disease end-points (such as communicable and non-communicable diseases and injuries) require similar actions for prevention and control, but also that specific strategies are developed for specific health issues that may change over time, depending on the state of knowledge. On this basis, there is a focus on common actions across health issues, as well as a recognition of the evolving nature of public health concerns.

Since the identification of key public health functions in Australia in 2000, similar work on defining core public health activities has been undertaken on a national level (such as in the United Kingdom) as well as on a regional basis (for instance, by the Pan American Health Organization and the Western Pacific Regional Office of the WHO).

Principles: The pride of the public health practitioner—values + pragmatism

Although public health issues are varied, drawing from widely differing spheres of knowledge, there are some key principles or shared features in public health practice that are considered to be defining qualities (Turnock 2001). Public health practitioners understandably have become proud of these qualities, listed in Box 1.5.

These principles encapsulate a concern to address the factors in society that might impede the fair distribution of benefits and burdens. Public health practitioners work to ensure that access to health resources is equitable, as well as to achieve equity in health outcomes. Given that poorer health is observed more in disadvantaged communities, public health practice is particularly concerned with strategies and actions that will improve the health of vulnerable populations.

To put the commitment to values in public health into practice, links with government are important, as government is the representative

> **Box 1.5 Key principles of public health practice**
>
> - A focus on prevention
> - A commitment to social justice and the fair distribution of benefits and burdens
> - Equity of access to health resources as well as equity in health outcomes and strategies focusing on improving the health of vulnerable population groups
> - A commitment to a dynamic agenda
> - An understanding of the need to balance science and society
> - A commitment to links with government and an appreciation that the process of achieving public health is inherently political
>
> *Source:* based on Turnock (2001).

institution of society responsible for social and economic development. This includes enforcing legislation (and therefore exercising the coercive powers of the state), facilitating and coordinating inputs and expertise from different parts of the community, and funding or providing specific programs to improve the health of the community. In different countries, this will vary according to history, culture, resources and the degree to which the government wants to intervene. All governments necessarily confront the dilemma of how far they should restrict the liberties of individuals in order to benefit the community.

The agenda of public health is expanding and evolving from the traditional domains concerned with control of infectious diseases and health hazards produced by poor sanitation, to encompass emerging issues that include chronic diseases and the promotion of healthy lifestyles. By the latter part of the twentieth century, warfare and HIV, along with substance abuse and health-care quality issues, presented new challenges to public health. While vigilance must be maintained over the 'traditional' interests of public health, it is likely that public health in the twenty-first century will expand and evolve to encompass issues that include climate change and biodiversity.

Prevention is a central value, objective and activity in public health. Prevention can be aimed at numerous issues—such as injury, specific disease, risky behaviour—and for numerous ends—such as quality of life, productivity and health-care resources. Ironically, when prevention is successful it is often invisible, and over time complacency can undermine prevention programs. Mass immunisation compliance, or the lack thereof, may prove to be a case in point.

The need to balance science and society relates to public health knowledge being derived from multiple sources. Medical and natural sciences inform the understanding of human biology, while micro-organisms and vectors contribute to environmental influences on health. Social and behavioural sciences inform the understanding of how society, culture and belief systems affect health perceptions and behaviours. Scientific knowledge is not absolute, however. Therefore, public health action often requires both assessment of the scientific evidence and an understanding of the community's expectations and aspirations. In their actions, public health professionals constantly need to strive for the right balance between the adequacy of scientific knowledge and an optimal social outcome.

Public health serves many communities, cultures and places. Inevitably, choices have to be made about what approaches would maximise the distribution of health benefits and health resources across society. At the core of these decision-making processes are differing expectations, values and perspectives, all of which must be considered and negotiated. Tensions and conflicts are difficult to avoid when choices and tradeoffs have to be made. Public health work is inherently political.

Public health achievements: Relevance to everyday life

Of course, pride in these characteristics of public health practice is meaningless if nothing is achieved by public health action. The effects of public health practice are not always immediate or dramatic—indeed, the benefits of public health initiatives may in some cases take many decades to emerge. Nevertheless, when the benefits do emerge, their effect is profound, and the health of entire populations of people is often improved substantially. For example, in the United States, the Centers for Disease Control and Prevention (CDC 1999) produced a list of the ten most significant health achievements during the twentieth century. They are listed in Box 1.6.

Australia has, of course, both benefited from the international dissemination of public health science and practice as well as contributed to that body of knowledge. In 2009 the Public Health Information Development Unit produced a report identifying public health actions that contributed to improvements in the health of Australians over the twentieth century. Some of the more prominent and recent measures are described in Box 1.7.

Basis of public health practice: An eclectic knowledge base

Significantly, all of these outcomes were achieved either in part or wholly by people and organisations 'doing' public health—that is, as a result of the key contributions that various disciplines add to the enterprise of public health. This includes, but is not limited to, epidemiology, psychology, sociology, cultural studies, political science, economics, organisational management, law and ethics, ecology and engineering (Naidoo & Wills 2001).

Epidemiology is the science of how often and why ill-health occurs in different population groups—that is, the who, what, where, when and how of disease causation. It is a starting point for public health intelligence. Epidemiological research has contributed to our understanding of the natural

---

Box 1.6 Ten of the most significant health achievements of the twentieth century

1 **Vaccination:** smallpox, measles, diphtheria, pertussis, rabies, typhoid, cholera and the plague are preventable.

2 **Recognition of tobacco as a health hazard:** smoking among adults has decreased.

3 **Motor vehicle safety:** deaths have decreased due to better engineering, wearing seatbelts, and decreased drinking and driving.

4 **Safer workplaces:** occupational diseases and injuries have decreased through safer production processes and control of work-related diseases.

5 **Control of infectious diseases:** the combination of clean water and antibiotics has contributed to improved health.

6 **Fewer deaths from heart disease and stroke:** smoking cessation, blood pressure control, early detection and better treatment have all contributed to decreased death rates.

7 **Safer and healthier foods:** micronutrient deficiencies have virtually been eliminated, and improved food hygiene and nutritional content have contributed to health improvement.

8 **Healthier mothers and babies:** infant and maternal mortality has declined significantly due to better hygiene, nutrition, access to health care and technological advances.

9 **Family planning and contraceptive services:** benefits have ranged from an improved social and economic position for women, to a decrease in infant and maternal deaths, to protection from sexually transmitted diseases (STD) and HIV/AIDS.

10 **Fluoridation of drinking water:** tooth decay in children, as well as tooth loss in adults, has been reduced significantly.

Source: Centers for Disease Control and Prevention (1999).

Box 1.7 Australian public health successes

• **Control of childhood vaccine preventable diseases:** As a result of specific vaccination programs since the introduction of the vaccination of children for diptheria in 1932, deaths from vaccine-preventable diseases have decreased by more than 99 per cent. In 2001, it was estimated that at least 78 000 Australian lives had been saved and substantial illness prevented through vaccinations for diptheria, whooping cough, tetanus, measles and poliomyelitis. The introduction of the Hib vaccine in 1993 has saved the lives of an estimated 100 children under the age of five. Although a vaccine for measles was included in childhood vaccination schedules from 1971, coverage rates remained low. As a result of national measles campaigns aimed at increasing vaccination coverage rates, measles notifications decreased from 4792 cases in 1994 to 45 cases in 2004, with only one death occurring during the period 1997–2004.

• **Control of adult influenza:** Following increased surveillance and vaccination programs, which commenced in 1999, hospital admissions and deaths rates from influenza declined, and influenza and pneumococcal vaccines for people aged 65 years and older were assessed as cost-effective.

• **Control of HIV/AIDS:** Following the first national HIV/AIDS strategy in 1989, infection rates slowed after 1994 and death rates fell from 6.4 males per 100 000 population in 1993 and 0.3 females per 100 000 in 1995 to one death per 100 000 for males and 0.1 death per 100 000 for females. The decline in mortality was attributed to safe sex and safer injecting campaigns, blood supply screening, infection-control guidelines and new treatments.

• **Preventing infant deaths from SIDS:** SIDS was the leading cause of death in infants in 1997–2001, peaking at 525 deaths in 1986. The number of SIDS deaths fell sharply from 11.4 per cent in 1997 to 7.5 per cent in 2001, attributed mainly to the change in prevalence of placing babies in the prone position to sleep. Public health researchers had identified that the sleeping position of infants was a preventable risk factor for SIDS, and an estimated 4084 babies' lives were saved after SIDS risk-reduction campaigns.

- **Road traffic safety:** Serious injuries and deaths resulting from road traffic accidents decreased substantially from the 1970s. In 1970, deaths from motor vehicle accidents peaked at 49 deaths for males per 100 000 population and eighteen for females, then fell to fourteen and six respectively by 2000. Serious injury rates decreased from more than five serious injuries per 100 drivers in crashes in 1964, down to two serious injuries per 100 drivers in crashes in 1995. Successful public health measures included compulsory seat belts from the 1970s, with enforced mandatory wearing of seat belts; mandatory wearing of motorcycle helmets (from 1973 for motorcycle drivers and their passengers) and of bike helmets (nationally from 1992); baby capsules and improved occupant restraints in motor vehicles; reductions in road speed limits, reduced speed zones (e.g. near schools), and traffic zones shared by motorists, cyclists and pedestrians; setting and monitoring blood alcohol limits (e.g. random breath testing, penalties and fines for drivers); driver education and testing; and road safety campaigns in schools and the mass media.

- **Reduction in tobacco smoking:** Since the 1970s, tobacco control measures have led to significant reductions in tobacco smoking rates and in tobacco-related diseases, contributing to increased longevity, improved quality of life, less disability and fewer deaths. Lung cancer deaths peaked in 1982, falling from 80 deaths in males per 100 000 population down to 50 deaths per 100 000 in 2000.

While there was a major decrease in the consumption of tobacco products from the mid-1970s, the death rates reflect the lag time evident in the relationship between tobacco consumption and the development of lung cancer. For females, death rates from lung cancer increased substantially after 1945 and have shown little evidence of the reduction seen in males. Regular daily smoking rates for those aged fourteen years and over fell by 40 per cent in the 20 years to 2004: from 29 per cent in 1985 to 17 per cent in 2004. Smoking rates for males have declined more sharply (by 43 per cent) than those for females (38 per cent), resulting in daily smoking rates of 18.6 per cent for males and 16.3 per cent for females in 2004.

Public health activities that have contributed to the long-term success in reducing tobacco smoking include identification and promulgation of the risks of active tobacco smoking (which had been known from 1957) and of passive smoking (the first NHMRC report on passive smoking was published in 1986); tobacco control legislation and bans; regulation and policing of sales to minors; QUIT programs, health education, promotion and social marketing campaigns; voluntary adoption of, and legislated, smoke-free premises—offices, restaurants, clubs and hotels, other entertainment venues and enclosed spaces; and monitoring and publicising information on population smoking practices (e.g. tobacco smoking rates, age of uptake and numbers of children in smoke-free homes).

Source: adapted from Gruszin et al. (2009).

history of disease and has enabled the identification and quantification of risk, thereby offering theories about causation. It contributes to the monitoring of population health trends and assists with public health action by providing the information base for targeting and planning interventions and their evaluation.

Psychology focuses on what people believe and

Box 1.8 The Sydney Olympics: A win for public health

How do you plan and implement public health services for Australia's largest sporting event, the 2000 Sydney Olympic Games? Some 11 000 athletes from 200 countries, 5100 officials, 11 000 media personnel and 100 000 visitors converged on Sydney for a two-week period. There was also an influx of 1.5 million people for the closing ceremony.

You begin five years beforehand by looking at the experience of previous cities holding summer Olympics. At previous Olympics, the major public health issues had been food-borne illness, heat-related illness and terrorist bombings. In 1997, New South Wales Health undertook a risk assessment that identified food-borne illness, terrorism, measles, rubella, pertussis, meningococcal and viral meningitis, tuberculosis, sexually transmissible infections, water-borne diseases and Legionnaire's disease as the potential major public health issues for the Sydney Olympics. The resulting public health action plan included:

- a comprehensive public health surveillance system for unusual patterns of injury and disease across Sydney
- Operation Foodwatch, which involved a systematic audit of Sydney's high-volume, tourism-related food outlets

- implementation of a broad environmental health program to maintain the highest standards for air and water quality, clinical waste management, sanitation, vector control and public contingency planning
- inspections of cruise ships moored in Sydney Harbour as hotel accommodation
- counter-disaster preparedness for biological and chemical hazards.

Approximately 800 people (including 400 ambulance officers) were involved in the delivery of public health services during the Olympics. Due to careful planning, trained staff, a comprehensive public surveillance system, strong inter-agency collaboration and clearly defined lines of reporting and communication, there were no outbreaks of infectious diseases or mass casualties reported. Overall, the surveillance system reported 12 754 presentations of public interest to sentinel hospitals, 930 notifiable conditions and 12 000 consultations at Olympic venue medical centres. Outcomes of this organised effort were that the strategies, linkages and structures developed for the Olympic Games may continue to exist in New South Wales, and knowledge was gained that could be valuable for organisers of large-scale sporting events in the future.

Sources: Jorm & Visotina (2003); Visotina & Hills (2000).

how they behave. *Health psychology* contributes to our understanding of the determinants and consequences of health and illness, as well as to the effective design of interventions. It does this by providing explanations about causality and control of health and illness, perceptions of risk, the motivation behind adopting beliefs and behaviours, and the role of communication and compliance in clinical settings. Theories and models of behaviour change have also been important in informing planning and evaluation of behavioural interventions in health promotion.

The social dimensions of health, illness and health care are explored in *health sociology*. Sociological analyses contribute to our understanding of the distribution of health and illness in people, and the place and time of occurrence, as well as pointing to the importance of the social context of health and disease. Health sociologists have a particular interest in differences between social groups. They examine the influence of ethnicity, culture, gender, migration, occupation and socio-economic status on health, and offer explanations about social inequalities in health. Sociological theories have also explained the experiences of the clinical encounter, of living with illnesses, patterns of health-care seeking, and the role of health professions. The study of social context and methods of social analysis is particularly important in planning community interventions and evaluating social impact (or distributional consequences) of interventions.

Cultures are systems of shared meanings, representations and practices that comprise the whole of social life and are expressed in religion, ethnic identity, diet, leisure, dress, behavioural norms and ways of interacting. The field of *cultural studies* has contributed to how we understand different cultural perceptions about health and illness, such as in relation to the body, gender, ethnicity and identity. Cultural studies points to the importance of subjectivity, and its methodological approaches have been important in elucidating the health issues confronting marginal and vulnerable groups. Understanding cultural representations of health in the media is also an important part of health promotion.

Public health policies and interventions are important mechanisms for change, and necessarily affect the positioning of interest groups and sources of power. *Political science* contributes to our understanding of institutional arrangements and interests in society in shaping health policy and decision-making, such as changing roles and tools of government and civil society, policy processes, interest group politics, exercise of power and effective advocacy. Understanding the political basis for decision-making enables the development and analysis of public health policies and their consequences. Understanding the dynamics of policy-making enables more effective engagement in policy advocacy.

Economics is concerned with how society chooses to employ finite resources to create various products over time and distribute them for consumption. Economists are also concerned with the costs and benefits of patterns of resource allocation. *Health economists* are interested in understanding resource allocation processes for health care and public health, including the use and effect of incentives, market forces and price signals, and the resultant distribution of costs and benefits. The tools of health economics are used to assist in priority-setting in investment decisions and to evaluate the costs and benefits of health programs, such as their cost-effectiveness.

Management approaches and organisational arrangements are central to the successful delivery of public health activities. *Management and organisational studies* helps us to understand the organisational factors—such as size, complexity, culture, environment and technology—that shape public health practice, guide program implementation and change management processes (covering finances, human resources, health information, leadership, motivation and teamwork). Systems theory and socio-technical systems approaches have been particularly important for informing health planning and health system development.

Those working in health are constantly confronted with life and death, with the appropriateness of interventions used to protect health and prevent disease, and with competing priorities for scarce public resources. *Ethics* and *law* contribute to improved understanding of the philosophical bases and debates in public health and help clarify societal and professional values. Legal studies also provides the theoretical frameworks for public health policies and their implementation, including informing legislative and regulatory strategies.

Ecology contributes to public health intelligence by helping us to understand interactions within dynamic systems: between natural and built environments, between species and between environmental factors. *Engineering* provides public health with the tools to ensure such things as a safe water supply, safe roads and safe workplaces. Microbiology, toxicology and industrial hygiene provide us with the basis for measuring and analysing hazards in the environment.

Because public health draws on different theories, concepts and tools from different disciplines, it can be a challenge for people from the various professions to learn each other's language and to work together. It has also contributed to debates among public health practitioners about what comprises public health. The ways in which these different disciplines have contributed to the public health toolkit will be described in Part II of this book.

A system to deliver the organised effort

Such a large array of health issues need to be addressed by a broad range of public health actions, often at local, state and national levels—if not on a global scale. Thus, mechanisms are needed for mobilising action. Not only will such mechanisms need to ensure well-planned and managed services are delivered, they will also need to support service delivery with appropriate scientific knowledge, sufficient financial resources and adequate workforce skills. A public health system with a number of key building blocks is required. The key elements of such a system are depicted in Figure 1.1.

The public health system is thus defined as the infrastructure for the delivery of public health services. The key elements of the infrastructure will be discussed in Part III of this book.

A local and a global endeavour

While much of early public health concerns were local—be they in the workplace or in the neighbourhood—the international dimensions of public health are not new. The issue of international health first arose in the late 1890s with concern about disease transmission due to shipping activities. Indeed, prevention of STDs among seamen was an important impetus for the creation of the US Public Health Service. In Australia, the first expression of national public health responsibility was the *Quarantine Act 1908*, thus the international health role was recognised early.

Institutional arrangement

In 1948, the World Health Organization was officially created as part of the United Nations system,

Figure 1.1 Public health system

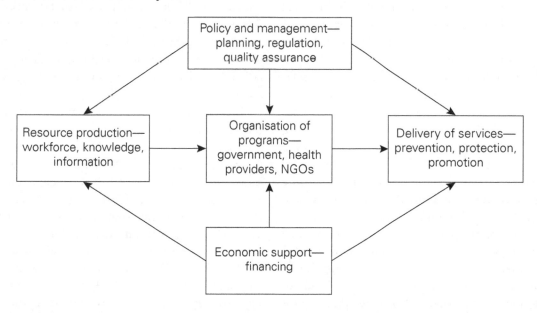

Source: Roemer (1991).

and it remains the 'world government' for health. All countries participate as member states and meet annually as the World Health Assembly. There are no private sector members, and NGOs (such as the World Federation of Public Health Associations) can become accredited but are not participants. Program operations covering such issues as communicable diseases, health promotion, environmental health and health information are implemented via six regional offices, each with its own annual regional committee meeting. Historically, the WHO has played an important role in providing technical advice, mobilising expertise in response to epidemics and guiding policy for health system development, particularly for developing countries. It has a particular role, as the global health governance body, in coordinating and setting international standards, such as for health information (International Classification of Disease), food (Codex Alimentarius) and radiation safety. The WHO also provides a symbolic and leadership role in projecting a vision for a healthy world. For example, in 1981 it called for countries to achieve 'Health for All by the Year 2000'.

Although the WHO is the official body for global health governance, there are other key agencies within the UN system that play important roles in international public health. The International Labour Organization is structured in a similar fashion to the WHO but deals with labour issues. Its work on labour standards has important implications for the WHO work on occupational health and safety. Similarly, global health issues are also touched upon by the activities of the UN Environment Programme and the Food and Agriculture Organisation. Organisations that focus on particular priority populations or health issues within a broader social framework include the United Nations Population Fund for population policies, family planning and assistance with population census; the United Nations Children's Fund for immunisation, maternal and child health, as well as education and family support; and the Joint United Nations Programme on HIV/AIDS, the coordinating body for addressing the global AIDS epidemic.

The 'development banks', such as the World Bank and Asian Development Bank, have been playing an increasingly important role in public health and health system development in the developing world. These bodies undertake desk studies to evaluate key health system issues, and offer loans for projects that address specific priorities. Examples of health projects include maternal and child health, control of infectious diseases, rural health services and health sector reform. Health has also been included as a component in other projects, such as poverty alleviation and urban development. The World Bank, in particular, has been influential in setting policy frameworks for health system development.

The US government has also occupied a particularly significant position in international health. The CDC is a world leader in disease surveillance and control, with sophisticated facilities as well as technical expertise. When outbreaks of new diseases occur (such as Ebola, Lassa fever and Bolivian haemorrhagic fever), CDC resources are called upon to act as the leading disease detectives. More recently, CDC has also placed staff within the WHO and the World Bank to provide technical support for other health initiatives, ranging from tobacco control to school health to behaviour risk factor surveillance for non-communicable diseases (NCDs).

For industrialised countries, the Organisation for Economic Co-operation and Development (OECD) often provides a preferred reference point for comparison, as OECD members comprise the industrialised countries of North America, Europe, Australasia, Japan and South Korea. Australia has taken a particular interest in the work of the OECD, as it is an organisation that benchmarks across countries comparable to Australia. However, the work of the OECD is focused more on health financing and health services utilisation, and has only recently begun to give consideration to the core public health activities.

How Australia participates

Australia has reaped enormous benefit from the international dissemination of public health science and practice. In recent years, Australia has drawn inspiration from the WHO, particularly from the 1978 Alma-Ata Declaration on Primary Health Care, the 1986 Ottawa Charter for Health Promotion, and the 2008 report from the Commission for Social Determinants of Health. The WHO work on the burden of disease, using the DALYs (disability-adjusted life years) methodology, has also been replicated in Australia.

Australia has also been celebrated for the contributions it has made to public health knowledge. For example, the Victorian Health Promotion Foundation, established under the *Tobacco Act 1987*, was the first organisation of its type in the world. It was funded from taxes on tobacco products, which were diverted to investments in improving the health of Australians. A review of health promotion in Australia (NHMRC 1997a) indicated that it was internationally recognised for its achievements in HIV/AIDS prevention and control, tobacco control and motor vehicle injury prevention.

From this position of substantial achievement, Australia participates in the efforts of the WHO as an active member of the Western Pacific Region. This is the largest and most diverse of the WHO regions, and includes a diversity of countries ranging from China to the Pacific Islands. Australia contributed A\$24.8 million to the WHO in 2010–11, as well as providing technical expertise. There were more than 43 Collaborating Centres (national institutions of excellence that have been selected and designated by the Director-General of WHO) in Australia by 2012, covering such diverse topics as women's health, malaria and influenza. Australia's achievement in public health has been recognised not only with numerous designations for Collaborating Centres, but also with the World Tobacco Day Medal in 2001 for work by the National Public Health Partnership on best practice guidelines for regulating passive smoking. The WHO Framework Convention on Tobacco Control (FCTC), ratified in 2004, was the first time that international treaty powers had been used, and Australia made a senior officer from the Commonwealth Department of Health and Ageing available to assist in the work. In 2012, Australia was again in the international limelight with the introduction of legislation requiring cigarettes to be marketed in plain packaging.

Improving global equity

Like other countries, Australia provides development assistance on a bilateral basis—that is, to specific countries and for specific projects. AusAID (the Australian Agency for International Development) has identified poverty alleviation as the main objective of the Australian aid program, and within that focus has included health as one of its priorities. Following the September 11, 2001 attacks on the World Trade Center in New York and the Pentagon, Australia—along with other developed nations—has now recognised the important links between poverty and globalisation, security and governance.

The connection between infectious diseases, poverty and human security is evidenced by the fact that most preventable infectious diseases, nutritional deprivation and maternity-related risks are concentrated among the world's poor. Poverty and health are also interconnected, as poor living and working conditions contribute to poor health, and health-care costs may lead people into poverty. Poor health also contributes to the reduced capacity for economic and social participation, reinforcing the inequalities that exist in society, including inequalities in health. When governments fail to invest in public health and basic health care, social inequalities can be exacerbated, leading to social instability. The legitimacy of governments also comes into question (Zwi, Fustukian & Sethi 2002).

In recognition of the complex, interrelated nature of health and development, the WHO established the Commission on Macroeconomics and Health in 2000 in order to persuade governments about the importance of investing in public health. In 2005, the WHO established the Commission on Social Determinants of Health to extend governments' understanding about the importance of paying attention to social and economic policies. The policy frameworks offered by the WHO consistently point to the need for cooperation between health and other sectors, and between government and civil society organisation.

Given the need for cooperation between the different sectors, the UN system has provided various processes by which governments and non-government bodies can formulate strategies to address global priorities. Major international conferences and treaties have been formulated in relation to:

- **women's status:** International Conference on Population and Development, Cairo (1993); Beijing Conference (1995); Convention on the Elimination of All Forms of Discrimination Against Women (CEDAW) (1979)
- **environment:** UN Conference on the Human Environment, Stockholm (1972); UN Conference on Environment and Development—the Earth Summit, Rio de Janeiro (1992); Kyoto Protocol to the UN Framework Convention on Climate Change (1997)
- **children:** Convention on the Rights of the Child (1989)
- **indigenous peoples:** Indigenous and Tribal Peoples Convention (1989); International Decade of the World's Indigenous People 1995–2004; Permanent Forum on Indigenous Issues (2002)
- **human rights:** Universal Declaration of Human Rights (1948); the European Convention on Human Rights (1950); World Conference on Human Rights, Vienna (1993); UK *Human Rights Act 1998*
- **tobacco:** WHO Framework Convention on Tobacco Control (2003)

Box 1.9 Non-government contributions to global health development

Development assistance may also come from the private, philanthropic sector. The Rockefeller Foundation has been important in establishing medical education programs and in supporting agricultural research to increase rice production, while the Ford Foundation has championed reproductive health and women's rights. More recently, the Bill & Melinda Gates Foundation has provided generous funding to support the Global Alliance for Vaccines and Immunization (GAVI) initiative as well as for specific health issues such as HIV/AIDS. International non-government organisations play a critical role in delivering public health services and in supporting development projects. Médecins Sans Frontières (MSF) won the Nobel Prize in 2000 for its public health and medical care work in conflict settings, such as refugee camps. In 1997, the Nobel Prize was awarded to the International Campaign to Ban Landmines (founded in 1992) and Jody Williams (USA) for advocacy in landmine removal. Humanitarian relief is provided by large organisations (such as Care International) as well as smaller missionary societies. NGOs (such as Oxfam and Save the Children) are more oriented towards community development and programs at the grassroots level.

- **people with disabilities:** Convention on the Rights of Persons with Disabilities (2007).

Since 2000, there have also been special UN general assemblies devoted to questions about children and the environment, HIV/AIDS and chronic non-communicable diseases (NCD).

In September 2000, the member states of the United Nations unanimously adopted the Millennium Development Goals (MDGs) (see Appendix B), further signalling a broad consensus for the need to reduce global inequities. Goals relating to health account for six out of the eleven MDGs, illustrating the fundamental contribution that public health efforts make to human development. Progress has been variable across countries, and the MDGs will be reviewed and updated in 2015.

Conclusion: Old and new public health

Because of the constantly evolving nature of public health concerns, and strategies adopted to address them, there have been numerous attempts to discard 'old public health' and adopt 'new public health'. Beaglehole and Bonita (1997) also suggest that public health has always been pulled in two different directions: towards a broad focus on the underlying social and economic determinants of health and illness; and towards a narrow focus on clinical conditions and biomedically based interventions. In Table 1.1, Lawson and Bauman (2001) suggest that this debate has emerged numerous times.

Continued debate, although valuable for honing professional practice and understanding, can lead people to miss the main point: that public health is an endeavour to provide the best health possible to populations of people. It is achieved through an 'organised effort' that encompasses not only public

Table 1.1 Chronology of the new public health debate

Time period	What's new
Antiquity	Roman aqueducts; Roman legal system*
1660	John Graunt 'Bills of mortality', demography*
1790s	Smallpox immunisation (Jenner)*
Mid-nineteenth century	Sanitary idea,* poverty, *Public Health Act 1848* (UK)
1850s	Epidemiological observations (Snow)
Late nineteenth century	Microbiology,* germ causation
Nineteenth–twentieth century	Decline in infectious diseases*
1920–1950	Rise of social medicine*
1950s	Era of mass screening,* immunisation
1960s	Increase in chronic diseases, non-communicable diseases; development of epidemiology and whole-population approaches to public health problems
1970s	Individual risk factor approaches predominate; use of health psychology and individual change models in public health; use of theoretically driven mass media campaigns
1980s	(WHO) Health for All (1978),* Ottawa Charter (1986);* notions of 'new public health' as structural and social change; leads to the development of contemporary health promotion
2000s	UN Millennium Declaration 2000, global partnership to address poverty as a determinant of health—time-bound targets deadline 2015, WHO Social Determinants of Health 2008, WHO Health in All Policies Statement 2010: requires a new form of governance where there is joined-up leadership for health across sectors and between levels of government

Note: * indicates another 'new' public health

Source: adapted from Lawson & Bauman (2001: 16).

health practitioners, but also a diverse range of government and non-government institutions and organisations, as well as the general population. The means by which public health practitioners achieve this purpose are many and varied, and always have the potential to expand or contract, depending on the nature of the health challenges facing populations of people—including available resources, current knowledge and the capacity of organisations and communities to work together towards a common goal. The knowledge base for these efforts is also diverse. Despite this fluidity, a number of core functions and activities are common to public health practitioners and across myriad health issues, wherever they may be.

Those who contribute their organised effort to achieving improved public health include an extraordinary range of people from diverse professions, with diverse skills and from diverse locations. They may work in government or non-government organisations, or in organisations concerned with particular illnesses or specific ethnic groups. They may work in the private sector. They may be chiefly concerned with health, or they may work in other sectors, such as housing, environment, agriculture or even meteorology. They may be employed on a high or low wage, or they may be trying to improve public health by voluntary action through a local community group. They may be statisticians, international development workers, doctors, nurses, community workers, men or women in a local service group, home-based parents with pre-school children who are concerned with the health of their community, or even politicians. It is by their *actions*

that we define their participation in public health, because it is by their actions that their values are put into practice.

Turnock's defining principles provide a useful checklist of those values. They embrace a commitment to social justice, to links with government, to a perpetually expanding agenda, to a focus on prevention and to the need to balance the contribution of science with community history, culture and expectations. Another characteristic shared and valued by effective public health workers is the courage to acknowledge the inherently political nature of the choices that have to be made if public health is to be pursued in the face of the competing expectations of individuals and groups.

Public health is concerned primarily with the health of populations of people, rather than with the health of specific individuals. As such, the success of public health practice is not measured by individual successes, but by the overall health of groups of people. Sometimes tough choices must be made in public health because there are simply not enough resources to ensure the health of everyone. Therefore, the health needs of large groups of people are prioritised over the health needs of small groups of individuals. Where there is conflict between the two, public health practitioners will always choose to assist the larger group, and so derive the best health benefit for the most people. While this is fair when both groups are considered as a whole, it can understandably appear to be very unfair to those people who miss out. Inevitably, political, moral and financial considerations are the everyday concern of public health practitioners.

2

The historical development of public health:
Landmarks in the field

Challenge

The flood disaster that began in the Northern Territory town of Katherine on 26 January 1998, when torrential rains from Cyclone Les caused flooding of the Katherine River, was a timely reminder of the lessons we have learnt from the history of public health. What is the first response of public health workers and disaster management authorities when the basic necessities of everyday life—such as clean drinking water from the tap, fresh food, gas or electricity for cooking, basic medical supplies, garbage collection and a functioning sewerage system—become inaccessible? Most residents had no shelter and their possessions disappeared in the floodwaters. When ponds at the sewage farm and those for wastewater at the dairy and abattoir overflowed, ideal conditions were created for an explosion in the mosquito population. Katherine was also cut off from its major supply routes (Hendy 1998).

How did the residents move from survival mode and begin to re-establish their daily lives? The organised response to this disaster revolved around the efforts of many groups and individuals. Community organisations established child care, evacuation centres and counselling; environmental health officers came from across the Northern Territory to help dispose of rotting food, putrefying chickens and other animals, and effluent-soaked fridges; while other public health staff cut short their annual holidays in order to provide assistance. The Australian Defence Force provided air transport to bring in supplies, trucks for distribution and assistance to the medical entomology teams to control mosquitoes. Power and water teams secured and maintained water supplies, sewage disposal and electricity to the intact part of Katherine. The state of disaster was lifted on 21 February 1998. (Hendy 1998)

As the incidence of floods, bushfires and cyclones is relatively common in Australia, how do we prepare for such occurrences?

Introduction

This chapter describes the origins of public health, including the important contributions made by the ancient world, and discusses how varying social and environmental contexts have shaped the development of public health practice. The chapter then outlines the beginnings of an organised approach to the threats of epidemic disease and the emerging role of government in public health, and examines the impact on public health of varying beliefs about the causes of disease.

The origins of public health as an organised effort by society can be linked with the emergence of agricultural societies from what were predominantly hunter-gatherer societies (Diamond 1997; McMichael 2001). The adoption of agricultural methods of production about 10 000 years ago was accompanied by an increase in the global human population; more complex administrative and bureaucratic systems of governance; specialisation in work, trade and commerce; increased social stratification; and urban settlements. Some commentators have observed that increased food supplies resulted in improved standards of living and a decrease in the incidence of infectious disease (Gordon 1976; McKeown 1979) but, despite these benefits, communal living in villages also brought with it fresh health hazards (Brockington 1958). Disease-causing microbes were able to spread more quickly, and to more people, simply because larger numbers of people were living in close proximity to one another, along with their domesticated animals (such as dogs and cattle) and uninvited guests (such as rats and mice). Infectious diseases like measles, smallpox and tuberculosis (TB) appear to date

from this early period of agricultural human settlement. Agricultural production required that people become sedentary (that is, live in one place), and emerging cities had new problems—such as overcrowding and the safe disposal of human waste—to deal with or (for a period of time) ignore.

The brilliance of ancient city systems

The challenges of living in cities were well understood by ancient civilisations. The ancient societies of early China, Egypt and India, and the Incas of South America, developed clever strategies to provide water, sewerage and drainage systems to their urban populations. Many equated cleanliness with godliness, and associated hygiene with religious beliefs and practices (Tulchinsky & Varavikova 2000). In particular, ancient Greece and Rome have been given a special place in the history of public health, and their legacy is still with us today in the use of such public health terms as 'hygiene', which comes from Hygeia, the Greek goddess of good health, and 'sanitation', which comes from *sanitas*, the Latin for 'health'. Many philosophies of health and illness that dominated European societies until the mid-nineteenth century were derived from ancient Greek philosophers, such as Hippocrates, who realised that health and diseases were the result of natural causes. In his book *Airs, Waters and Places*, Hippocrates systematically presented the causal relationships between environmental factors and disease. The rise and fall of epidemic diseases was linked to meteorological variations and the character of the seasons. This work was to be the basic epidemiology text and basis for understanding endemic and epidemic diseases for 2000 years, until the arrival of the new sciences of bacteriology and immunology in the nineteenth century. During the fifteenth century, Thomas Sydenham developed the theory of atmospheric contamination, based on the idea that the agents of epidemic disease were the poisonous effluvia, or miasmas, arising from organic matter (Rosen 1958; Porter 1999).

These ideas about the close relationship between the environment and disease were also stressed by Vitruvius, a famous Roman architect who probably lived during the reign of Caesar Augustus; he described how city sites must be considered carefully in order to avoid the corrupting effect of miasmas:

> For fortified towns the following general principles are to be observed. First comes the choice of a very healthy site. Such a site will be high, neither misty nor frosty, and in a climate neither hot nor cold, but temperate; further, without marshes in the neighbourhood. For when the morning breezes blow toward the town at sunrise, if they bring with them mists from marshes and, mingled with the mist, the poisonous breath of the creatures of the marshes to be wafted into the bodies of the inhabitants, they will make the site unhealthy. Again, if the town is on the coast with a southern or western exposure, it will not be healthy, because in summer the southern sky grows hot at sunrise and is fiery at noon, while a western exposure grows warm after sunrise, is hot at noon, and at evening all aglow. (Vitruvius 1960: 17)

Although some of their theories about the cause of disease and ill-health have been discarded today (at least in Western biomedicine), some of the measures taken by ancient peoples to ensure their health were quite similar to contemporary practice. The ancient Romans employed a number of techniques for the administration of their cities that might be described today as 'public health measures'. These included the construction of public baths, aqueducts for the delivery of clean water systems of sewage and waste

disposal, drainage of marshlands (which probably reduced the incidence of malaria) and (after some centuries) free medical care for the poor.

However, these 'public health measures' were not always evenly distributed among the inhabitants of Roman cities, and nor were they all regarded *primarily* as means by which people's health could be improved. The 'public baths', for example, were attended predominantly by people of influence and wealth, and not by Roman slaves or the poor. The slaves working in the baths were 'subject to many ills, dropsy, ulcers, abscesses—pale, sad, puffed-up, cachectic, and often attacked by the maladies of those upon whom they attended' (Brockington 1958: 122).

To Romans, attendance at the public baths was not so much a matter of hygiene as an important social event. Roman citizens would meet to discuss important issues of the day, enjoy sumptuous meals, bathe and exercise. Similarly, some activities that were once considered crucial to public health are not held in the same regard today—in ancient Rome, for example, temples were constructed for gods and goddesses to protect the people from specific illnesses and diseases. When Vitruvius described the ideal procedures for establishing a new city, sites for temples were allocated as soon as the city location and streets had been laid out, and *before* positions for aqueducts, fountains, baths and drains were decided upon. The amateur archaeologist Rodolfo Lanciani, who discussed the archaeology of ancient Rome in 1888, described some of these temples and their importance to Roman inhabitants:

> The clearest proof of the virulence of malaria in the first century of the history of Rome is afforded by the large number of altars and shrines dedicated by its early inhabitants to the goddess of the Fever and other kindred divinities. At the time of Varro, there were not less than three temples of the Fever left standing ... The Esquiline quarter seems to have been the worst of all in its sanitary conditions; in fact, besides

the Fever's temple, there was an altar dedicated to the Evil Eye (Mala Fortuna), and an altar and a small wood dedicated to the goddess Mefitis. Near the Praetorian camp, and near the modern railway station, I have found, myself, an altar consecrated to Verminus, the god of microbes; and lastly, in the very centre of the Roman Forum, there was an altar sacred to Cloacina, a goddess of typhoid, I suppose. It appears from the particulars just given that the primitive inhabitants of Rome, acting as men always do act when they find themselves exposed to the ravages of an unknown evil, utterly ignorant of its mysterious nature and of the proper way to fight and lessen its effect, raised their hands towards their gods, and actually increased the number of their divinities, and contrived new ones, imploring from heaven the help which they failed to secure with their own resources. (Lanciani 1967: 52)

After the fall of the Western Roman Empire and through the Middle Ages, there was a gradual decline in sanitation and hygiene standards in European cities (Winslow 1923), although in Islamic countries the hygiene practices of Rome and Greece were adopted and extended:

adding to the understanding of contagion by descriptions of smallpox, anthrax, measles and scabies. Hospitals became centres of learning, and medical schools, under such men as Al-Majusi, taught that the first art of medicine is keeping health in the healthy. (Brockington 1958: 122)

Trade, conquest and its consequences

Despite these early 'public health' techniques, knowledge about the causes and control of diseases remained limited. With trade and other population movements associated with events such as the Crusades, terrifying diseases, such as leprosy and bubonic plague, spread readily (Winslow 1923; Garrett 1994). Fear of new diseases and a lack of knowledge about the way they were transmitted often exacerbated the spread of epidemics. Nevertheless, people and governments did attempt to control disease, despite their limited (or often just plain wrong) knowledge about the causes of disease. Throughout the history of Europe, one of the most widespread tactics for disease prevention and control was to introduce quarantine practices and the isolation of sick or afflicted people. This was exemplified during the bubonic plague epidemic of the fourteenth century. Known as the 'Black Death', it caused an estimated 50 million deaths, half of them in Asia and Africa and the other half in Europe. Quarantine was first practised in Venice under the guidance of a sanitary council, and the term was derived from the Italian words *quaranta giorni*, which mean '40 days'. The effectiveness of quarantine at the time when modes of disease transmission were unknown is open to question (Brockington 1958; Porter 1999).

The Renaissance saw the flourishing of commerce, industry, shipping and cities. Epidemics continued to sweep across Europe along with the migration of large numbers of people. The transmission of infectious diseases also increased, and new diseases were 'traded' between continents, with devastating results on the health of indigenous communities in the Americas, the Pacific islands and, later on, in European colonies in Africa and Asia. These movements were associated with the expansion of European countries into the New World: the Spanish and Portuguese to South America (after 1400), the Dutch to South Africa (after 1700) and the English to North America and Australasia (1870–1920). Other activities associated with this expansion into the New World resulted in mass movements of people. Slavery is one example, accounting for the movement of 15 million people from Africa to the New World from the seventeenth to the nineteenth centuries (Brockington 1958).

Box 2.1 The Black Death: Pestilence, politics and public health

The Black Death swept through Europe between 1347 and 1351. A third of the population died, and the disease increased in severity as it moved north. The Black Death brought great social, political and economic upheaval, which helped to undermine the feudal system—basically by creating a shortage of labour. Whole villages were depopulated, the relationship between serf and master was broken, and many tenants moved to cities and towns. The plague's onset had been preceded by a period of climate warming that brought improvements in agricultural production and subsequent population increases. When the climate cooled in the early fourteenth century, famine returned; it was followed by malnutrition and starvation, leaving the population weakened and susceptible to disease. After the epidemic's outbreak (probably somewhere in the Crimea), it was spread by infected fleas that hitched a ride on those habitual stowaways, black rats (*Rattus rattus*). As a dense network of trade routes already existed from the Mediterranean ports to Northern Europe and Britain, the plague quickly spread inland. But, significantly, the pathogen mutated from bubonic to the pneumonic plague, which is spread by sneezing and coughing, and is thus a more efficient and deadly form of transmission (Bell & Lewis 2005).

Messina in Sicily was the first European city to be affected. The plague was brought there by visiting Genoan sailors. By the time attempts were made to drive them out of port, it was too late. A friar describes the symptoms:

At first [the boils] were of the size of a hazelnut and developed accompanied by violent shivering fits, which soon rendered those attacked so weak that they could no longer stand upright, but were forced to lie in their beds consumed by violent fever and overcome with great tribulation. Soon the boils grew to the size of a walnut, then to that of a hen's egg ... and they were exceedingly painful, and irritated the body, causing it to vomit blood. (quoted in Orent 2004: 116)

As one city after another succumbed, inhabitants who were able (usually the wealthier and more educated citizens) fled, leaving their possessions behind and their houses open. The sick were ruthlessly deserted, and the dead were left for collection and burial in communal pits. Fields were deserted and cattle wandered unattended.

City-states, such as Florence, set up temporary health boards to enforce existing sanitary legislation, such as street cleaning, the control of noxious trades, prevention of water pollution and bans on selling adulterated food. When Florence faced a fourth plague epidemic in 1383, many of the wealthy fled, while the poor who were forced to remain threatened to revolt. The measures taken to prevent the spread of plague were concerned more with preventing civil disorder and social breakdown. Thus, '[p]rotecting health was only considered in relation to the economic and political survival of the status quo ... Quarantine greatly interfered with trade and was vigorously resisted by merchants and their labourers, both groups being adversely affected.' (Porter 1999: 37)

By the early sixteenth century, the major Italian cities had established permanent health boards, which had the power to isolate victims and their families, and seize and destroy suspect possessions and merchandise. Port quarantine and military sanitary cordons dissuaded travellers and maintained public order, while the use of intelligence and surveillance measures limited the amount of damage an outbreak of plague could cause (Porter 1999). These measures became the model that was used throughout Europe to control plague.

As a feudal society, England lacked political structures for population control, and did not develop plague administration until the early sixteenth century. Early control measures were based on the house arrest of victims and their families, and caused revolt and civic disorder. The failure of these regulations thus contributed to the high mortality during London's Great Plague of 1665–66, which killed about 55000 of the city's half a million people. New public health measures were subsequently implemented to put victims into pest-houses and to isolate families for 40 days (Porter 1999). Plague disappeared from Europe after 1722.

At the end of the nineteenth century, another plague pandemic occurred which was an entirely new strain. It broke out in China and was spread by black rats to Hong Kong and then, via shipping routes, to India, South-East Asia, South Africa, the western United States, Australia and much of South America. In India, the plague claimed 12.5 million lives over the next 30 years. This pandemic was also the story of the researchers and doctors, such as Alexandre Yersin, who identified the plague bacillus as *Pasteurella pestis* or *Yersinia pestis*, an internal parasite of rodents that is transmitted from one host to another by fleas (Orent 2004). Plague remains an endemic threat, particularly in the United States and the Indian subcontinent, with several cases occurring every year.

The conquest of the Americas by Europeans can be attributed to the propagation of infectious diseases as much as to superior weaponry and military organisation. The Spanish and British explorers and adventurers, naturally immune themselves, carried with them a range of diseases—notably smallpox and measles—to which the indigenous peoples had no immunity (Bell & Lewis 2005). Conquest has its price.

However, the Enlightenment period saw further and rapid advances in science and technology, including medical knowledge. In this social environment of increased inquisitiveness, the vast devastation of diseases like the plague inspired some to carefully consider what was happening and attempt to identify patterns in the incidence of disease, which formed a basis for early epidemiology (Trostle 1986). In 1662, the Englishman John Graunt (1620–74) published one of the first analyses of vital statistics, *Natural and Political Observations on the Mortality*, and provided some of the earliest documentation on the relationship between mortality and living conditions (Brockington 1958).

Following Graunt, Ramazzini's treatise on occupational diseases in 1700, Sydenham's on malaria and clinical observation, Percival Potts' 1775 study of scrotal cancer in chimneysweeps and many more studies provided a basis for population-based investigations of disease causation (Brockington 1958; Trostle 1986).

Social change and public health: The sanitary revolution in nineteenth-century Britain

During the eighteenth and nineteenth centuries, the Agricultural (c. 1730–60) and Industrial (c. 1730–1850) Revolutions brought fundamental social, political and economic changes to European societies. The enclosure movement and the accompanying increase in farm sizes, along with the introduction of new farming practices, dislocated feudal communities and families. This forced destitute and unemployed peasants to migrate to rapidly growing industrial towns and cities. In England and Wales, the scale of this unplanned urbanisation meant that the urban population rose from 3 million (30 per cent) in 1801 to 28.5 million (nearly 80 per cent) by 1901 (Hamlin & Sheard 1998). Industrial cities like Liverpool and Manchester were described by Friedrich Engels as having 'streets [that] are generally unpaved, rough, dirty, filled with vegetable and animal refuse, without sewers or gutters but supplied with foul, stagnant pools instead' (Engels 1987: 71). Such an environment, coupled with a lowering of the bodily resistance of individuals to disease due to poor nutrition (starvation) associated with extreme poverty and little personal hygiene, resulted in epidemics of infectious diseases, such as cholera, typhoid and tuberculosis. Average life expectancy in Liverpool for the unemployed was fifteen years, and 35 years for an upper-class person (Hamlin & Sheard 1998).

Rapid economic growth, Simon Szreter (1997) has argued, brings about a disruption in a society's structures of authority, social relations and ideologies. The result during the second and third quarters of the nineteenth century in Britain was a period of political and administrative inaction in dealing with urban deterioration. It was against this background that the sanitary idea was brought to public attention by Edwin Chadwick (the architect of the 1834 Poor Law amendment, which was based on disincentives for obtaining public relief) and medical reformers. Chadwick believed that miasmas, the odours produced by organic decay, were the cause of disease epidemics, such as cholera and typhoid. In 1842, he published his famous *General Report on the Sanitary Condition of the Labouring Population of Great Britain*, which argued that it was filth and pauperism, rather than defects in character, that brought a decline in the moral behaviour of the working class (Flinn 1965). Hence, the guiding principle underlying his argument for sanitation reform was that the prevention of further environmental degradation was cheaper and more effective for society than continuing with expenditure on poor relief.

By focusing on the physical causes of disease, Chadwick was able to divert public attention from the views of other reformers who argued that it was the harshness of the Poor Laws themselves that caused such illness (Hamlin & Sheard 1998). In 1843, at Chadwick's request, the Royal Commission on the Health of Towns documented the sanitary conditions in 50 of the largest towns in England and Wales. Besides the technical and social data obtained, the commission reiterated the need for public health reform, and generally supported Chadwick's technical solutions of building networks of sewers,

providing constant water supplies and recycling (collecting and disposing of) wastes. But the job of putting together the policies needed to accomplish these changes was left to the central government.

The outcome was the *Public Health Act 1848* (UK), which has provided the basis for public health administration in many countries to the present day. Even though the Act did not contain a system for a comprehensive national sewerage plan or public health commissions, it did allow for groups of ratepayers (at least 10 per cent) to request the establishment of local public health boards. The Central Board of Health, with Chadwick as its first salaried commissioner, would then set one up if it was practicable. It could also impose a board in those areas where the death rate exceeded 25 per 1000. Where these boards were established, they were permitted, rather than required, to appoint medical officers. These boards were also given powers to undertake street cleaning and installation of sewerage systems and water supplies. The outcome was that local government began to acquire the broader powers and obligations that characterise many of its activities today. The appointment of medical officers became an obligatory function. Thus, by 1854 when Chadwick was forced out of office, the *Public Health Act* had been applied in 182 towns (Hamlin & Sheard 1998).

Opposition to the preventive measures arose from the emerging middle-class electorate following the *Municipal Reform Act 1835* (UK). Even though their wealth had increased and this 'shopocracy' of small property-holders were acutely aware of urban environmental degradation, they were not prepared to pay the taxes needed to fund these projects. Hence, this first attempt by the state in Britain to intervene in public health decision-making was at best tentative, and easily opposed by local political interests.

The threat of the spread of diseases also played a significant part in the sanitary revolution. While typhoid, typhus and diarrhoea were more devastating to the health of the working class, it was cholera (especially during the four epidemics in 1831–32, 1848–49, 1853–54 and 1866), and its unpredictable nature that sometimes saw it spread to middle-class suburbs, that was terribly feared. It was this spectre of cholera that 'brought together in one grand obsession, the preoccupations with the predicament and comportment of the poor, with the sanitary dangers these implied for the established citizens and with the need for urban sanitary and administrative reform' (de Swaan 1988: 124). Eventually people realised that the threat would remain until assistance was given to the poor to improve their living conditions and funds provided for the public works needed to ensure a safe water supply and sanitation system. Such a concern, or social consciousness, is a hallmark of a modern society (de Swaan 1988).

Thus, it was only from the late 1860s onwards that the public health/sanitation movement became genuinely effective. The passing of the *Sanitary Act 1866* (UK) gave all localities the sanitary powers that had previously been restricted to the local boards of health under the 1848 Act. As a result of the technological and civil engineering advances made during the preceding decades, most parts of London had covered sewers by the 1870s, and cesspools had been abolished. Between 1880 and 1891, urban authorities borrowed £7 738 522 for sewerage works and £3 225 500 for waterworks, and in the process transformed these services from being privately owned companies into public enterprises. The outcome was that the provision of such basic urban services became a true public good, and so was extended to all citizens. As these new sanitary arrangements were so effective and successful, they soon became uncontroversial and just a part of everyday life (de Swaan 1988).

In Britain, the growing public awareness of poverty and the increasing middle-class concern about the possibility of social revolution, as highlighted by the 1848 revolutions in Europe and the Paris Commune of 1871, eventually helped to force the state to include the working class in the democratic process. The result was the enfranchisement of urban and rural workers. Along with the growing influence of the trade union movement, this forced the state to mediate in the process of how the benefits of such rapid economic growth were being distributed within British society. This new alliance of interests brought with it the political will required to commit governments to invest in the public works needed to bring about sanitary reform and a more general improvement in the urban environment (Szreter 1997). This pattern of 'sciences influence[ing] public health decisions and conclusions, and politics deliver[ing] its programs and messages' (Koplan & McPheeters 2004) has become the hallmark of many of the public health achievements in the twentieth century.

What activities were involved in the sanitary reform?

The activities associated with the sanitary reform movement were focused on improving the environmental conditions in and around where people lived. Environmental hygiene is associated with the collection, transport and removal of refuse and general waste generated by homes and factories; the provision of drains to prevent the pooling of water that could become stagnant and breed insects like mosquitoes; and the construction of sewers to collect and transport human waste. The removal of waste was an effective form of pest control, particularly of rats and mice. These activities also included the development of regulations to ensure that buildings were weatherproof, well ventilated, well lit and provided with sanitary facilities, such as sinks and water closets (toilets). Places of public accommodation (boarding houses) were designed to prevent overcrowding. Eventually, food and water safety also became the subject of these activities.

Today, these activities are still provided by local councils, water and sewerage authorities, and this is why rates are levied against landowners. Regulations continue to apply to housing standards, accommodation premises, land-use planning, the discharge of waste by land or into the air or water, and hazardous industries. Before the construction of a new housing subdivision, drains, sewers, water supply, power, telephone and other services are designed and put in place. Public health laws in the states and territories of Australia still require that homeowners maintain their house and property in a clean and sanitary state.

Reports, insurance and the careful observation of events

As has been mentioned, Chadwick conducted a series of studies and documented life expectancy differences between gentry and labourers in his *General Report on the Sanitary Condition of the Labouring Population of Great Britain*. From a modern perspective, it is sobering to think that the gentry were found to have a life expectancy of only 36 years, and even more horrifying to discover that labourers could expect to survive, on average, just sixteen years.

These public health victories were not achieved solely on the basis of research and reports. In 1854, John Snow, a founding member of the London Epidemiological Society, investigated a series of outbreaks of cholera. He traced some 500 cholera deaths to the use of drinking water from the Broad Street pump. He eventually persuaded the authorities to take the simple remedy of removing the handle from the pump, which halted the epidemic in its tracks. However, the water companies' agreement to move their intake upstream away from the pollution reflected community concerns about the aesthetic quality of the water, rather than their understanding of the cause of the epidemic (Wilkinson & Sidel 1991).

Snow was one example of the so-called 'shoe-leather' epidemiologists. He used fieldwork to collect data to ascertain how the environment caused disease, as did many others, such as Panum and Farr (Trostle 1986: 39). The work of these pioneers provided a significant contribution to the

development of public health—particularly as part of their recommendations included a political agenda for social and cultural change (Trostle 1986).

The Australian experience: The colonial legacy

As mentioned earlier, as a result of exploration and colonialism, infectious diseases were introduced to susceptible indigenous communities around the world. In Australia prior to 1788, approximately 300 000 Aborigines had led a nomadic or semi-nomadic, hunter-gatherer existence for over 30 000 years on an isolated island continent (Cumpston 1989: 37). Thus, the nomadic tendencies, small population numbers and isolated environment were the protective factors for Aboriginal health. The most common health concerns related to eye diseases (associated with flies), skin sores, ulcers, pneumonia, diarrhoea and dysentery. Generally, it was held that most problems related to diet rather than infection (Goldsmid 1988: 28). However, between 1788 and 1791 typhoid, typhus, smallpox, influenza, diarrhoea and measles became a significant issue within the colony and, with the arrival of more colonists, these diseases became endemic within the population (Goldsmid 1988: 38). According to Goldsmid (1988: 38), 'Even at this early time the effects of diseases, especially venereal disease, smallpox and influenza, were disastrous for the Aboriginal population, with some tribes being completely destroyed.'

Syphilis, which was unknown in Aboriginal populations prior to European settlement, became so rife that it was thought that it alone would wipe out the Indigenous population (Goldsmid 1988: 37). The continued increase in European population resulted in changing the way of life of many Aborigines from a semi-nomadic to a more settled type of existence. This change in traditional life and culture then led to poor environmental hygiene and sanitation associated with settlements, and the inevitable epidemics of tuberculosis, pneumonia and typhoid (Goldsmid 1988: 39). The public health

Box 2.2 Engels: Conditions of the English working class

Friedrich Engels' report on the conditions of the English working class (published in Germany in 1845 and in England in 1892) is now viewed as part of a long tradition of writing about social inequalities in health. Born in Germany in 1820, the son of a textile manufacturer, Engels was introduced to the slum areas of Manchester by a young Irish working-class woman, Mary Fields, whom he later married. The report, based on Engels' observations, newspapers and contemporary documents, such as the report of the Factories Inquiry Commission of 1833, describes the squalid living conditions in the industrial cities and the condition of factory hands and workers in the textile, mining and agricultural industries. Engels wrote graphically about the slums that accommodated the workers:

Among them are mills on the river, in short, the method of construction is as crowded and disorderly here as in the lower part of Long Millgate. Right and left a multitude of covered passages lead from the main street into numerous courts, and he who turns in thither gets into a filth and disgusting grime, the equal of which is not to be found—especially in the courts which lead down to the Irk, and which contain unqualifiedly the most horrible dwellings which I have yet beheld. In one of these courts there stands directly at the entrance, at the end of the covered passage, a privy without a door, so dirty that the inhabitants can pass into and out of the court only by passing through foul pools of stagnant urine and excrement (Engels 1987: 88–9).

In order to gain an understanding of the effect of factory work upon the health of females, Engels argued, the work of children and the nature of that work must be considered:

The great mortality among children of the working class, and especially among those of the factory operatives, is proof enough of the unwholesome conditions under which they pass their first years … At nine years of age [a child] is sent into the mill to work 6.5 hours (formerly 8, earlier still 12 to 14, even 16 hours) daily, until the thirteenth year; then twelve hours until the eighteenth year (p. 171).

Especially unwholesome is the wet spinning of linen-yarn which is carried on by young girls and boys. The water spurts over them from the spindle so that the front of their clothing is constantly wet through to the skin; and there is always water standing on the floor … Another effect of flax-spinning is a peculiar deformity of the shoulder, especially a projection of the right shoulder-blade (Engels 1987: 181).

Engels then began to work with Karl Marx, building the foundations of the international revolutionary movement. The *Communist Manifesto* was published in 1848. While Engels' work was not unusual in describing the working and living conditions of the poor, what was innovative was that he argued that it was the poverty and deprivation from which the urban poor suffered, rather than the filthy living conditions, that led to the epidemics of disease and illness (Russell 2004).

In the United States, Lemuel Shattuck's *Report of the Massachusetts Sanitary Commission* (1850) documented differences in morbidity and mortality rates in different localities, and recommended a comprehensive, statewide public health system (Winslow 1923: 25–6). In 1869, the Massachusetts State Board of Health was established.

In 1883, Otto von Bismarck, the Chancellor of Germany, introduced legislation providing mandatory insurance for injury and illness, and survivors' benefits for workers in industrial plants, thus providing the first model of social insurance in the modern world (Winslow 1923: 62). The early champions of public health looked to deal with regulatory tools and medical services as appropriate responses to deal with health problems.

Box 2.3 Public health in British colonial India

In British colonial India, there was a strong association between public health and the British Army, particularly when the Royal Commission into the Sanitary State of the Army in India revealed the high levels of illness (morbidity) and death (mortality). There was also a disturbing imbalance between the health of British-born soldiers and Indian soldiers. Cholera was a leading cause of military and civilian deaths. These statistics provided medical officers with the opportunity to stress upon a previously indifferent colonial administration the practical value of sanitary reform and preventive medicine. The first steps were improvements in conservancy, water supply, drainage, and the siting and construction of barracks in the colonial cantonments in towns and cities.

Other public health measures adopted included providing smallpox vaccination to both British and Indian residents. Unfortunately, despite a professed intention that everyone should be vaccinated, limited resources meant that in practice vaccination was only provided to British residents, their Indian servants and others in regular contact with them. Although there was an element of humanism evident in the organisation of this vaccination program, the benefits were also understood to be financial. 'Every life saved [through smallpox vaccination] is additional revenue and an increase to the population and to the prosperity of the [East India] Company's territories in an incalculable trio.' (Arnold 1993: 136)

Prior to the 1890s, most public health programs operated in accordance with the 'miasmic' disease concept. When disease struck a military barracks or prison, the entire population of soldiers or prisoners would be evacuated to live outdoors in tents. Widespread attempts to reduce the incidence of disease did not occur until the 1890s, when British officials took extraordinary steps to prevent the spread of the plague. Bombay's municipal commissioner was authorised to enforce segregation and hospitalisation of suspected plague cases, and municipal officers were granted compulsory right of entry to infected buildings. A vast campaign of urban cleansing was initiated, and the colonial administration flushed drains, scrubbed stores and grain warehouses, and sprinkled disinfectant in side alleys and housing blocks. Hundreds of slum dwellings were destroyed. Later, these powers were extended, and placed under control of government and medical experts.

Justification for the colonial administration's new-found interest in the health of ordinary (city-dwelling) residents was only partially based on principles of humanism. Far more pressing was a resolution by the Western powers in the 1890s to place an embargo on any country that did not introduce strict disease-control measures to stop the spread of the plague. Thus, British authorities introduced public health measures primarily in an attempt to preserve trade, rather than from a concern for the quality of life of their Indian subjects. Also, they feared that if the plague arrived in Bombay and Calcutta, people would leave these cities in mass exodus, hampering trade and production even more. Despite the best efforts of the British administration, plague struck Bombay in 1896, and the effect on trade and production was profound. It has been estimated that 380 000 of Bombay's 850 000 residents fled the city between October 1896 and February 1887.

Source: Arnold (1993).

implications of this change due to colonisation have been recognised as having a diasatrous and ongoing impact on Indigenous people (Public Health Association of Australia 2010).

For Europeans settling in Australia prior to 1820, the geographical isolation, a small and dispersed population and the time taken to travel to Australia, which caused diseases to be short-lived and self-limiting, resulted in the major childhood infectious diseases being less prevalent than in the Old World. However, with episodes of immigration, infectious disease epidemics were introduced into Australia, and it was from this time that public health issues started to take a higher priority in the settlements. The period between 1838 and 1850 saw large socio-demographic changes in Sydney, with the small convict settlement of 12 000 being transformed to a busy city of 50 000 due to the inrush of immigrants bound mostly for the goldfields. Free immigration also resulted in young families settling in the colony, and this in turn altered the age and demographic structure of the population (Smith 1991).

The first legal public health order to emerge in the new colony of New South Wales was in October 1795, due to deaths from 'flux'. This order was proclaimed to prevent the pollution of the settlement's water supply (the Tank Stream). The fence along the stream had been removed, and pigs and other stray livestock gained access to and contaminated the stream. In 1832, the first statute pertaining to public health was enacted. It was called the *Quarantine Act*, and was copied from the 1825 English *Quarantine Act*. Further increases in immigration after 1850 saw rapid urbanisation and the subsequent environmental health problems of overcrowding, poor sanitation, contaminated food and polluted water similar to those seen in England and elsewhere in Europe. The overall result of immigration, unsanitary conditions, a large pool of susceptible people, poverty and non-existent public health preventive measures was the outbreak of epidemics in Sydney and other settled areas in Australia of childhood infections, such as scarlet fever, measles, diphtheria and whooping cough. After 1870, smallpox, tuberculosis, influenza, typhoid and bubonic plague followed. Although there was a high incidence of morbidity and mortality associated with dysentery, venereal diseases, bronchitis and gastroenteritis, it was the epidemics of smallpox and bubonic plague that caught the attention of the community and government.

Paradoxically, the epidemics of measles and scarlet fever which caused the highest mortality engendered the least public reaction, whereas outbreaks of smallpox and bubonic plague with comparatively less significant morbidity and mortality produced great public fear and hysteria (Smith 1991).

From the 1850s, Australian cities began to experience similar conditions to those that had led to the sanitary reform in England. In Sydney, the growth of the city ensured the continued deterioration of sanitary conditions, particularly in water supply and sewage disposal. Partly, this was also due to a system of private responsibility: the people responsible for the service—for example, waste removal—were not affected by a failure to carry out the service. The city provided few public services and refrained from construction of sewers because of the expense. Some sections of the community wanted sewers and others were not keen to pay for them (Beder 1989). An insight into the behaviour of the time can be gleaned from the following:

> The cesspits were emptied by private arrangement with 'night cart' men who would often dump their load on vacant land on the borders of the city or into the water reserve surrounding the water supply or they might sell it to the market gardeners. The uncleaned carts would return to the city in the morning, sometimes bring back garden produce from the market gardens, and remain in their smelly condition in the city all day. (Beder 1989: 27)

The arguments for and against the setting up of a central board to control water and sewerage continued until around 1875, when the fear of an epidemic provided further impetus. Conditions of the local environment were also found to be most unsatisfactory:

> at Rushcutters' Bay an extensive and stinking mud flat had formed which was exposed at low tide. At Woolloomooloo Bay a large bank had

formed and sewage floated on the surface of the salt water, oscillating back and forth with the movement of the tides. At Fort Macquarie a 'considerable bank' had formed and certain winds blew effluvia over 'a considerable area of the northern part of the city.' The water flowing from the Tank Stream into Sydney Cove was inky in colour, 'apparently putrescent, and floated on the surface of the Bay' for a considerable distance. (Beder 1990)

Finally, in 1888, the Metropolitan Water Supply and Sewerage Board was established (Beder 1989).

Similar circumstances were found in Perth: a growing population, the threat of epidemics, and municipalities that couldn't or wouldn't ensure sufficient sanitary services. A commission of inquiry established by the Legislative Council found that, despite an increasing population, little if any improvement was evident in urban sanitation:

> 'In Winter, most of the yards of Fremantle are one mass of filth' reported the municipal inspector. A bakery in High Street took the prize for squalor: 'the yard covered in large pools of animal filth and sewage, and the cesspit, which is in the corner of the stables, smelling foul: the well here is within fifteen yards of the cesspit'.
> (Hunt & Bolton 1978: 4)

On a previous occasion, it had been asserted 'that the citizens of Perth were living on a dunghill' and although resolutions were passed to address a sanitary system the council jibbed when the cost of the works was estimated (Hunt & Bolton 1978). Works eventually were begun on the extension and building of reticulated water supply systems in 1888 but, unlike in the eastern states, these were under the control of local councils. On one hand this suited the Legislative Council, which was ensuring protection of the rights of property owners from official interference, but there was concern and doubt that the Perth City Council could continue to

control water supply and sewerage for a metropolitan area that was expanding rapidly with the gold rushes. Eventually the government purchased the waterworks from the city and established a central authority, but it wasn't until 1912 that Perth had an operating sewerage system (Hunt & Bolton 1978).

The City of Melbourne was undergoing its own sanitary problems, particularly during and after the 1850s gold rush, with the increasing use of the Yarra River as the main sewer of the city. As Davison

---

Box 2.4 Conditions in working-class Melbourne in the 1880s

From their secure ramparts, upper-class Melburnians looked down over the river flats upon the inner ring of dismal working-class suburbs. Collingwood, Richmond and South Melbourne conspicuously lacked the fresh atmosphere, softening foliage and wide vistas of the hillside suburbs. Their low, flat terrain and soggy soil made drainage poor and enteric diseases a perennial hazard. Collingwood, the classic working-class suburb, was 'a sort of municipal Cinderella … low in more senses than one'; its blighted environment and endemic poverty gave it the highest death rate in the metropolis. But other parts of the flat were scarcely better— the riverside areas of South Melbourne were so beset with swampy ground, seasonal floods and an all-pervasive stench that visitors wondered, with more curiosity than concern, how people could bear to live there. Here, as in most parts of the unsewered city, household wastes and seepage from cesspools were permitted simply to run away through open drains into the river. In the inner suburbs, its flow was impeded by unfavourable topography, blocked drains and poorly designed streets, and in winter the river itself regularly broke its banks, depositing a noisome cargo over the lower reaches of the flat.

Source: Davison (1979: 150).

(1979) has observed, the inner core of working-class suburbs had become synonymous with dirt, disease and poverty.

Although the need for a deep system of sewerage was recognised as early as 1860, it wasn't until 1890 that a commitment was made to sewer the Melbourne metropolis. The need for this was made even more urgent with the introduction of a water supply without sewerage; subsequently, many thousands of people died from contagious 'filth' diseases attributable to the lack of sewerage (Dunstan 1984). The establishment of a central authority to develop and manage sewerage and water was not an easy task despite the effect on public health. There were many players in the politico-public health arena. Old and newer local councils, the Central Board of Health, the City of Melbourne, members of parliament who were variously for and against the role of the state (and the associated cost to it) and landowners all had positions on the issue, driven by differing motivations.

The Australian system of public health delivery began as a local activity, drawing on the framework offered by its British heritage. The earliest public health legislation was passed in Victoria in 1854, and was modelled on Britain's *Public Health Act* of 1848. The focus of concern—similar to that in industrialised England—was on local environmental conditions such as night-soil contamination and infectious diseases. The history of Australian cities also shows that progress in public health was slow and involved overcoming vested interests at the local and state political levels. This was particularly so in relation to the development of sewerage schemes. The rapid growth of cities also quickly outstripped the finite local resources, necessitating the eventual intervention of the state and thus central control of the expensive task of developing and maintaining infrastructure.

The development of the federal role in public health: A growing independence

The over-arching policy framework for public health, as for other areas of public policy, is derived from the Australian Constitution. When Australia was established as a federation in 1901, the Constitution prescribed particular powers for the federal (or Commonwealth) government. In other words, the Commonwealth could only exercise those powers conferred upon it by the Constitution. This means that the main powers of government, by default, rest with the states unless they are specifically allocated to the Commonwealth government by the Constitution. This is referred to as the principle of subsidiarity—that is, services are in principle provided by the particular level of government closest to the community in question.

Although local government is recognised as a crucial vehicle and setting for local public health activities, it is not recognised by the Constitution. As the Constitution only allows for two levels of government (state/territory or federal), the role of local government is determined by state legislation. The size and roles of local governments therefore vary enormously across the states and territories.

The federalist framework for government creates a number of complexities for health policy in Australia. The division of responsibility for financing and regulation (between federal, state/territory and local governments) can create enormous confusion in communities about where responsibilities and authority lie. Since Federation, however, the Commonwealth has become more and more influential in public health.

After Federation in 1901, the Commonwealth government did not immediately exercise its power regarding quarantine, which was its only public health responsibility under the Constitution. Eventually the *Quarantine Act 1908* was enacted, although it did not become operational until 1909. The Act was concerned with international or overseas maritime quarantine and the prevention of infectious diseases arising from the international movement of people and goods. Importantly from the public health administration perspective, there was agreement from the states that the functions of the Commonwealth included maritime quarantine, interstate quarantine, laboratory research into infectious diseases, collection of public health information and the establishment of uniform standards for foods and drugs (Cumpston 1989). This agreement laid the foundation for an expanded public health role for the Commonwealth government. Subsequently, the evolution of public health and health services delivery in Australia has marked a gradual shift from a local to a national emphasis.

The Commonwealth's involvement in public health began to expand in a tangible way with the establishment of the Commonwealth Serum Laboratories in 1916, the federal Department of Health in 1921, the Australian Institute of Tropical Medicine in 1910, and the National Health and Medical Research Council (NHMRC) in 1936 (Gordon 1976). Just prior to and after World War II, the Commonwealth government took some major steps in developing its role in public health. In 1936 Billy Hughes, the then Minister for Health and Repatriation, set up a fund for mothers and infants in response to concerns about the falling birth rate and high maternal mortality rate and under a policy of 'populate or perish'. One of the first resolutions of the NHMRC was to direct the attention of governments to the need for adequate supervision of the physical development of children before and during school age. In 1939 the first of the Lady Gowrie child-care centres was established, and these continue to the present day. At the same time, with war in the offing, a National Fitness Scheme was established to ensure physical fitness. These initiatives were important and heralded an incremental increase in the Commonwealth's public health role. In 1946, a referendum on the Constitution relating to the Commonwealth's powers in community services was conducted and passed, allowing the Commonwealth to pay benefits for pharmaceuticals, hospitals and nursing homes. This Constitutional amendment was seen as critical, as it laid the foundation for establishing national health insurance through payment of medical benefits. It also provided a platform for increased Commonwealth involvement in shaping national programs, which it achieved by offering matched funding to states.

An important post-war demand placed on the Commonwealth was the need to manage 500 000 immigrants from Europe. The Immigration Medical Service was established in 1947 to undertake this role (Department of Health and Ageing 2005b).

The role of the Commonwealth in health care continued to expand concurrent with its increased fiscal and taxation dominance. Some of the major health initiatives that were undertaken by the Commonwealth government ranged from legislating for the establishment and funding of health institutions (*Aged Persons' Homes Act 1957*) and the development of legislation such as the *National Health Act 1953* and the *Therapeutic Substances Act 1957*. Of particular importance was the initiation of national health campaigns such as the tuberculosis screening campaign in 1949, the introduction of Salk vaccine for poliomyelitis in 1956 and the National Standing Control Committee on Drugs of Dependence (1969). By the early 1960s, the Commonwealth Department of Health administered part or all of 22 Acts of Parliament, indicating the increased role and responsibility that had shifted to the Commonwealth. In 1967, after another referendum, the Commonwealth was able to make laws with respect to Indigenous Australians' welfare, and modest funding was provided to the states.

The election of the Whitlam Labor government in 1972 was a high point in the large and influential role of the Commonwealth in public health. In 1973, the government embarked on far-ranging health reforms with an emphasis on universal access to health care. The Community Health Program was one initiative at the time, followed by the

Medibank scheme and the establishment of the Health Insurance Commission (Department of Health and Ageing 2005b). Both these initiatives had far-reaching effects on the role of public health in Australia, and on the relationships between different levels of government—both at that time and up to the present day.

Conclusion: Civilisation and nation-building as a context for the organised effort

In this chapter, we have provided a number of historical examples of 'public health'. Key features of these public health measures are summarised in Table 2.1. Each example shows the clear relationship between ideas about the causes of disease and the focus of responses, and the impact of political and social considerations on the subsequent public health action.

In general, changes in public health practice have reflected changes in a number of features of modern nations and societies, with regard to both what illnesses and conditions occur and people's changing understandings of why they occur, and judgements about who is worthy of concern, what resources should be made available to combat illness and the purpose of combating disease. Technological and theoretical advances, not only in the understanding of human health and environments but also in the organisation and coordination of modern nation-states, have also had a profound effect on the implementation of public health practice.

Table 2.1 Key features of public health measures

Who, when, where?	What occurs?	Why is it thought to occur?	Who/what do health actions focus upon?	What action taken?	Why act at all?
Ancient Romans	Malaria (and other diseases)	Miasmas from swamps, corrupting winds	Environment and supernatural protection	City location, swamp drainage, construct temples	Keep citizens healthy (not specifically slaves or paupers)
Italian city-states	Bubonic plague	Miasmas and contagion from infected persons	Peasants, traders, religious leaders, houses and possessions, other cities	Quarantine, property destruction, embargo, movement restrictions	Preserve the health of aristocrats
British colonial India	Smallpox, bubonic plague	Miasmas, dirty conditions, contagious transmission	Environment and infected persons	Quarantine, property destruction, embargo, movement restrictions, limited vaccination, urban 'cleansing'	Protect and sustain colonial trade, British soldiers and British expatriates

As we have seen, the values and characteristics of modern public health have not always been acknowledged throughout human history. They are a result of changes in the way people perceive the relationship between citizens and the state—and indeed changing perceptions about who is considered a 'citizen' and therefore worthy of care. In the modern world, the trend is for more and more people to be considered worthy of care, and there is an increasing appreciation of the wide range of factors that contribute to people's health and well-being. Public health practice reflects these changes, and is a dynamic and exciting pursuit, promising great challenges and rewards to those who join this 'organised effort'.

3

Health in Australia today:
Health status, the health-care system and the place of public health

Challenge

You have been celebrating your great-grandmother's ninetieth birthday with family members of all ages. She brings out her photo album and reminisces about how hard life was for her family. One of her brothers died before she was born during the 1919 global influenza epidemic. Her oldest brother lost his factory job during the Depression and died of tuberculosis because he could not afford any medical care. His wife and three children then returned home to live with her parents and two youngest sisters. During the first ten years of her life, your great-grandmother's family lived in a two-bedroom house with an enclosed veranda. The toilet was down the back of the yard, and water was collected from a well. All the children walked several kilometres to and from school.

You are then surprised to learn that she was married at sixteen and actually gave birth to nine children, because your grandmother has only talked about her five aunts and uncles. One female infant died from pneumonia before her first birthday, while a boy of six died in an accident on the family farm. The third child was stillborn.

When your grandmother married after World War II, all of her four children survived childhood. But one of her brothers died in an industrial accident at an underground coalmine in New South Wales, while the other died ten years later of lung cancer. Your mother was born in 1958 and so is a member of the so-called 'baby boomer' generation—babies born in the period after the end of World War II.

Why has your mother's life been so different from that of your great-grandmother and grandmother? What were the most significant changes in and achievements for public health during their lives? What role did health care play in your mother's experience of a healthier and safer life than that of her ancestors?

Introduction

The current picture of health and disease in Australia is substantially different from that of 100 years ago. In the early 1900s, the (age-standardised) death rate for men was 1887 deaths per 100 000 males. By 2000, it had dropped significantly to 712 deaths per 100 000 (AIHW 2002). For women, the death rate fell more sharply—from 1516 deaths per 100 000 females to 450 deaths per 100 000 females, a reduction of 70 per cent. At the beginning of the twentieth century, infant mortality, maternal mortality and infectious diseases (such as tuberculosis, influenza, diarrhoea, typhoid, syphilis and diphtheria) were major health problems. Bubonic plague reached Australia in 1900, and particularly affected people living in Sydney and Brisbane. From 1900 to 1909, outbreaks of the plague occurred in many Australian coastal ports, including Adelaide and Melbourne. Parasitic diseases, such as malaria, schistosomiasis and filariasis (which can cause elephantiasis), were also introduced to Australia during the late nineteenth and early twentieth centuries, particularly when immigrants arrived in substantial numbers from diverse countries, many in search of a fortune on the Australian goldfields (Goldsmid 1988).

In contemporary Australia, and in contrast to some of the historical examples discussed in the previous chapter, the scope of public health action is extensive. Modern public health measures are concerned with all the conditions that affect people's health, including personal behaviour and the environments in which people live and work. The ultimate aim of public health is to ensure the health of all Australian residents, whether or not they are Australian citizens.

For a variety of reasons, public health action is driven primarily by altruistic and humanistic intentions, which regard all people as being equally entitled to good health and decent living conditions, an idea that is encapsulated in the UN Declaration of Human Rights. Public health is also driven by the achievement of economic goals, based on the

---

Box 3.1 Australia's people and their health

- 22.3 million people live in Australia, including about 557 000 Indigenous people (2.5 per cent of the total).
- 26.8 per cent of Australian residents are born overseas.
- Australia is highly urbanised, with over two-thirds of its population living in the capital cities.
- Australia performs well in quality of life measures, ranking among the top countries for many categories. Health, housing and governance are ranked among the top two countries, income is ranked fourteenth and work–life balance is marked 27th among industrialised nations.
- Average life expectancy at birth is 84.0 years for women and 79.5 years for men; it is much lower for Indigenous Australians—72.9 for women and 67.2 for men.
- Fertility rate is in decline, being well below replacement level—particularly for women aged less than 35 years.
- There are important differences in health status, health risk factors and health service access between rural and urban populations, between the general population and Indigenous Australians, and between people of different socio-economic backgrounds.

Source: adapted from AIHW 2012.

understanding that good health creates conditions for 'healthy' economies.

In this chapter, we outline the current health status of Australians. We show achievements and enduring challenges. We then consider the key features of the health system, including its historical development, which have been important in ensuring the health of the public. Finally, we consider the place that public health services occupy within the Australian health system.

An Australian picture of health: A good report card but improvements are possible

Changing patterns of health

Australians enjoy one of the highest levels of life expectancies in the world, just behind Japan and Switzerland and well ahead of comparable developed countries—the United States, the United Kingdom and Canada. The health profile of Australia is typical of industrial societies. The *World Health Report 2000* ranked Australia highly in terms of health status achieved (WHO 2000).

The picture of health in Australia has changed a great deal since the start of the twentieth century. Infant and child mortality has reduced dramatically since 1901, and has been the greatest contributor to the increased life expectancy of Australians (AIHW 2002). Mortality rates have not just reduced among young people, however. Across all age groups, death rates have declined substantially—a circumstance usually attributed to better living conditions, improved public health and safety initiatives and improved medical treatment. The data in Table 3.1 clearly show that the average health of Australians, at least when measured in terms of life expectancy, has improved over time. Another way of assessing health on the basis of life expectancy is to make comparisons between countries. Australia ranks highly among all nations in the comparison of life expectancy, including comparable countries in the OECD (see Figure 3.1). In 2009, Australia ranked

Table 3.1 Australian life expectancy (years) at birth, selected periods, 1901–2008

Year	Males	Females
1901–10	55.2	58.8
1920–22	59.2	63.3
1946–48	66.1	70.6
1960–62	67.9	74.2
1980–82	71.2	78.3
2000–02	77.4	82.6
2006–08	79.2	83.7
2008–10	79.5	84.0

Note: Since 1995, data on population and deaths have been averaged over three years to minimise year-to-year statistical variations.

Source: adapted from AIHW (2002, 2004a, 2010a, 2012).

sixth among OECD countries for life expectancy at birth for both males and females. The longest life expectancy was 79.9 years for males in Switzerland and 86.4 years for females in Japan. In Australia, life expectancy for the total population in 2008–10 was 79.5 years for males and 84 years for females. In comparison, for the Indigenous population in 2005–07, it was 67.2 years for males and 72.9 years for females (AIHW 2012).

While such data can offer public health researchers broad comparative information about the health status of Australians, they often want more detailed information about the factors that have shaped people's health. When looking at mortality rates, for example, public health researchers are most interested in finding out what people are dying from, so that they can begin to think (and act) practically about how to improve people's health. For this purpose, statistics on cause of death are used. See Table 3.2 for the major causes of death (mortality) in Australia in the period 2004–07.

Counting the number of deaths as a way of assessing the health of a population is well established in public health practice and dates back

Figure 3.1 Life expectancy at birth, top 10 OECD countries, 2009 or latest year available

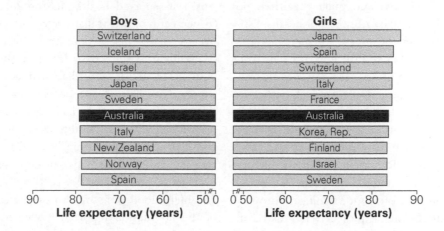

Source: adapted from AIHW (2012).

Table 3.2 Major causes of death, Australia, 2002, 2007

	Males				**Females**		
Causes of death		**% of all male deaths**		**Causes of death**		**% of all female deaths**	
		2002	**2007**			**2002**	**2007**
1	Coronary heart diseases (IHD)	20.1	17.2	1	Coronary heart diseases (IHD)	18.8	15.8
2	Lung cancer	6.9	6.7	2	Cerebrovascular diseases	11.7	10.4
3	Cerebrovascular diseases	7.2	6.4	3	Dementia and Alzheimer's disease	4.7	7.3
4	Chronic obstructive pulmonary disease	4.8	4.2	4	Lung cancer	3.9	4.3
5	Prostate cancer	4.1	4.2	5	Breast cancer	4.2	4.0
6	Dementia and Alzheimer's disease	2.1	3.4	6	Chronic obstructive pulmonary disease	3.5	3.3
7	Colorectal cancer	3.6	3.1	7	Heart failure and complications, and ill-defined heart diseases	1.9	3.1
8	Diabetes	2.6	2.7	8	Diabetes	2.4	2.8
9	Unknown primary site cancers	1.8	2.6	9	Colorectal cancer	3.4	2.8
10	Suicide	2.6	2.1	10	Unknown primary site cancers	2.1	2.5

Note: the rankings are for 2007
Source: adapted from AIHW 2004a and AIHW 2010a

to the pioneering work of John Graunt in the 1660s. Modern measurements of public health have increased in complexity, and public health is no longer measured solely by numbers of deaths. Estimates of 'the burden of disease'—which includes both death and disability—are now used. In this method, health conditions are ranked according to how many years of life are lost (either in duration or quality) due to the effects of specific diseases and health conditions, relative to average life expectancy. When this method is used, and when non-fatal conditions are included, the picture of health looks quite different: mental illness and chronic conditions account for a significant proportion of the health burden experienced by Australian communities. Table 3.3 shows the leading causes of burden of disease and injury in Australia in 2003.

There are, of course, many ways in which public health researchers measure the health of populations. In addition to mortality data, information about morbidity (non-fatal ill-health) is also collected and analysed regularly in Australia. Mortality and morbidity data usually are obtained from official or institutional records of various kinds, such as state government death registers and hospital admission records. However, these are not the only measures of Australians' health. The

Australian National Health Survey, for example, periodically collects information about Australians' self-reported health. In the 2011–13 survey, 56 per cent of Australians aged fifteen years and over reported their overall health to be very good or excellent, while 4 per cent rated their health as poor (ABS 2012b). More than 7 million Australians surveyed in 2007–08 (35 per cent of the population) reported that they had one or more of nine preventable chronic conditions including asthma, type 2 diabetes, ischaemic heart disease, cerebrovascular disease, arthritis, osteoporosis, chronic obstructive pulmonary disease (COPD), depression and high blood pressure. An estimated 2 per cent of the population reported having four or more concurrent conditions. The likelihood of having a chronic condition was seen to increase with age, as did the number of concurrent conditions. Fewer than 15 per cent of people in the 0–24 age group reported having at least one of the chronic conditions, compared with 78 per cent of people aged 65 or over. Chronic conditions were more prominent (four or more) in people aged over 45, and 8 per cent of people aged over 65 reported four or more conditions (AIHW 2012).

The factors that contribute to mortality and morbidity—risk factors—are often signposts to diseases that occur later in life. Risk factors have generally been thought of as those conditions (for example, hypertension) or behaviours (for example, smoking) that are associated with an increased probability (measured at the population level) of contracting or developing a disease or illness, or of dying. At a more fundamental level, risk factors also include genetics and exposure (even when in utero) to social, economic and environmental forces. These physiological and behavioural risk factors, as well as socio-economic and environmental factors, are important from a public health perspective, as they indicate the preventive action that should be undertaken. Table 3.4 contains a list of some of the commonly found physiological and behavioural risk factors in Australians.

Table 3.3 Burden of disease and injury (DALYs) by broad group cause, 2003

		% of total DALYS
1	Cancer	19
2	Cardiovascular	18
3	Other	14
4	Mental	13
5	Neurological	12
6	Chronic respiratory	7
7	Injuries	7
8	Diabetes	5
9	Musculoskeletal	4

Source: Begg et al. (2007).

Table 3.4 Risk factors for all Australians

	Male %	Female %	Associated conditions
Physiological			
Overweight	70.0	56.0	Coronary heart disease, type 2 diabetes, breast cancer,
Obesity	26.0	24.0	gallstones, degenerative joint disease, obstructive sleep apnoea
High blood pressure[a]	21.0	16.0	Coronary heart disease, stroke
High blood cholesterol level[b]	49.0	46.0	Coronary heart disease, stroke
Impaired glucose tolerance	9.2	12.0	Type 2 diabetes
Behavioural			
Smoking	18.2	174.4	Coronary heart disease, lung, mouth and cervical cancers (among others), stroke, chronic lung disease
Poor diet and nutrition[c]	4.5	6.6	Coronary heart disease, stroke, breast and digestive system cancers, type 2 diabetes, gallstones, osteoporosis, malnutrition, dental conditions
Excess alcohol consumption[d]	29.0	10.0	Coronary heart disease, liver and pancreatic disease, stroke, high blood pressure, cancers of the digestive system, accidents, mental illness, violence
Insufficient physical activity[e]	58.0	62.0	Coronary heart disease, stroke, type 2 diabetes, colon cancer, osteoporosis, bone fractures, falls, mental illness, obesity
Other drug use[f]	17.0	12.3	HIV/AIDS, hepatitis, renal failure, mental illness, suicide, violence, accidents
Not vaccinated[g]	8.2		Measles, diphtheria, tetanus, pertussis, poliomyelitis, *Haemophilus influenzae* type b
Excessive sun exposure[h]	24.0		Melanoma and other skin cancers, premature ageing of the skin
Unprotected sexual activity			HIV/AIDS, hepatitis, cervical cancer, infertility, pelvic infection, venereal disease

[a] Most recent available data 1999. Since 1980 prevalence more than halved (AIHW 2011c).
[b] Most recent available data 2000 (AIHW 2012).
[c] Percentage of adults with inadequate daily intake of fruit and vegetables.
[d] Aged eighteen years and over (drinking at sufficient levels to cause long-term harm).
[e] Aged fifteen years and over (less than 150 mins activity per week).
[f] Aged fourteen years and over.
[g] Children unvaccinated at one year of age.
[h] Adolescents with sunburn.

Source: adapted from AIHW (2002, 2004a, 2010a, 2011, 2012); ABS (2012b).

As with people in other industrialised countries, Australians experience a range of behavioural risk factors commonly associated with non-communicable diseases. Although smoking rates have continued to decline, with fewer than 17 per cent of Australians aged fourteen or over smoking tobacco daily, health problems related to alcohol, lack of physical activity and overweight/obesity are becoming increasingly evident (ABS 2012b). The ABS estimates that 44.7 per cent of adult Australians drink at levels that put them at risk of alcohol-related harm in the short term, by drinking more than four drinks in one session. Low physical activity levels had become more prevalent, but since 2007 these levels have decreased from 71.6 per cent to 66.9 per cent in 2011 for Australians aged fifteen years and over. However, young women (aged fifteen to seventeen years) are less active than young men, with 31.2 per cent of males compared with 11.8 per cent of females undertaking high levels of exercise and women twice as likely to be sedentary. Despite the higher rates of physical activity in men, more men are overweight or obese than women, and rates of overweight and obesity have increased for both men and women. Since 2007, the rate in men has risen from 67.7 per cent to 70.6 per cent, and in women from 54.7 per cent to 56.2 per cent in 2011. Rates of overweight and obesity in children aged two to seventeen years were also increasing, having risen from 22 per cent of children in 2000 to 25.3 per cent in 2007, although the rate was the same in 2011–12 (ABS 2012b).

By 2007–08, nearly every Australian aged 15 years and over (99 per cent) had at least one risk factor for chronic disease, such as obesity, high blood pressure or physical inactivity. The most common risk factor indentified was insufficient consumption of vegetables and the most common combination of multiple risk factors included an unhealthy diet and a lack of exercise—particularly for young adults aged fifteen to 24 years and males aged fifteen to 44 years (AIHW 2012). In relation to unhealthy diet, Australian Bureau of Statistics (2012a) data

from the 2011–13 National Health Survey showed that older people are more likely to consume sufficient fruit and vegetables (9.6 per cent of those aged 65–74 years compared with 4.5 per cent of those aged 25–34 years). In relation to physical activity as a risk factor, data from the report on determinants of chronic disease from the Australian Institute of Health and Welfare (2011c) show that people living outside major cities are more likely to be inactive (60.8 per cent of males and 64.7 per cent of females) than those living in major cities (55.6 per cent of males and 62.6 per cent of females).

Socio-economic status was shown to be an indicator for physical activity, with those who live in more disadvantaged areas more likely to be inactive (63.6 per cent for males and 67.4 per cent for females) compared with those who live in less disadvantaged areas (47.8 per cent for males and 55.2 per cent for females) (AIHW 2011c). Location was shown to be an indicator for alcohol consumption and smoking, rates of which vary between states in Australia. Western Australia had the highest proportion of adults who consumed on average more than two standard drinks of alcohol per day and Victoria had the lowest (25.4 per cent compared with 17.6 per cent). The highest daily smoking rates were recorded in the Northern Territory (23.9 per cent) and Tasmania (21.8 per cent), while the lowest rate was recorded in the Australian Capital Territory (13.4 per cent) (ABS 2012b). Income was shown to be an indicator of oral health, which improved along a gradient from the lowest income group to the highest income group. Adults on lower incomes were more likely to have missing teeth, experience toothache and avoid certain foods (6.1 per cent, 19.5 per cent and 24.2 per cent respectively) than adults on higher incomes (4.8 per cent, 11.3 per cent and 11.0 per cent respectively) (AIHW 2012).

Difference and diversity

Health patterns differ between men and women, as seen above, but patterns of health differ in other ways within the Australian population, as seen

---

Box 3.2 Health differentials in population groups

- The health status of **children** has generally improved, with a decline in the incidence of vaccine-preventable disease, deaths due to motor vehicle accidents and accidental drownings. The majority of children now use some form of sun protection. Overweight and obesity are on the increase, however.
- Adolescent mental health problems are more prevalent in **blended families** (families in which both parents have children from previous relationships), one-parent families, families with low incomes and families with one or more unemployed parents. Tobacco smoking, insufficient physical activity, alcohol consumption and illicit drug use are all matters of concern.
- **Immigrants** generally have lower death rates and hospitalisation rates than the general Australian population, but their 'health advantage' decreases as their length of residence in Australia increases. They also differ in rates of injury and disease, which tends to reflect immigrants' specific occupational and socio-economic circumstances, as well as health behaviour and health care-seeking patterns.
- Mortality rates for **Indigenous** Australians are higher for almost all causes of death. Hospitalisation rates are also higher for most diseases and conditions, indicating a higher occurrence of acute (brief and severe) illness. Chronic (long and continued) diseases (such as diabetes and kidney disease) and suicides are some of the leading causes of death for Indigenous Australians, while low birth weight, obesity, poor nutrition, use of alcohol and other drugs, poor housing and living conditions, and lower levels of health-care access are all major risk factors for poor health.
- People with **low socio-economic status** have higher rates of mortality and lower life expectancy at birth, are more likely to smoke, be more overweight or obese, and are less likely to be physically active.
- **Rural and remote** populations appear to have less access to employment and services, and tend to engage in behaviours that put their health at risk to a greater extent than urban (city) populations.

Source: drawn from AIHW (2002, 2012).

in Box 3.2, such as through the life course and in relation to social conditions.

The presence of health differentials across socio-economic groupings is a particularly striking feature in Australia, as well as in other developed countries. Rates are highest among people living in the lowest socio-economic areas and lowest among people living in the highest socio-economic areas for cardiovascular disease (23.8 per cent compared with 17.1 per cent) and type 2 diabetes (6.2 per cent compared with 2.9 per cent). Similar differences between people living in higher and lower socio-economic areas are also seen in relation to non-melanoma skin cancer, injuries among young people, depression and chronic respiratory disease. Rates of premature death among 15–64-year-olds are 70 per cent higher among those in the lowest socio-economic group compared with those in the highest socio-economic group. For cancer survival and self-assessed health status, rates are highest among people in the highest socio-economic group and lowest among people in the lowest socio-economic group (71 per cent compared with 63 per cent for five-year relative cancer survival rate) and 64 per cent compared with 48 per cent rate their health as very good or excellent (AIHW 2010a). People with disabilities aged under 65 are much more likely than people without a disability to report having long-term physical and mental health conditions, and to rate their overall health as fair or poor. Risk factors for chronic disease are more common among people with disabilities, including being overweight or obese, engaging in low levels of exercise and smoking daily (AIHW 2010).

Risk factors for chronic disease are more prevalent in people living in more disadvantaged areas. The rate of tobacco use among people living in the lowest socio-economic areas was 25 per cent in 2010, twice the rate among people living in the highest socio-economic areas. Similarly, people in the highest socio-economic group are the least likely to be overweight or obese (37.9 per cent). Interestingly, people in the middle socio-economic group are the most likely to be overweight or obese (42.7 per cent).

These differences between the most disadvantaged areas and the least are also reflected in use of health services. People living in more disadvantaged areas have relatively high rates of GP consultation and are more likely to be hospitalised with potentially preventable conditions, but are less likely to receive preventive dental care (AIHW 2012).

Understanding these differences is important for the formulation and targeting of intervention strategies. For instance, obesity has been framed as the latest epidemic but, as Table 3.5 shows, while rates of obesity among males and females are similar (26 per cent and 24 per cent respectively), the proportion of overweight males and females is higher, and males are more likely to be overweight than females (42 per cent and 31 per cent respectively). Obesity is also more of a problem in the Indigenous population (34 per cent) than the non-Indigenous population (18 per cent).

Although Australia compares favourably with other countries in terms of overall health status, the international comparison has been very poor when it comes to the health of Aboriginal and Torres Strait Islander (ATSI) populations. While the gap in life expectancy between indigenous and non-indigenous populations in Canada, the United States and New Zealand was reduced from 7–12 years during the 1970s to between 5–7 years in the late 1990s, it had remained at 20 years in Australia (AMA 2002; AIHW 2004a). By 2005–07 the gap in life expectancy between Indigenous and non-Indigenous Australians had reduced to 9.7–11.5 years (AIHW 2012).

Table 3.5 Overweight and obesity by socio-economic status and gender

	Overweight	Obese
Males	42	26
Females	31	24
Difference	**–9.0**	**–2.0**
Post-school qualifications	35.5	14.9
No post-school qualifications	33.3	19.0
Difference	**–2.2**	**4.1**
Employed	35.2	16.2
Unemployed	28.0	18.4
Difference	**–7.2**	**4.1**
Highest income 1/5	36.4	14.3
Lowest income 1/5	30.5	19.1
Difference	**–5.9**	**4.8**
Least disadvantaged 1/5	56	–
Most disadvantaged 1/5	66	–
Difference	**10**	**–**
Major city[a]	58	–
Other areas[a]	66	–
Difference	**–8.0**	**–**
Non-Aboriginal	33.6	18.0
Aboriginal	32.4	34.0
Difference	**–1.2**	**15.2**

[a] Overweight or obese.

Source: O'Brien & Webbie (2003: 21–2); AIHW (2011d; 2012).

The health gap between Indigenous and other Australians is of particular concern to public health professionals. In 2002, the Australian Medical Association (AMA) released the first of its two Public Report Cards on Aboriginal and Torres Strait Islander health. Titled *No More Excuses*, this report showed that the infant mortality rate for Aboriginal and Torres Strait Islander populations was three times higher than for the general population. Many communities, particularly those in rural and remote areas, were found to lack basic public

Box 3.3 A picture of Australia's children

Studies by the AIHW have found that over the last 20 years the lives of children have been influenced by the changing social context of Australia's development. Some of the findings were:

- Infant mortality halved from 9.6 per 1000 live births in 1983 to 4.8 in 2003, with a major factor being the declining rate of deaths from SIDS. Although the decline has continued, by 2010 the rate had levelled out to 4.13 per 1000 live births.
- Vaccination coverage rates had levelled out by 2011 at 93 per cent for children aged two; for five-year-olds, rates had improved to 90 per cent.
- In 2003, approximately 320 000 children aged from birth to fourteen (8 per cent) had a disability.
- Infants from least-advantaged socio-economic areas were twice as likely to die before their first birthday than those from the least-disadvantaged areas. Mortality rates in 2010 for Indigenous infants were significantly higher than for non-Indigenous infants (7.3 compared with 4.13 per 1000 live births).
- Between 1997 and 2006, injury, cancer and diseases of the nervous system were the major causes of death for children aged from one to fourteen years.
- The rate of sexual assault against girls was three times higher than that for boys.
- Asthma is a long-term condition for 12 per cent of children aged from birth to fourteen.
- One in eleven children (aged twelve to fourteen years) had smoked tobacco the week before the 2005 survey and 5 per cent had participated in risky drinking; since then, passive exposure to tobacco smoke for children has continued to fall, with the proportion of households with dependant children having someone smoking inside the home falling from 31 per cent in 1995 to 6 per cent in 2010.
- In 1998, 14 per cent of those in a study of 4500 children aged from four to fourteen years had mental health problems; results of a second national survey of child and adolescent mental health and wellbeing are anticipated in 2013.
- Almost one-quarter of children were developmentally vulnerable (below the tenth percentile) on one or more domains (health, emotional and behavioural development, education, identity, self-care skills, social presentation, and family and social relationships) at school entry, which suggests they may experience difficulty in Year 1.

Sources: AIHW (2005a, 2009, 2012).

Prevalence of overweight and obesity has been increasing among Australia's children and is now one of the highest among OECD countries, in 2007–08 one in twelve children was obese. This number has been estimated to be rising by 1 per cent per year, which could mean that by 2035, around 50 per cent of the population will be overweight. Data on physical activity indicates that in 2009 about three-quarters of children aged from five to fourteen participated in sport or cultural activities. There is a lack of recent data on mental health and for children from culturally and linguistically diverse backgrounds.

Source: AIHW (2005a: xi–xv); AIHW (2012).

health infrastructure—they did not have access to clean water, electricity and sewerage, and lacked adequate housing. Major problems with access to primary health care were also found, with little evidence of any improvements (AMA 2002). The ABS *National Aboriginal and Torres Strait Islander Health Survey* found in 2004–05 that a third of the 10 439 persons interviewed reported eye problems, one in seven (12 per cent) said they had asthma (which was most prevalent among people over 45 years), 12 per cent reported having long-term heart and circulatory conditions, and 49 per cent reported having consumed alcohol in the week prior to the interview (ABS 2006). There were also substantial inequalities between Indigenous and non-Indigenous men and women in rates of heart disease, stroke, injuries and poisonings.

Since implementation of the National Indigenous Reform Agreement endorsed by Council of Australian Governments (COAG) in 2008, access to primary care has increased, with 32 000 Indigenous patients registered for chronic disease care with a GP (Closing the Gap 2012). The report to COAG (COAG Reform Council 2012a) in relation to progress towards Closing the Gap targets during the period 2010–11 provides evidence of improvements in some aspects of Indigenous health; however, some targets were not met and rates for some indicators had worsened. Death rates improved significantly from 1998 to 2010 in Queensland as well as the Northern Territory, which was the only one of the states and territories on track to meet the 2031 death rate target. There has been no significant change in death rates in New South Wales and South Australia. Some indicators of child mortality have improved in some parts of Australia.

The Indigenous child death rate has decreased, with the rate falling from 252 per 100 000 children in 1998 to 203 per 100 000 children in 2010. This was a faster fall than for non-Indigenous child death rates, which decreased from 113 per 100 000 children in 1998 to 95 per 100 000 children in 2010. This means the gap is beginning to close between Indigenous and non-Indigenous child death rates (Figure 3.2). Infant mortality varied, from the lowest in South Australia (5.3 deaths per 1000 live births) to the highest in the Northern Territory (13.1 deaths per 1000 live births). The rate of Indigenous women smoking during pregnancy—which can be harmful to the foetus and infant—decreased in most states and territories between 2007 and 2009; however, the gap increased in Tasmania. The rate of low birthweight babies born to Indigenous mothers decreased nationally but increased in Victoria.

As there is a demonstrated link between education and health in the ability of populations to maintain health, the low school-retention rates for Indigenous students contribute substantially to

Figure 3.2 Child death rate, by Indigenous status, 1998–2010

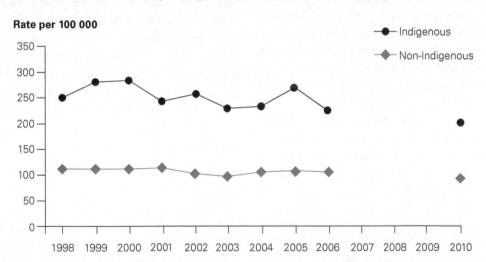

Children aged 0–4 years. Data are for NSW, Queensland, Western Australia, South Australia and the Northern Territory combined.

Note: A combined total is not available for 2007 to 2009 due to data quality issues in Western Australia.

Source: adapted from COAG Reform Council (2012a).

this health inequality. Retention rates reported in 2003 were 12.4 per cent lower for non-Indigenous students to Year 10; subsequently, rates have improved in some states between 2007 and 2010. However, attendance rates are decreasing in all states and territories in the later years of schooling. The greatest decrease in school attendance occurred in the Northern Territory, dropping from 69 per cent in 2007 down to 61 per cent in 2010. During this period, Tasmania maintained the highest school attendance rates, recording 83 per cent in 2007 and 82 per cent in 2010 (AMA 2003; COAG Reform Council 2012). Unemployment rates among Indigenous people have remained high, but by 2011 had decreased to 16.3 per cent as against 4.9 per cent, down from 20 per cent as against 7 per cent in 2004–05 (ABS 2012b). Rates of imprisonment for Aboriginal and Torres Strait Islander people have increased from 1746.3 per 100 000 compared with 115.5 per 100 000 non-Indigenous population, up to 1914 per 100 000 Indigenous population as compared with 129 per 100 000 non-Indigenous population. Rates of imprisonment in the Indigenous population further underline the systemic differences that are experienced by Aboriginal and Torres Strait Islander people in Australia.

What has changed and how?

As noted earlier, the current picture of health and disease is substantially different from a century ago, with achievements being made possible through a range of public health measures—many of which are still in use today. Key strategies for improving population health have included disease surveillance, contact tracing (where infected individuals are asked about other people with whom they have been in contact, and each person is successively and similarly followed up), screening, quarantine, environmental health inspections (for unsanitary conditions), the application of building and accommodation standards, and land-use planning. Many practices have long since become unnecessary or fallen from favour. For example, in the case of the bubonic plague,

bounties were paid to rat-catchers, who were required to kill the fleas on dead rats by dropping the rats into boiling water. As outbreaks of disease were sometimes met with fear and hysteria in the community, coercive measures such as compulsory quarantine became accepted actions for disease control. Legislation also became a major tool for public health action, and health education was introduced, which emphasised hygiene and patient compliance.

As the twentieth century progressed, new health issues emerged. Changes in Australia's demographic composition (caused by factors such as ageing and immigration), living conditions and ways of life meant that more attention had to be paid to chronic diseases and the special health needs of specific ethnic groups. Over time, changing socio-economic conditions brought attention to different groups and different health problems. For instance, occupational injury from mining has been an important consideration for public health during much of Australia's history, but has recently been overshadowed by the rise of occupational over-use syndrome associated with the widespread use of computers in the workplace. Increasing health differences between regions and population groups, according to socio-economic status, have also received more attention.

During the latter part of the twentieth century, groups within communities, such as women and people with disabilities, became more vocal and, by expressing their needs and concerns, drew attention to health issues specific to them. New technological possibilities also brought new hopes for better health (for example, a hepatitis B vaccine and neonatal intensive care) and challenges (such as the greater proportion of severely disabled children living to adulthood). Communities also became more aware of the potential impact on health arising from changes in environment, related in part to human activities, such as global warming. As new types of health problems gained in prominence (including those related to tobacco use, sun exposure, road accidents and unsafe sex), public health efforts had to respond by adopting new methods and techniques to deal with these problems, as will be seen in later chapters in this book.

Despite Australia's changing health profile, some health concerns persist. Health inequalities are the most notable and regrettable feature of the Australian health landscape. While disparities have always existed between groups due to biological differences (such as gender and the influence of age), there are other contributing factors. Therefore, it should be possible to reduce health disparities through various forms of action. Differences arising from social and environmental conditions—such as income, education, occupation and urban–rural residence—can be addressed through policy and program interventions. Most important in this regard are the large and persistent differences between Indigenous and other Australians, which pose a major challenge for public health action.

The Australian health-care system: A public health success story

The Australian health-care system has evolved during the twentieth century. From the early period of European settlement, when health care was primarily the responsibility of families and charitable organisations, the system is now largely professionally based and funded by governments. The Commonwealth government, through Medicare (the national health insurance scheme), provides funding for GP and specialist services, and subsidises the drugs approved for the Pharmaceutical Benefits Scheme (PBS). The Commonwealth government also subsidises private health insurance and residential aged care. Funding for public hospitals, home and community care, and some public health programs is shared between federal and state/territory governments, while states/territories are responsible for funding community health services and other public health programs. The states/territories also license private hospitals and nursing homes. Reflecting decades of change, the system resembles a complicated mosaic, but one that could

generally have a strong public health orientation (see Figure 3.3).

As Figure 3.1 shows, compared with many other countries, Australia has an enviable life expectancy. At the same time, it has managed to maintain relatively strong controls over health expenditure, compared with several OECD countries (see Figure 3.4). These general indicators show that Australian health policy can be regarded as an international success story.

Like many other industrialised countries, Australia has a strong tradition of government intervention to protect the interests and welfare of its population, particularly of vulnerable groups. Interventions have been in the provision of education, social security, family benefits, unemployment, child care and aged care. These services are well established in the mindset of Australians, who are so accustomed to this social policy that they are often not aware of it until specific services are undermined, begin to fragment or are seen to disadvantage specific groups. Australia's national health policy framework puts into practice the widely held value that everyone should have equal access to basic human services. In general terms, it is a redistributive system—that is, the system spreads the burden of paying for health care among all members of Australian society so that no one is excluded from the benefits of Australia's prosperity. The overwhelming public support for Medicare, an important safety net for health-care provision, is a particularly strong demonstration of Australians' beliefs about equitable access to health care.

Two components of social policy that have long served Australians are the (predominantly) public hospital system and the PBS, which ensures that essential drugs are made available at subsidised prices to those who need them. Medicare, the national health insurance system introduced in 1983, gives all eligible residents access to primary care. In transferring funds to the states for hospital services, the first Medicare Agreement (between the Commonwealth and state/territory governments)

Figure 3.3 Financing health care in Australia

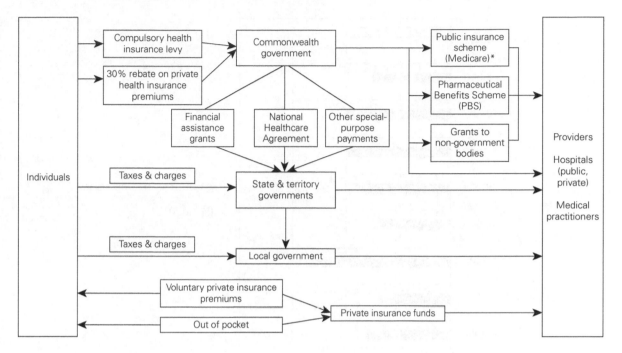

* Medical services.

Source: updated from OECD (1994) by Bloom (2000).

required that any eligible patient may elect to become a public patient, and so receive services without charge. Private health insurance became available as an optional adjunct to national health insurance.

The removal of financial barriers to health care—through universal health insurance—is one of the most significant public health features of the Australian health care system. In contrast to the United States, where over 40 million people (nearly 13 per cent of the population) do not have health insurance, Australians do not need to delay seeking medical care because of incapacity to pay, are generally able to obtain needed prescription drugs at a relatively low cost and can access a range of community-based health services for little to no cost. Preventive services are generally paid for by either federal or state/territory governments.

In addition to universal access to medical services and subsidised pharmaceuticals, the Australian health-care system displays other features that can be characterised as a public health approach to organising the health system. These include:

- a strong emphasis on reporting and monitoring, with a national health statistics agency (the Australian Institute of Health and Welfare), a variety of national health surveys, comprehensive hospital morbidity data collection and the development of uniform data-collection schemes in other areas of health services
- a strong emphasis on the planning and development of service networks, including planning guidelines for aged care that are based on access and equity, hospital role delineation around regional referral systems and, in some states, defined population catchments for health services

Figure 3.4 Percentage of gross domestic product spent on health care, 2000 and 2010

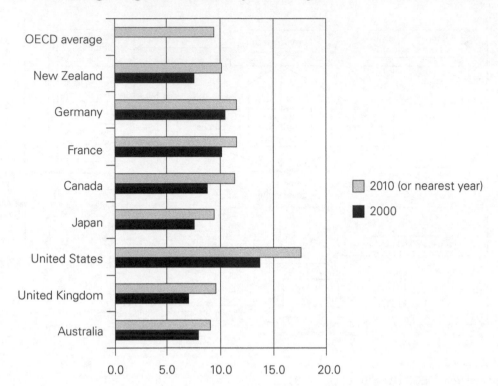

Source: OECD (2012).

- specified services for vulnerable population groups (such as women, immigrants and Aboriginal and Torres Strait Islander populations), particularly in recognition of the social context for health and health-seeking behaviours
- attempts to allocate resources—in some states/territories and for a range of national programs—on the basis of population health needs
- an interest in evidence-based approaches to health service delivery, moving from the adoption of best-practice guidelines by the National Health and Medical Research Council (NHMRC) to using cost-effectiveness evaluation criteria for benefit payments, to embracing the more recent evidence-based medicine (EBM) movement.

A review of the organisational structure of the Commonwealth Department of Health during the last century reveals how the focus of health policy has changed in Australia over time. In addition to previously established divisions with responsibility for acute care, aged care, pharmaceutical benefits and population health, among others, recent changes include the establishment of divisions devoted specifically to health protection, and to workforce and mental health (see Appendix C).

The passing of the Australian *National Preventive Health Agency Act* in 2010 and the establishment of the Australian National Preventive Health Agency in 2011 reflected a significant change in health policy focus to disease prevention, specifically chronic non-communicable disease.

Key priorities of the Commonwealth Department of Health and Ageing (DoHA 2012o) include:

- reforming funding and governance arrangements for hospitals, primary care and aged care
- improving access to locally based primary care services for chronic disease
- improving service delivery and early intervention for Aboriginal and Torres Strait Islander people to help close the gap in life expectancy between Indigenous and non-Indigenous Australians
- supporting people living with mental illness through integrated, effective and evidence-based mental health care
- reconfiguring service delivery in rural communities to improve health outcomes
- improving workforce capacity through expanding the roles of non-medical health professionals
- improving governance arrangements and reform of the national aged care system
- improving electronic infrastructure, such as personally controlled electronic health records.

Where does public health fit into the health system: Programs as well as a framework?

Public health services in Australia emerged from strong regulatory traditions. For most of the twentieth century, states had highly centralised Departments of Public Health or Public Health Commissions, which were responsible for environmental health, food safety, communicable diseases surveillance and control, radiation safety, occupational health and safety, control of drugs and poisons, health education, maternal and child health, immunisation, school nursing and school dental services, STD clinics and disaster management.

A review of the organisational framework for health administration in Australia indicates how public health concerns have evolved, and how the efforts of governments have been organised. As shown in Box 3.4, over the course of the twentieth century, governments' concerns have shifted from the management of infectious diseases to the payment of benefits for personal health care. Over the past 30 years, the public health presence within the Commonwealth government has been focused on new health priorities—such as HIV/AIDS, tobacco and illicit drugs, and now alcohol and obesity—which also reflect changing societal expectations.

From a budgetary viewpoint, public health programs under federal and state/territory health authorities have long been overshadowed by publicly funded personal health care (that is, hospitals and health insurance benefits). With the rise of community health services, it became possible for many public health programs to be integrated with personal health services delivery. Over time, services (such as maternal and child health), and health promotion have emerged as core components of the Australian health-care system.

Box 3.4 Evolution of the federal Department of Health

When the Department of Health was established in 1921, its main focus was on quarantine activities, and disease control and prevention. This was still generally the case by 1961, when the major concerns were the 12 847 notified cases of infectious hepatitis. As there was no vaccine available at that time, the public was informed of the 'need for scrupulous cleanliness in personal hygiene' (Department of Health 1961: 7). There were also 176 notified cases of poliomyelitis and the national tuberculosis drive continued. Some attention was being paid to population health through the National Fitness Movement, which was funded by the department through state councils and state Education Departments. Highlighting the increasing importance of vaccinations, the Commonwealth Serum Laboratories was established as a separate entity (Department of Health 1961).

By 1971, which marked the department's fiftieth anniversary, the focus of activities had become oriented towards the provision of services and benefits rather than being based more strongly on prevention. This is reflected in the health budget, which showed $160 million was spent on pharmaceutical benefits, $95 million on medical benefits and $73 million on hospital benefits. Yet communicable diseases were still a significant concern for the Public Health Branch, with 234 notified cases of malaria, 67 cases of leprosy and 7571 cases of infectious hepatitis. There were also 9562 new cases of gonorrhoea. A social and preventive medicine section, as well as a section for environmental health, had been added. The growing concern about the ill health caused by cigarette smoking was reflected in a revision of the voluntary code on tobacco advertising (Department of Health 1971).

During 1984–85, a major restructuring took place, and the new Health Advancement Division brought together those areas focusing on prevention and promotion, with new sections being established for drug dependence, health strategies, and social and community health. New programs included the Home and Community Care Program, a national campaign against drug use and measures to combat the AIDS epidemic in Australia. Given the greater role being played by the NHMRC and the TGA in public health, they became separate divisions. A sum of $500 000 was allocated to the National Health Promotion Program in the Health Strategies branch, targeting elderly and young unemployed people. Tobacco advertising was required to have four rotating health warnings, such as 'Smoking Kills' (Department of Health 1985).

By 1997, reflecting new policy directions, the Department of Health was being asked to focus more on consumer choice and outcomes, develop more sustainable financing, adopt evidence-based medicine, reduce service delivery through purchaser/provider separation and implement reform agendas across several programs. A new performance regime was also implemented across all departments, with performance indicators (such as effectiveness, equity and quality) and targets being established in advance.

The objective for the public health program had become: 'to promote and protect the health of all Australians and minimise the incidence and severity of preventable illness, injury and disability'. The main activities for the year were the development of national health priority areas, efforts to lift low immunisation rates, the establishment of the National Public Health Partnership, the Third National HIV/AIDS Strategy, the first collaborative national tobacco campaign and managing the newly described bat *lyssavirus* in Queensland (Department of Health 1997).

Since 1997, there have been significant changes in the structure of the Population Health Section, reflecting global trends as well as changing national health priorities. The Drug Dependence Section changed to the Drug Strategy and Population Health Social Marketing Section in 1999, which in turn had become the Drug Strategy Section by 2004. As a result of SARS and avian influenza outbreaks, the possibility of an influenza pandemic, the Bali bombings and threats from biological, chemical and radiological agents, the Biosecurity and Disease Control Section was established in 2004. Food and Healthy Living became a distinct section, reflecting the growing problem of overweight and obesity in the population. In 2006, Population Health was split into two: the Office of Health Protection and the Health Development Division. By 2012, Chronic Disease and Health in Social Policy had become distinct sections, reflecting a recognition of the need to address social determinants of health and the growing problem of preventable chronic diseases (see Appendix D).

Public health activities are often viewed as representing one component of the health service delivery system, since all health systems provide a set of programs that are aimed at prevention, protection and promotion. The scope of public health programs varies across countries. In Australia, the following areas are generally managed as public health programs:

- immunisation, HIV/AIDS and communicable diseases control
- surveillance, epidemiology and public health laboratories
- environmental health and food safety
- health promotion (applied in the areas of tobacco control, diet, physical activity, skin cancer prevention, injury prevention)
- drugs
- women's cancer screening
- maternal and child health
- school health
- refugee screening
- disaster management
- public health laboratories.

In present-day Australia, the delivery of public health activities partly reflects the historical origins summarised above, along with prevailing health concerns in Australia.

Public health programs often do not just involve components of the health care system, however. Many programs and activities are delivered by community organisations, professional bodies (such as the Cancer Council), schools and other government agencies—for example, in relation to environmental protection, occupational health and safety, or road safety. From this stance, public health programs are part of the health system as defined by government portfolio, but extend beyond the boundaries of the health authorities.

The major changes in the organisation of public health service delivery over the past few decades may be characterised as:

- *decentralisation*, with integration into the health care system (e.g. area-based public health units reporting to a manager of health services, rather than reporting to a Public Health Division in the state Health Department)
- *fragmentation*, with integration into other portfolios (e.g. the removal of specific policy and regulatory responsibilities from the Health portfolio into industrial relations, consumer affairs and primary industry portfolios)
- *increased participation* of stakeholders (e.g. the establishment of advisory structures with representation from industry interests, health professionals and consumers).

In the last quarter of the twentieth century, many areas have been shifted out of the Health portfolio as other portfolios have incorporated key public health functions. For example, responsibility for occupational health and safety has been transferred to labour and industrial relations portfolios, ostensibly in order to establish closer links with the broader public policy context for occupational health and safety. Police and road authorities have assumed responsibility for road safety issues, with much success. Recreational safety has become integrated with sports and recreation authorities. Environmental protection authorities have a revised and important role in environmental health. Water boards have a role in water quality. Finally, consumer affairs now play an important role in product safety.

The ways in which states and territories organise the public health service presence within their respective Health Departments is often subject to change. For example, in Victoria in 2009, the new Department of Health was established in order to focus on disease prevention and health promotion while maintaining responsibility for health services, but was separated from the Department of Human Services, which maintained responsibility for children, youth and families, and disability services. Maternal and child health services are the responsibility of the Department of Education and Early Childhood Development. In New South Wales, the Public Health Division is headed by the Deputy Director-General of Public Health as well as the Chief Health Officer, but in 2012 both of these roles were occupied by the same person. The division is divided into 'business units', including the Centre for Population Health, the Centre for Epidemiology and Evidence, the Centre for Aboriginal Health, the Centre for Oral Health Strategy and the Office of the Chief Health Officer. In Queensland, in order to integrate service provision, the Chief Medical Officer had assumed responsibility for population health and Public Health Units in sixteen locations across the state had responsibility for health protection and promotion. Reforms currently underway will place responsibility for public health units within seventeen newly established independent statutory authorities that also have responsibility for local hospital and health services.

There is often a tendency for the structure of state Public Health Divisions to change with relative frequency, due (among other things) to political considerations, new developments in the field of public health, current and emerging health issues and changed personnel (for example, when a new director is appointed, there is generally an expectation that they will 'make a mark' by reorganising the department). All of these contribute to divisional reorganisation and the descriptions provided here should therefore be regarded as a 'snapshot in time' of various Australian public health divisions.

Another area of change is the move towards specific regulatory authorities for particular issues, along with a goal of uniformity in national policy. National authorities have been responsible for the regulation of radiation and nuclear safety, therapeutic goods (pharmaceuticals and devices), food standards and gene technology. There are also new authorities governing blood supply and health workforce registration. These arrangements continue to mesh with state responsibilities in intricate ways.

With the integration of public health activities into the health-care system and into other portfolios, growth has occurred in the number and range of participants and stakeholders in public health. Public health delivery is no longer the sole concern of government, and is performed by many organisations outside of government. These service providers include local governments, health services that receive government funding, non-government organisations (NGOs) and consumer groups. The NGOs are diverse—ranging from large, disease-based organisations (such as the National Heart Foundation and Diabetes Australia) to small, consumer-based, self-help groups. In addition, professional organisations (such as the Public Health Association of Australia and the Australian Institute of Environmental Health) and tertiary education institutions are involved in policy advocacy, research and development, and professional development. Clearly, although particular public health programs are the full-time responsibility of particular people, the health of the population of a country like Australia depends on the interaction between a wide range of government and non-government groups.

The public health presence in the health system, furthermore, is not solely reflected in a set of programs. Public health knowledge and skills (such as epidemiology) also underpin the planning and operation of the health-care system—by providing analyses of health needs in the community, the informational bases for program planning and priority-setting, and the tools for evaluating impacts and outcomes of health interventions. Public health knowledge and skills further offer an approach to the design and management of the entire health system—by emphasising population health gain, cost-effectiveness of system design and interventions, community participation and mobilisation, and the value of links with other sectors that influence health outcomes.

A major challenge now facing the Australian health-care system is how to provide patient-centred primary care to meet the needs of the increasing proportion of the population living with chronic conditions. A study in 2011 of the primary care experiences of adults in eleven countries (including Australia, Canada, New Zealand, the United States and the United Kingdom), conducted by the Commonwealth Fund, shows that in the area of treatment of chronically ill and seriously ill people, Australia ranks reasonably well (see Table 3.6 for selected results). But the findings indicate that there are shortfalls in providing effective treatment to sicker adults in all eleven countries. In all countries surveyed, there was room for improvement in care coordination, system integration and engaging patients in care and self-management.

In Australia, there is room for improvement in several aspects of service delivery for people with chronic and serious illness. Patient safety could be improved—for 34 per cent of patients a pharmacist or doctor had not reviewed nor discussed their prescriptions in the past year and 19 per cent of people had medical, medication or laboratory test errors. Care coordination needs to be addressed too, as 55 per cent of survey respondents had experienced gaps in hospital or surgery discharge and 36 per cent had experienced gaps in the coordination of their medical care in the previous two years. Access to appropriate after-hours services is limited, with 56 per cent of those surveyed experiencing difficulty getting after-hours care without going to an emergency department. There is also room for improvement in doctor–patient relationships and communication: only 64 per cent of respondents who had seen a specialist in the past two years reported experiencing positive shared decision-making. Only 48 per cent of those with a chronic condition who had seen a professional in the past year reported overall positive experiences of being engaged by their health-care provider in discussing the management of their chronic condition. Only 59 per cent of those with a chronic condition could, between doctor visits, easily call a health professional to ask a question or get advice, and only 16 per cent had a health professional who contacted them to see how things were going.

Strengthening patient connection with primary care services is another area for improvement in

Table 3.6 Quality of treatment for chronically and seriously ill adults in five countries, 2011

	Australia %	Canada %	NZ %	UK %	USA %
Gaps in care coordination	36	40	30	20	42
Gaps in hospital or surgery discharge	55	50	51	26	29
Difficulty getting after-hours care without going to emergency department	56	63	40	21	55
Medical, medication or lab errors	19	21	22	8	22
Prescriptions reviewed	34	28	31	16	28
Positive shared decision-making with specialists	64	61	72	79	67
Positively engaged in care management	48	49	45	69	58
Can call a professional to ask question or seek advice	59	62	71	81	77
Professional contacts them to see how things are going	16	16	22	29	31
Has a medical home*	51	49	65	74	56

* Medical home—an accessible primary care practice that helps coordinate care.

Source: adapted from Schoen & Osborn (2011).

Australia: only 51 per cent of respondents who had a chronic condition had a regular doctor or place of care that was accessible and knew them, and helped coordinate their care. For people whose health care needs are more complex, having a medical home—an accessible primary care practice that helps coordinate care—is recognised as important in ensuring quality care. Patients who were connected to a medical home generally were shown to have more positive experiences, including better support for chronic conditions, better communication and better care coordination. Patients with medical homes were less likely to report medical mistakes and far more likely to rate their care highly. These trends are reflected in the higher rates recorded in Australia (shown in Table 3.7) for effective communication, coordination, quality, safety and patient satisfaction for patients with a medical home, compared with rates for patients without a medical home.

In order to ensure that the health system is performing effectively and meeting the needs of patients with chronic and serious health conditions, a switch to a patient-centred care approach is required in the delivery of primary care services. Reforms are required in the way resources are used, including reforms to payment and information systems and the redesign of health-care delivery

to support team-based care. The chronic diseases and serious illnesses that accounted for more than half of allocated health expenditure in Australia in 2004–05 (see Table 3.8) were cardiovascular disease (11 per cent of total health expenditure), oral health (10 per cent), mental health (8 per cent), musculoskeletal diseases (8 per cent), neoplasms (7 per cent), injuries (7 per cent) and respiratory diseases (6 per cent).

Conclusion: A work in progress

In this chapter, we have described the patterns of health that can be observed in the Australian population. We have described briefly how particular features of the health-care system have helped achieve this outcome. In particular, we have considered the place of public health services within the health-care system. We have observed that Australia has experienced enormous improvements in health status and compares well with the rest of the world, although significant health inequalities persist. Achievements have been possible, in part, because Australians have enjoyed a universal health insurance system for decades, so few financial barriers to accessing preventive services have existed. The downside of a publicly funded and organised health care system is that public health services

Table 3.7 Communication, coordination, quality, safety and patient satisfaction by medical home, 2011

	Has medical home* %	No medical home %
Positive doctor–patient relationship	79	52
Gaps in care coordination	31	41
Gaps in hospital or surgery discharge	49	63
Medical, medication or lab test errors	15	23
Positive patient engagement in managing chronic condition	56	38
Blood pressure under control	85	71
Quality of care rated as excellent or very good	79	56

* A medical home is an accessible primary care practice that helps coordinate care.

Source: adapted from Schoen et al (2011).

Table 3.8 Allocated health expenditure in Australia by disease group and area ($ million), 2004–05

Disease group	Admitted patients[a]	Out-of-hospital medical services	Optometrical and dental services	Prescription pharma-ceuticals[bc]	Community and public health[d]	Research	Total expenditure allocated by disease	Per cent of total allocated expenditure	Per cent of DALYs in 2003[e]
Infectious and parasitic	482	451	–	199	–	184	1315	2.5	1.7
Respiratory	1477	1039	–	725	–	69	3311	6.3	8.4
Maternal conditions	1539	116	–	4	–	12	1671	3.2	0.1
Neonatal causes	422	20	–	1	–	12	455	0.9	1.3
Neoplasms	2381	570	–	236	222	378	3787	7.2	19.4
Diabetes mellitus	371	288	–	275	–	55	989	1.9	5.5
Endocrine, nutritional and metabolic	448	500	–	1042	–	110	2100	4.0	1.1
Mental disorders	1411	538	–	854	1177	148	4128	7.8	13.3
Nervous system disorders	985	782	218	464	–	291	2739	5.2	11.9
Alzheimer's and other dementias	*169*	*32*	*–*	*91*	*–*	*35*	*327*	*0.6*	*3.6*
Other nervous system	*816*	*750*	*218*	*373*	*–*	*256*	*2412*	*4.6*	*8.3*
Cardiovascular	3009	1133	–	1636	–	164	5942	11.3	18.0
Digestive system	1849	447	–	764	–	48	3107	5.9	2.2
Genitourinary	1431	779	–	111	–	24	2345	4.5	2.5
Skin diseases	398	454	–	102	–	13	966	1.8	0.8
Musculoskeletal	2003	1181	–	680	–	92	3956	7.5	4.0
Congenital anomalies	209	24	–	2	–	54	290	0.6	1.3
Oral health	186	22	5064	6	–	27	5305	10.1	0.9
Injuries	2422	845	–	124	–	14	3405	6.5	7.0
Signs, symptoms, ill-defined conditions and other contact with health system[f]	3195	2712	–	919	–	22	6848	13.0	0.7
Total	**24221**	**11900**	**5282**	**8144**	**1399**	**1715**	**52660**	**100.0**	**100.0**

[a] Includes public and private acute hospitals, and psychiatric hospitals. Also includes medical services provided to private patients in hospital.

[b] Includes all pharmaceuticals for which a prescription is needed, including benefit-paid prescriptions, private prescriptions and co-payment prescriptions.

[c] Excludes over-the-counter medicaments, such as vitamins and minerals, patent medicines, first aid and wound care products, analgesics, feminine hygiene products, cold sore preparations, and a number of complementary health products that are sold in both pharmacies and other retail outlets.

[d] Comprises expenditure on community mental health services and public health cancer screening programs.

[e] Disability-adjusted life years (DALYs) comprise years lost due to premature death and years of 'healthy life' lost due to disability (Begg et al. 2007).

[f] 'Signs, symptoms, ill-defined conditions' includes diagnostic and other services for signs, symptoms and ill-defined conditions where the cause of the problem is unknown. 'Other contact with the health system' includes fertility control reproduction and development; elective cosmetic surgery; general prevention, screening and health examination; and treatment and aftercare for unspecified disease.

Source: AIHW (2010b:7)

compete with hospitals for limited resources, and often become the 'poor cousins' in the process.

In the following chapters, we will build on this broad context of public health in Australia, and answer the two questions in which students of public health are typically most interested: *How is public health done?* and *How do I do public health?* In Part II, we will begin to address these questions by describing some of the tools and theories used by people who practise public health, as well as some of the processes and dynamics that influence the way public health is done in Australia. By doing this, we hope to offer some practical tools and techniques to think about how to 'do' public health.

Public health has a long and complex history, which in many respects is a reflection of the complexities of its core concerns: namely, how to ensure that people are healthy, and how to achieve this aim across broad groups of people. Partly as a consequence of this long history, and the many diverse interests and activities that contribute to people's health, there is often considerable debate about where 'public health' begins and where it ends—is poverty, for argument's sake, a public health issue? Or is it an economic issue, or one of welfare? Even within the public health field, there are debates about what practices and approaches are similar or distinct—is health promotion a part of public health, or is it a different thing altogether? These kinds of conversations are ongoing in public health practice, and in the following chapters we will provide the tools to help understand these debates and why they occur. Despite—or perhaps because of—these debates, the practice of public health is alive and well, and the 'organised effort' of public health is able to develop in ways that make real and substantial contributions to the quality and length of people's lives.

Part II

Conceptual and analytical toolkit:
Key concepts and frameworks

4

Distribution of health and its determinants:
Changing concepts and models

Challenge

When a friend is unwell, you might visit them to offer comforting words of encouragement, some flowers and a 'get well' card. As you sit with them listening to their experience of illness, what are you thinking about their situation? Are you privately speculating that they are responsible for their illness? Do you hold them responsible for their own recovery? Occasionally, we all act as though becoming healthy is essentially under the control of the sick person—perhaps with some help from a doctor or other health-care provider. Depending on their health problem, you may encourage your friend to eat certain foods, swallow particular medicines or a herbal formula, resume gentle activity or keep warm. But if you reflect for a few moments, you may realise that it is not always the case that a person has much control over either developing an illness or recovering their health.

There are many factors that affect people's health. For example, a person who has a heart attack may come from a family with a predisposition to heart disease (geneticists and social historians have noted the tendency for specific groups to suffer from this condition). A person may have adopted risky behaviours like smoking in their teenage years because all their friends were smoking regularly (statisticians have repeatedly demonstrated how dangerous it is to smoke). After many years of working in the lowest status job in the organisation, a person may have been threatened with the loss of their job and eventually been made redundant (industrial psychologists have studied the impact of this kind of stress on health).

The factors that affect our health also go beyond those that are particular to individuals and families. For example, we also know that the incidence of heart disease has increased over the last 50 years as nations have become industrialised and populations have increased their dietary intake of saturated fat (epidemiologists, social historians and nutritionists have plotted this development). As we probe further, we discover that our bodies are not well adapted to eating large quantities of animal fat, and the fact that we do has contributed to the increase in non-communicable diseases noticed in industrialised countries (physiologists, biological anthropologists and evolutionary biologists have studied issues surrounding saturated and unsaturated fats in the human body). If we think about our ancestors' ways of life, we realise that sweet and high-fat foods, though desirable for energy, would have been hard to find—in fact, our ancestors had to spend a significant amount of time and effort obtaining them. Nowadays, while we desire them as much as our ancestors did, we have much easier access to them and consume too much. As far as our body mass index and heart health are concerned, our desires are better suited to life on the savannas than lunchtime at local cafes (psychologists have been particularly interested in behaviours associated with our modern patterns of consumption of these now easily available high-energy foods). We might also consider how our hurried modern lives contribute to our preference for fast, convenient and fried foods—all of which contain high proportions of fat (sociologists study the way such lifestyle changes occur with increased urbanisation). Finally, we may discover that selective breeding of livestock and modern food processing have led to a concentration of fat in our diet (McMichael 2001).

As the factors that affect our health can vary even more than those discussed above, what advice would you offer a friend who felt they were overweight and working in a stressful job? How might your views on the causes of and solutions to these issues contrast with the views of your friend or of doctors, naturopaths, family members, gym instructors or managers at the workplace? What would be a useful way to think about the causes of these health issues so that solutions could be discovered and pursued? What limits might your friend confront in understanding the underlying causes of the health issues facing them?

Introduction

Public health is concerned with improving the health of people. Therefore, it is potentially interested in all health issues that confront communities and population groups. This is potentially a large and complex effort, so it is necessary to determine the most important issues, pinpoint the issues on which it will be possible to

make a difference, and decide where an effective starting point might be.

If health is to be improved, it is necessary to understand the precursors and consequences of health problems so that appropriate action can be taken to prevent illness, promote health and ameliorate the consequences of disease and disability. On the basis of this knowledge, interventions to improve health can be designed, deploying a range of tools and focusing on environments, individuals, societies—or all of these contributors to health and well-being. The scope of health improvement is broad, so it often requires contributions from a diverse range of disciplines and professions.

This chapter is concerned with how we understand health and what tools we use to confront health problems. We begin with a brief overview of what 'health' is and how it is understood in the practice of public health. We look at the common methods by which we measure and monitor health and health determinants, and how we understand the complex patterns that emerge. We then review some of the theoretical or conceptual models that are used to explain the nature of health problems and look at how these models continue to affect the choice of public health strategies. The tools and explanations offered by different disciplines and professions to explain causation and tackling health problems will be explained in the next chapter.

Defining health: Not merely the absence of disease

> Health is a state of complete physical, mental and social well-being and not merely the absence of disease or infirmity.

As we have already noted, there are many definitions of 'health' circulating in the world today. However, the one above, first proposed by the World Health Organization (WHO) in 1948 and contained in the Preamble to its Constitution, is the one most often quoted by people writing about health and what it is. This broad and holistic definition is actually consistent with the earlier Latin phrase *mens sana in corpore sano* ('a sound mind in a sound body'), and can be contrasted with the synonymous use of the words 'sick' and 'evil' since the twelfth century (Young 1998: 3).

The WHO definition of health incorporates our historical understanding that the environments in which people live are important for health and well-being, countering the view—which emerged with the rise of biomedicine in the late nineteenth century—that 'health' could be understood *only* as the 'absence of disease or infirmity'—that is, to be healthy is *not to be ill*. The WHO definition of health—that health is not merely absence of disease and infirmity, but is concerned with complete physical and mental well-being—suggests that there are two things we need to consider when thinking about health: what causes disease and ill-health ('pathogenesis') and what creates health and well-being ('salutogenesis'). In fact, both of these considerations have been present, in one form or another, throughout the documented history of thinking about health. As biomedicine has increased in influence, however, European traditions have tended to focus on pathogenesis to the exclusion of salutogenesis, although this circumstance has slowly started to be redressed over recent years.

Understanding the distribution of health and illness: Counting, measuring and quantifying

Since the early days of the Greeks and Romans, when health and its possible determinants were first systematically documented, the picture of health has changed a great deal. Understanding these changing patterns and the factors responsible for them is a starting point for public health practice, research and policy. This task is at the core of the discipline of epidemiology, which in turn is one of the core public health sciences. Epidemiology is described by one of its more famous theorists, Mervyn Susser, as follows:

> Epidemiology is the study of the distributions and determinants of states of health in human populations. A determinant [of health] can be any factor, whether event, characteristic, or other definable entity, so long as it brings about change for better or worse in a health condition. (Susser 1973: 3)

As a support discipline for public health practice, the potential scope of epidemiology is very broad. There are no limits to phenomena that may be of interest to epidemiological study, as long as the phenomena in question affect people's health. And, given that 'health' is now generally understood to encompass 'physical, psychological and social' elements, the scope of epidemiology includes all of these concerns.

Monitoring health

As their major tool, epidemiologists use data that measures health status and possible factors that contribute to health and disease, and then analyse the relationship between these possible health determinants and a range of health outcomes. While the tools have become increasingly sophisticated, the principles have existed since antiquity. Indeed, since the time of Hippocrates, almost 500 years BC, the idea of observing, recording and collecting facts about health, analysing them and considering reasonable courses of action based on the results has been the work of many observers of health states (Teutsch & Churchill 2000).

The first application of systematic health monitoring was probably in the Roman armies, where doctors were employed on a per capita basis to look after the health of the troops. However, the first real public health action relating to surveillance probably dates back to the time of the bubonic plague in the fourteenth century. Ships nearing the port of Venice were boarded by public health authorities and persons with plague-like illness were prevented from disembarking. They were sent instead to the first quarantine station, which was run by monks on San Lazaretto island, in the lagoons near Venice. The ruins of the station are still in existence.

Population health measurement dates back to the late English Middle Ages, when causes of death began to be systematically ascribed and examined. John Graunt, a haberdasher and musician, published his *Observations on the Bills of Mortality* in the early 1660s.

In it, he summarised information that he had systematically collected from parish baptism and burial registers, enabling him to make inferences about causes of death in the seventeenth century.

In order to make any estimate reliable data must be obtained by researchers, epidemiologists and public health personnel. In public health practice, this data can come from a number of sources, including data already collected by other people or organisations (such as the routine reporting of notifiable diseases by medical practitioners). Where relevant or appropriate data is not available, research projects must be designed to obtain the information required by epidemiologists and public health workers. Some of the most common means and methods used to obtain this kind of data are listed in Box 4.1.

From the various sources of data, epidemiologists construct the rates of occurrence of different health events. These rates are a simple way of capturing and quantifying a complex event as well as a way of comparing these events across different population groups. Box 4.2 outlines the common measures of health used by epidemiologists. Unfortunately, despite a commitment to a broad definition of health (as per WHO), it is easier to measure death and disease than it is to measure health and well-being. Regular reporting—and monitoring—of health status thus frequently makes use of the measures listed in Box 4.2. In recent years, epidemiologists have begun to develop more complex measures in order to capture data on disability, social functioning and quality of life, and it can be expected that more of these composite health indices will be used in the future.

Public health surveillance

Health monitoring seeks to identify changes in the health status of a population or its environment. It is often intermittent rather than continuous, and does not involve intervention unless an important trend is occurring. Monitoring is carried out for a number of reasons, including to observe the effects of a new program (such as the introduction of a new

> ## Box 4.1 Sources of data for assessing the health of populations
>
> **Vital statistics:** Data about births, deaths, marriages and migrations are vital for understanding population dynamics. For instance, such data represent a starting point for assessing whether some groups have higher death rates than others, and whether a community is likely to experience the health problems of a young or old population.
>
> **Administrative data:** Data collected for purposes of administering programs can often be useful. For example, data collected by hospitals indicate the numbers and sorts of treatments used by all patients and identify which people are admitted to hospitals. This information can be very valuable for monitoring why people are hospitalised. Similarly, data about workers' compensation systems can indicate types of injuries that have occurred at work and their likely causes. Data can also be collected from a specific health program, such as an immunisation or screening program. For instance, a population sub-group may be prone to a particular disease, and a screening program for that disease in that population would monitor the trend in disease occurrence and use of preventive services.
>
> **Surveys:** Surveys use a set of predetermined questions to obtain information on specific topics. Usually, such data are obtained through research projects developed for a particular task, and are not routinely collected by organisations and institutions. However, ongoing surveys can also be done (such as the Australian National Health Survey and other state-based health surveys). Typically, survey participants are selected to be statistically representative of a whole population or a population group of interest.
>
> **Surveillance data:** Data about occurrence of specific diseases are routinely reported by doctors and/or laboratories under legislation. This is one of the basic duties of public health systems, and requires continuous scrutiny of all aspects of the occurrence and spread of diseases that might be relevant to their control and treatment. Surveillance systems can also be built around *sentinel events*, which are events that should not occur if preventive and curative care is appropriate. They are often avoidable deaths, such as those caused by medication errors or infections that occur in hospitals, and they may give the epidemiologist clues as to the source of an epidemic or to the circumstances leading to a disease or a death.
>
> **Qualitative data:** It is not always easy or possible to convert people's attitudes, beliefs and perceptions about health issues into numerical data (*quantitative data*). Interviews, focus group discussions and pictorial representations are some of the ways in which the quality of an experience or understanding about particular events are captured. Written or verbal responses to general or specific questions are important tools for understanding why an event happened, beyond the presence or absence of such an event. As is the case for surveys, this kind of data is not routinely collected by organisations and institutions.
>
> **Unobtrusive measures:** Sometimes it is possible to develop an understanding about health issues without collecting information directly from people. Unobtrusive measures are those—such as observation—that can be captured quantitatively or qualitatively without people being aware of it. This approach can be important in circumstances where the outcome of the study could be affected if the subject were aware of it.
>
> *Source:* Eager, Garrett & Lin (2001).

vaccine or drug), to assess quality control in research (for example, in medical trials) and to assess population changes as a result of the introduction of a new policy (for example, a traffic-calming intervention). In public health practice, however, the concept of surveillance—the idea that collecting and analysing data leads to action—is critical.

The techniques and study designs used to collect, store and analyse the data used for monitoring are often identical to those used in surveillance,

Box 4.2 Key epidemiological concepts and definitions

Age- and sex-specific rates: These are measures of health-related events that occur in a specific age or sex group in a given period, expressed as numbers per 1000 live population in that group.

Age adjustment: This refers to a procedure used to compare health patterns between cities or even countries. A standard population with a known age and sex composition is used as a benchmark to calculate, for each place, age-adjusted rates, which are then used to compare health between different places. This is often necessary because morbidity (illness) and mortality (death) affect age and sex groups differently, and if two places have different age and/or sex distributions, analysts may make the mistake of attributing differences in morbidity and mortality to location, rather than the age/sex composition of the populations in question.

Case fatality rate: This refers to the number of deaths per number of cases of disease. This measure is cumulative, so it is necessary to specify the time period to which it applies.

Disability-adjusted life years (DALYs): These are calculated as the number of disability-free years of life that might be lost as a result of premature death and disability due to a disease in a particular year. Based on expert evaluations of the degree of impairment resulting from particular diseases, this measure allows epidemiologists to obtain a more detailed understanding of health impacts than that achieved by a simple measure of mortality.

Disease susceptibility rate: This is the proportion of a given population who could be affected by an exposure. In chronic diseases, it reflects a combination of genetic susceptibility and other risk conditions and exposures, while in communicable diseases it reflects the non-immune population.

Incidence rate: This counts the number of *new* health-related events occurring in a population in a specific time period. It is calculated as a ratio of the total population at risk at that time, and expressed as the rate per a multiple of ten.

Infant mortality rate: This counts the number of babies who die between birth and 364 days as a fraction of the number who are born in that same year. It is expressed as the number of such babies who die per some multiple of ten, usually per 1000. For example, industrialised countries generally have an infant mortality rate (IMR) of less than nine per 1000, compared with developing countries, which generally have an IMR rate of more than 30 per 1000.

Life expectancy: This counts the average number of years a person at a given age may be expected to live, given current mortality rates.

Maternal mortality rate: This is the number of women who die while pregnant or within 42 days of termination of pregnancy. Included are deaths related to or aggravated by that pregnancy. Maternal mortality is closely related to the quality of prenatal, delivery and post-partum care.

Morbidity rate: This is the number of existing or new cases of a particular disease or condition per 1000 people.

Mortality rate: This is the number of deaths in a population. It depends on a reliable source, such as a system of mandatory reporting of deaths.

Premature mortality: This measure adds stillbirth rates to perinatal (around the time of birth) rates of death and calculates this measure as a ratio of total live births in the same year, expressed as numbers per 1000.

Prevalence rate: This is similar to counts of incidence. Prevalence includes *all* the individuals who have a disease, attribute or condition in a specific time period. As such, it counts both *new* health-related events *and* health-related events that already existed at the start of the time period in question. It is calculated as a ratio of the total population at risk during the same period.

Standard mortality ratio: This is calculated by dividing the observed number of deaths from a particular health event by the expected number of deaths (from a standard population) and multiplying it by 100. It allows cross-country comparisons of mortality rates.

Sources: adapted from Tulchinsky & Varavikova (2000); Lawson & Bauman (2001); Aschengrau & Seage (2003).

---

but because the data is not continuously collected there are qualitative differences in the ways it can be interpreted and used in subsequent health planning. The idea of surveillance has been at the core of public health practice, regardless of the type of disease or health risk.

Because infectious diseases used to be the main cause of death (and remain a major cause of death today in many developing nations), surveillance systems originally were concerned with acute infectious diseases. However, over time this has changed, and although many communicable diseases are notifiable, not all are communicated between people, and not all are acute. Diseases such as hepatitis B and C, as well as HIV infections, are today considered to be chronic diseases. Also, gradually some non-communicable and genetic diseases are becoming notifiable, such as Creutzfeldt-Jakob disease (one very rare communicable and genetic disease which is known as 'mad cow disease'), as well as various cancers and conditions involving glandular and eye disorders.

Current concepts of surveillance evolved from public health activities developed to control and prevent disease in the community. Four commonly used definitions of surveillance are:

- the traditional WHO definition: 'the systematic collection and use of epidemiological information for the planning, implementation and assessment of disease control' (WHO 1968: A.21)
- the US Centers for Disease Control and Prevention (CDC): 'Public health surveillance is the ongoing, systematic collection, analysis, interpretation, and dissemination of data about a health-related event for use in public health action to reduce morbidity and mortality and to improve health.' (CDC 2001)
- the National Institute of Occupational Safety and Health (NIOSH) of the US CDC: 'Public health surveillance is the ongoing systematic collection, analysis, and interpretation of health data for purposes of improving health and safety. Key to public health surveillance is the dissemination and use of data to improve health ... Surveillance includes both population- or group-based activities and individual-based activities.' (United States National Institute of Occupational Safety and Health 2004)
- a British textbook definition: 'Continuous analysis and interpretation and feedback of systematically collected data, generally using methods distinguished by their practicality, uniformity and rapidity rather than accuracy or completeness' (Eylenbosch & Noah 1988).

What features do these definitions of public health surveillance have in common? Clearly, surveillance is considered to be a systematic approach to monitoring occurrence of health and illness events, regular and routine analysis of this data, the estimation of disease and wellness rates and trends, and the use of this data for health-related program planning. There is no debate about what is meant by 'systematic' or 'regular' data collection: data may be collected on a continuous basis or by means of regular cross-sectional studies, as long as these are systematic and at intervals that are regular enough to be able to provide a sensitive measure of trends.

As we noted in Chapter 2, some of the first studies of health and illness in populations of people were conducted by men such as Graunt and Chadwick. They explored some of the issues and employed some of the methods that were later to become the concern of epidemiologists. While each increased contemporary understanding of the distribution of health and disease, it is also true that their areas of interest were limited by their understanding of what health was, and what its contributing factors were. For example, Chadwick was a firm believer in the miasmic theory of disease, and some of his most important contributions to epidemiology focused on the classic concerns of miasma theory— for example, by comparing populations that lived near swamps before and after those swamps were drained. A number of his colleagues (and those who followed) also focused on the effect of the *environment* on the health of populations.

Early public health practice was focused on case-by-case control of infectious diseases. Originally, the concept of 'surveillance' was associated with identifying individuals with serious infectious diseases to institute prompt isolation, and monitoring of contacts in order to detect early symptoms. The critical demonstration of a population approach to surveillance came from the field trials of poliomyelitis vaccine in 1955 (Teutsch & Churchill 2000), where daily surveillance identified cases of vaccine-associated paralysis that were related to a single vaccine manufacturer. By 1968, the WHO applied the term 'surveillance' to diseases themselves rather than to the monitoring of individuals, and included the implied responsibility of follow-up of cases to see that effective actions had been taken to prevent further cases in a population.

The contemporary purpose of surveillance is to be able to understand patterns of disease, to identify areas of high and low incidence, and to be able to identify differences within and between populations, as well as over time. The key uses of surveillance data (Hadden & O'Brien 2003) include estimating the usual and expected distribution, spread and magnitude of a given health problem or event in a population identified as being at risk:

- to understand the natural history of a health problem (disease or injury)
- to monitor changes in disease patterns and to detect and map outbreaks, epidemics and pandemics
- to identify groups at high risk for a particular disease
- to test hypotheses about aetiology (or disease causation)
- to identify potential control strategies
- to evaluate control strategies undertaken
- to monitor isolation activities
- to detect changes in health practice
- to identify research needs
- to facilitate planning of public health actions and resource prioritisation.

Hadden and O'Brien (2003) suggest five key characteristics of surveillance data: it is simple in nature because it needs to be very accessible; it is timely, recording events very soon after they occur; it is standardised in nature so that it is comparable with data from other places; it is ongoing; and analysis is easy, making feedback a routine rather than an arduous task.

There is no reason to restrict disease surveillance to either contacts of cases or the monitoring of infectious diseases. The concept of surveillance is now accepted as applicable to a wide range of health problems and risks other than infectious diseases— for example, accident and injury; several chronic diseases, especially cancers; and genetic disorders and birth outcomes. As well, service-oriented surveillance can be applied to iatrogenic disease (health problems that arise as an unanticipated consequence of receiving medical care), immunisation uptake, adverse drug reactions and hospital activity.

Understanding the determinants of health: Weaving knowledge with beliefs

Miasma, contagion and punishment?

The ancient Greeks and Romans thought diseases were related to emanations from the environment, or foul air (composed of malodorous and poisonous particles generated by the decomposition of organic matter). This theory of *miasmas* dominated European thinking about health protection and disease control well into the nineteenth century, and formed part of the basis for practical public health measures, such as sanitation, improved housing and improved urban environments.

In contrast to the miasma theory sat the contagion theory. Since the Black Death in the fourteenth century, many disease-prevention activities have been based on the idea that illness is contagious (Tesh 1988). The Venetians instituted the quarantining of ships during outbreaks of the plague, and some ports were completely shut down. On land, the sick were isolated from the well, and checkpoints were set up at entrances to cities to inspect travellers and their goods.

At the same time, throughout human history, much of the populace believed that diseases were caused by supernatural forces. In earlier societies, people attributed disease to evil spirits. In Christian

---

Box 4.3 Disease patterns

Surveillance tells us about incident cases, from which population attack rates can be calculated and compared. Disease patterns generally are thought of as *endemic, outbreak, epidemic* and *pandemic*.

Disease that is **endemic** is considered native to a defined population: a fairly similar (therefore having an expected prevalence) number of cases occurs in the same (age, sex) groups of people, in the same area, over a predictable time period. The number of cases of infectious diseases notified to any of the Australian state Health Departments or summarised at a national level can be found in the state and federal public health annual reports. For example, we expect to have between 4000 and 5500 cases of pertussis (whooping cough) each year (McIntyre et al. 2002).

If we understand the expected pattern of disease, we can identify **outbreaks**. An outbreak is a geographically localised unmistakable increase in cases of a specific disease, and is usually—though not always—limited by time (Last 2001). Taking the pertussis example above, the substantial 1997 outbreak of nearly 11 000 cases was easy to identify. Discussion surrounding the outbreak led to the subsequent revision of the national immunisation recommendations for pertussis.

The geographical context may be a definable area, such as a village, or may be associated with an institution. Outbreaks of listeriosis in the French Alps associated with soft cheese, for example, are sometimes quite prolonged, although confined geographically (De Buyser et al. 2001).

Epidemics are similar to outbreaks; however, while also defined by the classic epidemiological triad of people, place and time, they are usually transient, and often spread rapidly. Epidemics usually pertain to health events, but epidemics of health-related behaviours can also occur. An example of a common epidemic is the quite frequent occurrence of salmonellosis (a serious form of food poisoning) all over the world, including Australia, associated with unsafe food handling of mass-produced food—sometimes for wedding breakfasts or community celebrations, such as religious festivals, but also associated with some fast-food outlets (OzFoodNet Working Group 2003).

A **pandemic** is the term applied to a widespread outbreak of disease, distributed throughout a large region, country or even worldwide, which is usually quite prolonged. Influenza pandemics have occurred every few years for as long as it has been possible to diagnose it as a specific disease (Cunha 2004).

---

societies in the nineteenth century, most religious people accepted the view that disease was a punishment for transgression against God's laws (Tesh 1988). Because epidemics took a greater toll on the poor than on the rich, the supernatural theory allowed condemnation of the poor for their 'sinful behaviours'.

Influence of bacteriology

The emergence of the science of bacteriology in the nineteenth century had a major impact on our understandings of health and disease, and therefore on public health action.

Louis Pasteur introduced new techniques and ways of thinking about the patterns and transmission of disease among human populations, and a number of new and innovative theories about the causes of disease and illness began to emerge in European thought in the latter half of the nineteenth century. Pasteur refined his concept of the 'germ theory', which suggested that specific organisms caused specific diseases and symptoms, and that hosts (the persons or animals that these organisms attempt to infect) could become immune to these organisms. Robert Koch, a German physician, built on Pasteur's discoveries. He developed techniques to classify bacteria by their shape and their propensity to be stained by various dyes. In the process, he developed a set of rules (known as 'Koch's postulates') that led to the identification of tubercle bacilli as the cause of tuberculosis, which was the leading cause of death in Europe at the time. He then went on to identify another bacilli, *Vibrio cholerae*, as the cause of cholera. Koch's postulates provided people working in public health with a systematic framework by which to understand the effect of disease on human populations, and also indicated some ways by which disease could be controlled through public health initiatives (see Box 4.4).

With these criteria, Koch was able to lend considerable support to the germ theory of disease by providing a precise explanation for the occurrence of any particular (infectious) disease. The

> **Box 4.4 Koch's postulates**
>
> - The organism must be present in every case of the disease.
> - The organism must be isolated and grown in the laboratory.
> - When injected with the laboratory-grown culture, susceptible test animals must develop the disease.
> - The organism must be isolated from the newly infected animals and the process repeated.
>
> *Source:* Last (1995: 75–6).

importance of this idea to the practice of public health was that, for the first time, a demonstrable and certain chain of causality could be shown for infectious disease—that is, one could say that 'this particular organism causes this particular disease' and, furthermore, 'if we remove this organism (by destroying it), or negate its effects (by host immunity), this disease will not occur'.

The superiority of this idea over theories of miasma is obvious. Unlike miasmic theory, germ theory is specific. The incidence of disease in human beings was no longer mysterious, residing in 'evil airs' or the alignment of cosmic bodies, but due to identifiable organisms. Second, because specific agents of disease could be identified, so too could specific public health activities—such as slaughtering rats to prevent transmission of bubonic plague. Consequently, public health activities (particularly in European nations and their colonies) became far more systematic, and over time increased in scope as the causes (and cures) for an increasing number of health conditions were first identified (through biomedical and health research) and then acted upon (through public health interventions). This development, over time, has encompassed very diverse phenomena—no longer is public health practice solely concerned with disease control and sanitation, but also with non-communicable disease, injury, the health of groups within populations, effective legislation and so on.

Host–agent–environment

Over time, the key understandings of infectious disease provided by Koch, Pasteur and people such as Graunt and Chadwick were refined and applied in epidemiology in a model now called the 'classic epidemiological triad' (also known as 'host–agent–environment'). This model (see Figure 4.1) was important in recognising that, even if a pathogen exists, disease does not necessarily occur in all instances. To put it slightly differently, a person may be exposed to the agent but not necessarily become ill. Thus, this model suggests that a specific disease arises when a harmful agent comes through a sympathetic environment and into contact with a susceptible host. In a sense, this model brought together the miasma theory and the contagion theory (or the germ theory) and gave emphasis to the conditional nature of disease occurrence.

Later, the concept of a 'vector' was added to this model (see Figure 4.2), particularly as the complex aetiology (description of causes) of specific diseases (such as malaria, schistosomiasis, filariasis and many others) was discovered. The popularity of this triadic (three-way) theory of disease in epidemiology throughout the first half of the twentieth century can be explained partly with reference to the historical context of that period. The miasmic theory, which formed the basis of earlier epidemiological inquiry, with its emphasis on environmental aspects of disease causation, lent weight to the 'sanitation movement' of the late nineteenth and early twentieth centuries. Particularly in Western countries, this led to widespread concern about living conditions and sanitation, and subsequently the introduction of means for effective waste and sewage disposal, improved housing and food quality.

In the first part of the twentieth century, at least in Western countries, the greatest gains in public health were achieved through this understanding of the interaction between host, agent, environment and vectors. Public health practice focused on specific diseases and how they might be controlled, and public health programs expanded to focus on immunisation and vaccination initiatives (such as polio prevention), and made substantial gains in limiting mortality attributable to infectious diseases.

NCDs and the web of causation

The emphasis of public health and epidemiology began to shift again in the mid-twentieth century.

Figure 4.1 The classical epidemiological triad

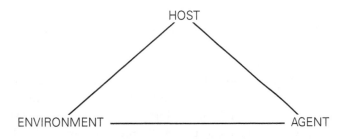

Host factors: The person at risk for a specific disease

Agent: The organism that is the direct cause for the disease

Environment: External factors that influence the host, the susceptibility to the agent, and the vector that transmits or carries the agent to the host

Figure 4.2 The expanded host–agent–environmental model

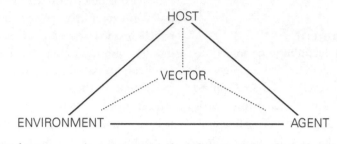

Host factors:	Age, sex, psychological state, education, lifestyle, occupation, genetics, social position
Agent:	Biological, genetic, nutrient, chemical, physical, mechanical hazards
Environment:	Physical, biological, social, economic, cultural

Source: adapted from Tulchinsky & Varavikova (2000).

With the great success of disease-control measures in industrialised nations, non-communicable (that is, non-transmissible, non-infectious or chronic) diseases have became increasingly evident in these countries. Such non-communicable diseases as heart disease and cancer became the major causes of mortality, and this increased incidence of non-communicable disease has forced epidemiologists to re-evaluate their triadic understanding of disease.

One approach was to incorporate factors such as personal behaviour, genetic makeup, social environment and so on into the basic structure of the triadic epidemiological model, as shown in Figure 4.2. In this way, the concept about what determined health remained the same, but more recent developments in our understanding of the factors that affect health would simply increase the complexity of this model.

However, what has become clear is that not all the factors listed above have an equal effect on the health of human populations. In terms of populations, 'health' is essentially an *aggregate* concept—that is, 'health' is a term used to describe the condition of an entire population by combining a plethora of factors that influence the health of

individuals and groups. While this can be a useful exercise when discussing large groups of people, its usefulness is limited when we attempt to improve the well-being of specific groups of people through public health measures. This is because, for different groups of people, and for specific diseases or health conditions, some factors will prove to be more important than others. For example, the incidence of teenage suicide will be reduced to a greater extent if public health programs focus on 'psychological' host factors, rather than 'genetic' host factors. While genetic factors may well play a part in *some* teenage suicides, far better results will be obtained from programs that allocate resources to psychological support for youth.

The expanded triad can provide a way of thinking, but it does not provide a precise view of the interrelationship between various factors; nor does it offer an explanatory framework for causation. Susser (1973), along with MacMahon and Pugh (1970), has therefore argued that agents and hosts are engaged in a continuing interaction with the environment, and that the notion of a web might better capture the complexity of these relationships. The 'web of causation' concept incorporates an understanding that some risk factors are more immediate (or *proximate*),

---

Box 4.5 Risk factors, protective factors and risk conditions

Risk factors: These are behaviours that, on the basis of scientific evidence or theory, are thought to influence susceptibility to a specific health problem. There are varied types and numbers of risk factors. The traditional categories have included:

- biological (from genetic endowment to ageing)
- environmental (from food, air, water to communicable diseases)
- lifestyle (from diet to injury avoidance and sexual behaviour)
- psycho-social (from poverty, stress, personality to cultural factors).

Many of these components are interrelated, and variations in one outcome (that is, a disease) may influence changes in others (such as well-being), depending on the mix of other factors that are present.

Epidemiological studies have linked specific risk factors to specific adverse health states. Tobacco, hypertension, diabetes and obesity are well-known risk factors for heart disease, while air pollution is a risk factor for lung cancer, pulmonary emphysema, bronchial asthma and chronic bronchitis (Turnock 2001).

Protective factors: These reduce the likelihood of a person suffering from a disease or can improve their response to a disease should it occur. They include such things as:

- high intake of fruit and vegetables
- a reasonable level of physical activity
- breastfeeding for at least three to six months
- social support and community networks.

Risk conditions: These are the situation/s and pre-existing state/s that might cause the condition of interest to arise. They are measured by a risk probability rate (per cent).

---

while others are more distant (or *distal*). Indeed, many proximate risk factors (such as smoking and diet) are related to a range of distal risk conditions (such as income and education). Contemporary models attempt to account for protective factors, risk factors and risk conditions.

The web of causation concept offered a more robust approach to thinking about the interrelationships between different determinants. It was, however, potentially too complex in that each health issue for each group might require somewhat different mapping of risk and protective factors. This would also require an enormous amount of data and research.

Recognising the importance of social and economic factors: A renewed appreciation of the environment

The health field concept

In 1974, a further breakthrough in public health thinking was achieved when the health field concept emerged from the Lalonde Report, *A New Perspective on the Health of Canadians*. This framework was simply a way of dividing up all the factors that contributed to health and illness into four major elements: human biology, environment, lifestyle and health-care organisation. It put the emphasis not so much on causation as on the different types of determinants on which one could possibly act. As such, this model was more helpful for public health practice.

The Lalonde model was supported by subsequent research. In a landmark study on the historical improvement in health, McKeown (1979) argued that the most substantial reductions in mortality since the 1700s occurred as a result of improved living standards, particularly regarding nutrition and hygiene. This put the emphasis on the importance of environment and public health measures. The work from the Alameda Population Health Laboratory (Breslow 2004) further added to our understanding about the importance of lifestyle, social support and socio-economic status.

Box 4.6 Health field concept

Human biology: This consists of all aspects of health that are developed within the human body as the result of the basic biology of humankind and the organic makeup of the individual—including genetic inheritance, ageing and internal bodily systems.

Environment: This consists of all aspects of health that are external to the human body and over which the individual has little or no control—including physical and social environment, safe products and urban infrastructure.

Lifestyle: This consists of the aggregation of decisions by individuals that affect their health and over which they have some degree of control—including personal habits.

Health-care organisation: This consists of the quantity, quality, arrangement, nature and relationships of people and resources in the provision of health care—including medical practice, hospitals, nursing homes, drugs, community care, ambulances and dental services (Lalonde 1974: 31).

Since then, other models have adopted a broader ecological perspective, giving emphasis to psycho-social environmental influences as well as linking mind, body and spirit with the biosphere (Hancock & Perkins 1985). Whitehead & Dahlgren (1997) proposed a similar model that put individuals with a set of fixed genes at the centre, surrounded by influences on health that can be modified. Layers include an individual's lifestyle, structural factors, like housing and working conditions, and then the over-arching socio-economic, cultural and environmental factors. They claim that any effective public health action has to approach issues at all of these levels.

Yet others adopt a model that places individual factors within broader social and economic contexts (Evans & Stoddart 1994), as seen in Figure 4.3. This model attempts to offer an explanation for the universal finding, across various nations, that mortality and morbidity follow a gradient across socio-economic groupings. It attempts both to recognise the underlying factors that influence susceptibility to disease and contextualise access to health-care resources.

The rise of 'social determinants'

While these models have been important in providing a framework for thinking about how the determinants of health interrelate, they do not necessarily explain what leads to health improvement or always point to what action should receive attention. To understand the dynamics of disease distribution requires monitoring over time, as well as specific epidemiological studies. As Geoffrey Rose (1992) points out, risks are usually distributed along a continuum, rather than being binary in nature. Small shifts in the distribution of risk throughout a population can make a large difference in the health status of the population. Thus, understanding the dynamics of disease distribution in populations is important in understanding disease aetiology. Such an understanding has now led to a heightened appreciation of the social determinants of health.

McKeown (1979), in analysing the historical decline in mortality since the 1700s, shows that the rate of decline was most significant in airborne diseases such as tuberculosis and enteric diseases spread by water, with food-borne diseases and vector-borne diseases being of lesser importance. He concludes that improved living standards—particularly nutrition and hygiene—have been the most important in contributing to the decline of mortality. Furthermore, the introduction of new crops, more effective agricultural techniques, mechanisation of farming and use of chemical fertilisers has provided the key to improved nutrition, and hence to a reduction in infectious diseases.

Since the 1970s, research attention has also shifted to examining people's location in different parts of the social structure, finding that it is of key importance in understanding why some people are more

Figure 4.3 Evans and Stoddart's model: feedback loop for human well-being and economic costs

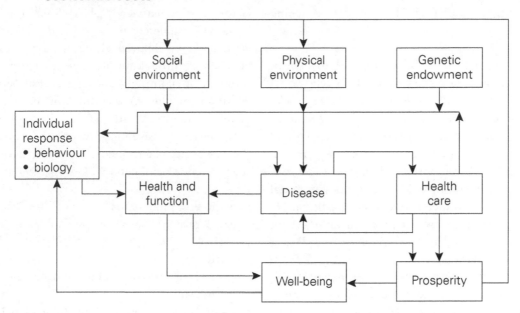

Source: Evans & Stoddart (1994: 53).

vulnerable to ill-health. Starting with Cassel's (1976) observation that social environmental conditions produce profound effects on host susceptibility, social epidemiologists have documented the link between poor health and the powerlessness brought on by social disorganisation, migration, discrimination, poverty and low support at work (Berkman & Kawachi 2000). At the same time, social support and family ties provide examples of the factors that might protect individuals from the deleterious consequences of stressful situations.

Furthermore, research since the 1960s has pointed to the persistent differential in health status across socio-economic groups. While the deprived conditions of the poor and industrial workers were described by early public health physicians and social activists (such as Virchow, Engels and Chadwick), there have been numerous statistical reports in the United States and United Kingdom in particular in which mortality from all causes of death has been shown to be consistently higher

for people with lower income and educational levels, and occupations with lower social status. The differential distribution of diseases across population sub-groups (that is, the persistent health inequalities) demands that health and disease be seen in their full social and historical contexts.

Research on health inequalities has been increasing at a rapid rate and across a large number of countries. The basic conclusions from the innumerable studies (NSW Health 2001) are as follows:

- Health increases along a gradient as affluence increases.
- Health inequalities have been described in all developed countries, at national/regional/local levels within countries, for almost all diseases and causes of death, for men and women, across the whole age range.
- Differences in lifestyle (such as smoking, diet and exercise) explain about one-third to half of the differences.

- The health gap between rich and poor is not decreasing. (Indeed, successful health-promotion campaigns may have led to some of the widening gaps.)

Two theories have been proposed to explain these patterns. One explanation—the psycho-social theory—stresses the importance of the social environment. On the negative side, hierarchical structures, social disorganisation, rapid social change, social isolation and bereavement all contribute to chronic stress and the loss of a sense of control. On the positive side, social cohesion, social support, social connectedness, social participation, resilience and civic trust can protect health. Stresses may be experienced at the community as well as at the individual level.

The alternative explanation—neo-materialism—posits that economic and political institutions create and reproduce income inequalities, which impact on individuals (through lack of resources and poorer access to services) and on society (through under-investment in human capital and social infrastructure). The increased health inequalities in the United Kingdom between 1970 and 1993 would appear to reflect the widening social inequalities in general.

These two contrasting explanations are probably not mutually exclusive. Underlying these discussions about the social determinants of health and illness, there needs to be a more fundamental analysis of the influence of culture, history, politics and social structures. In each society, there are distinct patterns of power relations, opportunities and dissemination of knowledge and information. Certainly from the viewpoint of developing interventions to improve health, both theories need to be taken into account, along with analysis of the particular contexts of societies and communities.

Adding to these debates are new findings about the life-course approach to chronic disease epidemiology. The Barker hypothesis (Barker 1992) suggests that many adult diseases have foetal origins. Subsequent research has validated the importance of the intra-uterine environment. Kuh and Ben-Shlomo (1997) further suggest that the focus on adult risk factors is a limited view. Habits acquired in childhood and adolescence persist into adulthood; deprivation in children also results in decreased life chances throughout life. The emerging theory is one of programming during a critical period of development plus an accumulation of risk from childhood to early adulthood.

Given an extensive and growing body of evidence, the key social determinants of health have been suggested by Marmot and Wilkinson (1999) to be:

- socio-economic status
- stress related to social and psychological circumstances
- early life
- social isolation or exclusion from the wider community
- nature of work—particularly occupational stress
- unemployment—or risk of unemployment
- social support from family and friends
- addiction to alcohol, drugs and tobacco
- the availability of good food
- a transportation system that encourages physical activity.

The social determinants of health act as both protective factors and risk factors.

Figure 4.4 illustrates how the Commission on Social Determinants of Health (CSDH) now has a focus on 'the fundamental global and national structures of social hierarchy and the socially determined conditions these create in which people grow, live, work and age' (CSDH 2008: 43), and their influence on the distribution of health and well-being.

Towards new measures of health and wellbeing: Taking the definition seriously

The new research about health and social inequalities across the life-course raises questions not

Figure 4.4 Commission on Social Determinants of Health conceptual framework

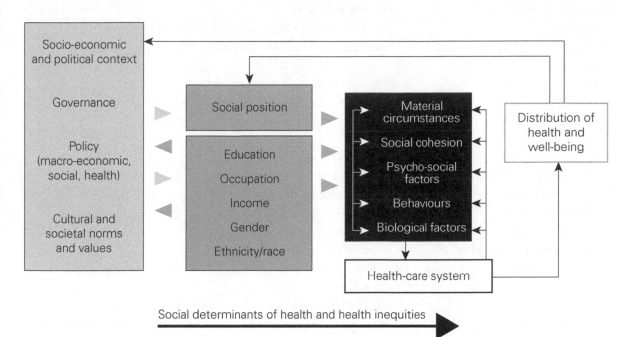

Source: CSDH (2008).

only about what creates health but also about whether the traditional measures of health—such as mortality or disease prevalence—are appropriate. Depending on the definition of health and the model of disease causation that one adopts, the indicators used may well be different, as seen in Table 4.1.

The traditional approach to health measurement focusing on measures of mortality and morbidity, including for specific population groups and specific health problems, remains important. However, the evolution of our understanding of disease causation has also placed a stronger focus on information about specific agents and susceptibilities (that is, both the biomedical determinants and the proximate risk factors) for diseases.

Contemporary public health approaches, on the other hand, critique both the biomedical emphasis and an 'illness-centred' focus on risk factors. The

evolving approach to understanding and measuring health therefore recognises that different groups of people have different definitions of health, and that each may imply a different way of *measuring* health. As our knowledge about risk factors expands, particularly in relation to factors in the social environment, the ways in which risk factors will be measured and monitored will also change.

Over the last decade, much international effort has been devoted to developing new ways of measuring and summarising health status. There is a need to develop a single health indicator that captures multiple dimensions of health (such as the SF-36 mentioned in Table 4.1), which recognises that notions of health need to be both multi-dimensional and to include subjective elements (like the experience of stress). Such an indicator is essential for meaningful comparisons across population groups and societies.

Table 4.1 Changing concepts of health and their measures

Concept of health	Possible indicators
Feeling good	Proportion of people reporting being able to do what they like
Physical, social and psychological well-being	Proportion of people reporting feeling well
Social role functioning	Proportion of people functioning well at work, in personal life
Good quality of life	Proportion of people judging quality of life to be high
Multi-dimensional (combined physical, social and emotional health, with both subjective and objective elements)	Medical Outcomes Study Short Form 36 (SF-36)
Healthy, disease-free lifespan	Health-adjusted life years (HEALYs)
Disability-free lifespan	Disability-adjusted life years (DALYs)
High quality of lifespan	Quality-adjusted life years (QALYs)
Good cardiovascular functioning	Blood pressure, heart rate, fitness
Endocrine regulation of stress	Secretion of stress hormones
Absence of disease	Disease morbidity (i.e. incidence and prevalence of health problems)
Length of life	Life expectancy
Absence of death	Mortality (of population or in relation to specific diseases)
Preventable deaths	Infant mortality rate, maternal mortality rate, death rate before age 65, potential years of life lost (PYLL), standard mortality ratio (SMR)

Source: adapted from Noack (1997).

The development of DALYs (disability-adjusted life years) is another attempt to have a common measure to assess relative well-being. Clearly, years spent with a disability should be differentiated from years of a fully abled life in an effective indicator of health: they should be registered as a lesser experience, regardless of the cause of such disablement. In addition, the use of the DALY does not distract the researcher with competing advocacies for the severity of any particular disease burden.

Community well-being indicators were developed in Victoria in 2006 for use by local government in policy-making in social, economic, cultural, environmental and governance dimensions (VicHealth 2006). Indicators fall under 21 distinct policy areas within five broad domains relating to community well-being: healthy, safe and inclusive communities; dynamic, resilient local economies; sustainable built and natural environments; culturally rich and vibrant communities; and democratic and engaged communities.

In recognition of the absence of participation and consultation with indigenous peoples in the development of the indicators in relation to the Millennium Goals, the United Nations has supported discussions in relation to the development of indicators of the well-being of indigenous peoples. Consequently, the UN Forum on Indigenous Issues has recommended that poverty indicators based on indigenous peoples' own perception of their situation and experiences be developed jointly with indigenous peoples, and also that further work be done on the development of cultural indicators in relation to the right to food and food security (UN Permanent Forum on Indigenous Issues 2006).

From the viewpoint of evolving public health knowledge, the ongoing challenge for health indicator development is the effective identification, capture

---

> **Box 4.7 Example of community well-being indicators**
>
> **Domain:** Healthy, safe and inclusive communities
> **Policy area:** Personal health and well-being
> **Indicators:** Self-assessed health
> Percentage of population who rate quality of life as average or better
> Life expectancy
> Physical activity (adequate exercise to derive health benefits)
> Nutrition: fruit and vegetable consumption per capita
> Obesity: body mass index (BMI) from self-assessed weight and height
> Illness and deaths from smoking, alcoholism and illicit drug use
> Incidence of psychological distress
> Prevalence of type 2 diabetes
> Gambling
>
> *Source:* adapted from VicHealth (2006).

and incorporation of social and cultural dimensions relevant to the population group of interest.

Conclusion: Distribution counts

In this chapter, we have introduced the internationally accepted definition of health and the approaches commonly used to measure and monitor the health of populations. We have also introduced different approaches that have been used over time to understand the patterns in the distribution of health and illness in society. We can see that monitoring health status and risks constitutes the basic tool that allows us to begin to understand the distribution and causation of health and illness. We can also see how concepts of linear causation have given way to the idea of a web of causation.

In tracing the evolution of public health models from a time when humans faced the terrors of communicable diseases to their concern today with the physical, social and psychological well-being of all individuals, we have seen that public health thinking has also accommodated social and cultural variations in the concept of well-being. Public health has come a long way from the fear of shadowy miasmas or punishments, moving through a focus on very specific bacterial agents and environments. Although many developing countries, and occasionally the non-vigilant developed ones, still face the challenge of communicable diseases, the rising incidence of non-communicable diseases has broadened public health concerns, first towards a web of known factors and then to a more open field of known and as yet unknown factors.

We now accept that health generally is determined by a combination of environment, lifestyle, health care and biology. We also accept that socio-economic differentials in health status are the most persistent pattern across developed countries. However, we still have a long way to go in truly understanding the pathway between the biological and the social.

Clearly, public health is an evolving field of inquiry, and the models and concepts that are employed in practice are always subject to revision as new situations and contexts are encountered. Modern public health is still concerned with basic priorities of sanitation and disease control, but as the complexity of health models has increased, so has the scope of public health (and epidemiological) interest. This is particularly apparent in recent times, with the attention paid to social determinants of health—how the social and behavioural lives of people can affect their health status. The next chapters in Part II discuss how different explanations are offered to explain causation, as well as how public health intervention strategies have been developed. Part IV of the book looks at a number of these concepts and tools in action, as they are applied to specific domains of public health in Australia.

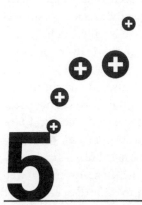

5

Explaining differences and determinants:
Environment, society and behaviour

Challenge

In October 2001, Rolah McCabe began proceedings for compensatory and exemplary damages negligence against British American Tobacco (BAT) in the Victorian Supreme Court. Her claim against BAT was based on several points: that she had been addicted to cigarettes manufactured by BAT since the age of twelve, and as a result had contracted lung cancer; that BAT knew that cigarettes were addictive and dangerous to health; that BAT's advertising targeted children to become consumers; that BAT took no reasonable steps to reduce either the health risks or the addictive nature of cigarettes; and that BAT has publicly decried research showing the health dangers of smoking (Hammond 2004).

Justice Eames awarded Rolah McCabe $700 000 in damages because BAT had 'subverted' the discovery process by willfully destroying documents that denied the plaintiff a fair trial. Following Rolah McCabe's death, BAT successfully appealed against the decision. A subsequent request for special leave to appeal to the High Court by her surviving family was rejected (Liberman 2002).

What types of evidence need to be presented to explain the causes of smoking addiction or lung cancer? What evidence is needed to establish who is responsible and to what extent they are responsible—especially where the development of a condition or disease involves personal behaviour? If the causative factors are complex and can be apportioned in numerous ways, how can people be educated about the actions that they could and should undertake for themselves as individuals—and for society?

Introduction

In the previous chapter, we looked at how we can understand patterns of health—how we can describe and monitor health patterns and design conceptual models to explain them. This chapter considers how we can investigate and develop explanations for health patterns, taking into consideration that they are influenced by a broad range of interconnecting factors, from physical environmental factors to the nature of individuals and society. The contribution of the health system to shaping health patterns will also be explored.

Public health knowledge draws from multiple disciplines. Organising the public health effort requires not only an understanding of the different tools and frameworks of thinking offered by these diverse disciplines, but also knowledge of how they can complement one another to form the basis for public action. This chapter starts with considering how causation can be investigated using epidemiological methods. Then the influences of physical, social and behavioural factors are discussed in turn, consistent with the broad models introduced in the previous chapter about determinants of health. The chapter concludes by suggesting that these theoretical perspectives are complementary and, when brought together, contribute to a systems understanding (or an ecological perspective) about health and illness.

Studying causation—the tools and methods of epidemiology: A basic science for public health

The concepts and models of health and factors shaping health discussed in the previous chapter are broad, and represent the possible array of influences on patterns of health and illness in populations. How do public health practitioners make sense of these factors and patterns in the context of the communities with which they work? How do they decide that, for any given group of people, *factor x* is the direct causative factor, and *factor y* is an underlying

factor? How do they decide that any particular group needs special attention? One way is to collect information about a population or a group of people, and to conduct studies that help to explain their differences—particularly in terms of what causes ill-health. This is the mainstay of work done by epidemiologists, who have adopted some of the core concepts, definitions and skills routinely used by people interested in the health of populations.

Data that already exist, often from complex statistical collections, can be valuable to epidemiologists and public health practitioners. However, in many cases new research must be conducted in order to obtain an adequate understanding of specific health issues, particularly in relation to their causes and what solutions work (in terms of either prevention or a public health response after the problem has emerged). To answer these questions, health researchers have adopted a range of approaches and methods to collect reliable data about the health of populations. They may collect data at a point in time, or over a long period of time. They may observe what naturally happens to people in their own environment, or they may devise an intervention to measure its effects. Box 5.1 lists the epidemiological approaches most commonly used for identifying what problems exist in a population, investigating what risk factors might have been responsible and evaluating the changes made by interventions to the level of risk or disease in a population.

Thus, while the expanded host–agent–environment model, the health field model and the determinants of health model all provide useful frameworks for considering the various factors contributing to health, they do not provide detail on the relative importance of specific factors to the health of specific groups of people. In order to achieve this, epidemiologists must tailor these frameworks according to their specific aims and objectives—and only after carefully considering everything they know about the disease or health condition in question.

Box 5.1 Common methods of population health studies

Cross-sectional surveys: the collection of data in populations or particular subpopulations to estimate occurrence of a health event in those groups.

Longitudinal surveys: the collection of data in a population over time in order to understand how health status and risk factors change over time.

Observational studies: undertaken to systematically measure a number of suspected factors and the occurrence of health events among members of a group or a number of groups of subjects. No intervention occurs except the observations of the subjects in their usual circumstances.

Ecological studies: use existing statistics to correlate the prevalence or existence of a disease with the frequency or trends of suspected causal factors in specific localities or over time. In these studies, however, the co-occurrence of factors related to a disease or problem does not necessarily prove a causal relationship.

Interventional studies: look at interventions such as immunisation, education, screening or treatment to examine their effectiveness when compared with a control group that did not receive the intervention.

Source: adapted from Detels et al. (1997).

As epidemiologists and health researchers are concerned with explaining the causes of ill-health, or explaining which interventions will result in better health, their research might adopt a range of strategies and study designs to answer their specific questions about causation and intervention effectiveness. Researchers could follow a population over a period of time, or select a population experiencing a condition and trace their past history of exposure. In order to isolate a specific condition or causative factor, researchers will generally want to have a comparison or control population and ensure that care is taken to control for any possible

bias. Researchers will also need a study population large enough, and sufficiently representative of the general population, to be able to confidently generalise about their study findings. Box 5.2 lists the commonly used types of study design.

Not all of these approaches and measures are appropriate for every research project—in fact, before research is conducted, researchers must carefully consider what kind of data they need to obtain, and select the best research methods to get the best data. Their choice will be affected by multiple considerations, such as the population they hope to study (for example, men/women, poor/wealthy, old/young or rural/urban) or the particular health condition or conditions (such as infectious/non-communicable or genetic/psychological).

It is important to recognise that populations are not *homogeneous* (that is, they are not all the same). Not all people in a given population have the same needs and expectations, experience the same living conditions or require the same assistance. Different factors will be important for different groups of people. It is also essential to distinguish between health factors that are *proximate* (affecting the health of people directly) and *distal* (underlying factors that create conditions for, or sensitise people to, ill-health but do not have a direct effect on health).

However, establishing which factors are proximate and which are distal is not always an easy task. While many studies might point to an association between a particular factor and a disease, the links between the conditions in which a disease is found and the disease itself are not always self-evident. (For instance, why do women smokers have a higher rate of cervical cancer?) Confirming the causative association is not always easy and the actual nature of the connection—including the causal pathway—may not be clear. Researchers need to be certain about whether a factor is causal or could be due to some other underlying—and perhaps unknown—factor. For this reason, epidemiologists will sometimes make use of some rules and principles developed by the British statistician Sir Austin Bradford-Hill to decide whether there is a causal relationship between any given factor and a particular disease, and if so whether that relationship is proximate or distal. These rules and principles are known as the Bradford-Hill criteria, and they are listed in Table 5.1.

The challenges in assessing and confirming causation are numerous. In real life, two people might be exposed to the same hazards but might not have the same disease outcome. This could be due to different levels of exposure to the hazard, or exposure under different conditions, or different underlying factors (such as genetic makeup) that increase susceptibility to disease. Thus, inherent in any attempt to understand causation is the need to assess level of risk. As well, if it takes a long time for a factor to have an effect on health, the visibility of a connection between a factor and its impact might be obscured. The key concepts involved in assessing health risk are listed in Box 5.3.

Risks to health—and also factors protecting health—can arise from the physical environment, social structures and environments, and the health system. As well, some risks and protective factors are unique to specific individuals, creating differences between individuals. It is to these different explanations that we now turn.

Influences of the physical environment: From simple causation to dynamic systems

Much of the early public health understanding about disease causation and determinants of health comes from early knowledge about the influences or impact of physical and natural environments on health. This traditional scientific paradigm (of linear causation and the epidemiological triad) has served public health practitioners well in helping to identify and quantify specific agents of disease causation—from mould in cold, damp housing to SARS to agricultural chemicals. Strategies for dealing with them are readily identified on the basis of such

Table 5.1 Bradford–Hill criteria

Strength	This is defined by the size of the risk as measured by appropriate statistical tests.
Consistency	The association is consistent when results are replicated in studies in different settings using different methods.
Specificity	This is established when a single putative cause produces a specific effect.
Temporal	Exposure always precedes the relationship outcome. This is the only absolutely essential criterion.
Dose–response	An increasing level of exposure (in relationship amount and/or time) increases the risk.
Biological plausibility	The association agrees with currently accepted understanding of patho-biological processes. This criterion should be applied with caution.
Coherence	The association should be compatible with existing theory and knowledge.
Experiment	The condition can be altered (e.g. prevented or ameliorated) by an appropriate experimental regimen.

Source: Last (1995: 77).

Box 5.3 Concepts for assessing health risk

Hazard: the probability of an adverse outcome.

Risk: an estimate of potential adverse health effects resulting from human exposure to hazardous agents or situations.

Dose–response curves: typically used to describe the effect of toxic agents on human subjects. The concept can be generally applied to indicate what amount of exposure to a substance will cause a response (be it physiological, clinical or behavioural). These are plotted with the magnitude of the dose along the horizontal axis and the magnitude of response along the vertical axis. Such curves are often S-shaped, with no observed response at the lowest dose, followed by the gradual development of an increasing response, finishing at a dose level at which no further response is observed.

Risk factors: increase the probability that an individual will develop conditions or diseases. These factors can include genetic, mental, physical, social, dietary or environmental factors. (Some people use the term **'risk conditions'** to refer to broader environmental risks, such as socio-economic factors.)

Protective factors: increase the probability that an individual will cope with stress, adapt to changing circumstances, be resilient and prevent conditions or diseases. These factors can be genetic, mental, physical, social, dietary or environmental. They moderate the negative influence on health of risk factors. As such, strengthening these factors is integral to health-promotion strategies.

Source: adapted from Detels et al. (1997).

---

knowledge, and tend to be directed at the environmental level (natural and built environments).

Factors in the physical environment that influence health are commonly described in terms of different types of agent (see Box 5.4). Concerns about the physical environment historically were focused on physical and biological agents. In the latter part of the twentieth century, concern shifted towards chemical agents. Just when society might have thought that medical science and engineering had provided foolproof protection from harmful environmental agents, the threat of bio-terrorism has again focused society's attention on biological and chemical agents. In the first decades of the twenty-first century, research investigating links between climate change and

> ### Box 5.4 Major types of agents of concern to health
>
> **Physical:** radiation, noise, heat, dust
> **Chemical:** solvents, pesticides, drugs, food additives
> **Biological:** bacteria, viruses, worms, fungi

health is revealing the wide range of impacts on agricultural, water, soil and other systems, and increases in associated risks to human health, from extreme heat, water-borne diseases and vector-borne diseases, such as malaria.

In trying to understand the relative importance of exposures to different physical agents, the first task is to determine the agent's toxicity or hazardous nature (that is, the inherent capacity of an agent to cause harm) and the actual or expected risk (that is, the probability that exposure to the agent under specific circumstances will cause illness). To assess whether a hazardous exposure will translate into a health risk requires an understanding about:

- the nature of the agent—the physical form, the concentration, any interaction with other agents
- the level of exposure—the dose, frequency, duration
- the nature of exposure—acute or chronic
- the route of exposure—skin contact, inhalation, ingestion
- the conditions of the subject/host—genetic susceptibility, general physical and mental health status, nutritional status, presence of other risk factors and protective factors.

A typical investigation about risks posed by agents in the physical environment consists of two interdependent phases—see Figure 5.1. The first phase is risk analysis. This is concerned with the identification of an agent (the source of health risk),

an understanding of the dose–response relationship, assessment of exposure (essentially quantitative), characterisation of the risk and the relative risks of a range of risk-management options (NHMRC 1994:56).

These steps lay the foundation for subsequent action in the second phase, which is related to risk management. Risk management is the process concerned with deciding what to do in response to the results of the risk assessment, within a context of community values and what is feasible—practically, economically and politically (NHMRC 1994:57). The focus of risk management (see Figure 5.1) is on avoiding adverse impacts by modifying environments, exposures and effects, or by directing efforts towards the mitigation of risk (Ewan et al. 1992:4).

The traditional environmental health paradigm, derived from the fields of microbiology and toxicology, is essentially built on early models of causation and biological plausibility—the idea that there is a single agent and that this agent will cause disease at a particular threshold of exposure. This model of causation also points to the importance of health protection as a key intervention—that is, prevention of exposure to the hazardous agent (or at least ensuring that exposure is below the threshold level).

In more recent times, environmental health research and practice have recognised that factors that cause diseases and conditions are linked in complex ways, and they exist (and interact) within a broader context. For example, what are the known causes of cancer? Cancers have been linked to a range of environmental factors, such as tobacco smoke, sunlight, heavy metals, naturally occurring or added factors in the diet, pesticides, nuclear radiation, asbestos and fumes emitted from industrial processes and internal combustion engines. In a given population, how do we identify and assess which of these agents (or combinations of agents, in cases such as mesothelioma) are responsible for the incidence of cancer? Which is the most hazardous agent? What is the most appropriate intervention? The need to answer these questions is

Figure 5.1 Relationship of risk assessment and risk management

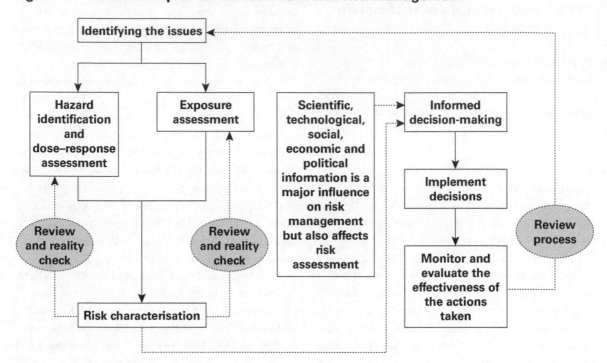

Source: DoHA & enHealth Council (2002: 17).

becoming more urgent as globalisation and increasing rates of population growth propel urbanisation and industrialisation in many parts of the world. Emissions of pollutants will increase, resulting in what McMichael (1993: 329) describes as 'complex ecological disruptions'. Consequently, it will become more and more difficult to repair damage to the natural physical environment (air, water and land) using technical solutions. It has become critical that processes are developed to predict and effectively manage potential environmental health risks before they become realities.

Table 5.2 provides an insight into the scope and complexity of potential risks in the environment that need to be assessed. The task of collecting and interpreting data for environmental risk assessments is complex and uncertain for a number of reasons. Due to the increasing complexity of both the physical environment and the causal relationships

between environmental risk factors and disease, not all data may be available to assess risks, or there might be uncertainties—about toxicological data variability in population factors (for example, uptake rates of chemicals into the body) or the sensitivity of individuals to various agents (which is affected by age, sex and general health status) (DoHA & enHealth Council 2002: 8–9).

In chemical risk assessment, the assessment of a hazard is based upon toxicity data from animal studies, and any application to humans (inter-species variation) comes from an extrapolation of that data. In addition, human populations are diverse (producing inter-individual variation), which raises more cause for uncertainty. In an effort to allow for uncertainty from a lack of full information ('imperfect information'), a margin of safety or 'uncertainty factor' has been incorporated as part of chemical risk assessment. Initially, experienced judgement

Table 5.2 Key factors in risk assessments

Hazard assessment	• Interactions with other agents in the environment • Immediate or delayed onset of health effects • Severity of health effects • Reversibility of health effects • Presence of clear thresholds for effects • Potency of agent
Exposure	• Duration of exposure • Frequency and consistency of exposure • Patterns of exposure • Past, current and future exposure • Timing of exposure • Exposure route (ingestion vs inhalation vs dermal contact) may influence outcome • Inter-generational exposures • Cumulative vs non-cumulative exposures • Failure of exposure controls • Quality of exposure data • Quality of exposure models
Population	• Genetic variability • Individual host characteristics (e.g. age, gender, body weight, pre-existing poor health, immune status, nutritional status, previous exposures, reproductive status) • Population characteristics (e.g. herd immunity and social behaviours for communicable diseases, social mobility for exposure to air and soil contaminants, recreational patterns of exposure to contaminated recreational waters)
Environment	• Intervention strategies (e.g. containment of contaminated soil, chlorination of water, pasteurisation of food) • Transport mechanisms (e.g. meteorological factors affecting air pollution, vectors for communicable diseases) • Factors affecting persistence (e.g. photolysis and volatilisation of chemicals, desiccation of micro-organisms) • Breakdown of public health measures (e.g. flooding affecting waste control and potable water treatment)

Source: DoHA & enHealth Council (2002: 9).

and intelligent guesswork were the basis for estimating the uncertainty factor (Interdepartmental Group on Health Risks from Chemicals 2003: 3), but now a number equal to or greater than 1 is used to divide exposure levels measured in animals to estimate exposure levels in human populations. There are two commonly used exposure levels: no observed adverse effect level (NOAEL) and lowest observed adverse effect level (LOAEL).

Uncertainty also exists when it comes to understanding and assessing the dynamics of environmental change. McMichael (1993: 6) observes that there 'is much that is uncertain or speculative about the causes and consequences of global environmental changes', but this is not an adequate reason to 'defer prudent social response. Scientists and policy-makers are going to have to learn to live with more uncertainty than in the past.'

Complexity and uncertainty are not only inherent in the source of risks and hazards in our physical environment, but in the way risks and hazards are assessed. This has led Weatherall (1994) to observe that it is not clear to what extent major current diseases are environmental in origin or how our genetic makeup is linked to our responses to new and changing physical environments.

Responding to this complexity and uncertainty poses new challenges. While the temptation might be to 'do nothing' because of a lack of conclusive evidence, policy-makers have been warned that 'an appropriate level of conservatism is important ... because, in general, underestimating a particular risk is likely to have greater health, environmental, economic and social losses than overestimating the same risk' (DoHA & enHealth Council 2002: 8). A second approach to uncertainty, brought about by a lack of data, has been the adoption of the precautionary principle, which essentially states: 'Where there are threats of serious or irreversible environmental damage, lack of full scientific certainty should not be used as a reason for postponing [preventive] measures.' (DoHA & enHealth Council 2002: 8)

In the future, progress can be expected in the use of technologies and science to further refine the techniques for risk assessment; however, risk management will continue to present many challenges. The Driving Forces, Pressure, State, Exposure, Effect, Action (DPSEEA) model (PAHO 1999) recognises the iterative nature of hazards, risks and health events (see Figures 5.2 and 5.3) while still

Figure 5.2 DPSEEA model

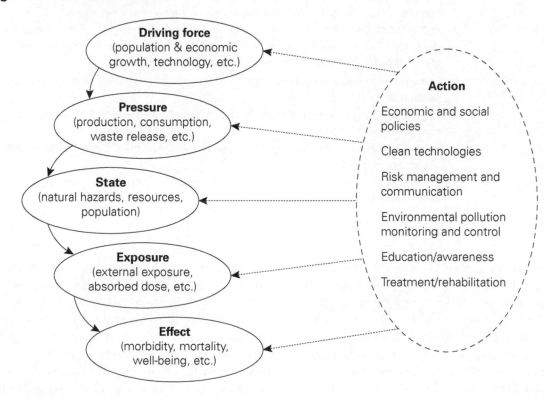

Source: PAHO (1999).

Figure 5.3 Example of the DPSEEA model

Imagine if a new agricultural industry were developed in a rural area that had small towns close enough to provide a workforce, and natural resources like land and water were available.

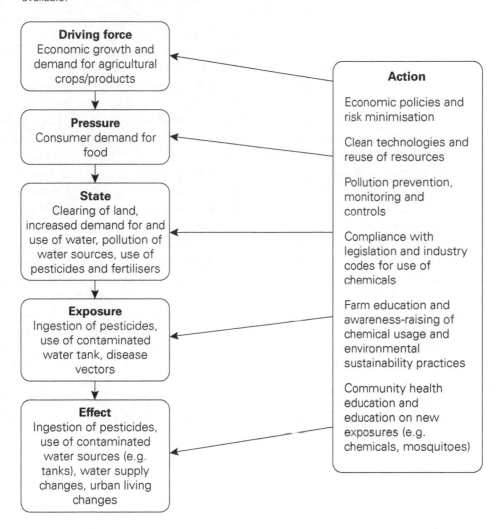

embodying a notion of causation that is grounded in the physical and biological sciences. Importantly, the model also incorporates the action component that is concerned with informed decision-making based on risk analysis and practical realities.

Influences of the social environment: Status and connections do matter

With the advent of the epidemiological transition in populations (that is, increases in non-communicable diseases relative to infectious diseases), a simple causation model to explain the determinants of health and disease does not work effectively, especially as there are multiple risk factors for each disease, and many diseases seem to share common risk factors. Furthermore, there is a clustering of diseases and risk factors in different sub-groups in the population. How could smoking be related to a number of chronic diseases, such as cancer, heart disease and stroke? And how could diabetes, kidney disease and heart disease have common risk factors? Furthermore, how could low socio-economic status be associated with nearly all causes of death?

Evidence about the socio-economic gradient in health status has pushed public health thinking not only into considering multiple risk factors but also the socially embedded nature of these factors. The interplay between social, economic and cultural environments is still being uncovered through research on social determinants of health—a body of research that has grown significantly since the 1990s. Public health intervention strategies derived from this understanding have been increasing in recent years, and tend to be directed at the social context in which people live and work (that is, at the community and societal levels).

The starting point for understanding health status in terms of social factors arises from the observation that, first, there are distinct patterns of ill-health related to age, gender and race/ethnicity and, second, these patterns are not simply biological but relate to the ways in which society is stratified by education, occupation and income (or socio-economic status). These patterns generally hold true whether they are related to causes of death, incidence of disease or lifestyles, or patterns of health behaviour.

Sociologists would see this persistent and universal pattern as a direct reflection of the social stratification that exists in society. Early writers such as Rudolf Virchow and Friedrich Engels began to shed light on this pattern, calling attention to how diseases can be direct outcomes of the political and economic structure of capitalist society. In particular, they believed that the organisation

of work and society reflected the requirement for work enterprises to create profits, and that certain groups would always be exploited, at the expense of others, in this quest for wealth. As a consequence, they asserted, individual biology is secondary to social structure. Later sociologists, such as Emile Durkheim (1970), in writing about patterns of suicide, would also suggest that social patterning of health status was related to the nature and level of social organisation (including social upheavals, social integration and social regulation). The poem by Bertolt Brecht in Box 5.5 provides another illustration of the concept of a social determinant of health.

There are different explanations at a more refined level for why this pattern occurs and persists. One school of thought is that the nature of the social environment is the critical factor. For instance, greater social support, social participation and social connectedness protect people against ill-health. Conversely, being socially excluded, being stigmatised and experiencing discrimination will contribute to (or result in) people having greater ill-health. Syme and Berkman (1976) showed that the lack of social ties or social networks predicted mortality from almost every cause of death. Kawachi et al. (1997) further demonstrated that individuals who are less socially integrated (that is, have fewer friends, are not in a stable relationship and have lower levels of involvement in community activities) experience a higher rate of mortality.

Box 5.5 'A Worker's Speech to a Doctor'

The pain in our shoulder comes
You say, from the damp; and this is also the reason
For the stain on the wall of our flat.
So tell us:
Where does the damp come from?

Source: Bertolt Brecht (1938) 'A Worker's Speech to a Doctor'

There is much debate about exactly how social environments shape health—what the pathways are that link social experiences to mental and physical health. Box 5.6 outlines some of the social factors that researchers believe are important, either as protective factors or as risk factors. For instance, participation in social networks can be conducive to health, while being socially isolated or unsupported can have negative health consequences. Social cohesion extends beyond support or participation by the individual, and refers to the extent of connectedness and solidarity among groups in society. It is sometimes used synonymously with social capital, and is concerned with the social norms (for example, how people value and relate to older people), networks and trust that facilitate cooperation within or between groups. Social capital can generate health benefits for society by promoting respectful and supportive behaviour, diffusing health knowledge or exerting social control over deviant health-related behaviour (Kawachi & Berkman 2000). However, some aspects

---

Box 5.6 Concepts associated with social determinants of health

Social capital: refers to those features of social structures (such as levels of interpersonal trust and norms of reciprocity and mutual aid in communities) that make resources, advantages and opportunities available to individuals and facilitate collective action (Pope 2003).

Social cohesion: refers to the extent to which society or a social group has strong social bonds and (conversely) is not ridden by latent social conflict. Socially cohesive groups share strong social norms, have abundant associations, and have available institutions for conflict management (Pope 2003).

Social norms: 'informal rules' that condition behaviour in various circumstances. Specific social norms include surrendering seats to the elderly on public transport and not littering, while generalised norms may include tolerance, behaving honestly and helping those in need. A key over-arching norm is that of 'reciprocity'—'do unto others as you would have them do unto you' (Pope 2003).

A social network: an interconnected group of people who usually have an attribute in common. For example, they may like a particular sport, or may share the same occupation or religion. At a more micro level, families and groups of friends will exhibit network characteristics. Different groups often have their own sets of social norms and levels of mutual obligation between group members.

Social trust: (or 'generalised trust') is a measure of social capital, which concerns the level of confidence people have that others will act as they say, or as they are expected to act, or that what they say is reliable. It refers to the general level of trust in a society—for example, how much one can trust strangers and previously unencountered institutions (Pope 2003).

Social exclusion: multiple dimensions exist, and can be experienced by successive generations. Social exclusion happens when people (or people in areas) are subjected to 'a combination of linked problems such as unemployment, poor skills, low incomes, discrimination, poor housing, high crime, bad health and family breakdown'. People most at risk of social exclusion are those who experience multiple disadvantages (Social Exclusion Unit 2004: 4).

Discrimination: a socially structured and sanctioned phenomenon, justified by ideology and expressed in interactions, among and between individuals and institutions, intended to maintain privileges for members and dominant groups at the cost of deprivation for others. Although sharing a common thread of systematic unfair treatment, discrimination nevertheless can vary in form and type, depending on how it is expressed, by whom and against whom (Krieger 2000: 41).

of social capital can have adverse effects, such as when strong internal group cohesion is associated with an intolerance of others. So exclusion and discrimination also become important explanations for the harms that social environments can exert. A conceptual mapping of relationships between social networks and health is represented in Figure 5.4.

Discrimination can occur in overt or covert ways, can be carried out in a verbal or physical manner and can occur in many settings, such as school (preventing entry to and affecting experiences at school), employment assistance, work, housing or health care (Krieger 2000). When individuals experience discrimination it is common for them to feel fear, anger and stress, resulting in physiological responses that contribute to physical and mental illness. When groups are discriminated against, poverty, poor housing, under-employment or unemployment, and lack of access to services can result, leading to worse health outcomes at the population level.

Another school of thought points to the economic environment—or the set of material conditions—as the key explanation for the social patterning of health status. The argument is that social relations between groups in society have a material basis, characterised by a control of resources, which can lead to the exclusion of less advantaged groups (Lynch & Kaplan 2000). When there is such a differential distribution of access to material resources in a population, a series of consequences might be predicted for disadvantaged groups. Poverty and low income result in poorer (if not inadequate) housing and nutrition, while poorer access to educational opportunities means people are confined to lower-skilled and more hazardous jobs. Conversely, adequate income can give access to the skills and labour of others, as well as other goods and conditions. Having more disposable income thus provides a buffer from many of the stresses of daily life. In the context of the city of Glasgow, Macintyre and Ellaway (2003) demonstrate that people with lower incomes live in neighbourhoods that provide fewer 'structural opportunities' for health improvement—that is, worse housing, less public transportation, more expensive and poorer quality food, fewer playgrounds and so on.

Social patterning of the health status of mothers is emerging as having particular significance, with associations now well established between the birth weight of newborns and the future development of adult diseases (for example, type 2 diabetes and coronary heart disease). 'Barker's hypothesis' or the 'fetal origins hypothesis' states that 'fetal undernutrition in middle to late gestation, which leads to disproportionate fetal growth, programmes later coronary heart disease' (Eriksson 2005). Not only does this theory shed light on the causes of disease, but it points to the need for shifts in social environment-type intervention strategies for primary and secondary prevention of disease which consider the full life-course—from events, experiences and environments before birth to late adulthood.

Still others argue that the more immediate psycho-social environments—within the family, the neighbourhood or the workplace—bring together key factors that determine patterns of health in populations. For example, Karasek et al. (1981) suggest that the two most important aspects of any job are the demands placed on the workers and the degree of control they have in making decisions in response to these demands. Workers with high psychological demands coupled with low levels of latitude in decision-making will experience job strain and consequent ill-health. The 25-year follow-up of the original Whitehall Study of British civil servants (Marmot et al. 1997) provided further evidence that 'sense of control' is a crucial explanation for differences in health status. Importantly, this study established that the variation in cardiovascular health status exhibited by workers was related to the gradient in their socio-economic status, supporting Rose's insight that both exposures and

Figure 5.4 Conceptual models of how social networks impact on health

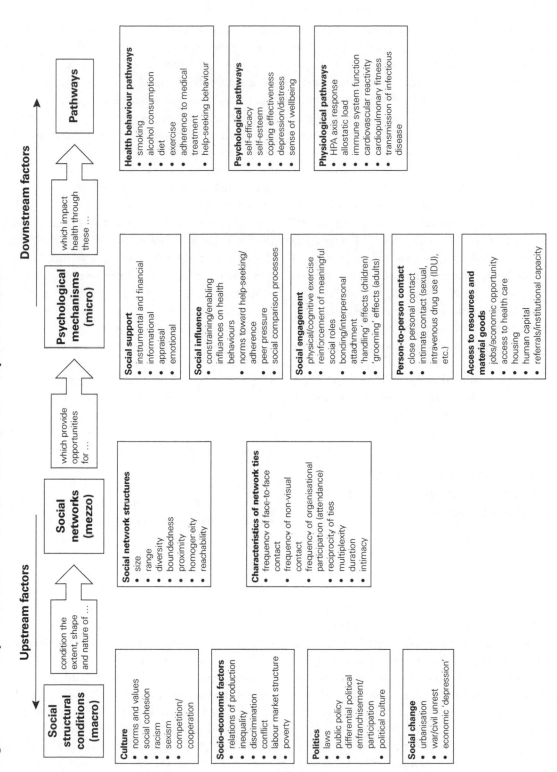

Source: Berkman & Kawachi (2000: 143).

health outcomes are distributed continuously in a population. A bio-psycho-social model helps explain the pathway to cardiovascular disease: psycho-social demands (or 'stressors'—ranging from daily hassles to specific stressful life events) combine with vulnerability factors (such as personality, coping responses and social supports) to produce a stress response, which is thought to affect immune system and metabolic function and, in turn, lead to disease states (Marmot 2000).

While different researchers place different emphases on social, economic and psychological factors, most will readily acknowledge that material conditions, social circumstances, psychological states and health behaviours are closely linked. Hence, those people who work in low-paid employment not only experience more job insecurity but also smoke more, exercise less, drink alcohol to excess more often, eat less nutritious diets and feel less hope for the future (Lynch, Kaplan & Salonen 1997). It is clear that further research on social determinants will entail understanding of how society (and the economy) operates, the natural history of diseases and psychological processes.

Influences of the health-care environment: Health care as a microcosm of society

Although many public health activities occur outside the health sector, health services remain an important determinant of health and well-being. The nature of the health system and the health-care environments in which care is delivered influence the health of individuals—and population groups—in a range of ways. While availability of services and access to them might be shaped by broader political and economic forces, a person's susceptibility and vulnerability to health problems and their ability to benefit from health services can be shaped by their experiences within the health system.

Access to relevant preventive services (such as screening for haemochromatosis or breast cancer) and good-quality acute or chronic care can affect the nature of health problems that might arise and how a person recovers from or manages a condition. The nature of clinical encounters and the extent to which a person's expectations of care match the actual service can affect trust, sharing of information, learning about treatment protocols and other aspects of consumer–health professional interaction. Each of these has consequences for health outcomes. The ways in which health services are set up and operated will influence an individual's experience of care and the extent to which they develop self-care skills. For example, asthma shared-care programs create close links between consumers, community health services, GPs and more specialised services. The profile of the health workforce can have a bearing on what resources (technical and knowledge based) are brought into the health-care process—for example, the levels and types of expertise and authority in a team of health workers. The health system represents a microcosm of the broader social environment—its structures, rules and resources shape the extent to which individuals and groups are able to take advantage of its various technologies to improve their health.

Transitions between states of health are not just biological processes but also have wider socio-cultural dimensions. Relationships between people (for example, with partners, adult and child family members, close friends or work colleagues) are changed when a person's health status changes. Consider how the following health conditions might transform such relationships: a healthy pregnancy, late-stage cancer, emphysema, obsessive compulsive disorder, a broken arm or depression. Although his methods and interpretations are debated, Parsons (1978) suggests that being ill signifies the breakdown in a person's capacity or desire to conform to social norms or expectations (that is, staying healthy). Individuals who are ill then adopt a 'sick role', where they can withdraw and retreat to a state of dependency on those who are caring for them. However, Parsons proposes that it is the medical profession that gives permission for (or legitimises) the adoption of the sick role, through its ability and power to arbitrate what is a genuine or non-genuine illness. Thus, an imbalanced power relationship exists between the doctor and the patients and, by extension, the health care system and consumers of health care.

Both the health system and clinical encounters tend to reflect a society's social stratification as well as the political economy. The authority of medical doctors relates to the preference given by the health system to medical knowledge and technologies that are consistent with a traditional scientific paradigm. This authority is reinforced by the hierarchical organisation of decision-making power along lines of expertise. This dominance is further underpinned by government policy (such as professional registration) that legitimises and secures the power of the medical profession over other professions (Willis 1989). The hierarchical arrangements seen in the broader health workforce reflect past and present divisions in society (on the basis of gender, ethnicity and class)—hence, nurses are typically women, and unskilled areas of work are carried out by minority/immigrant workers. Doctors' high incomes are not only sustained by their expertise and position of authority in the health system, but also by their links with the pharmaceutical and medical technology sector, whose profits depend on doctors' commitment to choosing their products.

The characteristics of patients also construct their experiences of the health system. Unequal treatment of women, adolescents, older patients and people of different racial backgrounds has been shown to be linked not only to their ability to pay for health care, but to their social characteristics (Institute of Medicine 2003a). While there are complex factors that contribute to this situation, the different treatment norms that exist contribute to the health inequalities seen in society.

Taking a wider view, the potential for health care to improve health relies not only on the clinical services, resources and opportunities provided to individuals in the health-care setting, but on aspects of the wider environment in which people must live and manage their health problems. Research into diabetes, for example (Fisher et al. 2005), suggests that the success of diabetes self-management will be influenced by the availability of, and access to, basic resources needed for disease management. These include healthy food choices, safe environments for physical activity, direct social support (whether face to face, via the internet or via social media) and social acceptance of self-management practices in workplaces, public places or schools. Where these resources are inadequate or unavailable (for example, in communities that are poorly served with fresh food outlets, or in workplaces in which workers of lower status face disincentives or discrimination for self-monitoring blood glucose levels or injecting insulin), benefits from good clinical care will be compromised and health will be at risk.

Influence of individual factors: Choice or chance?

Given similar social and economic environments, however, individual differences remain. What factors account for different health experiences for individuals within the same social group? If discrimination results in fear, anger and stress, and subsequent poor health, then how do some people overcome these assaults and even lead the fight against discrimination? If job demands and work stress contribute to a loss of sense of control at work and lead to poorer health outcomes, how do some people overcome those constraints or bypass the same sense of loss of control? Why is it that self-reported life satisfaction is predictive of better heath outcomes when people might objectively experience similar stressors or be exposed to the same risks? Subjective outlook and resilience are emerging issues to which public health researchers are paying attention as possible explanations for within-group differences.

Behaviour and lifestyle explain about 50 per cent of the mortality from the leading causes of death. Health psychologists have tried to understand how these health behaviours relate to personal beliefs—about causality, risk, illness and what they can control, for example—and how these might lead to particular patterns of health behaviour. Variation between individuals in beliefs about their illness might occur in terms of (Ogden 2001):

- identity—what label is given to the illness (symptom and diagnosis)
- perceived cause of illness—for example, whether biological, psychosocial or other reasons
- timeframe—how long the illness will last
- consequences—what the possible effects are or the impact of the illness on their physical, emotional or social existence
- curability and controllability—whether the illness can be overcome, and whether the outcome is within their control.

These different beliefs will combine to lead individuals to adopt different forms of behaviour, in relation to both preventing and managing illness.

There are additional factors that contribute to an individual's choice of different health behaviours. Attribution theory (Heider 1958) suggests that people want to understand what causes events, as this helps to make the world more predictable and controllable, and they can differentiate which health issues are outside their locus of control. However, individuals differ as to what they believe to be within their control. Bandura's theory of self-efficacy (Bandura 1977) adds to this perspective by suggesting that how confident an individual feels about adopting and maintaining certain behaviours is a key to behaviour change.

However, behaviours do not occur in a vacuum, and people respond to the reactions that others (such as family or peer group members) have to their behaviours. This means that behaviours can be reinforced by environmental conditions, just as they can be modified by changed environmental cues. Classical conditioning theory—which can be compared with the classical model of linear causation—proposes that a response can be trained by using a consistent stimulus (that is, Pavlovian behaviour). This is the basis for simple forms of rewards and punishments. Operant conditioning theory, however, suggests that people might display certain forms of behaviour on the basis that they will be rewarded. In regard to health education initiatives designed to change behaviour, this perspective would point to the importance of ensuring environments support and reward desired behaviour.

Given that public health services are delivered at both the individual and population levels, an understanding of an individual's beliefs, behaviour, responses, motivation, personality and important personal relationships remains important. Research—combined with awareness-raising about health practices related to gender, culture and age over the last two decades—has increased the likelihood that public health services will have strategies in place to better match the expectations and preferences of specific groups of service users—for example, women, Indigenous Australians and older people—with service features. While better awareness of diversity between population groups might have led to more openness and options—for instance, in birthing services (Small et al. 1999), chronic illness programs and palliative care (Kellehear 1999)—diversity within population groups at the level of the individual can remain under-recognised. Use of stereotypes to interpret an individual's needs, expectations and preferences in a health-care encounter can result, leading to impacts ranging from dissatisfaction with services to delivery of unsafe or inappropriate treatments.

Genetic makeup is a key factor responsible for health differences, and the Human Genome Project (see <www.genome.gov>) has stimulated many new questions and research themes. Important facts have been established that contribute to our understanding of the relative roles played by genes and the environment in shaping health patterns. For instance, particular genes can be expressed at different times in the course of a lifetime, and whether, or to what extent, they are expressed is strongly influenced by environmental conditions (Committee on Future Directions 2001). The fact that genetically determined traits are found—though not exclusively—in population groups (for example, Tay-Sachs disease among Jews, sickle-cell anaemia among Black Americans and thalassaemia among people from some Mediterranean countries) reflects continual adaptations by population groups to their environments; as a consequence, there are also population group differences in susceptibility to disease. Native Hawaiians, for instance, have a predisposition to diabetes (see Box 5.7) (Nabhan 2004).

As genetic differences are identified across populations and combined with the escalating knowledge related to genomics and to the environment, significant interest is being stimulated among researchers as well as the public in gene–environment interaction. Increasingly, a more integrative approach to understanding the production and improvement of health is emerging which spans levels of knowledge and inquiry from the molecular through to the environmental.

Towards an integrative perspective on health determinants: The sum is greater than the parts

Although determinants of health can be explored in depth through environmental, social, psychological and health-care system lenses, public health action requires that these perspectives are synthesised. Increasingly, each of the disciplines that contributes to public health is broadening its parameters, if not forging links with other disciplines. The bio-psycho-social model (Engel 1977) posits that there is a hierarchy of natural systems that spans the molecular to the global, and that all levels of the hierarchy are linked with and

influence each other. Within environmental health, the connections between the built and the natural environment are being explored within ecological models of health, including people–environment relations. These models are not inconsistent with earlier political economy of health frameworks in recognising that micro and macro, local and global, and biological and social analyses are not mutually exclusive (Higginbotham et al. 2001).

Given our understanding of human health as the outcome of complex processes that operate across physical, social and psychological systems, there is increased interest in what complexity science and complex systems thinking can offer for understanding determinants of health (see Box 5.8). In earlier chapters, systems were depicted as having an overall function and constructed from building blocks that are connected in various ways. The complex systems perspective suggests that the settings in which we live, work and play can be conceptualised as forms of interacting systems and that, together, they comprise a whole social (community) system. These component systems are in a constant state of flux, and move between order and disorder. They adapt in response to changes in their environment (that is, other systems) and evolve through interactions with other systems. There are times when the whole system is balanced and at equilibrium; at other times, a small change in one system can create predictable and unpredictable (desirable and undesirable) impacts on other systems and lead to transformations in the whole system. This way of thinking stands in contrast to linear, mechanistic thinking, and points to fresh ways to appreciate the nature of the determinants of health and health interventions. (Hunter 2009; Jayasinghe 2011).

From this complex systems perspective, we can see that optimal health might be the result of the self-regulation and maintenance of all relevant systems promoting physical, psychological and social well-being (Higginbotham et al. 2001), while ill-health might be due to the loss of the ability to self-regulate (at the individual, group or

Box 5.7 Taro for health: Genetics and the traditional Hawaiian diet

In 2000, Hawaii was statistically the healthiest state in the United States, yet one in five Native Hawaiians suffered from diabetes and 50 per cent were obese. Hawaii's Native inhabitants also recorded significantly higher rates of mortality than the national average from heart disease (two times), cancer (2.5 times) and infectious diseases (four times).

The Native Hawaiian Renaissance Movement of the 1970s was largely responsible for initiating efforts to confront the combination of loss of land, loss of culture and weight gain. The health problems of Native Hawaiians are the result of the combination of rapid dietary change and genetic makeup. Native Hawaiians (and many other indigenous populations) lack an enzyme that is required to efficiently metabolise fats. This has resulted in a special adaptation to the island ecosystem over many centuries that has fulfilled the special nutritional needs of Native Hawaiians. The outcome is that these health problems are now being addressed by reverting to a diet based on the many varieties of taro and the Hawaiian understanding of the laws of nature.

Taro is rich in calcium, potassium, iron, phosphorus, thiamine, riboflavin and several other B vitamins, as well as vitamins A and C. Significantly, taro does not contain any fat or cholesterol, but does have sufficient soluble fibre and amylase starches to make it a slow-release food. Taro roots are pounded into *poi* (mashed, cooked and peeled taro corms), which has been the mainstay of traditional Polynesian and Hawaiian diets. The decline in taro paddies has occurred in tandem with the rising incidence of diabetes and obesity. In the pre-colonial period, an estimated 20000–24000 hectares were planted with hundreds of varieties of taro, and these provided a staple crop for 250000 Hawaiians. By 1980, the taro paddies had declined to 200 hectares.

The establishment of the Cultural Learning Centre on the Waianae coast of Oahu in 1979 brought a revival of traditional Hawaiian values and customs, including the cultivation of taro. The outcome has been the 'Hawaiian Diet'™, which is high in complex carbohydrates and is based around *poi*, sweet potato greens, seaweed, native fish and fowl, fruits and fern shoots. It was devised using the results of the 1991 Waianae Diet study in which participants lost an average of 7.7 kilograms in 21 days, their blood sugar levels dropped 26 per cent and their cholesterol levels by 12 per cent. When the Hawaiian Diet™ was trialled with a multi-ethnic group of 22 people in 2001, the greatest improvements were found in the reduction of blood sugar and triglyceride levels of the indigenous participants.

The success of this return to a traditional diet is very much intertwined with the restoration of the Native Hawaiian culture and traditions. To achieve healthy bodies, it was necessary to have healthy communities and lands. Native Hawaiians are actively engaged with other indigenous cultures that are dealing with similar health problems.

Source: Nabhan (2004: 186–210).

community level) and the disintegration of support systems. To understand a state of health requires the mapping of all the causal influences and how they interconnect—it is akin to the epidemiological concept of 'web of causation'. To effect change in the state of health—for example, through health-promotion interventions—requires an understanding of how to exert influence on the system as a whole and not only on each of the factors, as altering one factor will influence others. These 'pushes and pulls' mean we need to maintain vigilance about the state of various systems—from microbiological, to individuals, to social systems and natural environments. Drawing on available evidence, a mapping of systems associated with obesity undertaken by UK Foresight (2007) points to

---

Box 5.8 Key concepts in complexity science

Complex systems:
- are made up of many agents that act and interact with each other in unpredictable ways
- are sensitive to changes in initial conditions
- adjust their behaviour in the aggregate to their environment in unpredictable ways
- oscillate between stability and instability
- produce emergent actions when approaching disequilibrium
- are dynamic and non-linear, and can rarely be explained by simple cause–effect relationships.

Source: Plowman et al. (2007: 342–3).

---

a diverse range of intervention points in 'the system' to reduce the incidence of overweight and obesity—from urban planning to changes in food supplies to promoting social capital.

As suggested by Bammer (2005) and Hunter (2009), understanding these dynamics—so that unfamiliar and new public health issues and problems can be tackled—will require theory and research methods to be drawn together and strengthened. The DPSEEA model goes some way towards incorporating ideas about complexity, and

reinforces the need to look into the variety of interacting forces shaping health so that effective interventions for improving population health can be designed.

Conclusion: Health is an emergent property of complex social systems

The central mission for public health practice is health improvement. Understanding how to improve health effectively requires an understanding of the factors that determine health and that cause ill-health to emerge, and how these factors connect and interact. Explanations about health and disease causation—which address factors in the environment, in society and within the individual—can be derived from various disciplines. These include epidemiology, microbiology, toxicology, physiology, sociology and psychology. At the practical level, the frames offered by different disciplines can be drawn together to ensure that each domain for public health action is informed by sound theoretical and technical underpinnings.

Health is a deeply personal and emotional issue, but it is also rooted in the social environment, and the socio-economic arrangements in society generally. These factors, and their interactions, are critically important to understand if one is concerned with improving the health of the public.

6

Public health interventions:
From quarantine to the rise of 'evidence-based practice'

Challenge

In your position as a research officer in the state government Public Transport Division, you are part of a team looking at what options are available to provide public transport to service a new housing estate. It is being built on a former industrial site, 10 kilometres from the central business district (CBD) of a capital city. This estate will contain a mixture of high-rise apartments, townhouses and public housing flats, a primary school, several day-care centres, an extensive shopping centre, numerous office blocks, a large sporting facility and a retirement village. This information tells you that your team must consider different options for the various groups of people who will live there.

What arrangements will be made for those people who travel to the CBD each day, for getting children to and from school, to enable the elderly and those without cars to get to the shopping centre and to social activities with friends? What evidence is available to enable your team to choose the best options and then to implement them?

One approach to planning new public transport services is to make an assessment of the needs of the prospective residents' groups by consulting with community organisations, the local council, prospective employers, the estate developers and the public transport companies, and by examining the options chosen for other recently established housing estates. What financial resources are available for any extensions to train and tram lines or bus routes? Is it a viable option just to rely on motor vehicles and a limited bus service?

Introduction

The previous two chapters explained how to understand patterns of health and ill-health in society, and the interplay between individual and system factors in explaining the causes and distribution of health and illness. These tools of 'discovery' form an important basis for public health 'delivery'. In other words, public health intelligence is the foundation for public health interventions.

This chapter is concerned with how we act on these patterns of health and illness, and how intervention approaches in public health have evolved over time. The chapter is divided into three sections. First, it examines the types of interventions that public health practitioners deploy, and how such interventions have changed over time. Second, it looks at how these interventions are planned and evaluated. Finally, it examines how the demand for evidence-based practice requires active efforts to transfer the evolving knowledge base into practice.

Public health interventions and the natural history of diseases: Horses for courses

The natural history of a disease is described in terms of the factors (contextual and individual) that lead to its occurrence, the clinical progression of the illness, possible treatments (that cure or ameliorate) and the long-term consequences (or sequelae). Interventions can occur at any stage along this pathway.

Public health interventions are those efforts organised at the level of a population—a community or society—that not only aim to maintain but to prevent a disease from occurring in a population, to stop a disease from becoming more prevalent and reduce its effects, or to rehabilitate and help prevent further deterioration. Depending on which of the above aims is to be pursued, interventions have been termed 'primary', 'secondary' or 'tertiary'. Table 6.1 lists definitions and provides examples of these different types of prevention.

Table 6.1 Aims of public health interventions

Levels of intervention	Stages of disease	Examples
Primary prevention Preventing a disease from occurring	**Wellness**	• Initiatives that prevent social isolation among elderly people • Programs that teach children how to care for their teeth to prevent dental caries
Secondary prevention Making early diagnosis and giving prompt and effective treatment to stop disease progress, shorten the duration of the illness, and prevent complications from the disease process	**Illness**	• Effective network of emergency services • Screening for complications that may arise from diabetes • Diet modification for patients with cardiovascular disease
Tertiary prevention Preventing long-term impairments or disabilities arising from disease, and restoring or maintaining optimal physical and social functioning once the disease process has stabilised	**Disability**	• Active rehabilitation following injury • A system for monitoring use of medicine by patients with chronic illness • Support for patients' self-help groups

Some people argue that most investments in public health should be concerned with primary prevention, and therefore prevent the initiation of a disease in a population. From the broader 'public health as an organised effort' perspective, the critical issue about secondary and tertiary prevention is the extent to which they are systematic, organised efforts that have a positive effect on the health of the population of concern. In other words, there are public health approaches to organising the delivery of health services that will ensure people can access services, as early as possible, for detection and treatment, or the support necessary to maintain their health and improve their quality of life.

The history of public health action has principally been concerned with disease control and prevention. A shift in the orientation of public health action towards promoting health and ensuring health equity has occurred in recent decades as many diseases have successfully been brought under control through targeted preventive programs. Nonetheless, knowledge about the causes and natural history of diseases remains fundamental to thinking about public health action.

Prevention as the focus: Defining the major strategies

Much public health action is concerned with primary prevention. This objective can be achieved in a number of ways, based on an analysis of the factors contributing to the problem and application of suitable intervention methods. The three major modes or strategies of prevention typically are categorised as health protection, disease prevention and health promotion. They can work on the levels of a whole population and population sub-groups, and can be distinguished by their overall aims.

Health protection is focused on ensuring that people are not exposed to hazards or risks in the environment. Traditionally, health protection has been concerned with hazards or risks in the physical environment, using legislation and inspection as the main tools for intervention. Typical examples include occupational health and safety, food safety, radiation protection and control of drugs and poisons.

Disease prevention is concerned with preventing the development or worsening of specific diseases or conditions. Strategies can be directed at changing exposure to environmental factors, such as removing a stagnant water supply that might contribute to mosquito breeding. They can also take the form of preventive services delivered to individuals in an organised way, leading to better health at the population level. Examples include immunisation programs and screening services (such as for breast, cervical and other cancers, hypertension, vision or hearing). The disease prevention approach is built on developments in scientific knowledge that explain the causes of diseases and conditions. In fact, the concept dates back to efforts to prevent the onset of diseases and conditions even when their specific cause could not be known because of the lack of scientific knowledge at the time. For example, Scottish physician James Lind in the mid-1700s tested various agents (such as oranges, lemons, vinegar and seawater) for treating British sailors who had developed a cluster of symptoms now commonly known as scurvy. He showed that sailors, whose diet primarily consisted of biscuits and salted meats, could recover their health and, moreover, prevent the onset of such symptoms when they ate citrus fruits (Tröhler 2005). This finding ultimately changed the opinion of professionals and authorities and led to the routine supplementation of sailors' diets with lemon juice.

Health promotion has roots in health education and social change traditions. Strategies can be directed to creating knowledge, attitudes, beliefs and practices among populations, which in turn lead to behavioural choices conducive to health. In tandem with this approach, strategies can be directed to changing environments so it is easier for people to make choices that maintain and enhance their health. Preventing specific diseases is neither the immediate nor even the main focus for health promotion. Instead, health-promotion theory emphasises the importance of increasing the capacity of individuals, communities and organisations to shape and implement agendas for action that are ultimately concerned with better population health outcomes. Even in health-care settings, a capacity-strengthening approach is relevant in work with people who are seeking to recover from or manage a disease.

Evolution of strategies for prevention: Increasing sophistication in public health action

From ancient times to the contemporary era, different strategies for prevention have been emphasised, in part because the main health challenges facing the community change. Awofeso (2004) argues that there have been several distinct eras of public health practice since antiquity, with each of these periods adopting different actions based on different understandings of disease causation and the availability and acceptance of certain interventions. These eras are discussed below.

Health protection: Quarantine, regulate, inspect

Health protection was the first strategy in public health practice. The earliest civilisations believed that diseases—which were mainly of an infectious nature—could be prevented by enforced regulation of human behaviour, whether this involved the adoption of community taboos or isolating diseased individuals from healthy people. As societies came to appreciate the importance of environmental factors in disease causation, legislated measures to ameliorate the physical environment were adopted as part of a health-protection approach. Standards were built into regulations for drainage, sewerage and refuse disposal.

While the scientific basis of public health has been changed significantly by the advent of bacteriology and acceptance of the germ theory of disease, many of the earlier tools for public health action remain relevant. Methods of preventing and controlling infectious diseases include increasing host resistance through improvements in general health and immunisation, breaking the chain of transmission of infection by detecting and treating cases; isolating infectious cases and quarantining contacts; controlling vectors and the environments that may harbour infections; using aseptic technique with patients; implementing sanitation and personal hygiene measures, including avoiding exposure to and limiting spread of diseases; and inactivating infectious agents through physical means (using heat, cold or radiation) or chemical means (chlorination or disinfection) (Chin 1986: 104).

Disease control: Detecting illness and preventing epidemics

Arising from the experience of infectious disease control and building on the classic epidemiological triad ('host–agent–environment'), the early part of the twentieth century saw disease control emphasised as a major strategy in public health practice. This reduced morbidity and premature mortality from specific diseases. Clinical preventive services became an important vehicle for implementing disease-control programs.

Disease control is effected through highly specified intervention measures directed to individuals through an organised approach, mainly involving primary health-care settings, such as general practices and health-care clinics. Individuals may be 'at risk' in terms of being part of an identified target group or having been exposed to risks. Early and continuing successful examples of this approach include childhood immunisation to prevent vaccine-preventable diseases, prophylactic immunisation for people exposed to risks (for example, meningococcal C or legionella), micronutrient supplementation to prevent malnourishment and oral rehydration therapy to inhibit severe diarrhoea. Screening for diseases or risk factors might precede clinical interventions—for example, screening for vision and hearing development in children, tuberculosis among immigrants and refugees, hypertension in middle-aged adults, cervical cancer in women by using Pap smears, and possible congenital malformation of foetuses by using antenatal ultrasound. Disease-control approaches rely on the application of expert knowledge. This strategy can be highly effective, provided there is sufficient population coverage, appropriate targeting of risk groups and cooperation by the population. For control of infectious diseases, coercive powers (provided through public health legislation) may be used to implement essential environmental and clinical measures. For monitoring of childhood growth and development (for example, parents taking their babies to the maternal and child health centre at the right developmental stage) and control of non-communicable diseases (for example, women attending a general practice for a Pap smear at the recommended screening intervals), compliance and therefore population coverage will depend on the extent of health knowledge in the target groups and the motivation and means to act on such knowledge.

Health education: Raising awareness and promoting behaviour change

Achieving willing cooperation with key measures (such as taking medicines or being vaccinated according to schedules) is the point at which the disease-control approach has often failed. Where knowledge, motivation and the means to act are not adequate, little voluntary health action will be undertaken. Health education thus developed to complement disease-control measures with the aim of increasing people's health awareness and developing attitudes, beliefs, knowledge and skills conducive to health. In contrast to the disease-control approach, which relies on experts directing health improvement activities, the health-education approach is based on an inherent assumption that health is a matter for which individuals have responsibility.

Health education aims to clarify values, provide information and develop essential skills so that people can make informed choices and adopt health behaviours that are believed by those delivering programs to be conducive to good health. The approach focuses on packaging health information and using communication methods that are meaningful to different groups. Health education is generally a targeted activity undertaken by governments, health services, educational institutions, consumer organisations and others with access to knowledge and influence. Some definitions of health education are as follows:

> Health education attempts to close the gap between what is known about optimum health practice and that which is actually practised. (Griffiths 1972)

> [Health education is] any combination of learning experiences designed to facilitate voluntary adaptations of behaviour conducive to health. (Green et al. 1980)

> Health education is not only concerned with the communication of information, but also with fostering the motivation, skills and confidence (self-efficacy) necessary to take action to improve health. Health education includes the communication of information concerning the underlying social, economic and environmental conditions impacting on health, as well as individual risk factors and risk behaviours and use of the health system. (WHO 1998)

Some critiques have suggested that health education processes can be controlling (authoritarian or paternalistic) in their approach, and do not lead to Green's 'voluntary adaptations of behaviour conducive to health'. A power imbalance in a relationship (created, for example, by health professionals having easier access to technical information and know-how compared with people using health services) can undermine the ability of people to use health information in making decisions based on their own beliefs, values and what they expect they can achieve. Concepts of partnerships (with individuals, groups and organisations) in the practice of health education emerged in response to power imbalances and to improve effectiveness.

The rise of primary health care

While infectious disease control and preventive medicine were the dominant foci of public health strategies during the nineteenth and twentieth centuries, the problems of health inequalities, and the social context that gave rise to these inequalities, were also receiving attention from public health researchers and practitioners. The early public health writers and activists (for example, Engels and Virchow) observed that health problems were differentially distributed across society. They observed that social context (including working and living conditions, and rights before the law) were important determinants of health and illness patterns. The social medicine movement that emerged in the twentieth century upheld this approach. Community health programs that developed in the United States in the 1960s (see Geiger 1984) and evolved in Australia in the 1970s stressed that medical services in the community should be moulded to respond to the prevailing health needs of the community, by being based on epidemiological analyses and the use of outreach and education as well as clinical preventive and treatment services. Additionally, community-oriented primary care (COPC) would focus on the determinants and consequences of health and illness. In doing so, it would be concerned with the environment and the family as well as with the individual, and with the provision of services as well as changing health behaviours (Starfield 1998).

COPC has gained acceptance in developed countries, particularly as an approach to health care in disadvantaged communities, and is represented in community health centres. At the global level, the concepts were comparable to the idea promoted

> **Box 6.1 Features of community-oriented primary care (COPC)**
>
> **Essential**
> - Clinical and epidemiological skills
> - Defined population
> - Defined programs to address community health issues
> - Community involvement
> - Accessibility to health care (fiscal, physical, cultural, etc.)
>
> **Desirable**
> - Coordination of curative, rehabilitative, preventive and promotive care
> - Comprehensive approach to behavioural, social and environmental factors
> - Multi-disciplinary teams
> - Outreach services
> - Community development
>
> *Source:* Tollman (1991).

by the WHO (2008c, 2012) that primary health care is the appropriate system for assuring adequate access to health care for all. Although ideas about primary health care or COPC have been around for some time, there are a number of forces currently driving still more strongly the development of this collaboration between public health and clinical medicine. First, with ageing of the population and the rise of chronic illnesses, there is an increased need for coordinated care. Second, changing technology, new knowledge bases and greater consumer expectations have meant that patient care increasingly is being shifted from hospitals into the community setting. Third, and perhaps most importantly, current economic and performance pressures on the health system favour the cost-effectiveness of prevention programs, which can only be achieved by such a collaboration.

The Alma-Ata Declaration, signed at the International Conference on Primary Health Care in

1978, represented a landmark in thinking about COPC and social medicine. The declaration framed primary health care (PHC) as not only a level of care provided by health workers, but a philosophy about community participation in health care. It specified service elements considered essential for a primary health-care system, such as education about how to prevent and control existing local health problems, family planning and immunisation. Equally importantly, it defined a number of principles for translation into different social and economic contexts:

- PHC is essential health care based on practical, scientifically sound and socially acceptable methods and technology.
- PHC is the first level of contact between individuals, the family and the national health system, bringing health care as close as possible to where people live and work, as the first element of a continuing health-care process.
- PHC evolves from the conditions and characteristics of the country and its communities, based on the application of social, biomedical

and health services research and public health experience.
- PHC addresses the main health problems in the community, providing promotive, preventive, curative and rehabilitative services accordingly.

Primary health care (like COPC) requires that the fields of public health and clinical medicine work in partnership, with shared responsibilities. A review of over 500 initiatives in the United States in the mid-1990s identified a range of possible synergies between the two fields (Lasker & the Committee on Medicine and Public Health 1997):

- improving services by coordinating care for individuals
- improving access to care by establishing frameworks to provide for uninsured populations
- improving the quality and cost-effectiveness of services by applying a population perspective to medical practice
- using clinical practice to identify and address community health problems
- strengthening health promotion and health protection by mobilising community campaigns
- shaping the future direction of the health system by collaborating around policy, training and research.

Emergence of health-promotion tools

The transition from disease control and preventive medicine to primary health care occurred alongside an epidemiological transition in the developed countries. In this transition, the leading causes of mortality shifted from infectious diseases to chronic diseases, and the simple linear model of disease causation seemed no longer to be applicable. Non-communicable diseases (NCDs) were clearly multi-factorial in causation, and involved a range of behavioural risk factors and environmental risk conditions to which clinical medicine, with its expertise in the treatment of disease and injury in individuals, was ill-equipped to respond.

Box 6.2 Essential primary health-care services

- Education concerning prevailing health problems and methods of preventing and controlling them
- Promotion of food supply and proper nutrition
- Provision of an adequate supply of safe water and basic sanitation
- Provision of maternal and child health care, including family planning
- Immunisation against the major infectious diseases
- Prevention and control of local endemic diseases
- Appropriate treatment of common diseases and injuries
- Provision of essential drugs

Source: WHO (1978: 2).

New strategies were needed to influence the increasing prevalence of NCDs. In addition, in recognition of the long latency period of NCDs, some argued that promoting positive lifestyles—the patterning of choices related to health concerning relationships, diet, physical activity and recreation, work, drug and alcohol use, and so on—had to start early. Services at the primary health-care level had new responsibilities to work with their communities to reduce exposure to behavioural and environmental risks associated with chronic diseases in particular.

Changing behaviour was emphasised over environmental change. Information, education and communication ('IEC') were adopted as the major approaches for fostering behaviour change. Drawing on a range of psychological theories (health belief model, theory of reasoned action, stages of change model and so on—see Appendix E) and also marketing theory, public health actions utilised leaflets and posters, individual counselling, school education sessions and community advisory messages via mass media (also known as social marketing). From the 1980s, in particular, health was starting to shape up as a lucrative new avenue for product development, with people becoming 'consumers' of a whole new range of health-related goods, services and programs to address diet, physical activity, smoking and other lifestyle habits. Marketing techniques typically used by the private sector became part of the public health toolkit.

However, some public health practitioners, particularly those working in disadvantaged communities, recognised that asking some groups to modify their behaviour was akin to 'blaming the victim'. Often, behaviours were predictable responses to impoverished environments or insufficient material resources, or natural responses to stressful life events. Consequently, practitioners adopted strategies to change environments so they were health enhancing, and naturally supported healthy choices and behaviours. Strategies drew on social change theory and included social planning,

community action to campaign for service and policy changes, and skills development of community members to solve problems that confronted them.

Yet such locally based community development efforts were time-consuming and resource intensive. Often the efforts and their results were not sustainable. They also did not deal with the reality that many features of lifestyles associated with chronic diseases were promoted by industry interests, such as the tobacco and alcohol industries and sectors within the food and entertainment industries. The social milieu created through industry advertising would influence the choices and behaviour of many more people than community development officers ever could. Similarly, policy decisions adopted by government—for instance, allowing such advertising, or planning urban environments that encouraged car use, or providing unequal access to education and human services—also created a larger context for health behaviours that locally based community development efforts could only weakly influence. The importance of policy and media advocacy was thus recognised by public health practitioners.

Increasing recognition of the complex social, economic and political dimensions of health led to a maturing of early (1970s) health-promotion activities that were strongly oriented towards changing lifestyles to prevent NCDs. Health promotion has now evolved to a more broadly encompassing concept that involves the adoption of multiple intervention methods. While lifestyles and NCD risk factors remain a focus for health promotion, it is now accepted that health promotion constitutes a set of strategies that can be applied to any health issue.

International consensus about the principles and strategies for health promotion was captured initially in the Ottawa Charter for Health Promotion in 1986 (see Appendix F). The five complementary strategies regarded as essential for preventing health problems and improving health are:

- developing and implementing healthy public policies
- creating living and working conditions that support health and healthy choices
- developing life skills in all population groups across the lifespan
- mobilising community action for social and environmental change
- expanding the mandate of health services, especially primary health care, so that they focus on the total needs of the individual as a whole person and contribute to the pursuit of health in communities.

These five strategies have since informed the design of public health interventions in many settings and for many issues, in Australia and elsewhere, and their application is more fully depicted in Chapter 15. Several theoretical understandings now inform a diverse set of actions for health promotion (as seen in Appendix E) and the list continues to expand (WHO 1986).

Vertical or horizontal strategies and programs? Tensions between health targets and community preferences

In Australia, the successes of tobacco control, HIV prevention and road safety have been attributed to the adoption of comprehensive health-promotion strategies (NHMRC 1997b). In particular, these achievements have been the result of a combination of legislative and policy interventions; social marketing to shift community attitudes and achieve support; active education programs directed at the general community as well as high-risk groups; and appropriate health services. Additionally, these successes have been underpinned by the development of technical capacity, strategic policy direction and structures for delivering programs at the community level.

Health-promotion thinking has also led to changes in the way public health legislation has

been designed. Instead of a sole focus on punitive measures, legislation (for example, in Victoria and Queensland) has been framed that encourages a proactive approach to health improvement, such as the development of municipal public health plans by local government. Recognising the importance of non-health sector influences on health, and therefore the need to work actively with other sectors, legislation (such as in Tasmania) has also required that health-impact assessments be performed on proposed projects or developments, in association with environmental impact statements.

Building on successes and community interests, Australia has adopted a large number of national public health strategies. These have been concerned with specific diseases (such as breast and cervical cancer, HIV and hepatitis C); particular risk factors (such as tobacco, alcohol and illicit drugs); key requirements for good health (such as nutrition and physical activity); a range of population groups defined by culture, gender or age (such as Aboriginal and Torres Strait Islander people, children and youth, women and older people); or programs in a series of settings (for example, schools or workplaces). Each of these strategies has combined a range of health promotion methods (including social marketing, community education and modification of environments) and has needed particular resources for implementation (such as workers with particular sets of skills and different forms of media).

The challenge for Australia in having adopted multiple public health strategies—short of a radical rationalisation of programs—is to ensure that they are implemented in such a way that resources, efforts and exposure to communities can be coordinated. This is especially important in light of the different priorities, levels of expertise, interest groups and public health-delivery structures across the federation. If each strategy aims to work—for example, in schools or Aboriginal communities— or to involve GPs, there can be problems of both 'reinventing the wheel' as well as placing substantial demands on schools, Aboriginal communities and

GPs. Similarly, if each strategy needs to be based on surveys of community attitudes and practices, then data-collection efforts will be duplicated in many communities and settings. Furthermore, the reality is that people often experience multiple health problems or are exposed to many risks at any given time. Hence, the preference of communities and patient groups will be for health strategies and programs to adopt a holistic approach to people's health and to community life, rather than just focusing on individual body parts or behavioural risk factors.

In the face of these concerns, models have emerged that demand a more integrated approach to public health practice. These are often based on a 'settings' approach—healthy cities, safe communities, healthy workplaces, healthy villages, healthy islands, health-promoting schools, and health-promoting hospitals and health services. The healthy settings idea has strong links back to the early history of public health, with action and

advocacy occurring in local contexts and the application of evidence continuing as key themes (see 'Application: Healthy settings' in Chapter 15).

The notion of 'settings' has been with health educators for a long time, cast as 'major social structures that provide channels and mechanisms of influence for reaching defined populations' (Goldstein & von Schirnding 1997). With the advent of the Ottawa Charter of 1986, 'settings' took on a new meaning, as the Ottawa Charter called for action to 'create supportive environments'. This recognition of socio-environmental influences on health led to the call for health promotion to have the objective of 'making healthy choices easy choices'.

More recent studies on community health and community-based interventions suggest that yet another element of the 'settings' concept is important. A setting is a context—and represents a complex set of relationships and structures—within which people live, work, trade or socialise. Settings represent social systems that are deeply

---

Box 6.3 Vertical, horizontal and diagonal programs

The debate between vertical and horizontal programs has been exacerbated by the extent of global investment in vertical programs, such as AIDS, tuberculosis and malaria since the early 2000s (Harris et al. 2011). With the realisation that disease-specific treatments cannot be successfully delivered without adequate health-care infrastructure and capabilities, there have been calls for health system strengthening (WHO 2007), including renewal of primary health care (WHO 2008c), as a renewed approach to horizontal programming. Considering that both strong delivery systems and targeted efforts are necessary to produce health outcomes, the 'diagonal approach' has been proposed as an alternative to vertical and horizontal programs. It has been used by researchers in Mexico to demonstrate the effectiveness in reducing child mortality of a

range of public health interventions bridging clinics and homes. Mexico had been recognised as one of seven countries on track to achieve the Millennium Development Goal regarding reducing child mortality, as during a 25-year period a decline in child mortality rates from 64 to 23 per 1000 live births had been achieved. This improvement in child mortality rates was attributed to a selection of highly cost-effective interventions, including investments in women's education, social protection, water and sanitation, a high level of coverage of public health interventions, leadership and continuity of public health policies, and investments in institutions and human resources. Using this diagonal approach, it was not possible to establish a causal link to the reduction on child mortality. However, researchers identified significant associations between the reduction in child mortality and the high levels of coverage achieved with public-health interventions, as well as the range of relevant interventions in place. (Sepulveda et al. 2006) binding, involve frequent and sustained interactions between people and are characterised by particular cultures and multiple forms of membership and communication. As a context for social relationships, settings also exert direct and indirect effects on health. For example, the Whitehall II study in the United Kingdom has shown that people at the lower end of workplace hierarchies have poorer health than people in upper-level positions of authority and decision-making because they lack control over factors such as their workload, which in turn influences perceptions and physiological responses (Marmot et al. 1997). Therefore, acting on community-level influences (such as in a workplace) will be as important as directing interventions to individuals (Kawachi et al. 1997; Birch et al. 1998; Kaplan et al. 1996).

The rapid diffusion, internationally, of the healthy settings approach in the 1990s partly reflected its appeal as a vision, with wide applicability and the potential to foster an integrated, practical approach to health protection and promotion. The evolving thinking of health promotion is that traditional boundaries between protection, prevention and promotion may no longer be relevant, and that the contemporary approach to public health intervention will require adoption and coordinated implementation of multiple approaches.

Planning and evaluating public health programs: Matching needs with action

The basic logic

The effectiveness of public health interventions is contingent on their design and implementation, both of which require effective planning. Planning is essentially a problem-solving technique used to assemble a series of activities in an orderly fashion in order to assist in the achievement of a desirable future state (Eager, Garrett & Lin 2001). In public health, the test of planning is whether there are improvements in health, health services delivery or

system performance. Whether the focus is on health or health services, each planning cycle is concerned with identifying key health issues and factors that pose risks or protect health, devising appropriate interventions, assessing options, setting priorities, implementing the selected program, and evaluating the process and outcomes.

The challenge in planning for health improvement—that is, for public health programs—is to discern all the relevant factors that are risks for health or that protect health (as seen in Figure 4.3) and then selecting the right mix of interventions. In efforts to prevent cardiovascular disease and diabetes, for example, a state government might implement a mix of interventions ranging from risk factor assessment and monitoring at the individual level, to environmental changes at the organisational and community level, to legislative changes (see Figure 6.1).

Common models

Models for health program planning have evolved over time as experience with public health programs has shown which elements are important to consider in designing, implementing and evaluating a quality program. Models vary in the specific steps they identify, the level of descriptive detail about how to undertake certain planning activities, assumptions about who will be involved in planning, use of theory and other features. However, the basic elements for health promotion planning, such as those described in Box 6.4, can generally be identified in most public health program planning models (see Table 6.2).

Green and Kreuter's PRECEDE–PROCEED model for health-promotion program planning (see Figure 6.2) is one of the most popular, with several hundred published examples of its use. The model has been tested and applied in a variety of settings, including schools, health services, workplaces and communities. It draws on a number of disciplines—epidemiology, social and behavioural sciences, education and health administration—and

Figure 6.1 Mix of interventions to prevent cardiovascular disease and diabetes

Individual focus ◄───────────────────────────────────► **Population focus**

Screening risk factor assessment Risk factor assessment and monitoring by general practitioner	Health education Skill development Healthy eating/ cooking demonstration Supermarket tours Education sessions about the benefits of physical activity	Social marketing Health information Local advertising campaign about the benefits of cycling to work 'Come and try' day at a local community house	Community action Community reference group to lobby council for safer facilities for physical activity Collaboration with local gym to offer off-peak rates for users	Settings and supportive environments Collaboration with major workplaces to introduce healthy staff canteen policy Collaboration with council and workplaces to provide facilities that encourage active transport (such as showers and bike racks)

Ensuring the capacity to deliver quality programs through capacity-building strategies, including:

Organisational development   **Workforce development**   **Resources**

Source: Victorian Department of Human Services (2004b: 9).

Box 6.4 Steps in health planning

- Select a health issue or population group of concern.
- Identify health needs (including key risk factors and groups at risk) by collating and analysing data from existing sources, and collecting additional information through interviews, surveys or focus groups (including information about perceived risks, health needs, and adequacy of current programs).
- Identify intervention options by considering which risk factors are amenable to intervention, and reviewing literature on what has worked as well as how current programs are working (the Ottawa Charter is a useful checklist for considering the different types of interventions that may be required).
- Select an appropriate intervention, set program goals and objectives, and ensure that the intervention selected is acceptable for the population group, and feasible within the timeframe and resources available.
- Develop implementation strategies and an action plan by defining all activities and their appropriate sequencing; set out a timetable for all actions on a coordinated basis.
- Implement and monitor to deliver the program; define key issues to be monitored and put into place a reporting or data-collection system alongside program activities.
- Evaluate to assess the impact and outcomes of interventions and determine whether the interventions have been effectively designed and delivered; the result of evaluation should inform future interventions.

Source: Eager, Garrett & Lin (2001).

Table 6.2 Health-promotion program planning models

Name of model	Author	Characteristics of model
Model for health education planning	Ross and Mico (1980)	Model represents six phases: initiation, needs assessment, goal-setting, planning and programming, implementation, evaluation. Each phase considers content, methods and process.
Planned approach to community health: PATCH model	Centers for Disease Control and Prevention (1987)	Model represents five elements: community members participate in the process, data guide the development of programs, participants develop a comprehensive health-promotion strategy, evaluation emphasises feedback and program improvement, the community capacity for health promotion is increased. Emphasises joint planning, implementation and evaluation between communities, authorities and agencies.
Cyclic nine-stage planning model	Ewles and Simnett (1990)	Model represents nine stages of planning in a cyclical model: identify consumers and characteristics, identify consumer needs, decide the goals of the program, formulate specific objectives, identify resources, plan content and method in detail, plan evaluation methods, carry out the program, evaluate the process and outcomes.
Program management guidelines for health promotion	Central Sydney Area Health Service and NSW Health (1994)	The program management guidelines aim to enhance quality of health-promotion program management. They are concerned with all phases of the program cycle (from planning to evaluation and sustainability) and present a series of questions to guide workers through the decisions required to manage programs effectively. The three components of the planning section are identifying a specific issue, target group, and focus for the program; designing the program; developing the action plan.
RE-AIM model	Glasgow et al. (1999)	Five-dimension model for planning and evaluating public health interventions: reach, efficacy, adoption, implementation and maintenance. The model proposes that these dimensions pertain to multiple levels (e.g. individual, organisation, community) and interact to determine the public health or population-based impact of a program or policy.
PRECEDE–PROCEED model	Two sets of phases work in tandem: Green and Kreuter (2005)	PRECEDE—acronym for Predisposing, Reinforcing and Enabling Constructs in Educational and Ecological Diagnosis and Evaluation; PROCEED—acronym for Policy, Regulatory and Organising Constructs in Educational and Environmental Development. Model proposes (1) multiple factors are involved in producing health and health risks and (2) because health and health risks are produced by multiple factors, efforts to bring about changes in behaviour, environments and society must be multi-dimensional or multi-sectoral, and participatory. Model evolved over four decades to increasingly emphasise social and environmental factors.

Source: adapted from Ewles & Simnett (1985).

Figure 6.2 PRECEDE–PROCEED model

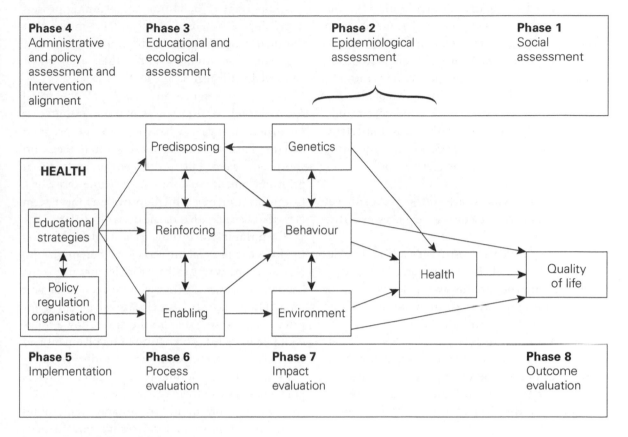

Source: Green & Kreuter (2005: 10).

emphasises a thorough assessment of the nature of a problem and its determinants as a basis for planning. The idea behind the model is that health and health risks are produced by a range of interacting factors and, as a consequence, interventions to bring about behavioural, environmental and social change must be multi-dimensional or multi-sectoral. The model begins with establishing desirable final outcomes (health and quality of life), and works backwards to discern the multiple dimensions of a problem, finally arriving at an understanding of the proximate and contributory causes. It encourages participation by the community being studied in a range of activities: finding its own definition of quality of life; defining its specific health goals and the way these

outcomes might be measured; identifying particular behaviours or environments that could be linked to these outcomes; analysing these behaviours and environments in terms of the factors (predisposing, reinforcing or enabling) that establish and maintain them. Following from this assessment is action—the formulation and implementation of solutions, including programs and policies—and evaluation.

Challenges in planning interventions

A common problem encountered in health planning is that plans and priorities that are determined on the basis of data are not always easy to implement in practice. For instance, different groups of people in the community are likely to have different views about which health issues and needs are priorities, or their stated needs may diverge from what the data suggest are priority problems. The literature on effectiveness of different interventions may not be applicable to the community or population group in question, or 'best practice' interventions may not be acceptable to the community, or feasible.

Various views exist about why community involvement in planning activities is important. From the equity or rights perspective, community involvement is needed for several reasons:

• Community voices are often unheard yet communities have distinct experiences, expertise and priorities.
• Planning should be transparent and accountable.
• Plans are more likely to be sustained when they incorporate the insights and understandings of the community, as they are more likely to be 'owned' by the community.
• Plans are more realistic and appropriate when they reflect community interests and priorities.
• Social assessment becomes important as the basis for understanding communities and how best to ensure that they benefit from health programs.

Community involvement also makes sense from a pragmatic, political perspective. The types of changes proposed in planning activities are likely to affect a range of individuals and groups, and not all of these will be fully supportive of proposed actions. Indeed, it is likely that there will be conflicting views as the interests of different stakeholders are inherently varied. As implementation requires the support of those affected by and involved in change, it is important to build into the planning process ownership of proposed changes. This means that the final program plan might contain a series of negotiated compromises, rather than what might be viewed as the technically ideal solution.

Social assessment—an analysis of the social and economic circumstances of a community—is important in laying a basis for realistic program designs. Finally, decision-makers often focus on short-term gains, but health benefits and societal priorities might require longer time horizons. Community members might provide a longer-term view that balances that of the decision-makers.

Community involvement in health planning might occur in different ways for different groups. Not everyone wants to be strongly engaged; some people are satisfied to receive information or give input. Others need to have close involvement, if not drive the process. Table 6.3 illustrates how groups could be involved. The nature of involvement and the nature of participants can vary during different stages of the planning process. Table 6.4 offers guidelines on who to involve and when.

Although community consultation can ground the planning effort in local realities and desires, in some cases it is reasonable to base planning on the best available evidence of what works, as long as the evidence is appropriate to a local context. Programs should also be informed by a logical model (or program logic), which sets out in a step-by-step manner which activities will produce what results and at approximately what point in time. Such a model will guide implementation planning

Table 6.3 Community involvement in planning

Level of involvement	Outcome of involvement	Community group of interest
Information	One-way information flow	Population as a whole
Consultation	Two-way information flow	Members of affected communities
Collaboration	Participative decision-making	Key stakeholder organisations
Ownership	Shared decision-making or transfer of control	Clients, staff, managers, decision-makers

Source: Eager, Garrett & Lin (2001: 155).

Table 6.4 Guidelines for identifying participants in planning

Core planning process	Who to involve
Needs assessment	Individuals, peak community organisations and stakeholders, self-help groups, community groups, members of affected communities
Setting goals and objectives	Nominees or representatives
Developing strategies	Self-help and community groups; stakeholders; nominees or representatives; members of affected communities
Establishing priorities	Nominees or representatives

Source: Eager, Garrett & Lin (2001: 156).

and ensure that all parts of the health program are coordinated. Programs can only achieve an impact if there is appropriate targeting, if the population coverage is substantial and if those involved in program implementation are appropriately skilled.

The program logic should also serve as the basis for monitoring and evaluation. Monitoring is a reflective activity whereby key participants track progress of and receive feedback on key indicators of performance. Indicators can be used to examine program progress in relation to planning, achievements of a program at different locations or for different population groups, or achievements relative to agreed standards—which may be national or international. Monitoring should be an integral part of the program-management process.

Evaluation

Designing how, when and by whom an intervention will be evaluated is as much a part of the planning phase as designing the intervention itself. Program resources need to be allocated to evaluation processes, and certain activities need to start even before program implementation (for example, assessing attitudes, behaviours or characteristics of the environment prior to the start of an intervention so that changes can be demonstrated).

Evaluations are usually required by funding agencies for accountability purposes. Of increasing importance from the point of view of strengthening the status of health promotion, evaluations of interventions also contribute to the knowledge base of public health practice, and support organisational learning. Without sufficient evaluation, the effectiveness of a public health intervention cannot be assessed and assured. With sufficient evaluation, the design and delivery of future interventions can be modified in the light of the successes and failings of past efforts, and can contribute to continued support and funding of initiatives.

Ideally, the approach to evaluating a program should be designed at the beginning, based on the program logic. Evaluation can be done early in a program to ensure it is on track—this is called process, or formative, evaluation. This type of evaluation can facilitate the ongoing improvement of intervention efforts, overcome resistance, build support and detect unforeseen challenges and consequences. It will ensure that the public health effort remains responsive to stakeholders. Impact, or summative, evaluation is undertaken at the conclusion of the program to assess its effectiveness (that is, did it work?).

Although early thinking about evaluation was focused on measurement of outcomes and assessment of whether program objectives were met, more attention is now given to process evaluation in order to gain a better understanding of why a program did not work or what factors truly contributed to program success. In addition, more recognition is being given to capturing the realities of different actors involved in the program (including program funders, implementers, recipients or participants), as each group is likely to have different perspectives and explanations of what is working and what is not. These different views can be fed

---

Box 6.5 Types of evaluation

Process (or formative) evaluation: is concerned with the strategies and processes that are used to implement programs.

Impact (or summative) evaluation: documents the immediate effects of programs and contributes to assessment of whether program objectives have been met.

Outcome evaluation: examines the long-term effects of programs and the extent to which program aims have been met.

---

back into action and the program activities can be adjusted to ensure that the program continues to meet the needs of the community.

Conclusions about the successes and problems of a public health intervention are difficult to draw if evaluation is only conducted at the end-point and only focused on the short-term outcomes of the program. It is important to assess how well the intervention was designed as well as delivered, in order to understand whether the idea was poorly conceived or poorly executed. Thus, evaluations need to cover the structure, process, impact and longer-term outcomes of interventions.

Evaluation experts adopt different approaches, depending on the question at hand as well as their general orientation. The earliest thinking about evaluation was to assess whether those who received interventions benefited more than those who did not. This is typically a 'pre-test' and 'post-test' situation, where a 'treatment' group is compared with a 'control' group. Randomised clinical trials, quasi-experimental studies and other types of comparative and controlled studies would be the preferred methodology. The program objectives are well specified, and the evaluation methods are usually quantitative.

The next generation of evaluation (Guba & Lincoln 1989) emerged when evaluators realised that program goals are not always neat and tidy, that programs might have multiple and complex components, and that they might deliver a range of intended and unintended consequences. Within this paradigm, it becomes particularly important to undertake formative (or process) evaluation, and examine program inputs and processes as well as outputs. Case studies are often used to illuminate how the program operates in specific organisational and social contexts.

A third approach to evaluation developed from the need to formulate professional judgements about programs against a preferred standard. Typically, outside experts make direct observations, interview program participants and review program documentation in order to assess strengths and weaknesses, and make recommendations about improvements. Standards can be quantitative or qualitative; they can reflect professional norms or be based on empirical research.

More recently, the political nature of evaluation has been recognised. That is to say, programs affect people in different ways, and their perceptions and opinions will often inform what position they take in relation to how a program should work. At the same time, one person's interpretation of reality is as legitimate as that of another person. Given this complex set of interactions, evaluators engage with all stakeholders and adopt a mix of qualitative and quantitative approaches.

Goodman suggests the principles listed in Table 6.5 for evaluation of community-based programs; these can be extended generally to most public health efforts (Goodman 1999).

Having a good logic model for a program is an important starting point for any public health intervention (see Figure 6.3). Logic models represent the reasoning behind a program, and visually communicate—through flow diagrams, for instance—the links between all elements of a program: inputs, processes and expected outcomes. The logic model, the planning model and the evaluation model should be consistent with each other. They help to

Table 6.5 Evaluation principles and tools for community-based programs

Principle	Tools
1 Evaluation of intervention should include an assessment of program theory	Logic models
2 Evaluation instruments should be adapted to each community	Questionnaires and surveys
	Social indicators
3 Evaluation should be guided by the key questions and often requires both quantitative and qualitative approaches	Experimental designs
	Qualitative designs
4 Evaluation should recognise the influence of complex social systems	Ecology and system design
5 Evaluation should involve stakeholders in a meaningful way	Participatory planning

Source: adapted from (Goodman 1999).

Figure 6.3 Components of a basic logic model

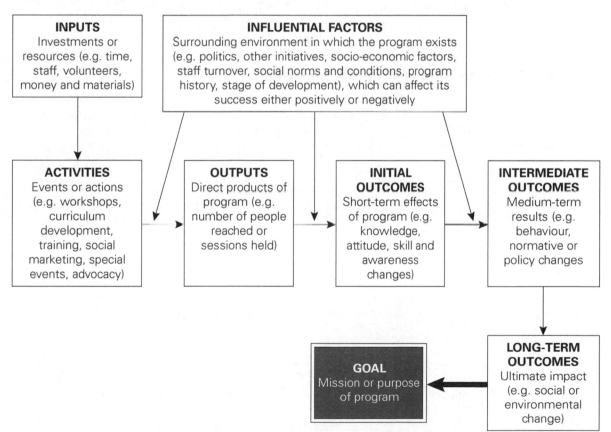

Source: US Department of Health and Human Services (2002: 15).

clarify the intervention strategy, assess the potential effectiveness of the strategy, identify appropriate outcome targets, set priorities for allocating human and financial resources, specify what evaluation questions are appropriate and point to the evidence base required. Most importantly, such models help build better programs.

Nutbeam's model of the hierarchy of health promotion outcomes is a type of logic model, contributing to our understanding of the links between health promotion interventions (education, facilitation, advocacy), their intermediate effects on determinants of health and their longer-term effects on health and well-being (see Figure 6.4). It emphasises the multi-dimensional nature of health promotion, and the complexity of the challenge in bringing about change.

Demand for evidence-based public health practice: Does it really work?

Program evaluation has become more important since the 1960s, as government funding in social programs has increased. Interest in the effectiveness of public health interventions has grown in more recent times, prompted by developments in technical knowledge, experience and the political context, and following the evidence-based medicine (EBM) movement. An evidence base for public health practice incorporates research into program efficacy and evaluation of the effectiveness of specific programs.

There are a number of reasons why the notion of evidence-based practice is as important for public health practice as for medical practice (Lin & Fawkes 2005a):

Figure 6.4 Outcomes model for health promotion

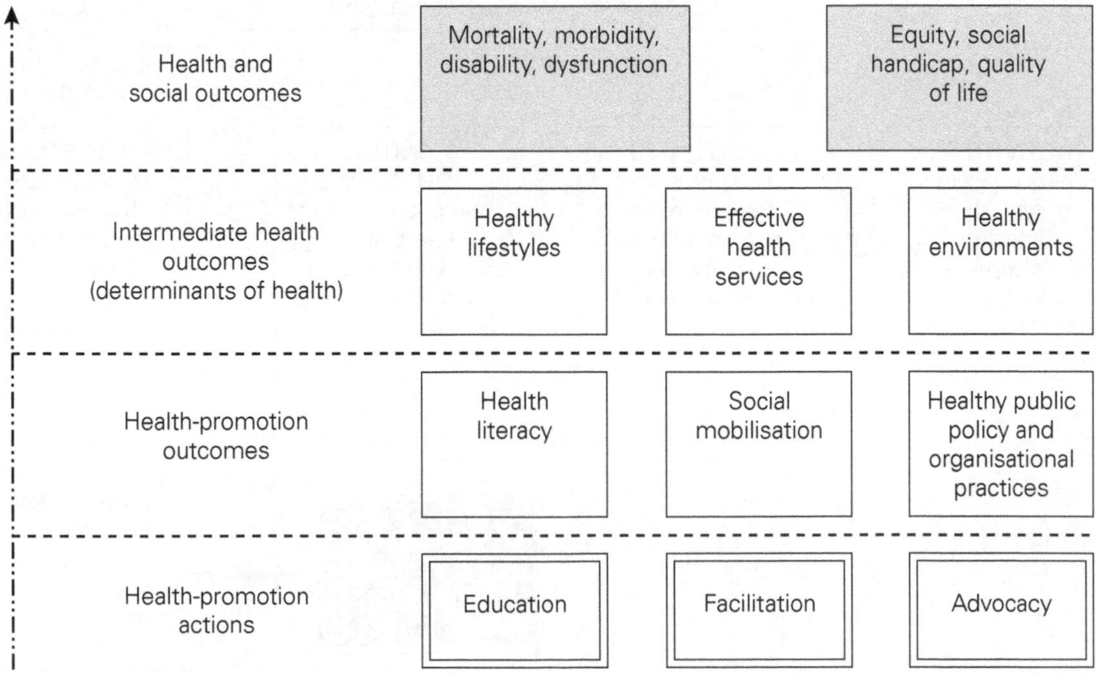

Source: Nutbeam (1996: 58–60).

- It is crucial to know whether interventions are doing more good than harm.
- Where resources become scarce, there is increasing competition between programs and services, and demand for cost-effectiveness considerations in investments. The costs and benefits of different approaches should be considered so that the best option and use of funding is adopted.
- The people who make the decisions about interventions, and those who are affected by the decision, should know the strengths, limitations and gaps in the available evidence.

What is evidence?

Evidence can mean different things to different people. Some adopt a general understanding derived from the dictionary—that evidence is anything that establishes a fact or gives a reason for believing something (Lin 2003b). In the discourse on 'evidence-based practice', however, proponents see evidence as information and knowledge derived from research.

The advent of EBM has promoted a particular approach to evidence-based practice in a range of health arenas, including public health. Arising from concerns raised by Archie Cochrane (1972) about whether medicine is practised on the basis of the best known evidence, EBM is defined as 'the conscientious, explicit and judicious use of current best evidence in making decisions about the care of individual patients' (Sackett et al. 1996). Reflecting Archie Cochrane's original vision, evidence for the use of specific clinical procedures and drug treatments is best generated by synthesising published primary research based on particular research methods, with a preference for randomised controlled trials (RCTs). Being able to attribute changes to a particular intervention is a key issue in producing evidence.

In the 1990s, clinical epidemiologists responded to Cochrane's call for more solid and proven evidence by setting up an international network collaboration on the systematic reviews of research on intervention effectiveness. The Cochrane Collaboration is now an international network of institutions that work together to undertake systematic reviews of intervention trials, and to disseminate the result of these reviews.

The production of evidence of effectiveness is a five-step process that can feed into collections of systematic reviews:

1 intervention
2 evaluation of intervention
3 published paper or report on intervention (primary research)
4 systematic review of multiple papers or reports (secondary research)
5 evidence of effectiveness of an intervention.

Systematic reviews of existing evidence are important tools for use by policy-makers, decision-makers and practitioners. They aim to give a thorough, unbiased search of the relevant literature, explicit criteria for assessing studies and structured presentation of the results. Their value lies in their attempt to avoid the bias that comes from single studies, while distilling the essential learnings for application in policy development, program planning and investment decisions (Joanna Briggs Institute 2004).

EBM strengthened progressively in the 1980s and 1990s, and has led to the pursuit of information about the effectiveness of all health interventions, which allows judgements to be made about their potential adoption.

In the late 1990s, government agencies in the United Kingdom and the United States (National Health Survey and Centers for Disease Control and Prevention respectively) began to develop guidelines for clinical preventive services and for community preventive services, covering such wide-ranging issues as immunisation, tobacco control, cancer screening and mental health. In Australia, the NHMRC began with the development of guidelines for clinical intervention research, setting out the criteria by which evidence should be evaluated. Recognising that guidelines differ in their purpose and formulation, the original criteria for evaluating evidence were revised (these included the level, strength, magnitude and relevance of the evidence) to include the evidence dimensions of all the studies relevant to the particular recommendation more broadly (NHMRC 2009c):

- the evidence base, in terms of the number of studies, level of evidence and quality of studies (risk of bias)
- the consistency of the study results
- the potential clinical impact of the proposed recommendation
- the generalisability of the body of evidence to the target population for the guideline
- the applicability of the body of evidence to the Australian health-care context.

In EBM, RCTs are ranked as the highest-quality, most robust method for attributing causes, as they control for bias in order to generalise. In the NHMRC's designation of levels of evidence in the area of clinical medicine (NHMRC 1999), a systematic review of all RCTs relevant to a research question (especially concerning drug treatments or clinical techniques) is therefore at the top of a hierarchy of study design and levels of evidence. Originally levels of evidence were assigned according to the particular study design utilised (NHMRC 1999). Subsequently, the levels of evidence were expanded to include additional levels of evidence in relation to the particular research question, recognising the importance of an appropriate study design to the type of research question. The additional levels of evidence are relevant to grading evidence for clinical guidelines for diagnosis, prognosis, aetiology and screening, where the study question may not lend itself to the use of a randomised controlled trial (NHMRC 2009c) (see Table 6.6).

Evidence for public health interventions

Public health researchers and practitioners were also challenged by the rise of the EBM movement. Based on the principles of EBM, Brownson et al. (2003) characterise evidence-based public health (EBPH) as the development, implementation and evaluation of public health programs through the application of principles of scientific reasoning. Tools for developing, collecting and disseminating systematic reviews of public health and health promotion include the Cochrane and Campbell Collaborations (international), *The Guide to Community Preventive Services* (USA) and the National Health Service Centre for Reviews and Dissemination (UK). The websites, purpose, audience and key features of each of these initiatives are included in the 'Useful resources' section of this book. For example, the Cochrane Collaborations today includes a public health review group, a consumers and communication review group, and an effective practice and organisation of care review group, as examples of areas of particular interest to public health practitioners. The recommendations of the Taskforce on Community based Preventive Services are summarised in Appendix G.

Using these tools has shed light on theoretical and practical issues about evidence, which have been centred on the hierarchy of evidence used to judge the strength of effectiveness and the types of outcomes to be assessed. Challenges in applying EBM to public health relate to the types of evidence and evidence availability, accessibility and applicability:

- Experimental designs that are narrow in order to capture evidence may not capture important contextual variables that influence outcomes at the community level.
- Decision-making contexts may vary, and so what counts as evidence may differ from location to location.
- Process evaluation is important to establish what aspects of a program work and why. It is

Table 6.6 NHMRC evidence hierarchy: Designations of 'levels of evidence' according to type of research question

Level	Intervention	Diagnostic accuracy	Prognosis	Aetiology	Screening intervention
I	A systematic review of level II studies	A systematic review of level II studies	A systematic review of level II studies	A systematic review of level II studies	A systematic review of level II studies
II	A randomised controlled trial	A study of test accuracy with an independent, blinded comparison with a valid reference standard, among consecutive persons with a defined clinical presentation	A prospective cohort study	A prospective cohort study	A randomised controlled trial
III-1	A pseudorandomised controlled trial (i.e. alternate allocation or some other method)	A study of test accuracy with an independent, blinded comparison with a valid reference standard, among non-consecutive persons with a defined clinical presentation	All or none	All or none	A pseudorandomised controlled trial (i.e. alternate allocation or some other method)
III-2	A comparative study with concurrent controls: • Non-randomised experimental trial • Cohort study • Case-control study • Interrupted time series with a control group	A comparison with reference standard that does not meet the criteria required for level II and III-1 evidence	Analysis of prognostic factors among persons in a single arm of a randomised controlled trial	A retrospective cohort study	A comparative study with concurrent controls: • Non-randomised, experimental trial • Cohort study • Case-control study
III-3	A comparative study without concurrent controls: • Historical control study • Two or more single arm study • Interrupted time series without a parallel control group	Diagnostic case-control study	A retrospective cohort study	A case-control study	A comparative study without concurrent controls: • Historical control study • Two or more single arm study
IV	Case series with either post-test or pre-test/post-test outcomes	Study of diagnostic yield (no reference standard)	Case series, or cohort study of persons at different stages of disease	A cross-sectional study or case series	Case series

Source: NHMRC (2009c:15).

important for sharing lessons but less available (less likely to be funded or published), and therefore less able to be accounted for in assessments of evidence.

- The ethical standards of research may preclude particular types of interventional research, and therefore the types of evidence available.

Even though RCTs are ranked in EBM as the highest-quality method for attributing causes, they are expensive. More importantly, RCTs are not appropriate for establishing evidence of effectiveness in multi-level and multi-strategy programs, such as those that look at the ways in which city environments can support health (sometimes known as healthy cities). Given the importance of social context and community preferences, Kohatsu, Robinson and Torner (2004) propose the definition of EBPH as 'the process of integrating science-based interventions with community preferences to improve the health of populations'.

Despite evidence that specific population health goals can be achieved with the right combination of strategies, support, effort and investments, generating good-quality evidence about health-promotion programs remains a challenge. The classic evaluation problem for health promotion is that measurable health outcomes require a long-term investment of possibly ten years or more. Being able to attribute other changes to a particular health-promotion intervention is a key issue in producing evidence.

A significant amount of work has been done internationally on suitable evaluation methods and tools, and on the identification of appropriate outcomes to measure impacts of health promotion (Rootman et al. 2001; Nutbeam 1996; Potvin & McQueen 2008). While evaluative efforts and the accumulation of an evidence base are important and necessary, effectiveness also depends on high-quality implementation. Intervention research that demonstrates the outcomes and costs of a program under ideal conditions to assess efficacy is a necessary prerequisite for research that tests the ability of a program to modify determinants of health in natural conditions in a variety of contexts.

Does evidence lead to effective public health action?

Despite its importance, planning is often done poorly, with inadequate attention to the full scope of factors (social, political, environmental, economic and technological) that have contributed to creating and sustaining a health issue or problem. Yet even good planning that applies appropriate theories and judiciously uses evidence does not guarantee effectiveness. High-quality implementation and the use of information from process evaluation are also essential.

The pathway from evidence to effective implementation to outcomes is complex and can take considerable time to be realised (Lin & Fawkes 2005a). This pathway is depicted in Figure 6.5. To achieve program effectiveness, the challenge is to translate theory into practice. Practice is made possible not only by having good information based on research and evaluation, but by having the right infrastructure (such as workforce skills, financial support, organisational arrangements and authority) and the right strategy for implementation (such as a mix of education, social marketing and community development) in the community of concern.

The most important component in planning for successful public health outcomes may be to involve key stakeholders, and to secure agreement and authority for implementation. The dissemination of evidence and the building of a coalition to advocate for public health action is well illustrated by the experience of tackling iodine deficiency around the world (see Box 6.6 and Figure 6.6).

The 5th Global Conference on Health Promotion, held in Mexico in June 2000, reinforced the importance of securing an infrastructure for health promotion. Moodie, Pisani and de Castellarnau (2000) argued there that future work to improve health would depend on two types of infrastructure. For the first type, new ways of working

Figure 6.5 Pathways from evidence to effectiveness

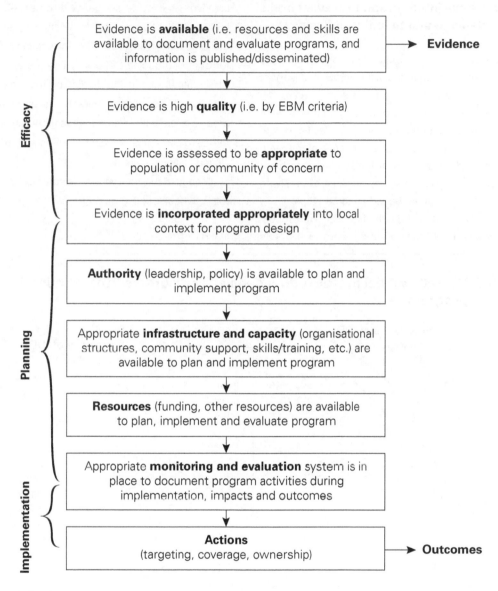

Source: Lin & Fawkes (2005a).

in partnerships with existing infrastructures would be required: 'synergies' must be found with groups like human rights lawyers, transport officials, city mayors and NGO officials. The second type represents an infrastructure dedicated specifically to the promotion of health: institutions like an 'Office or Commissioner of Public Health' or independent, publicly funded health-promotion institutions like VicHealth (see the story in Box 8.5) are mentioned. These institutions depend for their existence on a country's dedication to the value of health as a fundamental resource. As a manifestation of this

Box 6.6 Global intervention to prevent brain damage due to iodine deficiency

Iodine deficiency is the most common preventable cause of brain damage in the world today, and is most serious and irreversible when it develops in utero. An estimated 2 billion people are at risk, and it is a major problem in many countries of the Asia-Pacific region. During the last 25 years, a successful intervention strategy, based on the use of iodised salt, has been developed by Dr Basil Hetzel, an Australian Living Treasure, and colleagues, based on three steps:

1 the establishment of a scientific base, with reconceptualisation of the problem with a suitable acronym—the iodine deficiency disorders (IDD)

2 bridging the gap to a public health program, with the creation of an NGO, the International Council for Control of Iodine Deficiency Disorders, made up of scientists and public health professionals from a range of disciplines, available to assist national programs and with linkages to the world salt industry

3 the development of a global partnership though the United Nations system.

The success of this intervention is summed up well by Hetzel's wheel (see Figure 6.6).

Source: Hetzel 2004

Figure 6.6 Hetzel's wheel for the iodine deficiency disorders (IDD) elimination program

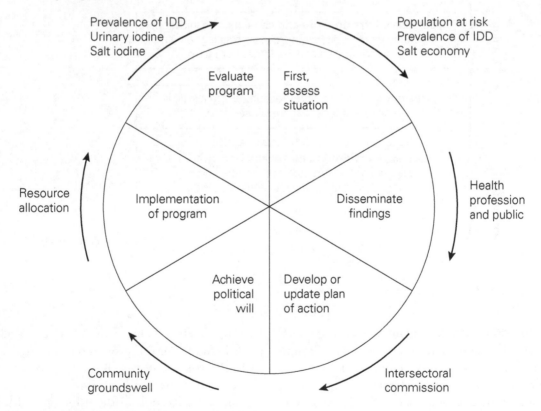

Source: adapted from Hetzel (2004).

value, public health needs to appear high on any country's political agenda.

The challenges in translating evidence into effective public health practice are substantial, although not insurmountable (Lin 2003a; Glasgow, Lichtenstein & Marcus 2003). Practitioners and policy-makers typically are driven by different imperatives from those who are involved with research and evaluation (Lin 2003b). Where the former groups want to achieve practical changes within a short timeframe, the latter group is interested in discovering how the world works. The former are willing to 'muddle through' and act on the basis of 'balance of probabilities', while the latter want proof 'beyond reasonable doubt'.

A number of approaches can be used to link up researchers and evaluators with practitioners and policy-makers (who are both users of evidence and creators of new evidence or realities). These can be implemented at the individual level, through training and workshops, audits and feedback, and decision-support systems (such as manuals or reminders). Organisational mechanisms can also be adopted—such as having a community liaison officer at a research centre, or a knowledge brokerage officer at a public health unit. Having a continuous partnership between practitioners and researchers, even at the stage of efficacy studies, and creating a climate for continuous learning will establish better conditions for ensuring that public health practice makes optimal use of relevant evidence.

Conclusion: An ever-growing toolkit

Improving the health of the population is the central *raison d'être* for public health. Over the history of humanity, the approaches for improving health have evolved from simple quarantine and isolation measures, to clinical preventive services directed at individuals, to a focus on behaviour change of individual risk factors, to intervening at multiple levels within a given context. The current wisdom is to pursue a selectively chosen, well-planned, evidence-based and coordinated approach to strategies directed at multiple levels.

The broad range of activities used in public health represents a 'methods toolkit'. These methods, identified in Table 6.7, are sometimes represented on

Table 6.7 Health-promotion intervention toolkit

Method, intervention or health-promotion action	Explanation	Examples
Screening	Systematic use of a test or investigatory tool to detect individuals at risk of developing specific disease that is amenable to prevention or treatment. A population-based strategy to identify specific conditions in targeted groups before any symptoms are apparent	Pap smears Blood pressure tests Mammograms Screening of migrants for specific conditions
Individual risk factor assessment	Involves a process of detecting the overall risk of a single disease or multiple diseases. Can include biological, psychological and behavioural risks	Living conditions Life history Dietary patterns Physical activity Body weight Tobacco use Drug intake

Table 6.7 Health-promotion intervention toolkit *(continued)*

Method, intervention or health-promotion action	Explanation	Examples
Immunisation	Aims to reduce the spread of vaccine-preventable diseases across targeted population groups	Tetanus Measles Polio
Health education and skill development (usually group activities to enhance skills for adopting and maintaining healthy lifestyle choices)	Provision of education to individuals (through discrete planned sessions) or groups, with the aim of improving knowledge, attitudes, self-efficacy and individual capacity to change	Offered proactively as part of a planned program (e.g. stress management) or offered as part of best practice direct-care services (e.g. antenatal program; secondary prevention programs, such as cardiac rehabilitation programs)
Social marketing and health information (coordinated communication strategies involving newspapers, radio, television, outdoor promotions and print communication, such as leaflets and newsletters)	Involves programs designed to advocate for change and influence the voluntary behaviour of target audiences, which benefits this group and society as a whole. Aims to shift attitudes, change people's view of themselves and their relationships with others, and change lifelong habits, values or behaviours	Coordinated use of a wide range of media: radio, television, newspapers, magazines, pamphlets, low-technology media, interactive technologies such as the internet, 'infotainment edutainment' May be combined with public relations and face-to-face communications Campaigns on HIV, destigmatisation of mental illness, road trauma, sun protection, farm safety Victorian state government 'Better Health Channel'
Community action (participation of community members and groups in advocacy and action for social and environmental change)	Aims to encourage and empower communities (defined by geographical areas and communities of interest) to build their capacity to develop and sustain improvements in their social and physical environments	Self-help and support groups involving women or future parents who wish to choose homebirth Community-led advocacy to improve road safety around schools; eliminate hazardous chemicals in local soils Employee groups acting to improve work conditions in their workplace

Table 6.7 Health-promotion intervention toolkit *(continued)*

Method, intervention or health-promotion action	Explanation	Examples
Settings and supportive environments (changes to policies, laws and regulations, physical and socio-cultural environments and organisations)	Includes: *Organisational development:* aims to create a supportive environment for integrated health-promotion activities within organisations, such as schools, businesses and sporting clubs	Employment of designated health-promotion worker to support colleagues in developing organisation-wide health activities
	Economic and regulatory activities: involves the application of financial and legislative incentives or disincentives to support healthy choices. Focus on pricing, availability restrictions and enforcement	Creation of incentives to increase take-up of immunisation—school entry and child-care payments linked to administration of childhood immunisation Pricing tobacco products to dissuade purchase by young people
	Advocacy: involves a combination of individual, peer and social actions designed to gain political commitment, policy support, structural change, social acceptance and systems support for a particular goal Includes direct political lobbying	Advocacy to increase the range of options for people with disabilities to use all public facilities, including sports and recreation programs

Source: adapted from Victorian Department of Human Services (2003).

a continuum, suggesting different scales of activity and loci for interventions, from the individual level to the population or societal level.

While intervention approaches have changed over time, and the advent of social media has created new possibilities, the notion of these efforts being organised has remained. The key ideas emerging from the sanitary movement that have been carried forward can be summarised as (Ashton 1992):

- the importance of working locally
- appropriate research and inquiry strategies
- the need for special skills and qualifications
- populism and health advocacy
- resourcefulness and pragmatism coupled with humanitarianism
- the value of producing reports on the health of the population
- public health as the responsibility of a democratically accountable body.

7

Health systems and policy:
Making sense of the complex mosaic

Challenge

Perhaps this is you—age 20, third year of university, working part time, sharing a house with a couple of other students, playing some sport when you have the time, a non-smoker and generally in good health except for the occasional cold or bout of the flu. One Sunday you are at your parents' house for a family birthday. When an advertisement for singles private insurance is shown on the television, your older sister suggests that you should consider taking out some health insurance cover. As a high-income earner on more than $90 000 per year, she has already signed up rather than pay the Medicare surcharge. She also receives a rebate from the government for having private health insurance.

Your father, who is a long-term supporter of the Australian Labor Party and believes in Medicare and the right of universal access to medical service, advises you not to waste your money. Your grandmother, who has an ongoing medical problem that requires elective surgery, and who relies heavily on her private health insurance, urges you to do so.

What factors will influence your decision? Your sister argues that, as there are queues at emergency departments in public hospitals and for elective surgery, you need private health insurance to be able to access effective care when you need it. But is this really fair? As you are already paying taxes, aren't you entitled to free health care? If you join a private health fund and do not need to use it for many years, aren't you effectively subsidising elderly people and those with ongoing health problems?

Your sister replies that as she has a high income and is in very good health, she should not have to pay an additional Medicare levy when her taxes are already being used to subsidise the health-care costs of the poor and disadvantaged. But should access to a health-care system be based only on a person's ability to pay rather than their needs? What would you decide?

Introduction

Because of the diverse ways in which the term 'public health' is defined and used, the relationship between public health and health services is often unclear. Public health is sometimes seen as separate from the rest of the health-care system, as a distinct set of programs either aimed at prevention or particular population groups at risk. There are, indeed, differing views about whether public health is one component of the health-care system, or whether health services are one aspect of the social enterprise of public health. In countries such as Australia, where Medicare offers universal access to medical and hospital care, public health is more frequently seen as a set of programs. In countries such as the United States, where nearly 20 per cent of the population has no health insurance, access to health care is seen as a core public health issue.

Regardless of the relationship, there is a need to understand health services, health systems and health policy from a public health perspective. Health services constitute one of the major categories of the determinants of health, and lack of access to essential services can contribute to poorer health outcomes. Furthermore, preventive health services are delivered through health care providers, and health promotion may be an important component of many community health services. How the health system is structured and financed may have significant implications for how public health activities are organised and delivered. Public health principles will also inform how a health care system should be organised and delivered.

Additionally, the health industry is a major part of the economy—it accounts for about 9 per cent of Australian gross domestic product (GDP). Health

services make up a large component of the health budget. With Australian states having constitutional responsibility for the delivery of services, health is an important portfolio for the government—typically a quarter of a state budget is spent on health, with the vast majority for hospital services. Public health programs often struggle for a slightly larger share of the allocated resources, and public health professionals often advocate for greater orientation towards prevention and population health needs in the health care system.

Although the types of personal health services and public health programs do not differ significantly across Australia—or indeed internationally—there are remarkable differences in the ways in which the health system is organised and administered across Australia and internationally. This chapter is concerned with the basic tools that assist us to make sense of the 'mosaic' of the health system, and its apparent lack of 'rationality'. In discussing the underlying dynamics of health systems and health policy, the assumptions and the core contribution of political science and health economics are revealed. The chapter starts with definitions of a health system, looks at how health systems have evolved and what they try to do, and the major typologies of health systems in the world. In discussing the role of government in health systems, a question is raised about who governs. Key concepts in health financing and resource allocation, health services organisation, health-care decision-making and health policy development are explained. The chapter concludes with a review of how health systems should be evaluated from a public health perspective—or what the critical tests are for judging how well a health system is able to serve the social enterprise of public health.

What is a health system?

Milton Roemer (1991) defines a health system as 'the combination of resources, organisation, financing and management that culminate in the delivery of health services to the population'. He identifies five major building blocks for a health system:

- production of resources (such as staff, drugs, facilities, knowledge base)
- organisation of programs (by a range of providers)
- economic support mechanisms (i.e. sources of funds)
- management methods (planning, administration, legislation)
- delivery of services (i.e. the range of health-care programs).

How the health system is organised is of fundamental importance for the health of the public as well as for the social enterprise of public health. A health system that does not provide affordable basic health services is likely to lead to many poor people delaying seeking care or falling into poverty because of health-care costs. A health system without appropriate quality standards or quality assurance processes may lead to poor health outcomes. Overcoming problems of financial, geographical and linguistic access as well as attaining effective health requires a well-coordinated, conscious, organised effort.

Historical development of the health system

Health services have not always been delivered on an organised basis. An organised approach to health care is a relatively modern phenomenon.

Early societies were conscious of the need for health care, although the origins of organised health care evolved gradually (Roemer 1991; WHO 2000). Medicine men or shamans were held in high esteem and supported by collective gifts. Chinese medicine can be traced back more than 3000 years. The city-states of Greece appointed physicians to serve the poor, and the physicians of ancient Rome were attached to the families of landlords. In medieval Europe, the church was the major repository of medical knowledge. It was during the Renaissance, with the rise of universities and the growth of cities, that doctors first set up shop as independent practitioners.

The Industrial Revolution transformed the delivery of health care, as well as society and economy in general (Roemer 1991). In industrialised countries, governments began to assume responsibility for some serious chronic diseases that were seen to be a threat to the community. Mental hospitals were first operated by government in Germany in 1859 and sanitoria for tuberculosis followed shortly after. With workers' health becoming a political issue, Bismarck, the Chancellor of Germany, enacted a law making health insurance and disability compensation coverage compulsory for low-wage workers. This was the first social insurance scheme in the world. The concept of employer liability for health insurance for industrial accidents gradually emerged across industrialised countries. Belgium adopted similar legislation in 1894, Norway in 1909 and England in 1911. As European nationals colonised Africa and Asia, medical systems were set up to protect European settlers and military forces, and these were slowly extended to the indigenous populations.

The pace of health system development accelerated in the twentieth century. The advent of the Russian Revolution in 1917 led to a free medical system for the entire population. This was the earliest example of a completely centralised and state-controlled health system, which was later adopted in Eastern European countries (Roemer 1991). The German model was more popular, however, with Japan introducing health benefits for workers in 1922, Chile establishing a scheme for all workers in 1924, France inaugurating its social insurance in 1928, and 90 per cent of the Danish population covered by work-related health insurance by 1935 (WHO 2000).

World War II damaged or destroyed the healthcare infrastructure in many countries. In doing so, it inadvertently paved the way for different types of health systems to be established. The Beveridge Report of 1942 identified health care as one of three basic prerequisites for a viable social security system (Roemer 1991); hence, in 1948, the British National Health Service was introduced to provide comprehensive health services to every resident. Social insurance was extended to entire populations across Western Europe and various forms of health insurance emerged in South American countries. Hospital expansion was seen in Scandinavia and the United States.

Health systems across the world today are modelled on the basic designs that have emerged since the late nineteenth century (WHO 2000). The major factors that determine the structuring of a health system include size of country, age of population and its geographical distribution, the political system, the economic resources available, history and culture, and values, ideologies and religion. Nonetheless, health systems today aim to promote access to health care through health insurance, with services provided by both public and private providers. The role played by government in a health system varies, but its direct involvement tends to be most extensive in health protection and disease prevention. The WHO defines health systems today as 'all activities whose primary purpose is to promote, restore, or maintain health'. This includes formal health services, home care for the sick, traditional healers, medication use, health protection and regulation—including environmental safety improvement.

The WHO Framework for health system strengthening (WHO 2007a) describes the health system as made up of six discrete and essential building blocks: service delivery; health workforce; information; medical products, vaccines and technologies; financing; and leadership and governance (stewardship):

- Good health services are defined as those that deliver effective, safe, quality health interventions, in an efficient manner, when and where they are needed.
- A well-performing health workforce works in a responsive, fair and efficient way, within available resources and circumstances, and staff are competent, fairly distributed and present in sufficient numbers.
- A well-functioning health information system produces, analyses and disseminates reliable and timely information on health determinants, health system performance and health status.
- A well-functioning health system provides equitable access to essential medical products, vaccines and technologies.
- A good health financing system provides adequate funds for required services and protects users from financial impoverishment related to fees for services, and provides incentives for providers and users to be efficient.
- Leadership and governance ensures strategic policy exists, combined with effective system design, coalition-building, management and regulation.

What does the health system do?

Health needs differ from country to country, as do expectations of what health care should be available and what health services should achieve. The WHO (2000) suggests all health systems have three major objectives:

- to improve the health of the population they serve
- to respond to people's expectations
- to provide financial protection against the cost of ill health.

These objectives do not mean that health systems must be alike in every country. Rather, the WHO suggests that health systems should strive to achieve performance targets that can be set according to a country's level of socio-economic development, as well as its cultural values. These objectives suggest that there are some basic interests that are shared across countries and cultures. If these objectives are not met, public dissatisfaction might become widespread and there may be economic losses for families and the economy. Thus, how well a health system functions is closely tied to social and economic development, as well as political support for government.

The WHO (2000) further suggests that four functions are required to meet the three major objectives listed above:

- service provision
- resource generation (e.g. workforce, facilities)
- financial mobilisation
- stewardship (i.e. looking after the system as a whole).

These functions approximate Roemer's (1991) building blocks (of service organisation and delivery, production of resources, economic support mechanisms and management methods), although the WHO gives particular prominence to the role of government (embedded in the concept of 'stewardship'), rather than the more generic term of 'management'. The relationship between the three objectives and the four functions is depicted in Figure 7.1.

Major types of health system

Given the importance of financing arrangements and ownership arrangements for service provision, health systems are often described by the extent to which financing and service provision is public or private. Table 7.1 shows examples of different types of health system according to these key dimensions.

Figure 7.1 Relationship between functions and objectives of a health system

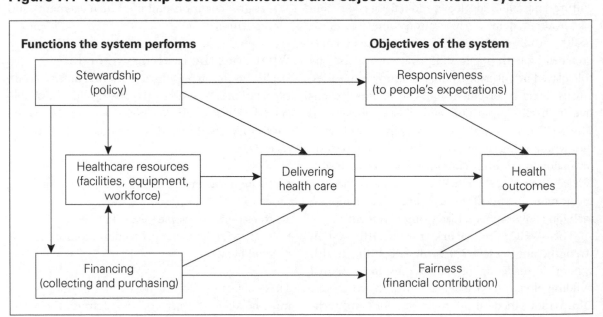

Source: adapted from WHO (2000: 25).

Table 7.1 Types of health system

	Public financing	Private financing
Public provision	UK—National Health Service	China—patient out-of-pocket payment for public hospitals
Private provision	Australia—Medicare + private doctors	US—private health insurance + private doctors

Each type has advantages and disadvantages. In the United Kingdom, there is apparent equity for all but limited choice and severe rationing. In the United States, there is a diametrically opposite system with substantial choice and access—provided you have health insurance coverage, which is typically employer-funded and based on your individual health-risk profile. Australia has a mixed system, which offers choice but is a complex

---

Box 7.1 How do patients experience different health systems?

A person with a chronic disease—for example, an elderly woman—would have widely varying health-care experiences, depending on the country in which she lives.

United States: She will need to decide which specialist to see—a cardiologist? an internal physician? an endocrinologist? a renal physician? The decision may be made by her health insurance company, since the company will have preferred providers. When she becomes an in-patient and when she is later discharged, the health insurer will be consulted about whether the various procedures and services are covered. She will find it challenging to locate private community support services, and they will be costly—unless she is over 65 years of age when Medicare will cover a set amount of services. Her drugs will also be a major expense for her, unless her insurance plan provides some coverage.

Australia: She will go to any GP of her choice, or several if she wishes to get multiple opinions, or will select one who will bulk-bill. If the GP refers her to a specialist and diagnostic investigations, Medicare will pay for most of the cost. Her hospitalisation will be free if she chooses to be a public patient. But she can opt to be under the care of a specific doctor, and then she can either pay out of pocket (i.e. be self-insured) or have her private health fund pay for a component of the hospital expenses. Medicare will pay for a portion of her specialist's expenses. She can be discharged home with support from a range of community-based services—from her local community health centre, local government or district nursing service, depending on where she lives. Her drugs will largely be covered by the Pharmaceutical Benefits Scheme (PBS).

United Kingdom: She will be enrolled with a designated GP, who will provide all aspects of care. If she is hospitalised, she will need to be on a waiting list for a bed in a National Health Service facility. It is free, as is the post-discharge nursing care, which is provided by the local council.

China: She will need to decide whether to go to (1) the major hospital outpatient department, which will cost her quite a bit of money but she will have greater confidence about the competence of the doctor, or (2) the local community health centre, which costs less but where the doctor has a low level of training. She won't know whether all the drugs she has been told to take are really necessary. She will be sent for technology-intensive investigations, which will cost her a lot, but she won't be certain about whether they are all needed. When she is hospitalised, her family will need to visit and bring food for her. Hopefully, her long stay in the hospital will not bankrupt her family—but she may need to borrow to pay the hospital bills as well as provide gifts for the doctor (to ensure that she receives prompt attention). When she is discharged, she will need to organise her own community care. It might be available from the local community health centre for a cost, or she may have to rely on her family.

system to navigate. In China, like many developing countries and transitional economies, access depends on capacity to pay, despite services being planned and run by governments.

Health systems can also be classified according to a number of other dimensions of the system or of the type of government (or economy or society):

- types of financing (tax, social insurance, out of pocket)
- dominant type of ownership/service provider (public, private, charitable)
- underlying political philosophy (socialist, capitalist)
- extent of government intervention/coverage (universal, poor)
- institutional arrangement for government (federalist, unitary)
- level of gross national product (high, low)
- level of economic development (industrialised, developing).

These different dimensions are often ways in which health systems can be compared for assessing the performance of any one country against peer countries.

Health systems differ because the decision about how to design health systems is ultimately a social and political decision—decisions are made in the policy arena about how resources will be used and shared, which reflects values and power distribution in decision-making. All countries need to have a system to mobilise financial resources for the health system. Some countries use taxation and social insurance as a basis for financing (so that there is subsidy across the population), while others rely on voluntary insurance or out-of-pocket payments (so that health care is an individual responsibility). How the funds are pooled is indicative of how health and financial risks are shared, which in turn points to the extent to which solidarity is an important social value. In Australia, lower income groups contribute less and are effectively subsidised by higher income

groups; younger people also subsidise older people as the latter are higher users of services. In the same way, healthier people subsidise those who are sicker. By contrast, countries such as the United States and China rely more on individual contributions than on the pooling of funds. The more individual out-of-pocket payments are drawn upon to finance the health system, the less equitable the access is likely to be. Individuals will also delay seeking care, thus prevention is likely to receive less attention.

All health systems also need to have a system for health service providers to be paid. Some countries pay their health-care providers on the basis of service provided (fee for service, case payment, etc.) while others provide a capped budget based on population (capitation) or on inputs. Systems that pay on a fee-for-service basis often encourage frequent attendance at the doctors or hospital, because there are incentives for providers to maximise their income. Systems that pay on a capitation basis theoretically have a greater incentive to deliver preventive services, because they are making the best use of limited resources. Many types of payment system have operated in Australia—including casemix (or the mix of diagnoses) payments for Victoria, capitation (or per head of population) in New South Wales health services. GPs across Australia are paid on a fee-for-service basis, and specialists provide services to hospitals either on a sessional or fee-for-service basis, depending on the nature of their contract with the hospital. This mix of different payment mechanisms (and therefore incentives) contributes to a great deal of the complexity within the Australian health system, although national reforms aim to pay hospitals on the basis of a national efficient price.

Containing health-care costs is a major concern for all governments. Some countries, such as Australia, control costs partly through 'gatekeeping' (such as making GP referrals to specialist physicians a condition of health insurance payment) or capped payments to providers (for example, public hospital budgets), while other countries use price signals to control the demand for services by patients (for example, co-payments). 'Gatekeeping' by GPs has the added advantage of providing a comprehensive primary care service.

In countries with strong public financing, such as Australia, public health services are more reliant on government. This means funding might be more assured, but is more politically influenced and has to compete with personal health care for resources. In these countries, access to basic health care is less likely to be a problem, as they are more able to provide or mandate universal coverage for health care. As a consequence, population health status is also likely to be less unequal.

Forms of financing and forms of organisation are important from a public health perspective, as they impose different incentives on the health service provider. This might not lead to beneficial impacts on population health. In a system where health service providers are highly autonomous, with limited public accountability and high degrees of market exposure and financial responsibility (that is, they need to earn revenue in a competitive marketplace), preventive services and health care for the poor are unlikely to be high priorities. In a system that is accountable to a highly centralised hierarchy, and with limited financial responsibility, the health service providers are less likely to be innovative and adaptive or responsive to local health needs. Achieving the right balance between autonomy, accountability and responsiveness is a major challenge for health policy-makers.

From the public health perspective, some of the key issues to consider when assessing a health care system are:

- *equity of access:* does everyone who needs health care have access regardless of income, race/ethnicity, gender, place of origin and beliefs?
- *population health gain:* does the health system produce good health outcomes?
- *cost-effectiveness:* are the resources available used to achieve the best outcomes possible?

- *community involvement:* do the patients and community members have a voice and influence to ensure services are responsive?

In other words, health systems might be compared against peer groups on any of the dimensions above (such as financing, service organisation, level of economic development or type of government). The public health interest transcends the specifics of each dimension, and imposes broad criteria about the overall performance of the health system.

What is the role of government?

The WHO (2000) suggests that the ultimate responsibility for how well the health system is serving the needs of the people always rests with the government. Governments have responsibility for the welfare of their populations, they have the capacity to influence all of economy and society, and they need to be concerned about the trust and legitimacy of their activities as seen by their citizens. The WHO suggests that key government responsibilities are:

- policy (i.e. defining vision and direction)
- intelligence (i.e. using information)
- influence (e.g. effective implementation of regulations).

The WHO (2000) criticises Ministries of Health as being too oriented to short-term results, having a narrow focus and giving insufficient attention to policy implementation. Governments are said to be more focused on the public hospitals and medical care, rather than other health-care providers or the health needs of patients and the population in general. They are said to pay more attention to writing rules and regulations than to policy implementation, including monitoring practices within the system. The WHO suggests that governments have to care about the longer-term development of people and society and that, to be effective, governments need to project a vision, be wise in using the best evidence possible in decision-making and adopt a range of policy instruments to effect positive changes in the health system.

There are numerous reasons why governments might be subjected to criticism such as that from the WHO. These explanations are provided from the perspective of different theories about the role of government. Historically, writers (from Plato, to Confucius, through the European Enlightenment philosophers, to today) have argued for different types of governing systems—meritocracy, democracy, technocracy, benign dictatorship—as being most appropriate for creating a good society.

Numerous views have been offered in more recent times as well. Institutionalists, such as James March and Johann Olsen (1989), suggest that the adequacy of formal processes of policy-making and the defined relationship between parliament/legislature and the bureaucracy form the key to understanding how well government manages its health system. However, pluralist theorists—for example, Robert Dahl (1982)—suggest that government mediates between different interest groups. They believe representative democracy allows for all interests to participate, although short election cycles can lead to a short-term orientation, and a focus on delivering benefit to particular interest groups. Public choice theorists, such as James Buchanan and Gordon Tullock (1962), believe that human behaviour is dominated by self-interest, so every player (politicians, bureaucrats, interest groups) seeks to maximise personal gain in the political marketplace. They argue for small government in order to maximise liberty. Elite theorists, such as C.W. Mills (1959), would argue that there is no such thing as a 'level playing field', and those with more wealth and power will ensure that policies maintain the status quo. Structuralists, such as Ralph Miliband (1969) and James O'Connor (1974), argue that the political institutions are supported by those with economic power, and an understanding of the role of government in health policy requires an understanding about the role played by the 'medical industrial complex' in the political sphere.

Regardless of the form and the role of government, there is debate about what government should do in relation to population health. There are, again, multiple perspectives. For those who see health as a right (such as Mann et al. 1999), government has a role to lead the multi-sectoral effort to ensure the best possible level of health is achieved. For those who believe health care is a right, the focus for government might be on ensuring basic health services are available, particularly for those who are vulnerable. For some economists who believe health care is a market commodity (for example, Enthoven 1997), governments have little role to play, as individual preferences and price signals will shape and drive the system. For other economists who believe governments need to ensure a productive workforce, investment in health is linked to the government's role in economic development (e.g. the Commission on Macro-economics and Health; WHO 2001c). Regardless of the philosophical position about health and health care, there is a general view that governments have a role to play in redistribution in order to correct the failings of the market; in regulation, to ensure the markets operate effectively; and in resource allocation, to ensure scarce resources are used appropriately.

Despite these differences of views, there is general acceptance that government must play a role in public health. Health economists (e.g. Drummond et al. 1997; Mooney et al. 1992) believe that there are a number of market conditions that cannot be satisfied in the health-care arena. Specifically, the problems of information asymmetry, merit goods, public goods, externalities and significant barriers to entry all call for government intervention in health care. Public health, in particular, requires government investment because the benefits are diffuse, externalities may be significant and public health programs are public goods (see Box 7.2). The seminal article that laid out the basic issues about applications of economics to health care is by the Nobel Prize winner Kenneth Arrow (1963).

Box 7.2 Definition of terms used by health economists

Information asymmetry: occurs when one party to a transaction has more or better information than the other party. Usually it is the seller or provider (i.e. the doctor) who knows more about the product or a service (i.e. health care) than the buyer (i.e. the consumer or patient).

Merit goods: goods (and services) where the benefits to a society exceed those for an individual. As individuals do not take into account the positive externalities (see below) that arise from the consumption of merit goods, the free-market system always under-provides them. One reason for this is that individuals find it difficult to make rational choices when the costs for such goods (i.e. payment of taxes that governments will spend on health-care programs) arise today and the benefits (i.e. improved access to health care) are only received in the future. Preventive services are the prime example.

Public goods: goods provided by the state, because in a free-market system private companies cannot charge the real cost of them. This situation arises because public goods have two particular characteristics. First, they are non-excludable—once the goods are provided, you cannot exclude people from using them, even if they haven't paid. Second, they are non-rival, which means that consumption of the goods by one person does not diminish how much will be available for the next person. An example is public health research—which becomes the basis for public health interventions.

Externalities: occur when one person's actions affect another person's well-being and the relevant costs and benefits are not reflected in market prices. A positive externality arises when a community benefits from a factory recycling its waste. But as the factory owner cannot charge the community members for these benefits, the waste may not be recycled as often as that community would prefer. A negative externality arises when one person's actions harm another, such as when a factory owner dumps waste that pollutes a nearby river and does not consider the costs such pollution imposes on others.

Barriers to entry: refers to obstacles that are placed in the path of a market participant who wants to enter a given field. They may refer either to an individual who is barred from entering some profession or trade, or to a firm—or even a country—that is barred somehow from entering an industry or trade grouping. Barriers to entry have the effect of making a market less contestable. An example is the high cost (including length of time) it takes to train health-care professionals.

How are health policies developed?

As can be seen from the above discussion, health systems and what governments do differ across countries. Federalist systems (such as Australia and the United States) and unitary systems (such as the United Kingdom and China) are different, but within each of those models health systems also differ. History, values and political ideology do matter. The perfect health system does not exist. Nor do health systems stay the same forever. The evolution of the health-care system has followed remarkably different pathways in countries with similar cultural backgrounds—such as the United Kingdom, United States and Australia. These differences reflect, in part, different pathways for policy-making.

Health policies might come in a variety of forms: as documents that state the intent of decision-makers, as pieces of legislation that lock a government's intentions into law, as budget statements that allocate money in line with policy, as a series of day-to-day decisions that produce a decision-making pattern. Health policies also cover numerous topics—from overall health system design, to structure of service provision, to method of financing, to specific health programs and services, to whole-of-government approaches to improve health and social well-being, to particular forms of industry regulation and consumer protection.

There are different theories about policy-making, which relate in part to different theories about the role of governments, but also about what informs decision-making.

Policy-making is typically a messy and circuitous process, but political scientists and public policy analysts often write about the policy cycle as a way to draw out the essential elements of the decision-making process. Although depicted in a number of different ways, the usual description of policy-making is a process that comprises a series of systematic and sequential steps (Bridgeman & Davis 1998; Edwards 2001):

1 issue identification—define why problems exist and what their impacts might be
2 policy analysis—collect relevant data and information, clarify objectives
3 policy instruments—consider options and proposals for solving key problems
4 consultation with stakeholders—canvass policy options with industry, professionals and community organisations
5 coordination with relevant decision-makers—that is, government departments at all levels
6 decision—agree to adopt a particular course of action
7 implementation—transplant policy to reality through legislation, programs, community education, etc.
8 evaluation—monitor progress and assess whether intended policy objectives were met.

This approach assumes that policy-making is rational and technical (and is comparable to earlier models, such as Easton's input–output model and Simon's (1955) model of rational decision-making).

Lindblom's (1959) early critique of rational decision-making pointed to the role of pluralist interest groups in shaping decision-making. With lobbyists targeting decision-makers at different points in time (or different stages of the policy cycle), he argued that 'muddling through' was a more common approach than rationalism.

Political pragmatism and electoral politics are also recognised as central to health care policy-making. Marmor and Christianson (1982) suggest that health policy goals are often political goals that are traded in a political marketplace, depending on what the participants in the marketplace expect to gain. The MBA thesis of former Australian Health Minister Dr Michael Woolridge documented an example of tradeoffs between economic policy and health financing policy during the years of the Fraser government, highlighting how health policies are made for reasons other than health needs (Wooldridge 1991).

Alford (1975) similarly recognised the importance of interest group influences in policy-making, but suggested that such viewpoints emerged from the social structures associated with interests. For health policy, Alford argued that the professional monopolists (for example, doctors, insurance companies, pharmaceutical companies) generally played a dominant role in policy-making and were opposed by health advocates (such as community groups); the corporate rationalists (who are often the planners, policy analysts and bureaucrats) often played mediating roles, depending on how the political forces were being played out. Lin and Duckett (1996) showed that the introduction of casemix payment in the Victorian hospital system—a radical reform in the Australian health system—was possible because the corporate rationalists dominated the political process.

The process of policy-making is thus generally seen as untidy. Sabatier (1988) suggests that policy advocacy coalitions—comprising people within and outside policy decision-making arenas who have shared values and interests—will drive policy decision-making. Competing policy coalitions may come to dominate policy-making when governments change, as seen in illicit drug policy (Fitzgerald & Sewards 2003). A less complimentary view of decision-making is suggested by the garbage can model of policy-making (Cohen et al. 1972), which posits a more random set of movements— that is, garbage in, and garbage out.

While different theories exist, it is clear that policy-making in a democracy does reflect political, economic and social interests, and progresses along a non-linear track. These policy processes may take simple pathways, such as when the government identifies a problem to be addressed, releases a discussion paper for consultation, issues a final policy statement, passes legislation and allocates funds for its implementation. More often, policy processes are subject to complex pathways. Multiple stakeholders may be involved in covert and overt lobbying. Alternative proposals may be developed and canvassed by different interest groups and political parties. The public statement of lofty goals and commitments may not be matched by the resources made available.

It is the view of many health professionals— including public health professionals—that it would be ideal if research evidence about health needs and strategies could drive policy formulation. The combination of epidemiological and economic data should lead to evidence-based policies. However, Australian health policy-making is, according to Sax (1984), 'a strife of interests'. Brown (1992) suggests that policies for health are an outcome of a synthesis of power relations, demographic trends, institutional agendas, community ideologies and economic resources. Professional dominance (Willis 1983) provides an underlying explanation for why the health-care system is the way it is. Evidence-based health policy is a rarity.

Given the strong role that government plays in investing in public health programs, public health policies are particularly susceptible to political influence, despite the profession's commitment to a strong scientific evidence base. The WHO's concept of stewardship points to the primacy of government in the governance of the health system, in

Case study 7.1
The politics of Medibank and Medicare

The political pragmatism and electoral politics of health policy-making can be seen in the history of Medibank and its successor, Medicare. The idea of providing a tax-funded universal-access national health insurance scheme has been one of Australia's most contentious political issues, because there are so many stakeholders involved in the distribution of financial resources for a public good. The first group of stakeholders comprises the service providers (as represented by the Australian Medical Association [AMA] and other medical groups) who want to preserve their high incomes and profits. The second group consists of the Australian public, which is concerned about being able to access affordable, high-quality medical services. The third group is government, for whom it is a

question of ideology, electoral support and restraining the escalating costs of funding a health-care system. As policy-makers are never able to satisfy all three groups at the same time, the stakes are high (Gray 2004: 11).

Therefore, when the Whitlam Labor government sought to introduce the radical Medibank legislation in 1973, the AMA was at the forefront of a bitter campaign built around the lobbying of members of parliament; the use of a public relations company to coordinate the placing of thousands of advertisements on TV, in newspapers and on radio; and the distribution of 16000 publicity kits (Gray 1984). To break the deadlock in parliament in order to pass the legislation in both houses, Bill Hayden, the Minister for Social Security, sought to negotiate with Catholic hospital administrators in the hope that they would influence the Democratic Labor Party senators to support the Bills. In the end, the Whitlam government was forced to a double dissolution election in 1974 and the Medibank Bills were passed at the subsequent joint sitting of both houses of parliament (Scotton & Macdonald 1993). Ironically, Medibank was introduced four months before the Whitlam government was dismissed on 11 November 1975.

As Medibank's 'basic principle was universal entitlement ... it has always been philosophically unacceptable to the Coalition' (Cassin 2003), so it was really no surprise that the election of the Fraser government in 1975 began the process of undermining that very universal nature. Medibank Mark II was designed to rein in costs, with a levy of 2.5 per cent, and the public was given the option of 'opting out' by purchasing private health insurance. Doctors were allowed to charge patients for the gap between the 85 per cent medical benefit they received from bulk-billing and the scheduled fee. These changes were seen as the first steps in dismantling Medibank (Scotton 2000) and moving towards the creation of a two-tiered health-care system. In May 1979, the 40 per cent benefit was abolished and replaced by a benefit of $20 for a single visit/service. The rates for private health insurance rose by as much as 42 per cent, causing many people to opt out. With the announcement of a new policy in April 1981, the universal entitlement was abolished and largely replaced with a voluntary health insurance scheme. Commonwealth payments were now being limited to those people who were privately insured, pensioners and the disadvantaged. Many interest groups voiced their concern about these changes because '[a] shift from public to private financing doesn't only increase barriers to access ... It also changes the burden of responsibility for health care costs, benefiting some groups but disadvantaging others' (Gray 2004: 65).

The Australian Council of Trade Unions (ACTU) organised a largely ineffective Medibank strike in July 1976, while the Australian Council of Social Services (ACOSS) and the Doctors' Reform Society strongly voiced their concerns. With the election

of the Hawke Labor government in 1983, the ALP restored its commitment to a universal health scheme and called it Medicare. Health Minister Neal Blewett was responsible for its implementation, but only after lengthy negotiations had taken place with the Australian Democrats, who held the balance of power in the Senate. Medicare was a return to Commonwealth-funded health insurance, with no option to opt out by taking out private health insurance. Medicare paid 85 per cent of the scheduled fee for those doctors who bulk-billed, and a levy of 1 per cent of gross income was applied to all taxpayers.

The election of the Liberal-National Party Coalition government in 1996 was to swing the health insurance policy back to private financing. Prime Minister Howard had actively opposed Medicare, as shown in his 1987 reply to the Keating Budget when he said that 'the government should have taken a knife to the expensive, failed Medicare system. Medicare is one of the greatest failures of the Hawke government.' (quoted in Ramsey 2003) The quandary for Howard, though, was that Medicare—in particular, bulk-billing—had always been popular with the Australian population. So Howard's response was several policy changes that incrementally undermined the universal entitlement of Medicare, as he sought to make individuals more directly responsible for their own health-care costs by introducing a private health insurance rebate.

The changes saw the introduction of a levy surcharge in 1996 for people earning $50000 or more a year, which was avoidable if they took out private health insurance. This was followed by a 30 per cent subsidy for low-income earners who had private hospital insurance, which was extended in 1999 to a rebate on all private insurance (Deeble 2003). With bulk-billing rates falling rapidly, the 'A Fairer Medicare' policy was launched in April 2003, leaving it as basically an insurance system for the disadvantaged and poor, as a safety net was introduced for card-holders who had to pay more than $500 per year for medical expenses (Gray 2004). These changes were strongly criticised by groups such as the National Medicare Alliance (comprising the ACTU, ACOSS, the Doctors' Reform Society, the Australian Nurses Federation, the Australian Women's Health Network, Public Health Association of Australia and the Health Issues Centre) along with the other political parties. Dr Kerryn Phelps, then AMA president, saw this package as 'an admission from the Government that it is not prepared to pay for Medicare … Targeting funding for particular groups is replacing the universal approach' (Phelps 2003).

As the government could not get the 'Fairer Medicare' package passed in the Senate, John Howard (rather than the Health Minister, Tony Abbott) formally announced the 'MedicarePlus' package in November 2003. It included new safety nets that started at $500

for cardholders and $1000 for everyone else. The Health Minister then released a media statement saying that this $2.4 billion package 'provides more opportunities for Australians to be bulk billed … [while] substantially increase[ing] the supply of doctors and nurses' (Abbott 2004b). This received support from the AMA, which particularly 'welcome[d] the removal of the compulsory bulk-billing of concession card holders' (Glasson 2003). The package passed the Senate when a deal was done with the independents to include dental cover. This package engrained a two-tier health-care system in Australia, '[b]ecause the poor are less healthy, [thus] a shift from tax funding to private financing represents a transfer of costs from the healthy and wealthy to the poor and the sick' (Gray 2004: 91). The contentious nature of health care policy-making will continue.

Case study 7.2
Medical devices, consumer protection and regulation: PIP breast implants

The Therapeutic Goods Administration (TGA) is the Australian government authority responsible for regulating medicines and medical devices collectively referred to as 'therapeutic goods'. All medical devices, including breast implants, must be subjected to review and will only be included on the Australian Register of Therapeutic Goods (ARTG) if they are successfully approved following a three-step process consisting of:
1 pre-market assessment
2 post-market monitoring and enforcement of standards
3 licensing of Australian manufacturers and verifying overseas manufacturers' compliance with the same standards as their Australian counterparts.
If a problem is discovered with a device, the TGA is empowered to take action, including withdrawing the product from the market (Department of Health & Ageing 2012c).

In 2010, the French medical device regulatory authority raised concerns about the Poly Implant Prothese (PIP) breast implant in regard to increased risk of rupture and the possible toxicity of the implant gel. In April 2012 non-implanted PIP implants were recalled by the TGA and they have not been available for use for breast augmentation since that time (Department of Health & Ageing 2102k).

It was relatively easy to recall non-implanted devices, but the alert raised questions about the safety of the implanted devices, and whether those implants should be removed. The media dubbed the implants 'Toxic Time Bombs', and there were calls for compensation because of the physical, psychological and financial costs suffered by women with the implants. The TGA advised that approximately 9054 PIP breast implants had been implanted by surgeons between 2002 and 2010, and it had received 37 reports of PIP implant rupture—that is, a rupture rate of 0.4 per cent over the past decade—a rate it stated was 'well within the expected rupture rate for silicone breast implants' (Department of Health & Ageing 2012k).

The TGA also advised that both it and their English counterparts had tested the PIP implants and found that the gel used was not toxic, and that the higher rates of rupture identified in France may have related to specific batches supplied in that country but not supplied in Australia (Department of Health & Ageing 2012k). Consequently, the TGA advised that patients with the PIP implants who had concerns should contact their treating physician for advice and follow-up (Department of Health & Ageing 2012k).

Regardless of the statements by the TGA a class action has been commenced involving 325 women (Brill 2012) against the manufacturer and related parties. Questions have also been raised as to the responsibility of the TGA. A Senate Inquiry was undertaken in regard to the management of the PIP implants by the TGA and the following key issues were raised:

- the critical need for the TGA to issue regular updates to consumers, medical practitioners and suppliers regarding device recalls, and the importance of including what information they know and what information they are developing, including what evidence is being gathered through further testing or follow-up with international regulators
- the importance of monitoring and following up conditions that are placed on sponsors when a medical device is included in the ARTG, not just when an issue is identified

- the need for comprehensive and accurate data collection when patients receive implants so this can be drawn on in the event of a device recall
- the necessity for post market surveillance to monitor the effectiveness of medical devices, and the role that everyone plays in this process—which is not always clear
- where consumers have raised issues, such as breastfeeding with implants, the need to address them in formal advice from the Australian government (Commonwealth of Australia 2012).

One of the recommendations made was that the TGA include in its advice that 'it is unclear whether PIP breast implants rupture more than other silicone breast implants and that further testing and investigation of PIP breast implants will continue to inform this advice' (Commonwealth of Australia 2012).

The Senate Committee had concerns about the way the TGA had monitored the PIP implant device and its effectiveness after its approval, the communication of information and its limitations, and the need to collect appropriate data to facilitate any recall of the device. Clearly, from these comments, the role of government as a regulator extends to monitoring the performance of the approved devices, and if the principle is to be applied consistently, extends to medicines and any other approval given by government. It also begs the question 'What if there is a failure in this responsibility?'

terms of steering the direction of its development. Yet public health is a social enterprise and is not the sole responsibility of governments. How the process of formulating public health policy should be governed is a key issue.

Instruments of and influences on governance: People, money and power

Beyond the specific characteristics of the health system, the formal structures (Cabinet, parliament) and processes (legislation, Budget) of government also influence how well the health system operates. For instance, the underlying tension within the Australian system can be traced to the involvement of both Commonwealth and state governments in health financing, and the involvement of both public and private sectors in health services provision. Although parliament and the political parties represented in it are the ultimate decision-makers, the critical decisions about how legislation is framed rest with government—including the Minister for Health and the Cabinet. These government processes are supported by the bureaucracy (that is, the Health Department).

The Budget is a similarly formal process, undertaken on a yearly basis. In this case, there is a dual process whereby the Health Department develops proposals for the minister's consideration, and at the same time, also works with Treasury. When agreements are reached between the two departments and accepted by the minister, the budget proposals are presented by the minister through the Cabinet approval processes. This typically takes about six months of each year, and a great deal of negotiation is necessary. This is because a Health Department usually wants to expand services, while Treasury is interested in minimising new expenditures. The political interests of government also might coincide with the views of officials in the Health Department about health needs and strategies. Furthermore, the political interests of the Health Minister may or may not coincide with those of other key members of Cabinet. Thus, the different imperatives that confront the Health Department, the Treasury, the Health Minister and other members of government constitute key influences on financial and other policy decision-making.

The positions taken by interest groups—be they health professional bodies, consumers and community groups, or industry associations— are also influential in the process of government decision-making. Alford (1975) suggests that the professional monopolists (doctors) seek a controlling influence on health policy, but they are challenged by corporate rationalists (such as the Health Department bureaucrats) who seek to promote rational planning and efficiency, along with the health advocates (such as consumer groups) who seek a voice in the policy process and argue against professional dominance in the health system. Interest groups track policy debates in parliament and in the media, participate in formal policy consultations (such as by making submissions) and lobby decision-makers, either in response to policy proposals or proactively in trying to set the agenda.

The media (newspapers, TV, radio, internet, social media) play a crucial role in mediating public debates and lobbying by representatives of interest groups. Politicians track media stories and debates to assess public sentiments on various issues. They also use the media to test public opinion and convey messages to the public. Investigative journalism can hold decision-makers to account. The media is often used by interest groups to create public debate and gain political attention. Media advocacy is becoming a core skill for public health practitioners, because of its power to influence.

Box 7.3 Human papilloma virus (HPV) vaccination policy

The human papilloma virus (HPV) is a highly contagious virus that is transmitted via sexual contact, with most people infected upon becoming sexually active. Around 80 per cent of people are infected with at least one genital type of HPV—which can cause genital warts and certain cancers in both women and men— at some stage in their life (Department of Health & Ageing 2012d).

In 1991, a research team based in the University of Queensland developed a vaccine for HPV, which is identified in 99.7 per cent of cervical cancer specimens. Clinical trials showed the vaccine to be 100 per cent effective in preventing HPV types 16 and 18, which were responsible for up to 70 per cent of cervical cancers. In July 2006, the TGA approved Australia's first HPV vaccine, Gardasil, for use in girls and women aged 9–26 and boys aged 9–15 (Cancer Council Australia 2008). The Australian government included Gardasil on the National Immunisation Program from April 2007 (Cancer Council Australia 2008), which meant the vaccine was free. The policy decision at that time was to make the vaccine freely available only for the vaccination of girls and young women, otherwise the cost of the vaccine for the required three doses would be $450.

The National HPV Vaccination Program currently provides the HPV vaccine to all females through school programs at age twelve to thirteen years. In New South Wales, Victoria, the Northern Territory and the ACT, students are vaccinated in Year 7 (age twelve) in high school. In Western Australia, students are also vaccinated at age twelve, but in the last year of primary school. In Queensland and South Australia, girls are vaccinated in the first year of high school, which is Year 8 (age thirteen). In Tasmania, vaccinations occur in the last year of primary school (Year 7, age twelve) or in the first year of high school (Year 8, age thirteen) (Department of Health & Ageing 2012i).

A change in policy occurred on 12 July 2012 when the Australian government announced that it would extend the current HPV vaccination program to include boys—specifically twelve and thirteen-year-old boys, who would also be vaccinated through school-based programs under the National Immunisation Program (Department of Health & Ageing 2012i).

So why did changes occur in policy and the government's willingness to subsidise the cost of the vaccine for boys, given the economic climate, a policy to return the economy to a surplus, and the fact that it will be some years before the cost benefit for the extended program will be known? Since the introduction of the HPV vaccination program, further research around vaccination rates and men's health identified the following at-risk groups:

- *Men who have sex with men (MSM):* the incidence of anal cancer in MSM is more than 30 times that in other men. The incidence is particularly high, with similar rates to that of cervical cancer prior to screening. HPV 16 is the predominant HPV type seen in male cancers, with HPV 18 having a lesser role. Together, these types account for 90 per cent

of all HPV-attributable cancers in males. It is likely that this at-risk group will gain the greatest benefit from the vaccine.
- *Unvaccinated women:* an estimated 28 per cent of women have not completed the full course of three doses of HPV vaccine. Coverage of 72 per cent is considered good, both in terms of international comparison and for a program delivered to adolescents in high schools, given that three doses are required.
- *Women not participating in cervical screening:* around 30 per cent of women do not participate regularly in cervical screening in Australia.
- *Aboriginal and Torres Strait Islander women:* this group has a higher incidence of cervical cancer than non-Indigenous women and lower participation rates for cervical screening.

Vaccinating boys against HPV infection is regarded as complementing the current vaccination program for girls by increasing herd immunity and providing indirect protection to the 28 per cent of girls who are estimated not to be fully vaccinated (Department of Health & Ageing 2012d).

This case study demonstrates the need to introduce public health policies and strategies on the understanding that further research and evidence will shape those policies and related strategies over time. Further, complex public health issues require the organisation and coordination of a range of strategies—in this case, screening, research to understand the issue and develop an effective vaccine, the development and delivery of a national vaccination program, program data analysis and policy change.

Note: The Nobel Prize in Physiology or Medicine 2008 was divided, with one half awarded to Harald zur Hausen '*for his discovery of human papilloma viruses causing cervical cancer*', the other half jointly to Françoise Barré-Sinoussi and Luc Montagnier '*for their discovery of human immunodeficiency virus*'.

Policy frameworks are thus not solely created by governments, but often occur with the input of interest groups, with the media playing a mediating role. The courts, in exercising their judgement on various legal cases, are also important in establishing rules and norms of behaviour across the society and the economy. Legislation might be tested in court, and court cases can establish precedents for how issues should be handled.

Given the varied contribution of different players in the system, it is evident that policy-making is not simply a technical exercise. Policy is not driven by research knowledge, nor does it develop solely through enlightened decision-makers (Short 1997). Decision-making is based on a combination of values, goals, scientific evidence, interest group pressures and organisational imperatives, which points to the importance of understanding who is actually involved.

Once policy decisions are made, there remains the challenge of how to ensure that the government's intentions are implemented. This is a core activity for Health Departments. Insofar as policy implementation often requires behaviour change on the part of health service providers and consumers, a series of 'policy instruments' will be needed. Policies can be implemented using regulation or administrative direction; funding; rewards and penalties; and social marketing, including using expert opinion for persuasion and appealing to people's interests (see Box 7.4). Many of the same skills involved in managing communication, the media and stakeholder participation during policy development also apply in policy implementation. The Intergovernmental Agreement on Federal Financial Relations is an example of a policy instrument designed to support the implementation of public health policy. For example, under this Agreement, the COAG Reform Council (2012b) reports regularly to the Prime Minister on the National Indigenous Reform

---

Box 7.4 Levers for implementing national health priorities

Australian Health Ministers have identified a number of national health priorities: heart disease, cancer, injury, mental health, diabetes, asthma, arthritis. So what? How will they ever focus people's attention on the fact that these are priorities? How will they get concerted action to tackle these as priorities? Some possible levers for the federal Health Department to use in policy implementation are:

- **National Partnership Payments and the Australian Health Care Agreement:** specify in the Commonwealth funding to states and territories that there is a 'base' payment for ongoing activities and 'reward' payments when specified targets are achieved.
- **Medicare Benefits Schedule:** price Medicare reimbursements to reward particular services that will have positive impacts on these conditions.

- **Pharmaceutical Benefits Schedule:** expand or restrict access to particular drugs in order to encourage use of the most effective means of managing these conditions.
- **Fund health promotion and preventive screening programs:** through the non-government sector, industry, and state and territory health authorities.
- **Social marketing campaigns:** direct messages to the community at large as well as specific target groups, to encourage uptake of health and health care-seeking behaviours.
- **Issue evidence-based guidelines:** through the NHMRC about best practice in prevention and medical care for these conditions.
- **Promote and fund professional training:** for a range of health-care practitioners to take up evidence-based guidelines.
- **Undertake monitoring and surveillance:** to track population health indicators as well as progress across the continuum of care.

Agreement. The report provides data that are used to conduct comparative analysis of the performance of governments in implementing policy to improve the health of the Indigenous population, in relation to the following priority areas:

- life expectancy of the Indigenous population
- mortality rates for Indigenous children aged under five years
- access for Indigenous Australians to education and employment in remote communities
- reading, writing and numeracy rates for Indigenous Australians
- school retention rates for Indigenous children
- employment rates for Indigenous adults.

Tools for evaluating policy options and supporting decision-making: Maps, compasses and sextons

Whether working at the macro level of policy or the micro level of program planning and delivery, decisions need to be made—about policy pathways, about program strategies and about priorities in general. Given the wide range of health issues that confront the community and for which interest groups demand government action, the assessment of different policy choices and intervention strategies is assisted by having specific criteria for appraising options. Clarity about criteria for decision-making also contributes to transparency and accountability.

Duckett (1990) suggests that four sets of criteria are commonly used for priority-setting in health:

- clinical/medical
- political/social
- ethical
- economic.

Medical criteria place primacy on clinical need—for instance, medical emergencies or life-threatening health events. Political and social criteria are concerned with the distribution of power and benefits to different groups in society. Ethical criteria for priority-setting focus on the relative needs of different groups of people. Economic criteria weigh up the costs and benefits of various interventions.

The Australian Health Ethics Committee of the NHMRC has suggested ethical guidelines for health-care resource allocation decisions, as outlined in Box 7.5.

In more recent times, with increasing government concern about 'value for money', economic evaluation is used with increasing frequency in public policy in general, and health in particular. Typical tools for economic analysis are shown in Box 7.6. In Australia, cost-effectiveness analysis has been used to determine whether new pharmaceuticals and new medical procedures should be subsidised by government.

However, these economic tools have not been used extensively in public health, despite the public health principles embodied in them. In part, this is because of the paucity of appropriate data and the difficulty in counting preventive action at the population level, and in part it is because most decision-making is based around changes at the margins of well-established funding patterns. Comparing costs across program funding options is the approach more typically adopted by decision-makers, often leading to tradeoffs being made between different programs.

Given the inherently political process of government policy and budgets, there will always be lobbying around increasing and decreasing funding when tradeoffs need to be made. More recently, administrative measures have been adopted or trialled in order to add rigour (if not transparency) to budgetary decision-making. Purchaser–provider contracting has been more commonly adopted, while program budgeting and marginal analysis (PBMA) has been attempted.

These measures have been adopted because they better approximate administrative decision-

---

Box 7.5 Ethical considerations relating to health-care resource allocation decisions

The following list of questions offers a way of checking the ethical implications of any policy or program of health-care resource allocation.

Justice and equity

- Is this policy/project/program just, fair and equitable?
- Are sections of the community being denied their fair share of basic health resources?
- Are health-care recipients being discriminated against on ethically irrelevant criteria of gender, age, race, nationality, religion, socio-economic status, 'social worth', geographical location, etc.?
- Are minority groups that lack the social power to press their claims being denied access to basic health-care resources?
- Are some groups considered to be effectively 'outside' the health-care system because of their socio-economic status or other factors?
- Has consideration been given to our obligations to meet the health needs of developing countries?
- Has consideration been given to the impact on future generations?

Autonomy

- Is the right of health-care recipients to control—as far as is feasible—their health care being respected?
- Is this policy or project medically or bureaucratically 'paternalistic' in that, in effect, it attempts to tell health-care consumers what is good for them without consulting them?
- Are health-care recipients being provided with effective information and counselling to enable them to give their informed consent and make informed choices about their health care?
- Are health-care recipients being given opportunities for choice so that they are enabled to make real choices about their health care?
- Are structures and processes in place to enable the community in a continuing way to have a say in the setting of health-care goals and their evaluation?
- Are the autonomy of professional health-care providers and professional standards appropriately ensured?
- Are there effective structures and processes in place to facilitate continuing input from health-care professionals, health-care recipients and the community at large?

Source: NHMRC (1993: 6).

---

making processes. Purchaser–provider contracting has been introduced widely as part of the public sector reforms of the 1990s. Although purchaser–provider contracting has been applied to personal health services, since an output-based funding formula can more readily be determined, health-protection and health-promotion activities continue to be historically funded, while public health authorities struggle to find new approaches to financing and resource allocation.

Program budgeting and marginal analysis (PBMA) has also been trialled at local and organisational levels to determine where incremental increases or decreases in resources might be shifted. The aim of this approach is to examine all the costs of activities within designated programs in order to decide whether reallocations within the program could generate an overall increase in benefits. Table 7.2 outlines where this type of economic evaluation technique has been used.

The economic analyses are increasingly coupled with 'burden of disease' analysis for priority-setting. Within this framework, the health of the population is analysed from the perspective of mortality and morbidity from acute and chronic conditions. The major diseases experienced in the community are often characterised in terms of DALYs, a composite measure of health status. Economic evaluation is then brought to bear in order to assess which interventions for the major diseases are most

Box 7.6 Types of economic analysis used for priority-setting

Cost-benefit analysis (CBA): by looking at one intervention on its own, or by comparing interventions, CBA aims to assess whether its costs outweigh the benefits. The specific methodology of CBA calls for all direct costs and indirect costs to be calculated, and for direct and indirect benefits to be translated into dollar terms. While CBA is the gold standard of economic evaluation, the limits of this approach include the difficulty associated with qualitative or subjective criteria, such as the value of health gain. The approach is used when the monetary value is seen as the dominant or single criterion for choosing interventions.

Cost-effectiveness analysis (CEA): by comparing two or more options with the same goals, CEA compares the costs and effects, and does not attempt to translate the effect into dollar values. While the costs are expressed in monetary values, the effectiveness may relate to a range of health outcomes, either as final health status measures or as intermediate outcomes and outputs. CEA is preferred to CBA in public health analysis as decisions may involve weighing many values, and health benefits need not be translated into dollar terms.

Cost-utility analysis (CUA): CUA is an extension of CEA that attempts to overcome the limitations of a single output measure. Using a common currency (such as PYLL, QALYs or DALYs), CUA compares interventions in terms of their usefulness in producing life years gained (PYLL—potential years of lost life), the quality of these life years (QALYs—quality-adjusted life years) or disability-adjusted life years (DALYs). To determine cost utility, analyses before and after the health-care program, as well as with and without the health-care program, need to be undertaken. Key to the notion of 'utility' is the statement of social preferences or a measure of satisfaction, and both QALYs and DALYs have been criticised for their inherent assumptions about valuation of life.

Source: Eager, Garrett & Lin (2001).

Table 7.2 Uses of economic evaluation

Scope of comparison	Examples	Analytical tool
Single intervention/disease/age group	Immunisation Family planning method	Cost-effectiveness analysis
Multiple interventions/diseases in single age group	Child health	Cost-utility analysis
Multiple interventions/diseases for multiple age groups	Public health strategy, health-care programs	Program budgeting and marginal analysis
Alternative delivery systems and interventions across the sector	Primary health care vs hospital Prevention vs treatment	Cost-effective analysis return on investment analysis
Health sector investment compared with investments in other sectors	Education vs health Agriculture vs health	Cost-benefit analysis

Source: adapted from Adhikari, Gertler & Lagman (1999: 17).

cost-effective. Priority-setting is thus done on both epidemiological and economic grounds. Box 7.7 illustrates how cost-effectiveness analysis might be applied to several conditions that pose major burdens to populations in order to determine the most appropriate intervention strategies.

Box 7.7 Cost-effectiveness of interventions

When policy-makers are making decisions about which interventions to choose, they have to consider whether a population-based or individual-based approach, or a combination of the two, is most cost-effective considering the available resources.

1 Cardiovascular diseases

To reduce the incidence of cardiovascular diseases, there are a number of interrelated risk factors to be considered, such as blood pressure, cholesterol and smoking.

Blood pressure: The two commonly used population-based interventions aim to reduce salt consumption. One is a voluntary approach that involves cooperation between government and the food industry to lower the salt content of processed foods. The second is the use of legislation to enforce such a reduction, accompanied by appropriate labelling. The individual-based approach uses drug treatment for people who already have the symptoms of hypertension. It is accompanied by an education program to guide their lifestyle and diet changes, and involves four visits to a health provider and 1.5 outpatient visits for health education.

The use of legislation is potentially the most effective way to reduce blood pressure for the largest number of people, as it will apply to all food being processed rather than relying on a voluntary agreement with the food industry. It is estimated to achieve a 30 per cent reduction in salt intake, while a voluntary code has a 15 per cent effect. Drug-based strategies are very effective for individuals, but they are more costly and increase the number of people suffering side-effects.

Cholesterol: Health education programs using mass media are very cost-effective, as they can produce an expected 2 per cent reduction in cholesterol levels across a whole population. Even more effective is the long-term effect over generations as cultural changes in diets can become self-reinforcing. Individual-based treatments using statins, which are now available at very low costs, are also very effective.

Combined interventions: The absolute risk approach is an alternative to focusing on blood pressure and cholesterol, and involves evaluating an individual's combined risk of a cardiovascular event over the next ten years. They are then offered treatment for multiple risk factors and engaged in health education. This is most effective for those people at greatest risk, but as the threshold is lowered for those less at risk, it becomes more expensive to achieve additional health benefit.

The most effective strategy to reduce cardiovascular diseases is one based on legislation to lower salt content and intakes accompanied by a mass media-based health education program focusing on ways to reduce blood pressure and cholesterol, and an absolute risk approach. When resources are limited, the most effective strategy is one of prevention and promotion, and the provision of clinical treatment to those individuals most at risk.

2 Addictive substances—smoking

In most countries, some form of government intervention to control tobacco consumption has been enacted; the major ones are population-based and involve legislation. The first type uses taxation to increase the cost of tobacco products, which in turn leads to a decrease in consumption and an increase in government revenue. The global average sees about 44 per cent of the price of tobacco products going to government revenue, which is often redistributed for health-promotion activities. Hence, for every 10 per cent increase in the price of cigarettes, consumption falls by between 2 and 10 per cent, particularly among young and low-income smokers. The second use of legislation is the banning of smoking in public places for reasons of food hygiene and to prevent the harmful effects on non-smokers of passive smoking.

Legislation can also be used to ban the advertising of tobacco products—which is based on the argument that it keeps young people free of the pressures to commence smoking—and to enforce the dissemination of information through health warnings on tobacco products and school-based health education.

The individual-based treatment uses nicotine replacement therapy (NRT), which has about a 6 per cent cessation rate in all smokers seeking to quit.

Results are estimated through the reduction in incidence of cardiovascular and respiratory diseases and various forms of cancer. Higher rates of taxation are therefore the most cost-effective intervention, and have the added bonus of providing governments with additional revenue. Greater improvements can be achieved by combining taxation with advertising bans and information dissemination. NRT is a costly consideration but improves effectiveness when it is part of a larger package of interventions.

3 Sexual and reproductive health: Unsafe sex and HIV/AIDS

The cornerstone of most approaches to the AIDS epidemic has been a combination of prevention intervention, the involvement of the affected communities, and appropriate care and treatment. Approaches have included population-based strategies, such as year-long mass media education programs; voluntary counselling and testing; school-based programs targeting 10–18-year-old youths; interventions for sex workers and MSM, where selected individuals are trained to interact with their peers; and programs to prevent mother-to-child transmissions (MTCT). Individual-based interventions have included using primary care facilities to provide treatment for sexually transmitted infections (STIs), mother-to-child transmission and anti-retroviral therapies (ARVs).

These interventions improve population health, while the use of ARV reduces morbidity and mortality for those individuals who are treated successfully. Depending on the resources of the country, consideration has to be given to determining which risk-reducing interventions aimed at unsafe sexual practices are the most cost-effective. While the treatment of STIs does have a higher impact on population health than other preventive interventions, it does not mean it is cost-effective. Offering ARVs to individuals with clinical AIDS does provide a substantial population health benefit, but the health gains are lower than those for prevention-based interventions. Depending on the resources available, evidence suggests that the best approach is a combined intervention based on peer outreach for sex workers, treatment of STIs, a mass media education campaign, school-based health education and interventions to prevent MTCT.

Consideration must also be given to the fact that the availability of treatment may encourage more people to voluntarily present for testing and counselling, which in turn can help break down stigma, denial and discrimination—barriers to effective treatment and to the scaling-up of prevention programs.

Source: WHO (2002: 114–27).

In an actual policy-making situation, such technical analyses might be used as one input, but will seldom form the full basis for decision-making. For instance, 17 400 premature deaths were averted in Australia because of lower tobacco consumption and the estimated total economic benefit to the community that year was $12.3 billion. The Australian national tobacco campaign cost less than $10 million (in 1999) and resulted in 190 000 people giving up smoking and the prevention of nearly 1000 deaths. On the other hand, the Commonwealth government subsidy for Zyban, a drug to help people quit smoking, cost $80 million per year (in 2001) and 80 per cent of the patients do not finish their treatment (Moodie 2004). It would also appear that a 5 per cent decrease in smoking levels could cut the PBS costs by 17 per cent over the next 40 years. So, should government subsidise Zyban or fund a tobacco campaign each year? The reality is that these decisions are made in different parts of government from the perspective of each program, and are not necessarily made side by side, as a health system-wide issue.

Assessing health system performance from a public health perspective: Health care as if people mattered

The public health perspective is a systems perspective. The public health approach to the health system is concerned both with whether the health system is providing the best health outcomes for the resources available and whether the resources and benefits are distributed in the most appropriate manner. Box 7.8 provides the key attributes that are used to assess the health system's performance from a public health perspective.

In a highly politicised environment, where interest groups lobby for their priority health problems, how do we know when the health system is performing well? Since the 1990s, report cards on government services have become increasingly popular. The *World Health Report 2000* was the first attempt to benchmark the performance of health systems. For this purpose, the WHO suggested three criteria and five key questions, as listed in Box 7.9 (WHO 2000).

These relate, of course, to the three objectives that the WHO has defined for the health system. It is interesting to note that, for the first two objectives, the WHO proposes both an absolute measure ('how good') as well as a relative measure centred around equity ('how fair'), but only the equity measure is proposed for the third objective. This is because the absolute level of financial contribution is not necessarily meaningful. Some countries are wealthy and invest more in their health systems, while others are poor and cannot afford a high

---

Box 7.8 Assessing health systems

Accessibility: How easy is it for the citizen to utilise the system; how many barriers are there to be overcome in gaining admission to an appropriate form of care?

Acceptability: How appropriate to the citizen's values and culture is the kind of care or treatment which is being offered?

Equity: Is each citizen or group of citizens needing to participate in the system able to access and use the treatment or care equally?

Quality: Is the care or treatment the best that can be provided; is it monitored by an independent assessor to ensure this quality is maintained; is it delivered with attention to the quality of the citizen's experience as well as to its completion in all its technical aspects?

Satisfaction: Is the citizen using the system registering satisfaction with the care or treatment in valid and reliable surveys or other consumer investigations?

Cost: What economic, social and environmental resources are being absorbed by the system and what resources do they return? Converting these three categories of resources to some empirical measure is becoming best practice in all accountancy systems. This process is called triple bottom line accounting.

Efficiency: Is it achieving the best effect on population health for the most economic use of resources?

Effectiveness: Is it making the biggest possible improvement in the health of the greatest number of the most needy in a population?

---

level of investment. So the key question around financial contribution, given finite resources, is how equitable it is. The combination of these questions translates into a focus on quality, equity and health system performance.

Box 7.9 Health systems performance

Criteria	Key questions
Health status	How good?
	How fair?
Responding to expectations	How good (responsive)?
	How fair?
Distribution of financial contribution	How fair?

Box 7.10 Key performance measures for a health system

Quality	= Level of health + level of responsiveness
Equity	= Distribution of health + distribution of responsiveness + distribution of financial contribution
Health system performance	= Resources in relation to level of goal achievement

---

While governments might argue that they have insufficient resources to achieve quality and equity, the WHO would suggest that performance is not related to the absolute level of resources, but rather is linked to the question of how well a country uses the resources that are available to it.

The World Health Report 2000 (WHO 2000) was the first attempt at a comparative measurement across health systems. It was a controversial exercise because many governments were not pleased with the outcomes and many researchers were critical of the methodology adopted. Australia performed well on quality and health system performance, but less well on equity—largely because of the gap between the health of Indigenous and non-Indigenous populations.

Although this report is an ambitious global attempt to provide comparative analysis, it is not the only approach for cross-national comparisons. Within the UN system, the UN Development Program has been publishing the *Human Development Index* (UN Development Program 2011) on a regular basis. It is a simpler index that provides a snapshot of human welfare at a broad level (for example, life expectancy, literacy and GDP per capita). The Millennium Development Goals provide more refined indicators across priority issues on which governments have agreed (such as infant mortality, HIV, education and women's empowerment). Many health indicators are included, underscoring the basic public health premise that health is both a basic condition necessary for social and economic development and a reflection of the human condition.

Among the developed economies, the Organisation for Economic Cooperation and Development has also spearheaded comparative analyses of health systems, with a focus largely on health financing. As this comparison is performed across countries with similar levels of economic development, there is less debate about the value, the methods and the uses.

Ultimately, the key questions are whether the ranking of health systems is valuable and useful and whether the disclosure of each country's performance is useful. Comparisons are probably a starting point for inquiry, rather than an end-point. Comparative analyses point to factors and issues that require closer examination, rather than providing definitive answers.

Conclusion: Balancing efficiency, effectiveness and equity

Public health activities occur from a base within a health system. A health system with a strong public health orientation will adopt a population and prevention focus. From a public health perspective, there are a number of critical factors that should be in place in a health system. These include access to basic services (including affordability), access to essential drugs, quality and safety, coverage of organised preventive services (such as immunisation, cancer screening), financing for cost-effective interventions and an appropriate regulatory framework for health protection.

The public health perspective is also concerned about sustainability of health systems—and therefore ownership and problem-solving capacity at the level of communities and health-care organisations. This translates into principles about participation, decentralised decision-making and an emphasis on capacity-building.

Health systems vary across countries, despite operating with similar principles. This is due to the inherently political nature of health policy decision-making. Competing voices and competing priorities, along with a variety of approaches to financing, administration and regulation, explain why Australia's health system can be depicted as a mosaic. Although our system encompasses the most basic public health principle—access to essential care and pharmaceuticals through Medicare—the strife of interests in health policy-making (relevant to public/private and Commonwealth/state systems) makes 'rational' public health policy decisions difficult to achieve. Various economic tools have become popular in recent years, but their use in public health programs is still limited, and their applications are problematic.

Australia's most significant public health challenge is health inequalities—between Indigenous Australians and the general community, across the socio-economic gradient, for particular culturally and linguistically diverse groups, and between rural/remote and urban communities. This is not something that health-care services and systems can fix readily. Public health policies, however, go beyond the health system. Given the large array of factors that influence health outcomes, most of which are outside the health system, public health policies require inter-sectoral collaboration, or a whole-of-government approach. This also means that public health policies are subject to numerous other considerations besides the health and well-being of the community. It makes public health policy-making particularly contentious and complex.

Part III

Public health infrastructure: Building blocks and the system of delivery

8

Who delivers public health?
Contemporary policies and players

Challenge

When you board an international flight, do you consider how many people are involved in your safe transportation from one place to another? First, there is the travel agent from whom you purchased your ticket, then the airport shuttle bus driver who gets you to the airport. At the airport are the check-in staff, the security, customs and immigration staff, the employees of foreign exchange and duty-free shops, and airport cleaners. To get the aircraft ready for departure requires the contribution of engineers, refuellers, baggage handlers, catering staff and cleaners. Then there are the pilots, other aircrew and cabin staff who ensure that your flight is safe, welcoming you and providing for your many needs while flying. Before you even get on to the runway, staff members in the air traffic control towers ensure your aircraft can safely share air space with other aircraft and also land safely. A similar number of people are involved at your destination and any stopovers in between.

Public health is a similar story, in that the length and quality of our lives depend, in part, on numerous interactions between many different people and organisations with complementary roles to play. One can think of a catastrophe being a test of the design and capacity of a public health system, but so are the changing standards and patterns of health and illness in a society. Designation of roles of who can be expected to be responsible for what matters is a key concern in public health, ensuring that the various people and organisations work together as part of a system, and if those roles are changing for whatever reason (for example, to increase efficiency or adapt to new technologies or social values), we need to be aware and ready to object if they are not in the interests of protecting our precious public health system.

What people, functions and organisations comprise our public health system? What tensions and challenges exist in making sure it operates and develops as an efficient and effective system? How does the system adapt to changing community values, new knowledge and know-how, or changing economic, social and political circumstances? How do members of the public play a role in developing, operating and assuring the adequacy of the system? What role is there for health organisations that seek profits from their operations or to satisfy the interests of specific population groups? How do they link in with the public health system?

Introduction

This chapter offers understandings of how we can contribute to building the public health system we want through the responsible agencies. By the 1970s, the major causes of death in Australia were traffic accidents, lung cancer, heart disease and suicide. The view that infectious diseases had been tamed (if not conquered) and the recognition of the multi-factorial nature of the new disease pattern led to calls for a new approach to public health. At the same time, the social movements emerging out of the late 1960s called for greater participation in health care and health policy from various groups within society. The women's movement called for enhanced family planning services and rights to legal abortion. The Indigenous rights movement led to a model of community-controlled medical services. Occupational health and safety (OHS) activists advocated for independent workers' health centres. Ethnic community organisations lobbied for improved equity and access in health care for immigrants.

It was within this lively climate that public health experienced a renaissance in Australia in the 1980s. This was seen through the development of numerous public health policy documents and national programs, and investment in new infrastructure for public health. These developments of the 1980s and 1990s not only provided the foundation for current programs in public health, but also set the framework for the future.

This chapter will review these significant changes in the direction of contemporary public health development. The new policy thinking of the 1980s (as the foundation of the current approach) will first be reviewed and the chapter will then examine the changing policy context of the 1990s and beyond. This policy discussion is followed by a survey of the approaches taken to develop national public health strategies and programs. The numerous organisations and players that drive and maintain the system will be described, along with the challenges in ensuring a coordinated and collaborative effort.

Innovations in community health policy and programs: A renaissance in public health begins

Major advances in public health policy and practice in Australia occurred at two key points: first, the rise of community health centres in the 1970s, and second, the development of a national infrastructure and program in the 1980s.

The election of the Whitlam Labor government in 1972 gave political voice and policy legitimacy to the social movements of the 1960s. The introduction of national health insurance—Medibank—was a response to the Henderson Poverty Inquiry, stimulating the removal of financial barriers to medical care. Medibank represented a major advance in a public health approach to health-care financing. The Community Health Program, introduced in 1973, offered a new model for health services delivery in the community, based on public health principles. These were essential building blocks for a public health approach to health system development.

While health services in the community (such as maternal and child health, school health and mental health) existed prior to the new program, the new vision was for a comprehensive range of primary health-care services, provided by multi-disciplinary teams with a population and geographical focus, and oriented towards prevention. The intent was that community health services would provide:

• information and counselling to improve personal habits and reduce adverse conditions and environments that often preceded disorders of health
• preventive measures, such as immunisation
• detection procedures to discover incipient or pre-clinical phases of disease
• motivation to seek care soon after departures from normal health were perceived
• diagnostic and therapeutic services during illness
• rehabilitation and supportive services
• assistance for those adapting to sheltered living or working conditions (Sax 1984: 104).

This program built upon a movement that had begun in the late 1960s with women's health centres, workers' health centres and Aboriginal medical services. It gave legitimacy to widespread investment in new types of health activities and health workers, and new ways of thinking about health services delivery. It also posed a challenge to hospital-based health care as well as to medical dominance in primary health care. As such, it was opposed by hospital and medical interests.

The Commonwealth offered funding to states to set up community health centres, but the approaches adopted within states varied substantially. In New South Wales, community health centres were placed across all health regions as a government health service, with a full range of

services (for example, child health, mental health, social work, health education, home nursing and dental services) but without primary medical care, as a result of opposition by the AMA. In Victoria, communities had to make submissions to obtain federal funding. As a result, there were fewer centres, and they tended to be concentrated in disadvantaged areas and to include primary medical care. They were also governed by community boards of management. Common principles underpinning these centres were:

> community health services are concerned first with the health needs of populations, and then with the individual as a member of the community. The implication is that services must be equally accessible to all individuals and that resolution of many individual problems can best be achieved by changes involving wider social and community groups. (Health Commission of NSW 1977: i)

The brief tenure of the Whitlam government saw the responsibility for the Community Health Program being handed back to the states, which displayed variable levels of interest and commitment to the ideals of the program. Nonetheless, the Australian community began to receive a wider range of health services, and a generation of health professionals became committed to the community health ideals that would subsequently inform the renaissance of public health in the 1980s.

The organisation, funding and foci of community health services have evolved over the past 30 years. They may be freestanding entities under community-based management, or they may be a division within an area health service. In whatever form, they remain a major vehicle for the delivery of public health services—be they health promotion and health education, screening and preventive services, outreach to vulnerable population groups, or continuing care for the aged and disabled.

> **Box 8.1 Goals of community health services**
>
> The seven goals for community health services were:
> 1 prevention
> 2 self-help
> 3 participation
> 4 integration
> 5 area responsibility
> 6 accountability
> 7 teamwork.
>
> *Source:* Health Commission of NSW (1977).

The rise of new forms of health care in Australia was consistent with international developments. Concepts of 'social medicine' had been embodied in multiple forms of health services delivery in different countries, ranging from neighbourhood health centres in the United States to barefoot doctors in China. These developments culminated in the 1978 International Conference on Primary Health Care and the World Health Organization's (WHO's) Alma-Ata Declaration. The call for primary health care as the main approach for health system development has influenced health policy in many countries, and has been an important reference point for the development of public health in Australia. This approach was considered to be the most effective way to provide public health programs to dispersed communities, by encouraging local groups to assume some proportion of responsibility for their own health needs. 'Vertical' health programs—those run by 'from-the-top' *centralised* authorities, such as the state—were not proving very successful, as they failed to deliver appropriate services to whole populations, and were very expensive to run. It was thought that by *decentralising* public health programs (that is, by giving communities a greater role in the way that health services were provided), more people would receive the benefits of those programs, and that the cost of

health services programs to nations and centralised organisations would be reduced.

Innovations in public health institutions: The enlightenment continues

When Labor was returned to government in 1983, national health insurance was reintroduced, now called Medicare. During the period that Dr Neal Blewett was the federal Health Minister (1983–90), substantial investments were made to develop new infrastructure that supported new approaches to health policy, and many new national public health programs were initiated. The 1988 Medicare Agreement also saw additional funding provided to states for expanding community health services.

Additional institutional presence was needed to bring ideas into reality. During the 1980s, public health infrastructure was created as follows:

• The Australian Institute of Health (now the Australian Institute of Health and Welfare, or AIHW), as the national health statistics agency, was established as a statutory authority of the Commonwealth of Australia in 1987.
• The Consumer Health Forum was funded in 1987, both as a national voice of consumer organisations and to enable participation in policy development.
• Secretariat funding was provided to support non-government organisations, such as the Public Health Association and the Australian Community Health Association (which then was abolished by the Howard government), to assist their participation in policy formulation and professional development.
• Postgraduate training programs in public health were set up to enable rapid expansion of the public health workforce in all states through the Public Health Education and Research Program, which was disbanded in 2010.

- The Public Health Research and Development Committee was established within the National Health and Medical Research Council (NHMRC) to ensure public health research had secure funding (but the function of this committee has since been absorbed into a general health and medical research committee, which also covers public health).
- The National Occupational Health and Safety Commission was legislated in 1985, in the Industrial Relations portfolio, creating a national focus for OHS.

One of the first major developments in public health policy was the establishment of the Better Health Commission in 1985. Seen as Australia's response to the WHO's call for 'Health for All by the Year 2000', the Better Health Commission was, according to Health Minister Neal Blewett:

> the first concerted national effort to change the basic direction of health policy in this country. For far too long, the emphasis on health care in Australia has been on illness treatment rather than prevention. Not enough attention has been paid to the encouragement of a healthy environment and lifestyle. (Better Health Commission 1986: xii)

Comprising mostly prominent citizens, including well-known media and sporting figures (as opposed to public health professionals), the commission's report suggested that there was more Australia could do to improve its health status. The report nominated nutrition, heart disease and injury

Table 8.1 Chronology of key public health development to 2000

1973	Establishment of Community Health Program, an example of the strong preventive aspect of public health policy
1974	Establishment of Health Insurance Commission (HIC) to operate Australia's first universal health insurance scheme, Medibank
1975	Establishment of Medibank, the tax-funded universal health insurance scheme
1984	Establishment of Medicare (National Health Insurance)
1985	Establishment of Better Health Commission to report on the health status of the Australian population and to recommend how to address national health problems
1985	Establishment of National Campaign Against Drug Abuse
1986	Independent Review of Research and Educational Requirements for Public Health and Tropical Health in Australia (Kerr White Report) published
1987	Establishment of AIHW
1988	Report of the Health Targets and Implementation (Health for All) Committee delivered; led to the National Better Health Program to oversee the development of national strategy to improve health status and inequities
1989	Establishment of National Women's Health Program and National Aboriginal Health Strategy
1989	The first National HIV/AIDS Strategy published
1991	Establishment of BreastScreen Australia and National Cervical Screening Program
1996	Australian Health Ministers' Conference (AHMC) endorses the concept of the National Public Partnership, which represents a transition in public health to a more general concern with a 'whole-of-system' approach

Source: NPHP (1998e).

prevention as national health priorities, and raised the importance of intersectoral collaboration in making gains in population health.

Reports, as we well know, do not necessarily lead to policy action or automatic Budget authorisation. In order to ensure that there was commitment by health officials to adopt public health action, the Health Targets and Implementation Committee was subsequently set up, with all states/territories and the Commonwealth participating. Its 1988 report, *Health for All Australians*, nominated health goals and targets across a range of diseases and risk factors, and recommended funding for the National Better Health Program as a Commonwealth–state cost-shared venture to address five health priorities (hypertension, cancer, injury, nutrition and health of older people).

The Commonwealth was not the only jurisdiction moving forward in the 1980s with a bold public health policy agenda. The Cain Labor government in Victoria embarked upon a series of ministerial reviews—of community health, health promotion and public health legislation. The *Tobacco Act 1988* was an international landmark in requiring a specified portion of tobacco tax to be spent on health promotion, buying out of tobacco sponsorship of sport and arts, and setting up the Victorian Health Promotion Foundation (also known as VicHealth). The Victorian *Health Act 1958* amendments that year instituted municipal public health plans for local governments, along with health impact statements (although the latter element was never proclaimed). Community health services were expanded, and district health councils were set up as a novel mechanism to establish community accountability for health services and community development in health.

In South Australia, also with a new Labor government, a Social Health Branch was created within the South Australian Health Commission, signalling a broadening of the health policy agenda and framework for health services delivery. Similar reviews were undertaken of public health legislation and local health, and Welfare Councils were

also set up. In New South Wales, even in the final days of a Labor government, the health-promotion budget was doubled in 1986 from \$5 million to \$10 million. A 1986 review of public health in that state led to the establishment of an expanded central capacity in health promotion, along with a new Epidemiology and Health Services Evaluation Branch. Despite government change in 1988, New South Wales proceeded to create Area Public Health Units, introduce a practice-based trainee program, and encourage joint appointments between area health services and universities in public health.

Health-promotion activities generally received a big boost. Social marketing was discovered by the public health sector (pharmaceutical companies had been using forms of social marketing for years), as campaigns were run to encourage people to improve heart health, reduce fat intake, eat more fruits and vegetables, immunise children against measles, quit smoking, seek Pap smears and so on. At the same time, community development was being practised in community health centres. Multilingual health information and health service access was provided by newly created ethnic health workers. Outside the health sector, all states and territories initiated major campaigns to reduce road deaths. Non-government organisations, such as the National Heart Foundation and Cancer Councils, also became strong advocates of public health.

This proliferation of program and institutional building activities reflected efforts to put in place the fundamental underpinnings of a modern public health effort, which had yet to be established in Australia.

New strategies and programs in the 1980s: A hundred flowers bloom

The series of new public health policies, strategies and programs devised in the 1980s brought many more players into the public health arena. Researchers, community activists and professional bodies became enmeshed in the government's participatory policy

Box 8.2 Industry partnerships: Issues to be considered

Benefits

- Industry partnerships can create new ways of financing/promoting public health initiatives.
- They can help the development of better working relationships between jurisdictions and industry.
- They can create opportunities for industries to promote the goals of respective public health jurisdictions (for example, the production and marketing of sunscreen to reduce skin cancer incidence).
- A jurisdiction can receive an injection of resources by having a company sponsor awards, conferences, staff positions, publications, research and product development, and data registries.
- Industry can receive the exposure of being a supporter of public health activities through the use of a logo.

Potential risks for jurisdictions

- Does the potential industry partner have such things as good workplace practices? Do they have a good environmental and health record and ethical investments?
- Will the use of a government logo give that company a potential unfair advantage?
- Will the partnerships create inappropriate industry expectations, particularly if the sponsorship arrangement involves purchasing goods?
- Will the partnerships create a potential conflict between sponsorship and regulatory functions, such as data confidentiality or sustainability of the sponsorship arrangements?

Source: NPHP (1998b).

processes. In 1986, the National Women's Health Policy was released following a year-long consultative process that involved women across Australia. Reflecting the expanded public health thinking, this policy stressed the importance of understanding health in a social context. Priorities nominated by women tended to be less oriented towards clinical conditions.

In 1989, the National Aboriginal Health Strategy was released, following a two-year period of analysis and extensive consultation with Indigenous communities and organisations and non-Indigenous organisations throughout Australia. A historic document, it recognised that the poor state of Indigenous health was linked to colonial settlement and consequent Aboriginal dispossession. It adopted a holistic view of health, including spiritual well-being. The strategy also placed community control of health services at the centre of the policy agenda. Other priorities identified included the need to train more Indigenous health workers, to develop culturally appropriate health promotion and prevention strategies to overcome specific health problems, and to build effective inter-sectoral collaborations (National Aboriginal Health Strategy Working Party 1989). Subsequently, tripartite forums were set up in all states, comprising Commonwealth, state and community organisations, to oversee the implementation of the strategy.

The renaissance of public health, following this initial period of infrastructure and policy development, then shifted to creating myriad special-purpose payments to the states and territories for Commonwealth–state cost-shared programs (that is, the Commonwealth put up 50 per cent of funding for a national program, provided the states and territories matched it). To some extent, these programs reflected interest group prowess, while other programs were created to address emerging needs widely recognised by the public. In addition to women's health and Indigenous health, major programs set up in the late 1980s to early 1990s included breast screening, cervical screening, HIV/AIDS, a national campaign against drug abuse, immunisation, innovative services for homeless youth, the National Better Health Program and a national mental health strategy.

Involving stakeholders became a key feature of public health policy development and program implementation in the 1980s. Clinicians and consumers were directly involved in the piloting of breast cancer screening programs and an organised approach to cervical screening. The implementation of the Innovative Health Services for Homeless Youth program came under the aegis of committees that included Commonwealth, state and youth organisation representatives. The National HIV Strategy was particularly notable for its inclusion of the affected community, along with its bipartisan support.

In 1995, the Health Advancement Standing Committee of the NHMRC undertook a review of health promotion in Australia, to ascertain the factors contributing to successes and to identify barriers to further progress. The efforts related to HIV prevention, tobacco control and road safety were identified as leading examples of public health achievements. Indeed, these achievements have been recognised internationally for their public health successes. The committee identified three elements that were important in all three efforts: strategic policy direction, technical capacity and supportive structures. In the case of HIV, there was an elaborate network of national committees that brought together government, community organisations and researchers, as well as bipartisan political support. Substantial funding has been invested in epidemiological, social and biomedical research, and in a range of community programs, including needle and syringe exchange, condom promotion and other approaches. Law reform has been a central part of the national response as well. With the combination of these efforts and resources, Australia has largely contained the epidemic within the community of men who have sex with men.

In relation to tobacco control, a multi-faceted strategy has also been adopted, consisting of epidemiological and behavioural research, legislation/regulation (ranging from advertising/sponsorship bans to warning signs to smoke-free workplaces), price signals (that is, tax), community education and personal health services. The fall in smoking rates has been one of the most dramatic and sustained internationally. The experience in relation to the reduction of road accidents points to the success of a similar multi-faceted approach: a combination of engineering (roads and cars), regulation (speed cameras, blood alcohol tests, seatbelts) and mass education, all supported by strong research.

At the beginning of the 1990s, the financial mood of governments changed across Australia. Although new national public health strategies continued to be developed (for such issues as food and nutrition, injury prevention and health-promoting schools), there was less and less funding available to seed initiatives. Interest groups may have felt a sense of recognition for their cause, but the resources available for implementation were in decline.

Over the period 1996–98, Australia's Commonwealth, state and territory governments negotiated two public health reforms: the 'broadbanding' of program funding so that the states/territories received one block grant from the Commonwealth rather than specific program dollars; and the establishment of the National Public Health Partnership (Lin & King 2000). The latter is explained in more detail below.

Reforms of the 1990s: Rationalisation reigns

In the 1990s, a wave of neo-liberal reforms swept through Australian jurisdictions, with ramifications for public health. Starting with the election of Jeff Kennett and a Liberal government in Victoria in 1992, governments moved to disinvest in areas that were seen as unproductive, inefficient or a drain on government expenditure. New public management approaches were introduced across the public sector—such as contracting out, corporatisation, privatisation, benchmarking and purchaser/provider split.

In the health sector, funding approaches aimed at promoting technical efficiency were introduced, such as casemix funding (for hospitals) and competitive tendering or output-based funding formula for other health services and programs. Figure 8.1 shows government expenditure under the Public Health Outcomes Funding Agreements (PHOFAs) from 1999. The 2007–08 peak was due to the National Human Papilloma Virus Vaccination program. The increase in expenditure in 2008–09 was due to selected health promotion (15.8 per cent) and screening programs (12.7 per cent). Public health funding was particularly vulnerable to these policy decisions for a number of reasons. For one thing, prevention is difficult to fund from an output perspective, and health-promotion activities in community health centres began to wither (Walker et al. 1996). For another, newspaper headlines announcing a 'crisis in the hospital system' were politically more damaging than problems with those services that

did not return an immediate benefit. Furthermore, little work had been done to suggest what constituted core public health activities and at what level they should be funded. Finally, the locking in of dollars for Commonwealth–state cost-shared programs meant that state-funded public health infrastructure was the easiest target. Public health services were either left behind by the health sector reform agenda or were the victims of savage budget cuts.

The renaissance of the 1980s had led to a proliferation of programs, defined in a range of ways, that reflected the numerous interest groups and specialties in the field. When the health system began to contract in the 1990s, the number of strategy documents continued to grow, with little funding attached. By the end of the 1990s, Australia had nearly 30 national public health strategies,

Figure 8.1 Total government expenditure on public health activities, constant prices, 1999–2000 to 2008–09

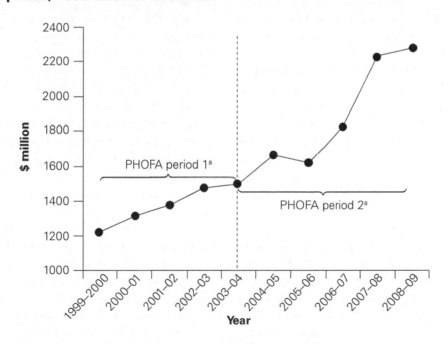

[a] The first PHOFA period in this report was from 1 July 1999 to 30 June 2004; the second was from 1 July 2004 to 30 June 2009.

Source: AIHW (2011e).

covering population groups (Indigenous health, ageing, women), risk and protective factors (tobacco, physical activity, nutrition, alcohol), diseases (breast cancer, diabetes, HIV infection) and settings (schools). Some were well-funded programs, others brought stakeholders together for periodic meetings, and still others lobbied for more attention. These 'stove pipes' competed for scarce resources more often than they built alliances for common action.

At the same time, Australian Health Ministers declared four health priorities, beginning in 1993; these were heart disease, cancer, injury and mental health. Following the election of the Howard government in 1996, diabetes was added as a fifth national priority. In 1999, asthma was also added to the list. In 2002, arthritis became the seventh national priority. Although these priorities had their genesis in the National Better Health Program, the evaluation of the program suggested that a strong focus on health promotion did not appropriately engage with the mainstream of the health system, in particular the clinical interests that were important components of the continuum of care. The difference between 'public health strategies' and 'national health priorities' was not always clear, partly reflecting the bureaucratic location of these policies within the Commonwealth department. Nonetheless, during the second half of the 1990s, specific funding was made available to newly declared national priorities, in part due to strong lobbying efforts by non-government and clinical interests to have the disease with which they were associated declared a priority.

Reflecting the move towards national approaches to public health, a number of reports have been written that identify public health priorities in Australia. The 1986 Better Health Commission report, *Looking Forward to Better Health*, identified three public health priorities (injury control, cardiovascular disease and nutrition) and stimulated the National Better Health Program. The priorities under this program (hypertension, preventable

cancer, injury prevention, nutrition, the health of older people) were subsequently taken up when the national health priority areas (NHPAs) were formally designated. These priorities reflected work previously undertaken (cardiovascular disease, cancer, injury prevention) as well as new national priorities (such as mental health). The 1993 report *Goals and Targets for Australia's Health in the Year 2000 and Beyond* (Nutbeam et al. 1993) identified additional areas for goal-setting, such as health literacy and health skills improvement, which might lead to reductions in prevalence across a range of specific diseases. Four focus areas were identified in the *1994 Better Health Outcomes Report*: cardiovascular disease, cancer, injury and mental health) (Duckett 2000). Since 1996, five additional national health priorities have been adopted: diabetes, asthma, musculoskeletal conditions, obesity and dementia. These priorities coincided with new studies on the burden of disease. A chronology of these developments is provided in Table 8.2.

Despite the apparent political commitment that accompanied the growth of public health funding in the 1980s, and a proliferation of national committees and working groups on specific issues, public health activities were still not uniformly appreciated or visible. Indeed, public health crises—particularly related to infectious diseases—have often provided the opportunity for new investments. For instance, when the country's largest outbreak of Legionnaire's disease occurred in Wollongong in 1988, it directly led to the investment of resources into area-based public health units across New South Wales. In 1997, a series of food-borne disease outbreaks in Victoria led to the consolidation of whole-of-government responsibility for food safety within the health portfolio. Crisis-led funding is not necessarily the most appropriate financing avenue, yet in the absence of an agreed approach for infrastructure and program development, public health officials had to rely on crises to find the opportunities.

In 1996, Australian Health Ministers signed a memorandum of understanding to establish the

Table 8.2 Chronology of national health priorities

Year	Report
1985	Better Health Commission established
1986	*Looking Forward to Better Health* report published
1988	*Health for All Australians* report published
1991–92	Review conducted into the goals and targets approach
1994	*Better Health Outcomes* report published
1995	Better Health Outcomes Overseeing Committee (BHOOC) established by AHMAC
1995	National Health Goals and Targets Program reviewed by BHOOC
1996	National health priority area initiative commenced (the priority areas were cancer, mental health, injury and cardiovascular disease; diabetes was added later in the year as the fifth priority area)
1997	National Health Priority Committee established
1997–99	NHPA baseline reports published
1999	Asthma added as sixth priority area
2000	National Health Priority Area Council (NHPAC) established
2002	Arthritis added as seventh priority area
2005	National Chronic Disease Strategy endorsed at Australian Health Ministers' Conference
2008	Obesity added as eighth priority area
2012	Dementia added as ninth priority area

National Public Health Partnership (NPHP) as a mechanism for system-wide coordination of public health, reporting to the (AHMAC). The proposal emerged from informal discussions among Chief Health Officers, who saw the benefits from a more collaborative approach to policy development that adopted a longer-term view of the needs of the system. In the memorandum of understanding signed by all Health Ministers, the aims of the partnership were stated to be 'to improve the health status of all Australians, in particular population groups most at risk, through improved collaboration in national public health efforts, better coordination and sustainability of public health strategies, and strengthened public health infrastructure and capacity nationally' (NPHP 1998a). The NPHP group comprises one senior representative from the Commonwealth and each of the states and territories, along with the director of the AIHW and the chair of the Health Advisory Committee of the NHMRC. The initial priorities

of the NPHP, under the 1997 *Memorandum of Understanding* (NPHP 1998a), focused on public health infrastructure development: information, legislative reform, workforce development, research and development, planning and quality assurance, and coordination of national public health strategies. The emphasis on infrastructure development reflected in part the outcomes of the NHMRC review of health promotion in Australia (NHMRC 1997b).

The NPHP has had a commitment to the cross-cutting agendas of addressing health inequalities, improving the quality of public health practice, engaging with key stakeholders, strengthening the evidence for public health interventions and enhancing economic arguments for public health, integrating key risk groups and areas into all work programs, promoting collaboration and priority-setting through public health research, and achieving regulatory reform. The NPHP undertook a series of works to improve planning and resource allocation for public health activities, including a public health expenditure study (AIHW 2001), a study with the aim of defining core functions for public health (NPHP 2000c), a planning framework for public health (NPHP 2000a), a review of resource allocation for public health (Deeble 1999a) and a schema for using evidence in public health (Rychetnik & Frommer 2002).

During the late 1990s and early 2000s, public health continued to be funded poorly and unsystematically. Consistencies occurred across all jurisdictions in approaches to tackling national health priorities. Breast cancer, SARS and hepatitis programs received funding, but funding for primary care was limited to services provided by general practitioners. Meanwhile the strategic framework for chronic disease adopted in 2001 by the NPHP still lacked a federal policy and budgetary response. Despite 2004 being an election year, public health policy was not visible and the Budget was narrow, apportioning $33 million to address emerging risks, such as disease surveillance and incidence response, compared with only $5 million to address previously recognised national priorities, such as chronic disease and related risk factors (Lin & Robinson 2005).

Reinvigorating public health, or health promotion

After the 2007 election, the Rudd Labor government embarked upon further reforms to give attention to prevention. Agreements for National Partnership Payments for Preventive Health were struck with states/territories so that substantial incentive funding was made available for the achievement of agreed public health targets. The Australian National Preventive Health Agency (ANPHA) was also created under legislation to lead national efforts in prevention. Table 8.3 outlines the strategic direction of ANPHA, while Box 8.3 explains the six broad-ranging goals that will be pursued and that

Table 8.3 Australian National Preventive Health Agency (ANPHA)

Vision

• A healthy Australian society, where the promotion of health is embraced by every sector, valued by every individual and includes everybody.

Mission

• To be the catalyst for strategic partnerships, including the provision of technical advice and assistance to all levels of government and in all sectors, to promote health and reduce health risk and inequalities, and to initiate actions to promote health across the entire Australian community.

Values

• **Catalyst**—initiate, foster, broker, promote and add value to prevention and health-promotion efforts throughout Australia
• **Collaboration**—build and strengthen effective and lasting partnerships across all levels and all relevant portfolios of government and with the health system, the research community, industry, media and the non-government and community sectors
• **Credibility**—support and produce well-researched and high-quality policies, programs and advice, based on the best available evidence and expertise
• **Innovation**—facilitate solutions that go beyond the traditional silos and boundaries of institutions and sectors and actively seek new approaches to connect research with policy and practice
• **Integrity**—be accountable for all facets of ANPHA's work, acting with honesty and transparency in all work
• **Learning**—foster continuous learning and development.

Box 8.3 ANPHA strategic plan, 2011–15

Goal 1: Healthy public policy

Promote and guide the development, application, integration and review of public, organisational and community-based prevention and health-promotion policies.

Goal 2: Health risk reduction

Provide policy advice and program leadership to support the development, implementation, evaluation and scaling-up of evidence-informed health promotion and health risk-reduction strategies for population groups across the lifespan and in a range of settings, with an initial focus on obesity, tobacco and harmful alcohol consumption.

Goal 3: Knowledge management

Drive the development of dynamic knowledge systems that enable evidence-informed policy and practice in prevention and health promotion across Australia.

Goal 4: Information and reporting

Guide improvements in national surveillance systems for prevention and health promotion, and ensure that information on the progress of prevention and health-promotion strategies is made readily available and is regularly reported.

Goal 5: Capacity-building

Build broad and comprehensive prevention and health-promotion capacity.

Goal 6: Organisational excellence

Establish ANPHA as an innovative, reliable, transparent and accountable organisation, highly regarded by governments, partners, staff and the community, with a strong national identity.

Source: ANPHA (2011)

Table 8.4 Chronology of new developments in health promotion

2006	Australian Better Health Initiative
2008	Closing the Gap: National Indigenous Reform Agreement
2008	Healthy Communities Initiative
2009	National Preventative Health Strategy
2009	Indigenous Chronic Disease Package
2009	Healthy Workers
2010	Australia's first Male Health Policy
2010	National Indigenous Tobacco Initiative
2011	Healthy Children

provide the basis for a national and systematic approach to health promotion.

The players: A conceptual map

As an organised effort, public health requires the contribution of many and varied players. Governments provide policy, including legislative frameworks, as well as resources to support public health services delivery. Services are provided by practitioners in various settings—community health centres, hospitals, general practice, NGOs, schools, workplaces, industry and so on. The technical expertise that forms the basis of public health interventions is also found in diverse institutions—government authorities, universities and research institutes, NGOs and health service providers, to name a few. The efforts of these players need to be mobilised and coordinated if public health action is to be effective and resources used judiciously.

While public health action occurs at multiple levels, many issues and their solutions have a local character, such as the encouragement of physical activity using local facilities or the management of land contamination. Most of the time, however, health issues are not contained by borders, so regional, state and national actions are required to tackle communicable disease outbreaks, food safety, tobacco control and injury prevention. Indeed, local issues may well have links to global dynamics, as populations, products and workforces move between countries. Mechanisms for mobilising public health action are required at different levels for different issues.

Australia's public health system is complex. Organisational players operate at various levels, reflecting partly the complexity in the health system and the structures created by federalism. An effective, well-coordinated public health system requires a number of key building blocks, each drawing on the specific expertise of various players yet mutually reinforcing. The key government roles of policy and investment are accompanied by the '3 As': analysis, advocacy and action. Figure 8.2 provides a conceptual map to help situate these organisations and their respective roles in public health practice. While organisations often play roles beyond those identified in the simplified diagrammatic representation shown, each of these functions is usually located within a few key types of organisation.

Policy and investment

In Australia, public health investment and direction (through policy) typically is determined by a number of government bodies. Governments, representing the interests of citizens, enact legislation to provide a framework for health protection, disease prevention, health promotion and other public health activities. Governments also invest in public health infrastructure—through information systems, workforce or research—and develop policies and strategies for dealing with current issues of concern to the community and emerging issues for health. These investment and policy decisions are then translated into programs that are delivered through different organisations, in different settings and for different population groups.

Historically, governments have been the most important providers of health-protection services. Partly, this is because public health activities improve the health of populations, rather than assuring health for every individual in society. Sometimes this concern of government for the well-being of populations of people can mean that the autonomy of individuals must be constrained in order to protect the interests of the larger population—and, on occasion, the individuals affected by governments' concern for the whole population are not willing to forgo their own desires and activities in deference to the 'greater good'. For this reason, the implementation of public health legislation and the enforcement of regulation occasionally require the exercise of various forms of coercion—and the state is, in most circumstances, the entity best equipped to enforce policies that affect large groups of people (most commonly through various law enforcement bodies).

Analysis and capacity-building

Effective public health programs depend on sound knowledge and a skilled workforce. For this reason, the analytical and capacity-building

Figure 8.2 A conceptual map of the public health system

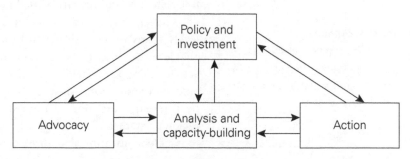

functions of public health must be closely and carefully coordinated with public health action. Universities, professional organisations and large non-government organisations are dominant players in analysis, research and capacity-building. Analysis and research provide the knowledge base for much public health action, and undergraduate and postgraduate courses in core public health disciplines—such as environmental health and multidisciplinary education in public health—build public health system capacity by increasing the number of skilled people who are able to work in the field. Support for public health research has increased significantly since the late 1980s, through investment by funding bodies both inside and outside government, and as part of Australian national public health strategies. Large non-government organisations, such as the Cancer Councils and the National Heart Foundation, are also important funders of prevention research.

Advocacy

Public health policy directions are determined by advocacy as well as by research. Changes in policy might be advocated by many stakeholders, including groups of citizens, professional and community groups, and industry lobbies. Advocacy also comes in many forms—letters and petitions, stories and comments transmitted through mass media, and delegations to ministers and officials. Advocacy efforts are often sustained over a period of time and achieve multiple incremental changes, such as in the case of tobacco control and public health policies around smoking. Advocacy and consumer groups are effective because they present a unified voice to politicians and people working in public health, and this coordination of effort and message often has a greater likelihood of success in effecting policy change.

Public health action

Public health action often involves more than just acting within the policies, procedures and duties outlined by the state. Often, effective public health action requires public health workers to anticipate what is required and take the initiative, and make contact with and use of people from outside the world of 'public health' as it is defined by the state. Thus, while governments often define the roles and procedures of public health activities and define public health 'workers' as those people employed in organisations specifically nominated as 'public health organisations', in practice effective public health action involves people and agencies from outside these state-defined public health bodies. Public health action is eclectic, and increasingly it involves communication and a coordinated effort with players from a diverse range of disciplines and sectors.

While governments have had a strong role in direct service delivery during much of the twentieth century in areas such as maternal and child health and immunisation services, the trend has been towards funding external health service providers to deliver public health services. In the public sector, community health services (including such specialist services as women's health centres and Indigenous medical services) represent the primary vehicle for health promotion and preventive services. In Victoria, Primary Care Partnerships, established across the state in 1999, served to coordinate community-based agencies (Health Issues Centre 2008). With the development of Divisions of General Practice in the 1990s, GPs played an increasingly active role in public health, by focusing on the population covered in their practice and systematic approaches to monitoring and improving health status (see Gray 1997). The introduction of the Medicare Locals networks commenced in 2011, to identify gaps in primary health care services at the local level, focusing on high-need and under-serviced groups. The Australian Medicare Local Alliance was introduced in 2012 to coordinate state-based functions of the Medicare Local networks. Medicare Locals are accountable to local communities, to better target services to respond to local needs, whereas the role of the Alliance is to ensure Medicare Locals function as a cohesive group, responsive to changing national government priorities.

The players: Public sector arrangements

Local government

Historically, local government has played a most important role in public health. This is because many of the early public health problems (including waste management and infectious disease) were local occurrences. The specific roles and responsibilities of local government (including public health) have varied across Australia, depending on the legislative framework of the respective state/territory.

Traditionally, local government activities have been concerned with infrastructure required for community living and economic development—that is, 'roads, rates and rubbish'. The role of local government in public health typically has focused on environmental sanitation and food safety, as prescribed in early public health legislation. The majority of its workforce were referred to as 'health inspectors' and 'food inspectors', whose job was to check premises to ensure public health legislation was not breached. Other important local government public health roles concerned the regulation of building standards and standards of public accommodation (particularly in the latter, to prevent overcrowding in boarding houses). Building professionals, town planners, engineers and other local government officials therefore had a key role to play in public health.

Since the 1980s, both public health and local government legislation have undergone major reviews in all jurisdictions. Consistent with contemporary thinking about public health legislation, local government roles have expanded to fit with a broadened concept of public health, and this expansion has been complemented by the increased positive powers allocated to public health activities in

contemporary legislation. For example, the responsibility to develop municipal public health plans, which would incorporate the full range of public health strategies required to maintain and improve the health of a local community, was introduced in Victoria in the late 1980s. At the same time, workforce training systems for environmental health officers also shifted from vocational education to higher education, and today the workforce usually is referred to as 'environmental health officers or practitioners'. More recent legislative changes have enhanced the requirements of local government in relation to health planning. In Victoria, amendments to the *Health Act 1958* and the subsequent enactment of the *Public Health and Wellbeing Act 2008* require that public health and well-being plans are based upon an examination of data about health status and determinants of health in the municipal district, and also include the input of people from the local community in the development, implementation and evaluation of the plan. The plan must also specify how the council will work together with the state government health department and other agencies involved in public health activities in order to achieve the goals of the plan (Victorian Department of Human Services 2009).

With changing community expectations, the role of local government in other spheres of community life has also broadened, so that local government is often referred to as 'community government', the level of government closest to the people. Community development, environmental and land-use planning, waste management, economic development, recreation, environmental and heritage conservation, home care, Meals on Wheels, child care and community transport are some of the key activities of local government that contribute to health and well-being. A diverse workforce carries out these functions. The evolving practice of municipal public health planning brings together these diverse strands of local government and calls for local leadership in intersectoral coordination, particularly in health promotion.

Box 8.4 Statutory role of local government in public health

Victoria

Victorian local councils have responsibility to implement the *Victorian Public Health and Wellbeing Act 2008*. The functions of local councils in relation to public health include:

- creating supportive environments for health and strengthening the capacity of the community and individuals to achieve better health
- initiating, supporting and managing public health planning processes at the local level
- developing and implementing local policies for health
- developing and enforcing up-to-date public health standards
- facilitating and supporting local agencies with an interest in local public health
- coordinating and providing immunisation services
- maintaining the municipal district in a clean and sanitary condition.

The new Victorian *Public Health and Wellbeing Act 2008* replaced the previous Victorian *Health Act 1958*, strengthening the role of local councils in taking appropriate action to protect the public from perceived risks and hazards while at the same time protecting the rights of citizens.

South Australia

Local councils in South Australia have responsibility to implement the new *Public Health Act 2011* with staged implementation, due to be completed by mid-2013, when the Act will completely replace the concurrent *Public and Environmental Health Act 1987*. The public health functions of local councils will include:

- preserving, protecting and promoting public health
- identifying and reducing or eliminating risks to public health
- assessing public health impacts from activities and development, or proposed activities or development
- providing or supporting the provision of immunisation programs
- preparing a regional (local) public health plan that assesses the state of public health in the region, identifies public health risks, develops strategies to address these risks and identifies opportunities to promote public health
- providing a two-yearly report to the Chief Public Health Officer that provides a comprehensive assessment of the extent to which the council has succeeded in implementing the regional public health plan.

Sources: Victorian Department of Health (2010); South Australian *Public Health Act 2011*.

State government

As dictated by the Australian Constitution, states/territories have all the powers not prescribed for the Commonwealth government, although they may choose to delegate some of these powers to local government via state legislation. Typically, state/territory health authorities are responsible for:

- provision or supervision of health-protection functions (such as environmental health, food safety, drugs and poisons, and radiation safety)
- disease prevention and control (surveillance, contact tracing, health education, outbreak investigation, immunisation, sexually transmitted infections [STIs], tuberculosis and refugee screening, cancer screening)
- strategic direction for health promotion (tobacco, nutrition, physical activity, women's health, maternal and child health, injury prevention, and drug and alcohol).

In addition, public health divisions within the health authorities provide a range of functions to service these programs and other aspects of health policy development. These often include epidemiology, health program evaluation, research, workforce development, inter-sectoral policy development and coordination, and clinical service guidelines.

The organisational arrangements for public health, as described in Chapter 3, vary between states and territories. Some are strongly centralised, with the head office taking direct responsibility for service delivery, although service units might be placed in a range of locations. Other states have developed strong decentralised structures—for example, each area/district health service in New South Wales has had a public health unit since the 1980s. In Victoria, the delivery of public health is undertaken by a wide range of organisations, including local government, community health services and NGOs, such as Cancer Councils and the Heart Foundation.

The role of the Medical Officer of Health was central to the early public health framework, and remains important to this day, with all state health authorities having a Chief Health Officer who exercises statutory responsibilities. Early legislation gave the Medical Officer of Health responsibilities for the control of communicable disease—particularly epidemics and outbreaks—and additional health-protection duties, generally of a regulatory and enforcement character, developed over time. Today, the Chief Health Officer is often the face and voice that advises and reassures the public in times of public health crises, such as food poisoning outbreaks.

Not all state/territory-level public health responsibilities are vested in state/territory health authorities. In Victoria and Western Australia (and previously in the ACT and South Australia), for example, there are statutory health promotion organisations that report to the Health Minister but are not part of the departmental framework. Table 8.5 outlines how health-promotion services are organised. There are also areas of public health that may, or may not, be located outside the health portfolio, or be defined for different jurisdictions. For example, Food Safety Victoria is located within the state health authority, while Dairy Food Safety

Table 8.5 Organising health promotion

New South Wales	Victoria
• Decentralised—area health services	• Strong local government role
• Limited local government role	• Multiple health services providers involved
• Limited NGO role	• Strong NGO role
• No health promotion foundation	• VicHealth and Department of Human Services

Box 8.5 Health-promotion foundations

In 1987, the Victorian parliament passed the *Tobacco Act*—the first Act of its kind internationally—setting aside a portion of the tax on tobacco sales for health-promotion activities (Galbally 2000: 267). The passage of the legislation was achieved with active lobbying by a broad coalition, led by the Anti-Cancer Council of Victoria, and underpinned by substantial health and economic research and public opinion surveys. The Act banned advertising of tobacco products at public events (with limited exemptions, such as the Grand Prix) and, as a tradeoff, the arts and sports sponsorship was 'bought out' by VicHealth. In doing so, VicHealth required art and sporting organisations to enter into partnerships with health sector organisations to promote health messages. In addition, VicHealth funded community-based health-promotion programs and public health research.

Western Australia, South Australia and the ACT have passed similar legislation and established equivalent bodies. In 1996, the tobacco industry was successful in having the High Court declare the state taxation arrangements to be unconstitutional. As a consequence, the tax is now collected by the Commonwealth and transferred to the state treasuries, which then provide the foundations with their budgets.

South Australia and the ACT no longer have health-promotion foundations.

Victoria reports to the Minister for Agriculture. In New South Wales, however, Safe Food NSW is within the Agriculture portfolio.

There are other areas of public policy that are critical for public health and for which relatively uniform government portfolio arrangements can be found. Some of the key policy partners are listed below:

- **Environmental protection:** All states have an independent authority that is responsible for safeguarding the cleanliness of air and water. In most states, responsibility for sustainability and climate change lies within the state government department responsible for environmental management. However, Sustainability Victoria has the statutory authority to facilitate and promote sustainability in the use of resources in Victoria. The Queensland Climate Change Centre of Excellence (QCCCE) is the only state-based climate science research centre in Australia.
- **OHS:** Most states transferred this function from public health authorities to the industrial relations portfolio in the 1970s. At present, the prevention function is typically integrated into workers' compensation and vocational rehabilitation systems (for example the WorkCover Authority).
- **NSW Road and Traffic Authority** and **Victorian Transport Accident Commission:** The highly successful campaign in Australia to decrease the road toll has been led by the authority responsible for roads or for transport, working in conjunction with the police.
- **Consumer affairs:** Consumer product safety is particularly important for injury prevention, and is generally located with other consumer protection functions.
- **Sports and recreation:** The promotion of physical activity is increasingly being recognised as essential for the prevention of chronic diseases, and Sports and Recreation Departments across Australian states/territories have primary carriage,

in partnership with the health authorities, for the national strategy of 'Active Australia'.
- **Education:** The school system has long been an important setting for health education and promotion, not only through the personal development or health education curriculum, but also because schools are where such health promotion programs as 'Sun Smart' are implemented, and because the school environment itself contributes to health.

In addition to these whole-of-population policy areas, there are state/territory authorities that contribute to public health objectives through programs targeted to specific population groups and/or communities. For example, health outcomes and access to health information and services might be affected by the extent to which the Department of Multicultural Affairs is successful in assisting ethnic communities, or the Departments of Housing and Community Services are effective in securing better living conditions and services for the disadvantaged. Thus, increasingly, public health is seen as a whole-of-government responsibility.

Federal government

As discussed in Chapter 2, the role of the Commonwealth historically has been limited. Its traditional public health role has been in international health, with the *Quarantine Act 1908* the first expression of national public health responsibility. Since the early decades of the twentieth century, the Commonwealth has become increasingly involved in health financing, alleviating financial barriers to health-care access and using the power of the purse to entice state/territory health authorities to adopt common approaches to policies and programs. As Table 8.6 shows, the Commonwealth's role in public health has grown significantly since the 1970s.

At the national level, specialist agencies have also been set up over time for regulatory purposes. Key regulatory agencies within the Commonwealth Health portfolio include:

Table 8.6 Commonwealth initiatives in public health

Year	Commonwealth initiatives
1973	first grants to the Aboriginal Medical Service
1973	establishment of the Hospital and Health Services Commission and subsequent development of the Community Health Program
1975	introduction of Medibank and establishment of the Health Insurance Commission
1978	establishment of the Migrant Health Unit
1983	development of the Medicare Scheme
1985–86	establishment of the Home and Community Care Program
1985	testing of all blood supplies in response to the AIDS pandemic
1985	establishment of the National Campaign Against Drug Abuse
1986	enactment of the Disability Services Act
1987	merger of the departments of Health and Social Security into the Department of Community Services & Health
1989	enactment of the new Therapeutic Goods Act
1989	development of the National Aboriginal Health Strategy and establishment of the Aboriginal & Torres Strait Islander Commission
1990	use of casemix for the allocation of resources in hospitals
	establishment of Divisions of General Practice
	establishment of the National Safety and Quality Control Council
1991	establishment of the Australia New Zealand Food Authority
1996	development of the National Immunisation Campaign
1997	establishment of the National Tobacco Campaign
2001	establishment of the National Drugs Campaign
2005	commencement of National Primary Care Collaboratives (NPCC Phase 1) to address chronic disease
2005	commencement of the National Skin Cancer Awareness Campaign
2008	commencement of Australian Primary Care Collaboratives (NPCC Phase 2)
2007	commencement of Encouraging Better Practice in Aged Care to support uptake of evidence-based best practice
2009	establishment of National Partnership Agreement on Essential Vaccines to increase immunisation rates
2010	launch of first National Male Health Policy to address health inequalities for males
2010	development of new National Women's Health Policy, first new policy in twenty years for women's health
2011	establishment of ANPHA for chronic disease prevention
2011	launch of Health Heroes Campaign to attract more ATSI people to work in indigenous health roles
2011	launch of 'Swap It, Don't Stop It' Campaign, to reduce risk factors for chronic disease
2012	launch of the national e-Mental Health Strategy
2012	launch of National Binge Drinking Campaign, introduces replacement for alcohol sponsorship of sporting clubs

Source: DoHA (2005b, 2012j)

- the **Therapeutic Goods Administration**—responsible for safety of pharmaceuticals and other therapeutic devices
- **Food Standards Australia New Zealand**—responsible for national and trans-Tasman food standards and regulation
- the **Australian Radiation Protection and Nuclear Safety Agency**—responsible for the safe operation of nuclear and radiation plants and devices.

Each of these authorities has taken on roles that have historically been the responsibility of the state/territory governments, and a process of harmonising regulatory frameworks or referring powers to the Commonwealth continues. These authorities also sit between, or juggle, the national and international industry interests and the interests and priorities of the state health authorities.

The players: Outside government

General practice and other health services

General practitioners form the foundation of primary care in Australia. Traditionally, GPs have provided office-based services that respond to people presenting with specific health symptoms and complaints. This form of service delivery is

---

Box 8.6 Role of the public service

The public service at both federal and state levels is a key component of the policy-making process and has three main roles to play:

- supporting the development of policies and steering them into practice
- overseeing the delivery of the services associated with those policies
- providing ministers with advice for policy-making.

Traditions in the public service stem from the Westminster model: it is a professional or career service (public servants have the skills and capacity to serve different governments and ministers), it is politically neutral, appointments are merit based and tenure is permanent. These conditions of employment have been eroded over the last 20 to 30 years as governments have implemented reforms to reduce the size of the public service, introduce greater workplace flexibility (Mulgan 1998), privatise service delivery, achieve greater accountability and 'manage for results'. This new public management approach is more consistent with a private-sector approach. It was implemented in moderate forms by the Hawke and Keating Labor governments and more radically by the Howard Liberal government (Johnston 2000). While short-term contracts may bring some benefits, there can be long-term ramifications. To function effectively, even a scaled-down public service needs permanent employees who have specialised skills and judgement built up over time. These include skills to do research and write policy, monitor contracted services and provide independent advice (Davis & Rhodes 2000).

The public service has also lost its monopoly on providing advice to ministers, and now has to compete with a variety of alternative sources. Foremost is the bevy of advisers that most ministers now employ, who are very policy-oriented and largely unaccountable. Such competition for advice raises the question of 'whether the public service is achieving the right balance between responsiveness to the government of the day and maintaining the appropriate degree of independence' (Keating 1996: 9). Therefore, when government Health departments are developing policy, expert advice from key stakeholders has become critical. Building partnerships with academia, research institutions and the community and private sectors, and thereby enhancing capacity for strategic policy-making as well as policy implementation, are among the goals of the reform agenda for the Australian Public Service commenced in 2010 (Department of the Prime Minister and Cabinet 2011).

---

reinforced by the fee-for-service reimbursement from Medicare. GPs have been a central feature of health services in the community, and are often the pivotal point for ensuring patients' access to a range of health and social services. During the 1980s, many public health strategies recommended that GPs be better educated or skilled for prevention.

In 1993, as part of the GP Strategy, the Commonwealth established Divisions of General Practice in all states and territories. These were loosely arranged networks of GP practices that were encouraged and supported to extend primary care into the community. Grants were provided to conduct community needs assessment, which formed the basis for developing multi-disciplinary programs for prevention and rehabilitation.

In 1999, the GP Partnership Advisory Council (advising the Commonwealth Health Minister) and the National Public Health Partnership agreed to consider how GPs might become more active contributors to public health activities. Although GPs do not cover a specified population (Australians are free to choose GPs under Medicare), there was agreement that GPs could be more systematic in the way they addressed the preventive health needs of their patient population. 'SNAP' (smoking, nutrition, alcohol and physical activity) has been recommended as a core population health focus for GPs, and today Medicare Locals, as the new primary care organisations, have been formally charged with responsibilities for improving population health.

Other health services contribute to public health in a range of different ways, mainly through secondary or tertiary prevention. Hospitals, rehabilitation services and aged-care services cooperate to assist in restoring or maintaining health and quality of life for people who are ill and disabled. Their effectiveness in achieving public health objectives relies in part on strong links to GPs and community health services, and on systematic attention to early detection. In addition, these institutional health services can adopt an orientation towards health promotion principles, ensure enhanced knowledge and skills for individuals, and increase the involvement of communities and families in public health objectives. Table 8.7 illustrates how different public health services are supplied by different providers within the health system, each with different target groups and health objectives.

Laboratories form a crucial component of the public health service delivery system, although they are not particularly visible to the community. They examine samples and conduct tests to provide confirmation of suspected health problems

Table 8.7 Public health service delivery in the health system

Service strategy	Level of prevention	Focus of concern	Target	Common providers
Health protection	Primary	Health	Community	Government
Health promotion	Primary	Health	Community or population group	Government Community health services
Preventive services	Primary	Health	Individuals	GPs Community health services
Screening and early detection	Secondary	Health and suspected illness	Individuals	GPs Hospitals
Rehabilitation and palliation	Tertiary	Illness and disability	Individuals	Community health services GPs Hospitals

Source: adapted from Turnock (2001).

or health hazards, such as Legionella, food-borne diseases, cervical cancer or lead poisoning. The reports they provide of notifiable diseases form the foundation of infectious disease surveillance.

NGOs, advocacy groups and professional organisations

Although the public sector plays a dominant role in funding, if not delivering, public health programs, non-government and professional organisations also play important roles—in community education and service provision, research, workforce development and political advocacy. Governments can work closely with NGOs to enlarge the resource base—both human and financial—for public health. At the same time, NGOs might be involved in 'keeping government honest' or in promoting their own interests. The balance of these relationships might also shift over time.

Large national and state bodies, such as the National Heart Foundation and the Cancer Councils, have had a strong involvement in public health through sophisticated research and intervention programs related to tobacco control, sun protection, women's cancer screening, and food and nutrition. For example, national programs in cancer prevention and cancer screening have been tested and evaluated by cancer organisations prior to their adoption. Cancer bodies have also been vital to successful lobbying for, and the passage of, tobacco-control legislation.

Other NGOs are more directly involved in service delivery, or may be more local in operation. The Family Planning Association, for example, provides local clinical services as well as training for clinicians. The Association is present in all states, although its services profile varies. By contrast, not all states have a service such as the Multicultural Centre for Women's Health, situated in Melbourne—which offered health education to immigrant women workers through factory outreach services and operated until 2011, when the unique state-based organisation joined the new national program, Multicultural Women's Health Australia.

Professional bodies—such as the Public Health Association of Australia (PHAA), the Australian Health Promotion Association, the Australian Epidemiology Association and the Faculty of Public Health Medicine in the Royal Australasian College of Physicians—lobby on behalf of the workforce and offer opportunities for professional development, as well as advocating particular public policies. The *Australian and New Zealand Journal of Public Health*, for example, published by the PHAA, is a highly respected international journal. Environmental Health Australia accredits courses across Australia and assures the educational standards for environmental health officers when they enter the workforce. The Council of Academic Public Health Institutions of Australia (formerly the Australian Network of Academic Public Health Institutions) brings together the heads of the Schools of Public Health across Australia, and has worked on such issues as quality assurance and learning outcomes.

While many of the NGOs and professional bodies are active in lobbying for their own interests, there are also advocacy groups that lobby on behalf of the community, or for particular groups within the community. Local governments join to form the Australian Local Government Association and through that body advocate positions about public health. The National Aboriginal Community Controlled Health Organisation argues for financial support for Aboriginal medical services and for other policies and strategies to improve Aboriginal health. The Consumer Health Forum was established in 1988 as a peak body for consumer organisations concerned about health, and its representatives have been involved in the formulation of a number of national health policies, with particular contributions to debates surrounding chronic illnesses and pharmaceuticals. Consumer advocacy bodies may be state oriented as well, such as the Health Issues Centre in Melbourne (which conducts

Case study 8.1
Men's health: A new national priority

Australian men are more likely than Australian women to get sick from serious health problems, and they die in greater numbers than women from almost every non-sex-specific health problem (Better Health Channel 2012):

> Male deaths outnumber female deaths in every age group apart from the over-65 years, and only because so many men die before reaching retirement. Compared to women, men visit the doctor less frequently, have shorter visits and only attend when their illness is in its later stages. (Better Health Channel 2012)

So why are women seemingly healthier than men? Several theories have been proposed, including the concept of an Australian culture that supports the stereotypic tough and independent Aussie male. In terms of mental health and well-being, 78 per cent of suicides in 2008 were men, with one out of every six men suffering from depression at any given time (Better Health Channel 2012). According to the Department of Health and Ageing, the high level of male suicide and substance abuse indicates that mental health disorders may be under-recognised, under-diagnosed and under-treated (DoHA 2012a).

In 2010, the federal government developed the National Male Health Policy, which is the first time that men's health has become a priority at the national level. The policy is focused on raising awareness about preventable health problems and targeting males with the poorest health outcomes. The six policy priorities are:

- optimal health outcomes for males
- health equity between population groups of males
- improved health for males at difference life stages
- a focus on preventive health for males, particularly regarding chronic disease and injury
- building a strong evidence base on male health and using it to inform policies, programs and initiatives
- improved access to health care for males through initiatives and tailored health-care services, particularly for male population groups at risk of poor health.

Funding of $16.7 million over four years was also allocated to the policy (DoHA 2012a), and has been used to:

- undertake Australia's first national longitudinal study on male health over four years
- support the Men's Sheds program
- produce regular statistical bulletins on male health
- develop a range of health-promotion materials for males.

Although the funding level of the policy is comparatively small, one aim of the policy is to integrate with existing policies and initiatives—for example, Men's Sheds. Importantly, the policy provides a focus, framework and support for men's health-promotion initiatives of other organisations—for example, Movember. This policy has the potential to organise the effort on men's health.

policy research with a focus on the state of Victoria), the Health Care Consumers Association in the ACT and the Health Consumers Council in Perth.

Not all NGOs and professional organisations agree on public health priorities or strategies. Non-government and professional organisations often compete with each other for resources, and for political and professional influence. They can come together in alliances to pursue similar goals—such as the 'Friends of Medicare' campaign (comprising PHAA, the Doctors Reform Society and Australian Council of Social Services (ACOSS) in the 1990s, but might also find their goals or philosophy opposed to one another. They reflect shifting cultures, disciplines and ideologies, which are the constants in the field of public health.

Teachers, journalists and other professionals

Public health services are also provided outside the health sector, although not all professionals who contribute to public health might identify themselves as public health providers. Health professionals often need to work in partnership with other professionals to achieve public health objectives, particularly for primary prevention.

Health education and personal development are important parts of the school curriculum, and teachers play instrumental roles in their delivery. Schools also adopt policies that are health promoting, such as sun protection in the playground, no smoking on school grounds and healthy food choices in canteens. Thus, schools are important places in terms of where health knowledge is gained, healthy behaviour is encouraged and health skills (including the '3 Rs' of reasoning, relationships and resilience) are developed.

Health information is provided to the general public by journalists, whether by radio, the internet, TV, newspapers or magazines. News stories about health issues are reported on a daily basis, and journalists are very influential in terms of how knowledge is transmitted, popular beliefs and attitudes are developed, and health policy debates are framed.

Architects, engineers and urban planners are also critical contributors to public health through the way they plan and build houses and urban infrastructure (such as roads and bridges), and structure the environment in which people live, work and play. They need to ensure safety in their designs and construction. They can also contribute to health through attention to environmental management and sustainability, the psychosocial impact of designs and access to services.

Industry: enemy and/or partner?

How the public health enterprise should work with industry has been a matter for debate, and historically there have been mixed opinions on the matter. For example, internationally, pharmaceutical and pesticide producers have been important in the battle against particular epidemics, such as malaria. At the same time, their product development, pricing and access policies have sometimes created major concerns for public health advocates. Another example is anti-retroviral therapy (ARV) for people with HIV, which has been priced beyond the reach of patients in countries that are unable to provide subsidies. Inappropriate use of pesticides and antibiotics has also led to the emergence of drug-resistant mosquitoes and bacteria—although this situation is not always directly attributable to the actions of industry.

In all countries, various segments within the food industry have played contrasting roles in relation to public health, ranging from those with an interest in producing and promoting healthy products (such as fruits and vegetables) to those whose products may harm health (for example, some processed foods and fast foods). Similarly, mining and manufacturing interests (such as in the case of asbestos) have both harmed the environment and workers' health, while others have made an explicit ethical commitment to contribute to healthy environments and workplaces. The tobacco industry, though, has been one of those industries working actively against public health over a long period of time.

For these complex reasons, public health advocates have been cautious when it comes to questions of industry sponsorship or industry partnership. At the same time, public health advocates also recognise that partnerships with industry can be helpful in persuading policy-makers to act differently. As well, industry itself can adopt more appropriate policies and investments.

Coordination and priority-setting in public health: Creating a semblance of order

NHMRC and AHMAC

The growth of new programs and strategies, along with the myriad players, requires increased efforts in coordination, as well as financial negotiations. One of the challenges for any federal system is to balance national interests with local ones. Commonwealth–state/territory relations are an under-current in all aspects of health policy, and managing or coping with these dynamics may be an integral part of public health practice in Australia.

Public health policy in Australia during the twentieth century has been characterised as having three phases (Duckett 2007). The early stages of public health and health promotion reflected a period of medical dominance. The NHMRC has played a key role as an authoritative standard- and priority-setting body since its inception in the early part of the twentieth century. During the 1960s and 1970s, community-based approaches to public health and health promotion emerged as interest groups articulated dissatisfaction with the existing health services. Community approaches have had some success, notably the involvement of the gay community in HIV-prevention activities in the early 1980s. By the late 1980s and 1990s, there were attempts to develop national approaches to public health and to coordinate health policy. This was accompanied by an attempt to provide economic justification for investing in prevention.

One of the earliest frameworks for health governance at the national level was the Federal Health Council, established in 1926, which was expanded in 1937 and renamed the National Health and Medical Research Council (NHMRC). Despite its longevity and national profile, the NHMRC composition was not defined by statute until the passing of the *National Health and Medical Research Council Act 1992*. The NHMRC's principal committees are comprised of representatives from communities, consumer and professional organisations, and governments, and have ministerial-appointed chairs. The core work of the NHMRC is conducted through its principal committees: in 2006 there were five, including Research, Health Advisory, Health Ethics, Human Genetics and Licensing. The strength of its voice, came largely from the medical researchers;

however, since the recommendation of the 2009 review of the NHMRC to increase the focus on public health priority areas, in 2012 an additional committee, Prevention and Community Health, was created (NHMRC 2009a, 2012b).

If the NHMRC was dominated by the medical profession, then the bureaucracy found its voice through other structures that focused on policy development and coordination. The Health Ministers of all jurisdictions meet twice per year as the Australian Health Ministers' Conference (AHMC). Its deliberations are supported by the Australian Health Ministers' Advisory Council (AHMAC), which comprises the chief executive officers of all the state and territory health authorities, with the chair of the NHMRC in attendance as observer. The AHMAC also supports other cross-portfolio ministerial councils, including the police and the National Food Standards Council. Agreement about policy and program priorities is achieved through the AHMAC and then formally adopted by the AHMC, often through multilateral agreements.

The AHMAC sets up many ad hoc committees to deal with issues as they arise. This has resulted in an ever-increasing number of working parties, taskforces and sub-committees, which are then periodically streamlined or terminated. Public health-related working groups established in the mid-1990s included the Communicable Diseases Network of Australia and New Zealand, the National Immunisation Committee, the Australian National Council on AIDS and Related Diseases, the Australian National Council on Drugs, the National Mental Health Strategy Working Party, the National Health Priorities Committee (NHPC) and the National Health Information Management Group.

These AHMAC sub-committees exist in addition to those committees that are appointed by the Commonwealth Minister for Health to oversee national strategies and programs. In 2005–06, AHMAC conducted a review of sub-committees and working groups in order to streamline the number of sub-committees within the structure provided by the principal committees. A further aim of the review was to establish criteria for closure of sub-committees when the terms of reference or agreed work program were effectively completed. In 2012, the principal committees are the Australian Health Protection Principal Committee, the Community Care and Population Health Principal Committee, the Hospitals Principal Committee, the Mental Health and Drug and Alcohol Principal Committee, the Health Workforce Principal Committee and the National Health Information and Performance Principal Committee. The NPHP has had a commitment to the cross-cutting agendas of addressing health inequalities, improving the quality of public health practice, engaging with key stakeholders, strengthening the evidence for public health interventions and enhancing economic arguments for public health, integrating key risk groups and areas into all work programs, promoting collaboration and priority-setting through public health research and achieving regulatory reform. The NPHP undertook a series of works to improve planning and resource allocation for public health activities, including a public health expenditure study (AIHW 2001), a study with the aim of defining core functions for public health (NPHP 2000c), a planning framework for public health (NPHP 2000a), a review of resource allocation for public health (Deeble 1999a) and a schema for using evidence in public health (Rychetnik & Frommer 2002).

Coordinating public health strategies

A brief review of the history of institutional arrangements for public health in Australia shows the dynamism of the field. Coordination mechanisms reflect both the shifting health issues of concern to governments and changing approaches to public administration. When the National Public Health Partnership group was created, this was the first time that a national policy coordination (rather than a financial negotiation and program delivery coordination) had been undertaken.

Given the numerous national public health strategies, one of the challenges is how national strategies could be coordinated better, particularly as many of them enunciated similar actions—that is, all these national strategies proposed to work in schools, in Aboriginal communities, in general practice settings and for data collection. In 1999, the National Public Health Partnership released a set of 'best practice guidelines for strategy development' (see Table 8.8).

The NPHP then set out to consider, given the burden of disease posed by chronic diseases, how it might take on the preventive aspects of the National Health Priorities, with a framework that suggests working across diseases and on common underlying risk factors (be they behavioural, psycho-social or socio-economic). In typical public health fashion, the aim was to foster partnerships—across and between governments, NGOs, specialists and advocates.

The strategic framework proposed by the NPHP identified a 'cluster' of modifiable risk and protective factors, biological risk factors (or markers) and preventable conditions, broadly aligned with the National Health Priority Areas, which could act as the focus of the prevention effect (NPHP 2001: 3). A model was developed (see Figure 8.3) to illustrate the opportunities for prevention and health promotion at each stage in the development and progression of chronic disease. While highlighting the need to integrate planning for the prevention and control of chronic diseases across the health system, such a model also suggests that it could be the basis for partnerships and joint planning between public health workers, allied health workers and clinicians with respect to the contribution they make to health improvement (NPHP 2001).

Given that the Review of National Health Priority Areas in 1999 pointed to the need for nationally coordinated efforts and a stronger action orientation, it was something of a surprise that this proactive effort from the NPHP encountered strong resistance from disease-based interests (such as clinicians concerned with stroke, heart disease, etc.), and from bureaucratic managers with program responsibilities.

Table 8.8 Best practice guidelines for strategy development

Public health importance	• Does the matter/issue pose a threat to the health of significant population groups across the country? • What is the impact of the condition/health issue on the community in relation to the burden of illness; cost; variability in terms of access to preventive, diagnostic or treatment measures? • Does a national approach provide potential to address the needs of disadvantaged groups?
The views of affected communities	• How important is the issue to the affected community(ies), in relation to risks, morbidity and the mortality of their constituency? • Where does the issue rate as a priority across the broader community?
The available evidence base	• What does the available evidence base indicate about the capacity to act on the issue in a way that will lead to improved and cost-effective health outcomes and health gain? • Is there evidence to support alternative interventions or to discount the effectiveness of existing interventions?
Is more information required about the problem?	• Are there any barriers to using available validated interventions? • Are there strategies to overcome these barriers? • Are there other steps to be taken, prior to or of higher priority than initiating a national strategy, such as research or further community consultation?
The views of states/ territories	• Would states/territories find a national approach beneficial? • Does the health issue cross state/territory boundaries? • Is there multilateral support for the initiative? • Is the maintenance and consistency of national standards integral to the optimal effectiveness of the proposed intervention(s)?
The value adding of a national approach	• Does a national approach provide potential to address inequities in state/territory capacities? • Can efficiencies be gained and duplication avoided through a national approach? • Are there potential benefits through improved coordination of infrastructure (e.g. use of expertise, information, workforce development, disease response, research, best practice dissemination) and intervention coordination?
Capacity for evaluation	• Is it an issue for which national participation is required to aggregate sufficient data to evaluate change and trends in the condition/risk factor? • Is the impact of the proposed national activity measurable?

Source: NPHP (1999: 14–15).

However, by 2005 a National Chronic Diseases Strategy was adopted by Australian Health Ministers, building on these public health foundations.

The political interest and support for vertical programs (also referred to as 'stove pipes' or 'silos' because they do not link with other programs) may be a permanent feature of the policy landscape. From a public health practice perspective, what may be more important is to make programs work in an integrated or seamless fashion at the point of service delivery. The National Public Health Partnership also initiated an examination of integrated public health practice around Australia (see NPHP 2000e). Integration made sense from a number of perspectives—it made more efficient use of resources, addressed the social context of people and communities, and avoided reinventing the wheel. Integration may be approached in a number of ways: combining risk factors or working

Figure 8.3 Comprehensive model of chronic disease prevention and control

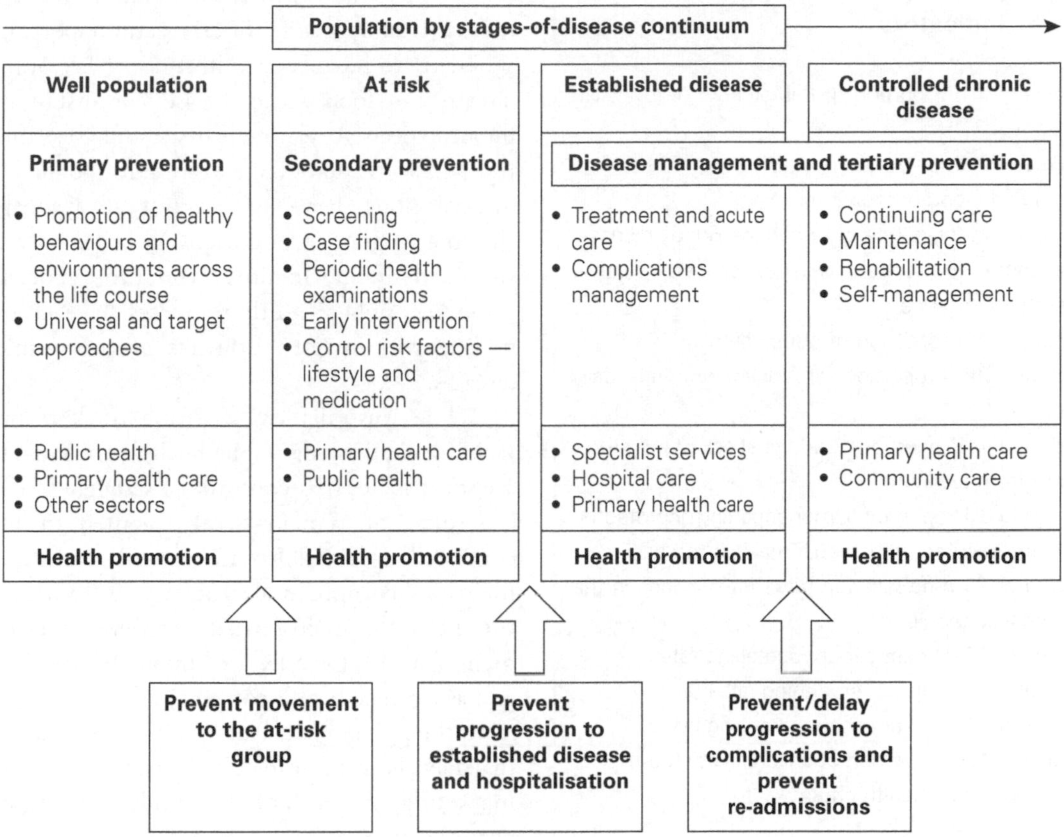

Population by stages-of-disease continuum →			
Well population	**At risk**	**Established disease**	**Controlled chronic disease**
Primary prevention	**Secondary prevention**	**Disease management and tertiary prevention**	
• Promotion of healthy behaviours and environments across the life course • Universal and target approaches	• Screening • Case finding • Periodic health examinations • Early intervention • Control risk factors — lifestyle and medication	• Treatment and acute care • Complications management	• Continuing care • Maintenance • Rehabilitation • Self-management
• Public health • Primary health care • Other sectors	• Primary health care • Public health	• Specialist services • Hospital care • Primary health care	• Primary health care • Community care
Health promotion	**Health promotion**	**Health promotion**	**Health promotion**
	⇧	⇧	⇧
	Prevent movement to the at-risk group	**Prevent progression to established disease and hospitalisation**	**Prevent/delay progression to complications and prevent re-admissions**

Source: NPHP (2001: 6).

across population groups or geographical communities. Examples of integrated approaches were most often found in programs that adopted a 'healthy settings' approach to health promotion (such as health-promoting schools and healthy cities), which have now been adopted as part of the national preventive health reforms. The outcomes of these community-building projects, though, are more often defined in terms of changes in capacity, participation or collaboration than in changes in health status.

The developments in local integrated public health practice are consistent with new emphases by new governments on a range of initiatives that focus on communities rather than individuals. Variously termed 'community strengthening', 'social capital',

'place management', 'joint ways of working' or 'integrated governance', these approaches fit well with public health practice principles.

Since the development by the National Public Health Partnership of a chronic disease-prevention framework in 2001 as an integrated response to the national health priority initiative (NPHP 2001), prevention has now become a major national policy plank across the health system, with the adoption of the Australian Better Health Initiative by the Council of Australian Governments (COAG) in 2005, the appointment of a Preventive Health Task Force in 2007 by the Rudd Labor government, and now ANPHA as a statutory body charged with leading the prevention effort.

Box 8.7 Health-promotion performance indicators

- Indicator 1: Proportion of babies born of low birth weight
- Indicator 2: Incidence of sexually transmitted infections and blood-borne viruses
- Indicator 3: Incidence of end-stage kidney disease
- Indicator 4: Incidence of selected cancers of public health importance
- Indicator 5: Proportion of obese persons
- Indicator 6: Proportion of adults who are daily smokers
- Indicator 7: Proportion of adults at risk of long-term harm from alcohol
- Indicator 8: Proportion of men reporting unprotected anal intercourse with casual male partners
- Indicator 9: Immunisation rates for vaccines in the national schedule
- Indicator 10: Breast cancer screening rates
- Indicator 11: Cervical screening rates
- Indicator 12: Bowel cancer screening rates
- Indicator 13: Proportion of children with fourth-year developmental health check

Source: ANPHA (2012).

However, under the COAG Reform Council (established in 2007), performance indicators have been agreed for each of the six National Healthcare Agreements in relation to health care, education, skills and workforce development, disability, affordable housing and Indigenous reform. There are thirteen agreed indicators for health promotion and disease prevention (see Box 8.7). These suggest that vertical public health programs will continue to be the focus for governments across Australia.

Public health at the crossroads

Contemporary history shows that social movements and reformist governments have been important in the expansion of public health efforts. Yet, at other times, the norm is for public health efforts to be driven by a series of crises and opportunities. When there have been outbreaks of Legionnaire's disease and food-borne disease, for instance, the public expects government to act and governments respond with additional investments. Public health interventions, however, do not always capture the imagination of politicians in order to receive sustained funding. In more recent times of declining resources, public health resources have increased in line with major outbreaks of communicable diseases.

While Australia has a strong track record of tackling challenging public health problems, there are some issues that continue to struggle to receive attention, or remain firmly planted in highly contested grounds. Ironically, with the development of environmental protection authorities and the rise of the environmental movement, environmental health (as a field of public health practice and as a public health concern) largely disappeared from the public agenda and public consciousness. It may have been a case of complacency, or poor social marketing, or a lack of clear understanding about portfolio responsibilities. Hepatitis C also has failed to receive public attention, despite its potential to affect a large portion of the population. In this case, public attitudes towards marginalised groups, such as drug users, may contribute to political diffidence in addressing the looming epidemic. In contrast, the problem of illicit drugs falls into the too-hard basket for seemingly different reasons. Although illicit drugs are not the major culprits in substance abuse (tobacco and alcohol affect more people), the drama, the myths, the human tragedies and the fear of criminal activities appear to touch a nerve in the population. The unresolved debate over the past two decades continues to be whether the right policy emphasis should be harm minimisation or law and order. In that sense, the response remains one of reacting to the problem, rather than being concerned about prevention. Despite the apparently divergent issues and contexts, it would seem that societal values and community anxieties are at the heart of what drives a public health policy agenda.

This review of the contemporary history of public health in Australia points to political influences and interests as significant drivers. In the 1990s, the rural vote began to fall away from the traditionally preferred conservative political parties. The reasons are complex and relate to structural change in the economy, rural decline and a host of other factors. Nonetheless, rural health became a top priority. Not only have a large amount of resources gone into setting up new university departments of rural health around Australia, but many funding programs now suggest that preferential consideration would be given to project proposals that target rural and regional health needs. Given the battle for the rural vote, rural health is likely to remain a priority for some time.

Crises and political flavours of the month come and go, but some public health challenges have been persistent. Inequalities in health status, particularly between Indigenous and non-Indigenous Australia, are yet to see improvement. Inequalities in health status between people of differing socio-economic status also persist. Since the late 1990s, governments have begun to implement geographically based, integrated social development strategies—known variously as community strengthening, place management and neighbourhood renewal. In particular, the increasing prevalence of non-communicable chronic diseases (NCDs), more prevalent in lower socio-economic groups, is now receiving necessary priority attention from all levels of government. To combat the growing problem of NCDs, in addition to social factors, environmental influences on health will need to be addressed. If these efforts receive substantial enough investments, for a sufficiently long period of time, and are skilfully implemented, then there may be hope that this most fundamental of public health challenges can be tackled successfully.

Conclusion: A more complex landscape

The 1980s saw a renaissance of public health in Australia. Investments were made in public health infrastructure, and a large array of joint Commonwealth–state public health strategies/programs were implemented. These have laid the foundation for public health practice today. They also provide the context for many players—inside and outside government, and inside and outside the health sector—involved in public health activities. Coordination and negotiation are a crucial part of the organised effort of public health.

A review of the contemporary history of public health in Australia shows that the combination of reformist government and social movements has been an important factor in the public health renaissance of the 1980s. However, the expansionary approach could not be sustained in the 1990s, given the changing political ideology about the role of government. In this increasingly complex world of competing priorities, in the face of shrinking resources and economic rationalist reforms, the question for public health policy was whether to persist with an expansionary agenda, led by interest groups and defined around population groups, risk factors and diseases that often overlapped with each other. In other words, should public health strategies simply reflect and respond to the myriad community and professional interests—however they wish to define themselves—or should a more coherent and coordinated framework for achieving health gain and investing in programmatic action be developed?

The first decade of the new century has seen the unprecedented development of infrastructure for the promotion of public health, with the incumbency of reformist governments at both federal and state levels, and new legislation directed specifically at disease prevention, health promotion and well-being—and, most significantly, legislation designed to address the social and environmental determinants of health. The framework has been set for future developments in public health practice.

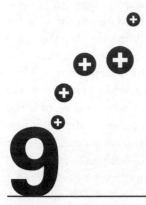

9

Legislative authority for public health action:
How governments and societal expectations intersect

Challenge

A chest x-ray of a young Chinese man on a student visa in Australia revealed he had TB. Treatment for the TB was commenced, but it was later determined that he had a multi-resistant strain of the disease and he was admitted to hospital. After six weeks in hospital, he was discharged and treatment continued on an out-patient basis. However, the young man started to neglect the treatment regime and he couldn't be located easily as he did not have a permanent address.

The Department of Immigration and Citizenship (DIAC) was notified and they put a trace on his mobile phone. A public health order was also issued by the public health authority and, when he was eventually located, the order was served by the Medical Officer of Health using a telephone interpreter service. The young man was confined to a locked hospital room with a 24-hour security guard. He refused to eat and was losing weight, but it was decided that he would need a total of eighteen months of therapy. Meanwhile, DIAC officers reported that there were irregularities with his visa application and the suggestion was made that he be placed in custody at Villawood Detention Centre. Not long afterwards, the young man escaped from hospital and could not be found. (Senanayake & Ferson 2004: 573–6)

You have just been appointed the new Director of Public Health and the minister has requested your advice on the key issues and your recommendations. What advice would you give the minister?

Introduction

Public health law is one of the chief organising forces for public health, and it provides the government authority, the policy framework and the accepted mechanism by which the state is able to intervene in the everyday lives of citizens on the grounds of protecting the health, security and well-being of the community. Although the basic responsibility of government is to protect its citizens, government interventions are not without controversy, and are often a source of debate within the community—particularly if these interventions interfere with the individual privacy and rights of citizens, and with the economic interests of businesses. What, then, is the role—if any—of government in protecting the community from public health threats? Should this role include coercive powers, such as the power to intern and treat individual citizens, or the power to close down businesses? When do the rights of a community outweigh the rights of a citizen? These questions have been raised ever since the enactment of the English *Public Health Act 1848*, which has provided the basic rules of modern public health practice in Australia.

With these questions in mind, this chapter examines a number of the basic features and concepts associated with the law, law-making and the administration of law, including reasons why we make laws and how they are made. The features of public health law and the traditional regulatory tools associated with public health law are also described and discussed. The latter part of the chapter examines the continued use of legislation as a public health tool for the management of contemporary and emerging public health issues.

Sovereignty and legislation

The concept of sovereignty or being sovereign is described as being free and independent. The sovereign nation-state has total jurisdiction over people and property within its territory. 'Sovereignty refers to that organ or actor within the state which possesses no legal limits to its competence.' (Jaensch & Teichmann 1979: 216). In Australia, parliament is sovereign as it, and no other, has the ability to make laws.

There are, however, some problems with this notion of sovereignty equating to 'total jurisdiction' and 'autonomy'. There is an argument that in a federal system of government, like that of Australia, there is no one organ with total jurisdiction, as the Constitution provides for shared responsibilities and law-making. In the international arena, treaties and international laws constrain the nation-state and limit autonomy and absolute freedom. The United Nations was established to restrain the exercise of sovereignty.

In democratic systems of government, laws are made, changed and removed at the initiative of the government of the day (or the body responsible for legislative decision-making). At elections, the political parties will develop and publicise their policy platform to the electorate and criticise the platform of their opponents. In other words, the party will tell the people what priorities it has and what it will do to address the issues of the day. If elected, the party forms the government and has a mandate from the people to implement its policies. These policies may have a minimal or substantial impact on citizens and business—for example, the level of personal taxation, requirements for greenhouse gas emissions, or changes to hospital and medical rebate schemes.

Policy implementation may take the form of a legislative program, including a budget, so that resources are allocated to implement the legislation. Although the government of the day has a popular mandate to govern, laws can only be made by the legislature (parliament) or by delegation of parliament.

The rule of law: Equity before law

Stories from history portray the reigning monarchs of various countries making and breaking laws to suit themselves. Often these laws were made or broken to achieve some advantage for the monarch. A notable example was Henry VIII of England, who wanted a divorce but was unable to obtain annulment from the Catholic Church. Subsequently he set in place, through parliament, a number of laws to replace the church laws that were then in force. These particular laws made Henry the Supreme Head and King of England and also the Head of the Church of England, and marked the beginning of the English Reformation. Henry then divorced his wife.

The rule of law removed the divine right of monarchs to do as they pleased, and institutionalised the principle that every person is subject to the same law. In 1885 A.V. Dicey further developed our understanding of the rule of law as it operates within the Westminster system of government. He explained that the rule of law consists of three linked ideas:

1   **The supremacy of regular law rather than arbitrary power:** no one can be punished or lawfully interfered with by the authorities except for breaches of law established in the ordinary legal manner before the ordinary legal courts of the land; governments cannot exercise arbitrary power through secret, arbitrary or retrospective laws.
2   **Government under the law and equality before the law:** ministers of state and government officials are subject to the law and accountable for their actions before the ordinary courts of the land; there is a consistent application of the law and legal processes regardless of position or status.
3   **The protection of individual liberties by the common law:** free access to the courts of justice is a sufficient guarantee for civil liberties and against injustice.

In Australia, the rule of law is a principle underpinning our system of government, although it is not defined within the Constitution. However, it can be argued that it provides citizens with certainty by clearly identifying the conduct required by the law and by requiring the government to act according to the law (Palmer 2005).

Why regulate?

The word 'regulation' can often have negative connotations of unnecessary restrictions, police powers and government control. Regulation at its broadest means influencing the flow of events. The traditional rationale for government lawmaking is an economic one—to ensure the market operates effectively, to correct market failure or to prevent harmful effects of economic activities. Economic theory suggests that regulation should cover the structure of the market—that is, the conduct of buyers, sellers and providers and the performance of the market, particularly their impact on welfare and living standards. Regulation also shapes norms and the functioning of social institutions (such as schools, churches and community organisations). Regulation therefore contributes to defining what behaviour is acceptable in society.

Government and regulatory authorities often justify their regulatory decisions as being in the 'public interest' or the 'common interest', and this includes ideas of 'consumer protection'. There is a presumption that public policy is to be undertaken in the interests of the entire community and not one section of that community. According to the Government of Canada's External Advisory Committee on Smart Regulation (2004), there seem to be five approaches to understanding the public interest:

1 **Process:** the public interest arises from, and is served by, fair, inclusive and transparent decision-making procedures.
2 **Majority opinion:** the public interest is defined by what a reasonably significant majority of the population thinks about an issue.
3 **Utilitarian:** the public interest is a balance or compromise of different interests involved in an issue.
4 **Common interest:** the public interest is a set of pragmatic interests we all have in common, such as clean air, water, defence and security, public safety and a strong economy.
5 **Shared value:** the public interest is a set of shared values or normative principles.

Unfortunately, there are a number of views on what is in the public interest. Often there is not one single public interest but rather a mixture of public interest considerations. The regulator is then placed in a position to determine the balance between such considerations. The use of genetically modified food provides a good example of the balance of public interests. There is a public or common interest in both food safety and in economic growth generated by technology. Thus, regulation will depend on the balance of safety (social) and economic considerations (External Advisory Committee on Smart Regulation 2004).

The traditional regulatory tools of public health authorities have included the following controls of individuals and businesses:

• commercial land use, premises and businesses through licensing or registration of the premises or business activities conducted on the premises, such as liquor licences, restaurant registrations, town planning permits, aged-care and child-care business registrations. These controls extend to inspections to ensure compliance with standards, including the identification of unsanitary conditions, unsafe environments, and impure or dangerous products.
• specific health professions through licensing as a way of setting standards for entering a field, such as medical practitioner registration, or setting standards for qualifications in a field, such as environmental health officers
• hazardous or risky commercial activities, such as tattooing and acupuncture, responsible service of alcohol, and prohibition of activities that may cause uncontrolled pollution
• any activities carried out on private property that may give rise to unsanitary conditions, unsafe environments and nuisances
• standard enforcement through court action, seizure or impoundment of goods; issuing of notices, including notices to cease operations, directions or penalty infringement notices; quarantine of goods and individuals; and suspension of registration or licence.

The exercise of any of these regulatory tools may lead to controversy. Public health regulators are often placed in situations where they need to consider the risk to the public from the activities conducted by individuals and businesses, and then use the correct regulatory tools to manage the hazard. Criticism can be levelled for being 'heavy-handed' or for failing to act effectively or quickly.

Types of law: The ABCs

The federated government structure of Australia means that we live with two legal systems, two parliaments and two judicial systems. There are two sets of laws—federal and state. There is no one place where law, including public health law, can be found, as laws develop at different times in response to different issues. Four different types of authority can be located:

1 **Constitutional law:** derived from the Constitution of Australia, which defines the powers, duties and limits of the federal government.

2 **Legislation or statutory law:** Acts and statutes enacted by parliaments at the federal and state levels. They represent government policy choices and include how state powers are to be exercised, program authorisation, government agency responsibilities, and relationships to organisations receiving public funding. Local laws or rules developed by local government and statutory authorities made under various state statutes are included in this category.

3 **Administrative law:** the decision-making processes of government agencies and statutory bodies. This category includes not only the implementation of legislation and regulation, but also administrative practices by various public-sector bodies.

4 **Common law:** previous decisions of federal and state courts, as well as legal custom or precedent.

Acts of parliament are statutes, which is the type of law made by our elected representatives in federal or state parliaments. Acts of parliament are the highest form of law, and they usually contain the intent of the legislation and the broad key legislation to be implemented. A minister is usually made responsible for the administration of specific legislation, as part of their portfolio, and they are assisted by a government department or statutory authority to administer the legislation. Acts of parliament usually provide for the making of regulations and orders. These regulations, orders and rules are referred to collectively as subordinate legislation.

Subordinate legislation provides a greater level of detail than is needed to implement or administer the provisions in the Act. An example is the regulation-making powers under the South Australian *Radiation Protection and Control Act 1982*, which allowed the governor-in-council to make regulations for the granting, issuing or giving of licences; or regulations in relation to the medical examination of persons exposed to radiation. These regulations would provide the operational processes and requirements for departmental officers who have been delegated the responsibility for implementing the legislation, and for industry and others who must comply with the legislation.

How legislation is made

The development of legislation is a formal parliamentary process that involves the scrutiny, debate and discussion of the proposed legislation at predetermined stages. This formal process is outlined in Box 9.1.

Box 9.1 How laws are made in the Westminster system

Legislation is proposed: Legislation may come from different sources, including ministers, their staff, backbenchers, recommendations of commissions and parliamentary committees.

The proposal is refined: Government agencies and ministers will be involved and public input may be sought through the release of discussion papers.

It goes to Cabinet: Usually Cabinet approval is needed for the proposal to proceed.

Party approval is sought: This is a good point of influence for advocates because backbenchers (who support your issue) can request changes to the proposal.

The Bill is introduced: The Bill is read a first, second and third time. During the second reading, the Bill may be debated in detail and amendments presented and voted on.

Royal approval is given: The Governor-General (on the Queen's behalf) gives royal approval to the Bill—it is now an Act of parliament.

Source: Public Interest Advocacy Centre (1996).

Public health law

At a conceptual level, public health law—although linked to the fields of law, medicine and health-care law—is a distinct discipline with a theoretical and practical differentiation from other disciplines (Gostin 2000a). Public health law is concerned with the health of the public, which means it is intended to avert a risk of serious harm to other persons, to protect the welfare of incompetent persons, and to prevent a risk to the person from themself (Gostin 2000b). Public health law can be defined as:

> The study of the legal powers and duties of the state to assure the conditions for people to be healthy (e.g. to identify, prevent, and ameliorate risks to health in the population) and the limitations on the power of the state to constrain the autonomy, privacy, liberty, proprietary, or other legally protected interests of individuals for the protection or promotion of community health.
> (Gostin 2000b)

According to Gostin et al. (2003: 9) this definition suggests five characteristics of public health law:

1 **Government:** Public health activities are primary responsibilities of governments. Government creates policy and through the parliamentary process laws are enacted. Thus, public health law is generally statutory (that is, it is contained within an Act of parliament or regulations made under such an Act). These laws may regulate particular behaviours and activities in the community that may impact detrimentally on the public's health, and they also allow for the development of the infrastructure required to regulate, research and manage public health activities, such as the establishment of health authorities, laboratories and research projects.

2 **Populations:** The focus of public health is on populations. Governments ensure a focus on populations by setting out the intent or sometimes the objectives of legislation within the legislation itself. For instance, in New South Wales, the objects of the *Public Health Act 2010* are:

- to promote, protect and improve public health
- to control the risks to public health
- to promote the control of infectious diseases
- to prevent the spread of infectious diseases.

In Tasmania, the full title of the *Public Health Act 1997* is '[a]n Act to protect and promote the health of communities in the State and reduce the incidence of preventable illness' (Government of Tasmania 1997). Both pieces of legislation clearly indicate the intention of parliament in enacting the legislation. The *Tasmania Food Act 2003* has both a long title—'[a]n Act to ensure the provision of food that is safe and fit for human consumption and to promote good nutrition and for related matters'—and a set of objectives that aim to ensure food for sale is both safe and suitable for human consumption, and to prevent misleading conduct in connection with the sale of food (Government of Tasmania 2003).

Governments also ensure a population focus by defining the purposes of public health authorities. An example is the functions of Victorian municipal councils as set out in the *Public Health and Wellbeing Act 2008*: 'The function of a Council under this Act is to seek to protect, improve and promote public health and well-being within the municipal district.'

3 **Relationships:** Public health law forms a connection between the state and individuals within the community who might place either themselves or the community at risk. These laws enshrine the responsibilities and rights of both the state and the individual.

4 **Services:** A number of services are provided by government and the private sector that are essentially organised on a population basis. Classic examples are childhood immunisation

services, screening services (such as breast cancer screening) and radiation safety services. In a number of cases, government plans and provides the resources for services but does not directly provide the service.

5   **Coercion:** Public health law provides public health authorities with the power to coerce individuals and businesses to comply with the legislation rather than relying on voluntary compliance. The exercise of these powers is also controlled through the use of processes required to be followed when enforcing legislation.

Reynolds (2011: 11) observes that the legislative scope of public health has expanded from its original focus on insanitary conditions and noxious environments to include:

- requirements for the reporting and control of diseases and the concerns regarding pandemics, such as avian influenza
- food safety laws that were first focused on food adulteration and now underpin national standards for food safety
- drug laws that originally regulated 'patented medicines' and now regulate the pharmaceutical industry and therapeutic goods (medical devices), blood and blood products
- laws that are directed towards mortality from lifestyle diseases, such as control of the sale of tobacco, and requirements for reporting of cancers and birth abnormalities.

State powers

Public health legislation gives the state the authority to intervene in public health matters in the interest of the public. Legislation sets the ground rules for industry to operate, while protecting public health and safety. Historically, it was accepted that the state should have Draconian powers so that it could control infectious disease and tackle other severe public health problems. Legal power to detain a person has been used to protect the public from the

spread of communicable disease, to protect vulnerable persons and to restrain violent persons. These powers are often referred to as the 'police powers' of the state. Gostin, Koplan & Grad (2003: 14) provide one definition of police powers:

> the inherent authority of the state to enact laws and promulgate regulations to protect, preserve and promote the health, safety, morals, and general welfare of the people. To achieve these communal benefits, the state retains the power to restrict ... private interests—personal interests in autonomy, privacy, association, and liberty as well as economic interests in freedom to contract and uses of property.

Box 9.2 Traditional areas of public health law interfering with liberty

- Licensing of health professionals (e.g. osteopaths, nurses, dentists and Chinese medical practitioners)
- Vaccination of individuals, and the isolation and quarantine of goods and individuals
- Registration and accreditation of health institutions (e.g. hospitals and nursing homes)
- Registration and inspection of food retail and manufacturing businesses
- Registration and inspection of businesses that provide personal health services (e.g. skin and body piercing, body art and colonic irrigation)
- Regulation of air, water and land pollution and contamination, including the abatement of unsanitary conditions on private property
- Development of labelling and compositional standards for food, including health claims
- Regulation of public drinking water supplies (including fluoridation)
- Regulation of land use through zoning of commercial and residential areas

---

It should be remembered that public health law does not reflect the existence of a coercive state. Rather, it should be seen broadly as the authority and responsibility of government to ensure the conditions necessary for preserving the health of the public. This then means that there are times when tradeoffs are required between the rights of individuals and the interest of others in society. This includes economic liberty, as well as individual autonomy and privacy.

The powers of the federal, state and local governments to police and protect the health of their citizens are contained within the Constitution as well as in a wide range of statutory, administrative and judicial decisions in both civil and criminal jurisdictions.

Origins and early issues of Australian public health law: A patchwork

The first legal public health order in the new colony of New South Wales was proclaimed in October 1795. It related to the prevention of pollution of the settlement's water supply, the Tank Stream, which had resulted in cases of 'flux' (Smith 1991). Several attempts were made to introduce and implement quarantine regulations from 1800; however, the first statute pertaining to public health was the *Quarantine Act 1832*, which was copied verbatim from the English *Quarantine Act* of 1825. Other statutes pertaining to registration of marriage and burials (1825), nuisances (1830 and 1833), slaughtering of cattle (1830 and 1834), building standards (1837) and adulteration of bread (1838) were passed (Cumpston 1989). The discovery of gold in Australia and the rapid social changes that followed resulted in the threat of epidemic disease, so on 19 December 1854 the Victorian colonial government passed 'An Act for Promoting the Public Health in Populous Places in the Colony of Victoria'. This was the first health Act passed in Australia and 'health Acts' were passed in the other states from 1872 to 1896 (Cumpston 1989: 233, 390). Various disease epidemics resulted in the passing of specific legislation in response—for

example, smallpox in New South Wales in 1881 and Tasmania in 1903, and plague in New South Wales in 1921 (Cumpston 1989: 391).

With Federation, the states continued to exercise their legislative and administrative controls in public health while the Commonwealth passed the *Quarantine Act 1908*. According to Bidmeade and Reynolds (1997), the state public health laws, although consolidated and added to, remained largely unaltered through most of the twentieth century until reforms were needed from the 1970s. These reforms were in response to new public health challenges of illicit drugs; demands for national uniformity in food, therapeutics and poisons; infection control and HIV/AIDS; and tobacco control.

The evolution of public health legislation reflects the various stages of social and economic development of Australia. In the early days of the colony there was a need to protect the basics of life, such as water supply. As a destination point for convicts, travellers and gold-seekers, it became necessary to protect the colony's population from diseases brought into the settlement; hence, quarantine laws were developed. As the colony grew in population it became necessary to control activities that were annoying (nuisances) or could otherwise negatively impact on health (such as building control, environmental hygiene and food safety). The making of and subsequent amendments to these laws were strongly influenced by the English legislation and the threat of epidemic disease. These laws were stringent, requiring enforcement by authorities and compliance by individuals, reflecting 'a top down process, imposed by sanitary reformers on those in want of sanitary reform' (Bidmeade & Reynolds 1997). A further trend seen in the evolution of public health legislation is what Cumpston (1989: 391) refers to as the 'dissociation of many public health activities'.

Public health legislation has been broken up into specialised laws that are administered by other organisations outside of the health bureaucracies (for example, occupational health and safety, environmental pollution, food safety, water supply and water catchment management). More recent approaches to legislation have reflected concerns with a broader approach to health issues and the need for specifying processes for addressing health concerns, such as health plans, health impact assessment and the active involvement of the community in these processes. The way in which this legislation is framed includes positive or enabling actions, and is different from the framing of the traditional compliance-type provisions.

The evolution of Australian public health laws has resulted in a mix of old and new laws, which may or may not have been reviewed regularly and thus may or may not reflect contemporary public health concerns (Bidmeade & Reynolds 1997); however, according to Reynolds (2011: 2), since 2004 there have been new approaches to public health legislation with five of six states and one territory embarking on new legislation reflecting these new approaches. These new approaches included finding new ways to deal with old problems and reworking old ways to deal with new problems. According to Reynolds (2011: 9), they indicate a renaissance in public health law. Appendix H shows clearly the dates of some of the major public health legislation in each state and territory. There is a large range in the age of some legislation, reflecting earlier issues, such as the Commonwealth *Quarantine Act 1908*, and later legislation reflecting new issues, such as the Commonwealth's *Gene Technology Act 2000*. Subsequently, this age range of the legislation raises issues pertaining to the consistency of legislative content, as each piece of legislation would reflect the current policy approach and contemporary public health concepts within the six states and two territories.

Dilemmas in public health legislation: Balancing local and national interests

There are a number of features associated with public health legislation and its administration by eight jurisdictions in Australia. The following provides an insight into some current issues associated with public health legislation.

Reacting to public health threats

The history of public health legislation shows how it evolved in a reactive fashion. Take, for example, the outbreak of bubonic plague in 1900 in Victoria, Queensland and Western Australia. This disease is highly communicable, and at the time there was no effective treatment. Hence, the disease had a high mortality rate—463 people (38 per cent) died out of 1212 who contracted the disease (Cumpston 1978). Reacting to this threat was understandable. Reactive legislation development continued to be a feature of public health up until the turn of this century— for example, the outbreak of Legionella at the Melbourne Aquarium, which resulted in changes to the legislation (*Victorian Health Act 1958*) to include the registration and assessment of cooling towers. However, as Reynolds (2011: 308–9) notes, the advent of wide-scale public health threats—such as pandemic influenza, which is easily transmissable and spread rapidly—has changed the focus of public health legislation. This change has moved from a narrow focus of the risks associated with individuals within the context of a disease to the development of broad emergency powers contained within the public health legislation, which will allow interventions to be put in place 'when an emergency has occurred, is occurring or is about to occur' (Section 87, South Australian *Public Health Act 2011*). An example of these broader powers can be seen in the recently enacted South Australian public health legislation, which states:

> On the declaration of a public health incident or public health emergency, and while that declaration remains in force, the Chief Executive must take any necessary action to implement the Public Health Emergency Management Plan and cause such response and recovery operations to be carried out as he or she thinks appropriate. (South Australian *Public Health Act 2011*, s. 89)

The other issue behind the need for emergency public health powers is the concern with public health threats associated with terrorism.

The legacy of history

Another inherent feature of public health legislation is what Gostin (2000a: 317) coins a 'problem of antiquity'. As has been mentioned, some statutes have been enacted comparatively recently, but many public health statutes were originally framed in the nineteenth century and have been amended a number of times since. The original framing of older legislation reflects the scientific understanding, legal standards and community norms at that time. Amendment of only parts of the legislation raises the potential of differing values and understandings within a piece of legislation. Similarly, reforms of public health legislation need to include all legislation pertaining to public health and not just one Act of parliament. Thus, a reform of legislation requires the examination of the legislation that pertains to public health, food safety, environment protection and occupational health and safety, so that the reasons and values of the reform are reflected in all relevant legislation.

State variation, consistency and public health law reform

A federal system of government poses a major challenge for the development and administration of public health law. As has been discussed, public health legislation has been developed independently within each state since around the early to mid-1800s in response to the local state situation.

As economy, society and health problems are not confined by state borders, there is a need to make the existing legislative frameworks consistent so as to respond effectively to contemporary public health threats. Health threats such as SARS and HIV/AIDS extend beyond the scope of one jurisdiction, and many hazards and diseases pose risks for the nation or whole regions of the globe (Gostin et al. 2003: 10). The ease of international travel, worldwide markets

for food and drugs, international treaties, pollution, global warming and bio-terrorism have changed the scope of public health issues from essentially local to global issues, which demand unified action at national and international levels.

As the economy and trade became national and international in scope, multiple and differing regulatory regimes were seen as an impost on business. The existence of multiple regulatory regimes in Australia has been seen to be a significant impediment to the competitiveness of Australian business and industry in the world economy.

Food safety standards have been an issue for legislative uniformity in Australia since 1905 (Smith 2001), and the lack of uniformity was:

> a significant impediment to the development of an efficient and competitive export industry, and the current administrative mechanisms were costly in terms of time and resources ... [and] these mechanisms ha[ve] reduced the efficiency and competitiveness of the Australian food industry through increased costs and impediments to product innovation and adoption of new technologies. (Smith 2002: 335)

At the domestic level, there had been constant industry criticism of the lack of uniformity as:

> [T]he existing system of non-uniform *Food Acts* and non-uniform control renders it impossible to institute throughout Australia uniform food standards. This is completely unsatisfactory from both a public health and economic viewpoint. It also creates great difficulty for the food industry to meet the varying requirements of the respective State and Federal Authorities involved. (ANZFA 1998: 4)

The problems of differing public health regulatory frameworks across state borders—whether concerned with environmental health, food safety, drugs and poisons, infectious diseases or tobacco control—became more contentious as industries became national, if not global, in scope. In addition, Australia entered into international agreements on various issues—such as the General Agreement on Tariffs and Trade, whereby Australia agreed in 1994 to conform with international food safety standards (Smith 2002).

The question of how to achieve national uniformity, or at least to harmonise the regulatory approaches across state boundaries within a federal system of government, has become an increasing preoccupation in the latter part of the twentieth century. Uniformity was not only a matter of tidiness or reducing the cost of doing business, but it was also a question of whether citizens' entitlements and rights should be comparable, regardless of where they lived. An examination of public health legislation across Australia showed that Western Australia still operated under the *Health Act 1911* but had enacted the *Food Act 2008*, and a number of states were still operating under legislation enacted in the 1970s and 1980s but at the same time had more recent legislation (for example, food safety legislation), which would reflect contemporary societal values (see Appendix H). This then poses difficulties in providing consistency of administration when the policy intent, legal concepts and principles underpinning each statute may be quite different.

The role of the federal government

In the 1980s, Australia began moving towards national uniformity in public health legislation by working incrementally on the issues of the day. A number of different approaches have been taken to achieve 'harmonisation'. For scheduling of drugs and poisons, the powers have been transferred to the Commonwealth, with a national committee advising on the national approach. For food safety, states and territories agreed in November 2000 to the establishment of the Australia New Zealand Food Standards Council (ANZFSC) and the development of an inter-governmental agreement that contained a clause stating that no state or territory

would by legislation amend a food standard other than in accordance with the agreement (Smith 2002). Another example in relation to consumer rights and complaints about health practitioners is the Australian Health Care Agreement (Medicare Agreement 1993–98), that became the vehicle to require states and territories to pass legislation to formally adopt the Medicare principles and to establish complaints mechanisms. Clause 4 of the agreement requires the establishment of complaints bodies that are independent of the public hospital system to resolve complaints, and by 1995 most states had either enacted or were in the process of enacting legislation (Government of Tasmania 2005; Government of Victoria 2005b).

In recent years, the Council of Australian Governments (COAG), the peak inter-governmental forum in Australia, has become pre-eminent in further establishing the federal government's authority and role in developing nationally uniform legislation. However, persuading states to adopt uniform legislation is not easy, so the Commonwealth has resorted to using its financial levers to achieve this end. This persuasion was formalised through the Intergovernmental Agreement on Federal Financial Relations, which commenced on 1 January 2009. It sets the rules for the Commonwealth's financial relations with the states and territories (COAG Reform Council 2008) and underpins the COAG reform agenda. The public health legislative priorities within this reform agenda include:

- **Occupational Health and Safety:** a model Work Health and Safety Bill was agreed to on 11 December 2009, but some states have since made variations away from the model thus putting at risk the achievement of national legislative uniformity.
- **Health workforce:** an earlier inter-governmental agreement was signed by the states and territories in May 1992 to implement a mutual recognition scheme through legislation. This was superseded by the Intergovernmental

Agreement for a National Registration and Accreditation Scheme for the Health Professions, which was signed in March 2008. The scheme applies to chiropractors, dental care professionals, medical practitioners, nurses and midwives, optometrists, osteopaths, pharmacists, physiotherapists, podiatrists, psychologists, Aboriginal and Torres Strait Islander health practitioners, Chinese medicine practitioners, medical radiation practitioners and occupational therapists.

• **Food regulation:** on 3 November 2000, the Intergovernmental Agreement on Food Regulation was signed by COAG. The aim of the agreement was to deliver a more streamlined, efficient and nationally focused food regulatory system for Australia. Part of the completion of the reform was the signing of a further Intergovernmental Agreement on 13 February 2011 to establish a centralised interpretive advice function in Food Standards Australia New Zealand (FSANZ). COAG now considers that reforms around food regulation have been completed. (COAG Reform Council 2012)

Clearly, the federal government has had a role in bringing about consistent legislation within Australia so as to ensure the rights of citizens, reduce costs and restrictions on business, improve international competitiveness and achieve specific public health goals. However, one of the hallmarks of a federal system is difference, and the challenge is to balance the goals of unity and difference and not seek uniformity for its own sake. The Centre for Comparative Constitutional Studies (1999) has suggested that there is a spectrum of uniformity that goes from complete uniformity to no uniformity, but in between there is a range of choices—including harmonisation, reciprocity, coordination of policy and legislation, and exchange of information between governments. The extent of uniformity depends upon cooperation between the jurisdictions, and this is where support mechanisms

come into operation: ministerial councils, intergovernmental agreements and central administrative bodies.

Ministerial councils, such as the ANZFSC mentioned earlier, carry the authority of their respective governments and are able to make decisions in their field of responsibility concerning the development of legislation. Intergovernmental agreements are the means by which an understanding that has been reached between governments is written down, and this includes the role, functions and processes of ministerial councils. Examples include the registration of the health workforce and food safety standards mentioned earlier. Central administrative bodies or national authorities usually are established to implement the government's decision and develop the required administrative apparatus. Examples include the FSANZ, Therapeutic Goods Administration and Australian National Training Authority (Centre for Comparative Constitutional Studies 1999). The important role of the Commonwealth that it has evolved, and is continuing to do so, is as a facilitator of both policy and legislation (Reynolds 2004).

Challenges to traditional public health legislation: Community and individual rights, and social and economic fairness

Public health law can be criticised for not keeping pace with economic and social changes. It tends to react with specific legislation to issues that arise so that, over time, the legislation resembles a patchwork. The Draconian powers that are embedded into traditional public health laws have been adapted to ensure regulatory activities are carried out under principles of social and economic as well as procedural fairness. Regulation inevitably depends on the exercise of discretionary authority, and such authority can be exercised in a discriminatory fashion—whether deliberately or inadvertently. In recent years, there have been increasing constraints on public health officials, such as avenues for redress, to reflect community concerns about the exercise of discretionary authority.

The advent of HIV, in particular, called into question the balance between human rights and the punitive powers of the state. Since 1989, there has been a large amount of legislation enacted in response to the disease, and this in turn has generated debates about the regulation of private sexual behaviour and attendant issues of discrimination and drug use (ANCARD 1999b: iii). Australian governments, however, recognised that an effective response to the HIV epidemic would require strategies that went beyond the traditional and punitive public health remedies of abatement, control, notification and isolation. This response would need to respect human rights and, by doing so, 'protect those who were vulnerable and marginalised, establish trust for efforts to access populations that are hard-to-reach, promote confidence in health services, and secure the cooperation necessary for preventing further transmission' (Clayton 2010: 97). To achieve these outcomes, it was recognised that there was a need for law reform, and this was pursued through a Legal Working Party under the Intergovernmental Committee on AIDs (IGCA). A critical task was to formulate: 'public health legislation which would balance individual human rights with the need to protect the wider community'. A reform program was developed that included HIV-specific laws, such as notification of cases, confidentiality of information and sanctions for transmission, but also reforms to help create an enabling environment for HIV prevention (Clayton 2010: 10).

Laws criminalising the sex industry have attracted similar arguments from human rights and public health advocates, who argue that such laws would impede public health outcomes. Mandatory health tests and the identification of sex workers are seen to be discriminatory, and prevent the participation of the industry in public health strategies designed to ensure safer sex practices and broader legislative reform. To ensure participation, it may be better to decriminalise sex work so that sex workers are treated in the same way as workers in any other industry, and provided with the same entitlements of holiday and sick leave and superannuation, as was recommended by the Legal Working Party of the IGCA. Unfortunately, the legislation and its administration around the sex industry have remained diverse. New South Wales and the ACT have recently decriminalised prostitution but this is not so in other juridictions. In those states that maintain criminal laws against prostitution, it appears that the law is infrequently policed (Donovan et al. 2012: 9), so the legislative patchwork continues.

During the 1980s, public health law reformers also began to consider what positive powers should exist, beyond the punitive powers. How can the state assure the conditions for people to be healthy in a positive way rather than only reacting to public health threats? Consideration was given to widening the scope of activities that could be undertaken by health authorities to enable them to include planning and assessment as part of their usual activities. The ability to conduct health impact assessment of public policy proposals, to develop municipal public health plans and to fund health promotion activities through ear-marked tobacco tax (also known as hypothecation) were some of the leading Australian achievements during this period. This contemporary view of public health law also saw regulatory powers as a complementary tool to health education for improving public health—indeed, as an essential component of a health-promotion strategy. Notable examples of this approach include successful campaigns to reduce road traffic accidents and to control tobacco. The review of public health legislation in Victoria in 1987, as outlined in Box 9.3, provided a good example of enabling the state Health Department and local councils to extend their respective roles in improving conditions for health with the introduction of health impact statements (HISs) and municipal public health plans.

Box 9.3 Developments in Victorian public health law

Health impact statements (HISs)

Two major processes were introduced under the 1987 legislation. The first provided for people to apply for a formal inquiry into any activity or proposed activity that might constitute a danger to human health. If it were determined that an inquiry was to be conducted, then public consultation was to be undertaken and a discussion paper prepared. The discussion paper was to contain all scientific, medical, sociological, economic and other relevant perspectives and a reasonable time provided for public consultation. In the *Public Health and Wellbeing Act 2008*, public inquiries can only be initiated by the Minister of Health or the Secretary of the Department, and the terms of reference and timelines for such an inquiry must be published in the *Government Gazette*.

The second process was the development of an HIS by the department after consultation, and based on the evidence collected about the activity or proposed activity. The HIS also was to contain the assessment of the dangers to health posed by the activity and any recommendations. All HISs were to be tabled in parliament. Under the 2008 legislation, the Minister of Health has the power to direct the Secretary or Chief Health Officer to conduct an HIS. There is no requirement to provide a report on the assessment.

The more recent public health legislation has limited the initial and innovative legislation, which introduced inquiries and an HIS by vesting the authority for initiating such processes with the minister or secretary of the department.

Municipal public health plans (MPHPs)

Municipal councils are well placed to ascertain and respond to local public health issues within their communities. The legislation reflected this feature and introduced, as an innovation, the public health planning role of municipal councils where each council, in consultation with the Secretary [of the Department of Human Services], prepared a municipal public health plan that would identify public health dangers affecting the municipal district, and would outline strategies to prevent those dangers. The requirement for a Public Health and Wellbeing Plan was continued with the 2008 legislation but, importantly, a further innovation was included: that the council must also integrate the public health plan issues and strategies into the Council Plan. This innovation raises the standing of public health and planning for public health, and ensures that a budget is allocated for public health strategies.

Although HISs were written into the legislation, the provisions were never proclaimed and implemented in Victoria, but they were introduced into Tasmania. The concept of local-level public health planning contained in municipal public health plans (now known in Victoria as Public Health and Wellbeing Plans) was also introduced into Queensland and South Australia (where they are known as Regional Public Health Plans).

The introduction of municipal public health plans (MPHPs) and HISs into legislation was seen to be innovative. Both of these innovations were concerned with managing and controlling future risks to health rather than reacting to crises. The more recent legislation extends the initial legislative requirements for Public Health and Wellbeing Plans to include the involvement of the community and how the council intends to work in partnership with the department and other agencies in the pursuit of public health objectives. In terms of local planning, there is a requirement to ensure that public health planning, council planning and the municipal strategic statement (local policy for development and planning) are consistent with one another.

According to Reynolds (2004: 85) the new approach to public health law, which started in the 1980s, had these characteristics:

- the creation of comprehensive areas and approaches within public health law in fields such as food, drugs or tobacco
- a mix of Commonwealth and state involvement in these fields
- a focus on regulating corporate activities in the interests of public health
- a more obvious competition between potentially conflicting interests—where protecting public health must sit with facilitating local industry or providing consumer protection, with legislative requirements to formally take account of those interests
- penalties that are significantly higher than they were in the previous public health laws.

Implementation of legislation: Carrots and sticks

Traditionally the implementation of legislation has been based on what has been described by Braithwaite (2003) as the 'classical deterrence approach'. In this approach, the assumption is that compliance with legislation comes from the fear of punishment—that is, fines and other penalties. However, the effectiveness of this approach has been questioned (Braithwaite 2003). One reason is that regulatory agencies are not as powerful and efficient as they need to be to make the deterrence model work. It is not possible to have sufficient resources to monitor every operator and every transgression. Furthermore, there may be high rewards for non-compliance and low penalties (if caught).

Compliance seems to be higher if the regulatee wishes to maintain legitimacy with government, industry peers and the public, and also if there is a relationship of trust between regulator and regulatee. Informal sanctions (such as negative publicity, public criticism, embarrassment and shame) also

seem to have a greater deterrent effect than formal sanctions of fines, compensation, and cancellation of licences and registration. It is interesting to note that Western Australia, New South Wales and Victoria have established a public 'name and shame' register of people convicted on food safety offences. Ayres and Braithwaite (1992) propose a regulatory hierarchy (see Figure 9.1) as a more effective and efficient form of implementing regulation.

Alternatives to the deterrence approach are being examined, and these include the need to build the capacity of institutions to develop citizens who are self-regulating, and who understand and practise democratic virtues. Restorative justice ideas about using bottom-up collaborations between state, business and society actors to solve specific compliance issues would mean moving away from a punitive model to one of collaboration between state, market and civil society (Braithwaite 2003). These ideas would represent a fundamental shift away from the model of regulatory implementation that has been in place since the beginning of public health Acts.

The advent of biosecurity threats associated with the release of chemical, biological or radiological agents, or a communicable disease like avian influenza, has initiated a more comprehensive and integrated package of responses by government. One new measure has been the establishment of the National Emergency Medicines Stockpile, which contains, among other things, a reserve of essential vaccines, antibiotics and anti-viral drugs, and chemical and radiological antidotes, to ensure adequate medical supplies in the event of a pandemic (Murnane & Cooper 2005). A range of other measures have been established to prevent the entry of pandemic disease, including increased border control. In the event of an escalation of overseas pandemic influenza events, aircraft commanders will be required to declare the health of passengers via the use of health declaration cards, which will be checked by Customs officers. In this way, any passenger incubating the illness can be

Figure 9.1 Pyramid of regulatory strategies

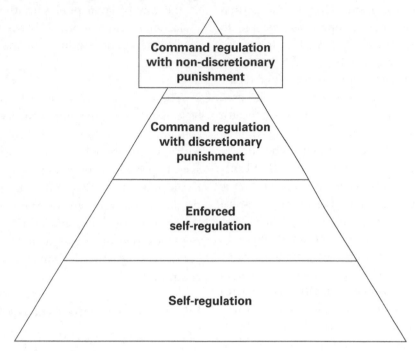

Source: Ayres and Braithwaite (1992: 35).

identified. Other measures include increasing social distance in the general community through the closure of schools, and restricting mass gatherings so as to prevent the spread of influenza between people (Department of Health and Ageing 2005c). The rapidity with which pandemic influenza can spread has meant that increased restrictions have been imposed on travellers specifically, as well as on the general community, to prevent the entry and spread of the disease. These measures also heighten ethical issues concerned with constraints to individual freedoms.

Evolving thinking about public health law

Public health law has been an important tool of public health in the past, but what of the future? What sort of public health laws do we need that will assist in ensuring conditions in our communities that will protect and promote health, particularly with new and emerging public health threats? Gostin puts forward seven models for legal intervention designed to prevent injury and disease and promote the public's health (Gostin 2000b, 2004). These models form a useful framework for thinking about how public health law could and should be deployed.

- **Model 1—The power to tax and spend:** This power supports public health infrastructure and public health programs. The power to tax and the power to grant tax relief can provide inducements and disincentives for certain behaviours. However, some taxation schemes can disproportionately benefit the wealthy or disadvantage the poor. It would be interesting to consider Australian taxation laws from a public health perspective, and in terms of their effect on the social determinants of health (DoH).

- **Model 2—The power to alter the informational environment:** The government has tools at its disposal to encourage people to make more healthy choices. Via law, it can also require information to be given to consumers, such as labelling of product ingredients or health warnings. Such powers can be used to address the social determinants of health indirectly by encouraging and funding research and community discussion about such issues.
- **Model 3—The power to alter the built environment:** This power is relevant to the development and encouragement of social capital through planning and zoning laws, deciding on the location of toxic disposals, planning for communities that encourage more active lifestyles and increasing social interaction.
- **Model 4—The power to alter the socio-economic environment:** This power can be used to bring into effect social policy objectives, such as to redistribute wealth and address material disadvantage. It can undoubtedly affect the social DoH, given that income inequalities are one of the most powerful indicators of health outcomes. The reduction of socio-economic status disparities should be a political—not a health—decision, but the decisions should be guided by evidence.
- **Model 5—Direct regulation of persons, professions and businesses:** This traditional power is used to set clear, enforceable rules to protect workers, consumers and the population at large. Regulation is typically used to curb the excesses of entrepreneurial activities.
- **Model 6—Indirect regulation through the tort system:** Civil litigation can redress different kinds of public harm, including environmental damage, exposure to toxic substances, hazardous products and defective consumer products. Litigation can be costly for individuals, businesses and society as a whole, but can also serve as an incentive for people to engage in safer and more socially conscious behaviour.
- **Model 7—Deregulation:** Laws may get in the way of good public health outcomes. For instance, criminalising activities may drive such activities underground and make them more difficult to regulate.

The application of some of these elements can be seen in Box 9.4, relating to obesity. The examples contained in Box 9.4 show that much can be done with government policies supported by legislation to assist in providing conditions for health within the community. They also show, among other things, the direct links between government economic and financial management and other policies, and the need for supporting strategies in these areas as these policies form part of the conditions for health in a community.

Deregulation, risk and rights

The changing framework for public health legislation is related not only to the evolving roles of the Commonwealth and the states, but also to changing views about the role of government in general. The risk of serious harm to other persons and protecting incompetent persons 'in their own best interests' has long been the justification for public health regulation. Contemporary debates about public health legislation, however, raise such questions as how much room there should be for individual liberty, what responsibilities should be borne by industry, how paternalistic government should be, how much risk is too much risk, how different forms of risks (and risk for different population groups) can be traded off, and how certain the risk might be. As Table 9.1 shows, for every public health activity, there can be a debate about the public benefit and the rights of the individual.

In the 1990s, there was a trend towards deregulation as well as increased valuing of individual rights and liberties. Deregulation is intended to allow the market to work freely or unencumbered by government regulation and, in theory, the result would be

---

Box 9.4 How can law be used to address obesity?

Obesity is considered a significant public health issue and the subject of some debate within the community. How can legislation be used to support a public health policy in relation to this issue? Reynolds (2003) suggests that the following provide a range of options for legislation.

Taxation and spending

- Should the tax system play more of a part in promoting good nutrition, apart from excluding fresh fruit and vegetables from the Goods and Services Tax?
- Should there be an increased tax on high-fat foods?

Product regulation and information

- Foods need to have accompanying information that allows for healthy choices—for example, nutrition panels on packaged foods—but what about takeaway foods?
- Should foods have maximum levels of fat, sugar, salt, etc. so there is no consumer choice?
- Should there be restrictions on the advertising and promotion of certain types of food (those high in fat, sugar and salt) or restrictions on the advertising

of certain foods at certain times, such as children's television viewing times?

- How should governments approach sponsorship or promotional deals with schools? What about schemes such as high-energy food wrappers returned for sports equipment?

The built environment

- What can government do in terms of the built environment to support opportunities to exercise? How can environmental and planning controls be structured to encourage more physical exercise? What are the associated factors that need to be considered—for example, design and isolation, modes of transport and safety?

Review of government policy

- Should there be an introduction of sustainability criteria across all portfolios—for example, transport policy—which encourage activity and exercise?
- Should there be a review of taxation policy, removal of tax advantages for the increased use of cars and the introduction of a tax for car parking?
- Should there be reform of liability legislation and legal indemnities to support organised sport and recreation?

---

increased commercial performance by the market and therefore benefits to the consumer.

The balance between the precautionary principle and industry interests as a core issue in public health regulation can be seen in the emergence of gene technology, particularly the use of genetically modified organisms (GMOs). The precautionary principle provides a guide for decision-making so as to prevent harm—in this case, to human health—the 'it's better to be safe than sorry' approach. However, there are issues around probability of harm and the level of evidence required for the application of the principle.

The newer public health challenges of tobacco, GMOs, global warming, acid rain, avian flu, influenza and so on also point to the increased importance of international conventions and treaties. The UN system provides various processes by which governments and NGOs may formulate strategies to address global priorities.

International conferences, such as the Cairo Conference on Population (1994) and the Beijing Conference on Women (1995), have been important vehicles for negotiating shifts in understanding about reproductive rights and women's position in society. The Rio Environmental Summit (1992), the

Table 9.1 Public health regulations: Public benefit vs individual rights

Public activity	Public benefit	Private rights
Surveillance and monitoring	Monitor health, control disease outbreaks	Health information privacy, doctor–patient confidentiality
Screening and case finding	Education, treatment and support services	Personal autonomy, health information privacy
Immunisation	Disease prevention	Religious freedom, personal autonomy
Prohibition against smoking and illicit drugs	Protect health of others, reduce social and medical costs	Freedom of action, personal autonomy
Requirement to wear safety protection	Prevent personal injury, reduce social and medical costs	Freedom of action, personal autonomy
Product safety design	Prevent personal injury, reduce social and medical costs	Business interests, consumer cost, freedom of contract (manufacturer–consumer)
Environmental regulation	Prevent acute and long-term risks to health and environment	Business and property interest, consumer cost
Occupational health and safety regulation	Reduce acute and long-term risks to health, reduce medical and social cost	Business and property interest, consumer cost, freedom of contract (employer–employee)

Source: adapted from Gostin (2000b: 86–7).

Kyoto Conference on Greenhouse Emissions (1997) and post-Kyoto protocol negotiations were similarly important for addressing global warming as well as environmental sustainability. The UN General Assembly Special Session meeting on HIV/AIDS in 2001 adopted a global intersectoral action plan to tackle the AIDS epidemic. Yet few of these are enforceable agreements, as legal frameworks would simultaneously constrain national sovereignty and free trade.

The Framework Convention on Tobacco Control represents the first time that the World Health Organization (WHO) has used treaty powers for public health purposes (see Box 17.11 in Chapter 17). It can be expected that legal frameworks and treaty powers will become more important for public health practice in the twenty-first century, just as local public health ordinances have evolved into national legislation during the twentieth century.

International health regulations: Creating a new world order

In 1951, the World Health Assembly adopted the International Sanitary Regulations (renamed the International Health Regulations in 1969), with member states automatically becoming parties to the regulations. The regulations were adopted to monitor and control six infectious diseases: cholera, plague, yellow fever, smallpox, relapsing fever and typhus (Brockington 1958: 216–17; WHO 2005c). The WHO approved a new set of regulations in May 2005, which constituted a legally binding international agreement on the 192 member states, the aim of which is to manage the international spread of diseases that pose a threat to global health security. The need for the new regulations and a more coordinated international response was demonstrated with the outbreaks of SARS in 2003 and avian influenza in 2004–05. Under the new regulations, countries have broader obligations to detect and respond to public health emergencies, and the WHO has a new role and responsibility to assist countries to respond to the emergency (WHO 2005c; Public Health Agency of Canada 2005).

The important idea underlying the International Health Regulations is that the regulations extend the obligations and responsibilities of WHO member states (194) beyond the citizens of their own country to the citizens of other countries (WHO 2005c; Public Health Agency of Canada 2005).

Conclusion: What society expects from government

Governments play a leadership and an enabling role in public health practice. Historically, law has been a critical tool for public health action, and many of the first efforts by early public health advocates were about obtaining government support for the enactment of laws to protect the community. Public health law is very much tied to the needs and values of populations and the services they require; it is also the manifestation of active intervention by the state in the everyday lives of individuals and businesses, with the purpose of regulating activities so as to provide conditions in the community that will protect and promote health. In setting out rules by which citizens and businesses should behave, public health legislation can be quite controversial and a hotly debated topic within the media and the community. Public health laws represent an agreed authority framework, at a particular point in time, for public health interventions to occur.

Evolving community values and expectations, along with unexpected health threats, often prompt a rethink about the legislative framework. The HIV epidemic forced reconsideration of public health legislation to reflect societal norms about human rights. The expectation that governments are less interventionist and less punitive has promoted both deregulation and greater emphasis on law as a positive tool.

Public health laws are an important tool today and for the future in terms of assisting in securing conditions for health. Gostin (2000a) has observed that public health and public health law are both highly political, and are influenced by social, cultural and economic forces that shift and reflect different ideologies and social conditions over time. The challenge for Australian governments is to actively ensure that public health law both reflects and is consistent with current government policies, and that there is clear accountability for its administration.

10

Public health intelligence:
Information and the research base for action

Challenge

After many years of saving, you and your partner are now able to obtain a bank loan to build your own home. You have been interested in building a house that is environmentally sustainable and have been researching options for many years. You have attended home shows, read magazines, watched 'do-it-yourself' programs on TV and visited several locations where land has been for sale. When deciding on which block of land to purchase, you must find out which one is suitable for your proposed home—does it have a northerly aspect for solar power, does it have a water supply, would it be exposed to prevailing winds?

Then you must find out what regulations apply to the building of an environmentally sustainable house. One of the first issues is the building material you will use: timber and brick, or alternatives, such as mud brick or straw bales. Perhaps you'll build semi-underground or with a rooftop garden. What type of heating system will you choose? Are you going to generate your own electricity and put the excess back into the grid? Will you install a grey-water system?

Then there is the question of how to find a builder with experience in using unconventional materials. Do you need an architect to draw up the plan? If you decide to build your own home, what regulations apply? Perhaps you could join a group of people with similar interests, or consult the Housing Industry Association for information on builders and trade contractors.

In undertaking any new project, one of the key tasks is to utilise data and information to both define the problem to be solved and decide on how to approach it.

What do we need to know? Where can the most reliable sources of research data and information be found? How can these sources be accessed and how should they be used to make decisions and take action?

Introduction

Roemer (1991) defines a health system as 'the combination of resources, organisation, financing and management that culminate in the delivery of health services to the population'. The delivery of any service depends on infrastructure for delivery—that is, the building blocks, the basic materials and the capacity to carry out its main functions. Public health is no different: public health infrastructure is the underlying foundation that supports the delivery of public health activities (CDC 2001). Public health infrastructure thus comprises all the boxes in Figure 1.1, which depicts a public health system, including the people and their skills, the funding to support people and activities, the required physical stock (such as buildings and equipment), the service provider organisations, the knowledge base, the means by which information is generated and transmitted, and the relationships that exist between these different elements.

Chapter 8 reviewed the organisations and players in this system and Chapter 9 examined the public authority basis of their work. This chapter will review the information and knowledge base (or 'public health intelligence') that public health practitioners and organisations require for delivery of public health activities, while Chapter 11 considers the human and financial resources required to maximise the translation of the knowledge base into action. In describing the current systems within Australia for public health information development and public health research, this chapter will consider how data and research findings become information or intelligence that is useful for policy and practice, and the challenges for transforming information into appropriate decision and action.

Public health information sources

Information requirements

To plan and provide the public health infrastructure that is needed, we must know about the demand for, and use of, various services. There must be an organised effort to obtain the information required to budget and plan public health projects. As we have already demonstrated, public health is a complex and multifaceted activity. Information must be derived from a variety of sources and analysed in a number of ways to help make appropriate decisions about public health infrastructure.

The information resources required to support public health practice are potentially vast. The National Health Performance Framework outlines various aspects of health status, determinants of health (DoH) and health system performance to be considered (NHISSC 2009)—as outlined in Figure 10.1. There are a number of different ways of collecting information about the health of populations. These include:

- routine notifications of specific diseases—for example, *Salmonella* food poisoning cases
- health-event diagnosis-related identification—for example, a diagnosis of breast cancer
- condition-specific data collections—for example, diabetes registers
- recording of specific interventions—for example, immunisation registers
- collection of data on routine events—for example, birth notifications
- collection of data related to compensation for health problems—for example, workers' compensation
- collection of information on unusual or accidental events—for example, data from the Coroner's Courts

Figure 10.1 The National Health Performance Framework

Health status
How healthy are Australians? Is it the same for everyone?
Where are the best opportunities for improvement?

Health conditions Prevalence of disease, disorder, injury or trauma or other health-related states	**Human function** Alterations to body, structure or function (impairment), activity limitations and restrictions in participation	**Wellbeing** Measures of physical, mental and social well-being of individuals	**Deaths** Mortality rates and life expectancy measures

Determinants of health
Are the factors determining good health changing for the better? Where and for whom are these factors changing? Is it the same for everyone?

Environmental factors Physical, chemical and biological factors such as air, water, food and soil quality	**Community and socio-economic** Community factors such as social capital, support services, and socio-economic factors such as housing, education, employment and income	**Health behaviours** Attitudes, beliefs, knowledge and behaviours such as patterns of eating, physical activity, smoking and alcohol consumption	**Bio-medical factors** Genetic-related susceptibility to disease and other factors such as blood pressure, cholesterol levels and body weight

Health system performance
How does the health system perform? What is the level of quality of care across the range of patient care needs? Is it the same for everyone?
Does the system deliver value for money and is it sustainable?

Effectiveness Care/intervention/action provided is relevant to the client's needs and based on established standards. Care, intervention or action achieves desired outcome	**Safety** The avoidance or reduction to acceptable limits of actual or potential harm from health-care management or the environment in which health care is delivered	**Responsiveness** Service is client oriented. Clients are treated with dignity and confidentiality, and encouraged to participate in choices related to their care

Continuity of care Ability to provide uninterrupted, coordinated care or service across programs, practitioners, organisations and levels over time	**Accessibility** People can obtain health care at the right place and right time irrespective of income, physical location and cultural background	**Efficiency and sustainability** Achieving desired results with the most cost-effective use of resources. Capacity of system to sustain workforce and infrastructure to innovate and respond to emerging needs

Community and health system characteristics

Source: NHISSC (2009).

- collection of information in periodic national surveys—for example, the Census
- sentinel surveillance—for example, the sentinel chicken program (whereby chicken blood is analysed for the presence of antibodies of Murray Valley encephalitis) and the influenza surveillance programs.

The challenge for the public health practitioner is to make sense of this mass of data, and to use the information to inform public health action.

Population and health status information

Data about people, the economy and society represent the starting point for understanding communities and their contexts. Australia has an enviable array of information with which to work. The Australian Bureau of Statistics (ABS) is the national agency responsible for the collection of population, economic and social statistics. It conducts a national Census once every five years as well as a range of other surveys. Statistics about births, deaths and marriages are maintained at the state registries. These basic statistics form the foundation for health policy and programs. The demographic data, in particular, help public health practitioners plan their services, as health needs are likely to differ according to age, sex and ethnicity.

Data about health events (other than births and deaths), on the other hand, have relied on a range of mechanisms and have been slower to achieve national coverage and uniformity. A comprehensive picture of health and illness is not possible, as information about disease incidence has been less comprehensively covered, and collecting of information about health and well-being (rather than disease) is seldom carried out. A description of population health status is often more readily achieved at the state level, as health data collections typically are maintained at that level.

Historically, it has been important to record cases of contagious or communicable diseases, such

as cholera and tuberculosis, to monitor their spread and progress, and to try to contain them. Even now, doctors are required by law to notify the authorities when they treat patients for some communicable diseases. These illnesses are therefore known as 'notifiable diseases'. Historically, GPs have been given a small sum to reimburse them for the time and effort they put into reporting the notifiable disease to the authorities (such as the Health Protection and Surveillance Branch of the Australian Department of Health and Ageing, or DoHA). Due to the administrative effort involved in filing a notification (the written report must be sent by post or facsimile), and also sometimes due to a lack of training about this process, some GPs are disinclined to follow through. Under-reporting by doctors and hospitals has been documented as a problem, but notification rates have improved since the law requiring notification has also applied to pathology laboratories.

Registries are another important source of information about disease incidence. All states have cancer registries that capture demographic and clinical details of each new case of cancer, helping to identify geographical areas or types of cancer that might need further investigation. The first national stroke registry was established in Australia in 2009. National disease registries have also been established in Australia for diabetes, Creutzfeldt-Jakob disease, muscular dystrophy and other diseases. In addition, registries were developed to underpin cancer screening programs in the early 1990s, so that information about all cervical screening and breast screening tests is now recorded and women are reminded every two years about re-screening. A similar concept was applied to the Australian Childhood Immunisation Register in the mid-1990s, whereby parents are now reminded in accordance with the National Health and Medical Research Council (NHMRC) immunisation schedule to bring their children to immunisation clinics. These program-based registries are useful for providing information about access to and use of public health services.

Box 10.1 National list of notifiable diseases

Acquired Immunodeficiency Syndrome (AIDS)

Alphavirus and flavivirus

Anthrax

Australian bat lyssavirus

Barmah Forest virus infection

Botulism

Brucellosis

Campylobacteriosis

Chlamydial infection

Cholera

Creutzfeldt-Jakob disease (CJD)

Creutzfeldt-Jakob disease—variant (vCJD)

Cryptosporidiosis

Dengue virus infection

Diphtheria

Donovanosis

Gonococcal infection

Gonorrhoea

Haemolytic uraemic syndrome (HUS)

Haemophilus influenzae serotype b (Hib) (invasive only)

Hepatitis A

Hepatitis B—newly acquired

Hepatitis B—unspecified

Hepatitis C—newly acquired

Hepatitis C—unspecified

Hepatitis D

Hepatitis E

Highly pathogenic avian influenza in humans (HPAIH)

Human immunodeficiency virus (HIV) infection—individuals less than 18 months of age

Human immunodeficiency virus (HIV) infection—newly acquired

Human immunodeficiency virus (HIV) infection—unspecified individuals over eighteen months of age

Influenza (laboratory-confirmed)

Japanese encephalitis virus infection

Legionellosis

Leprosy (Hansen's disease)

Leptospiriosis

Listeriosis

Lyssavirus (not elsewhere classified)

Malaria

Measles

Meningococcal infection (invasive)

Mumps

Murray Valley encephalitis virus infection

Ornithosis

Pertussis (whooping cough)

Plague

Pneumococcal disease (invasive)

Poliomyelitis (paralytic and non-paralytic infection)

Q fever

Rabies

Ross River virus infection

Rubella

Rubella (congenital)

Salmonellosis

Severe acute respiratory syndrome (SARS)

Shiga toxin- and verocytotoxin-producing Escherichia coli (STEC/VTEC)

Shigellosis

Smallpox

Syphilis (congenital)

Syphilis (infectious—primary, secondary and early latent—and less than two years' duration)

Syphilis (more than two years' or unknown duration)

Tetanus

Tuberculosis

Tularaemia

Typhoid

Varicella zoster (chickenpox)

Varicella zoster (shingles)

Varicella zoster (unspecified)

Viral haemorrhagic fevers (quarantinable)

West Nile/Kunjin virus infection

Yellow fever

Health service statistics

In the absence of comprehensive information about disease incidence and prevalence, health service utilisation data is often used as a proxy for understanding what the health needs are in the community. Australia has comprehensive information about hospital discharges, including special data collection about births. Information is not only available by the service location (the hospital), but is also available about the patient—age, sex, country of birth, Aboriginality, postcode of residence and diagnosis (as coded according to the International Classification of Disease, or ICD). For mothers and babies, information is also available on birth weight, previous pregnancies, type of labour and birth, perineal status and maternal medical conditions. However, this hospital morbidity data is of limited use for describing the health or health needs of the community, because unmet needs are not captured, and the same patient attending different hospitals or the same hospital multiple times will be counted as separate individuals, rather than an individual requiring a high level of care. Data are now collected on out-patient attendances, but this did not happen until 2005, when data recording was established for 24 particular types of clinics.

On the other hand, some comparative analyses can be undertaken which point to issues requiring additional investigation. For instance, analysis can be done by geographical area of residence or by country of birth to compare whether some procedures are over or under used, whether birth weight is particularly low, and whether some people are being admitted to hospitals for conditions that could have been managed in the community setting, as illustrated in Box 10.2.

Information about contacts with the primary health care system—for instance, with medical practitioners and community health services—is important for knowing about the less serious health problems (that is, problems that can be managed without hospitalisation), but these are not covered as well as information on vital statistics or hospital morbidity collection. While Medicare Australia (formerly the Health Insurance Commission) has data about GP and specialist visits, the information is more useful in helping us understand the use of health services, rather than for analysing health conditions. State health authorities have adopted a range of approaches to collecting information about contacts with community health services, but national harmonisation is made difficult by differing administrative structures and service definitions, as well as less adequate infrastructure for information technology and data collection. Nonetheless, it is possible to obtain data about community health visits from state health authorities. The Bettering the Evaluation and Care of Health survey, launched in March 1998, continuously collects data from general practices across Australia on morbidity and treatment, and can reveal activities within that primary care setting.

Information about population health risks

Information about population health risks, as well as about people's health knowledge, attitudes and behaviour, is less well covered. The ABS has undertaken regular National Health Surveys (NHS), along with surveys of ageing and disability, mental health and nutrition. These surveys are conducted on the basis of household interviews and provide information on the self-reported perception of health and health services use.

Non-government organisations have conducted biomedical surveys designed to gather health information about the population. For example, the National Heart Foundation collected information about cholesterol and blood lipid levels, which offers insights into heart health, diet and obesity. National public health strategies (such as those related to HIV, drugs and tobacco) have also invested in their own surveys of key risk groups or behaviours (such as smoking, alcohol consumption, safe sex and methadone use). State health authorities (such as Departments of Health), in order to obtain more

Box 10.2 Ambulatory care sensitive conditions

Ambulatory care sensitive conditions (ACSC) are those conditions where hospitalisation can be avoided through the application of prevention-oriented care and early disease management. Health literacy enhancement measures might be especially important for a number of conditions. Therefore, better access to primary health care increases the use of ambulatory care and generally improves the health status of the population. Based on the objectives of primary care, there are three categories of ACSC: vaccine-preventable (i.e. influenza, bacterial pneumonia, tetanus), acute (i.e. dehydration, gastroenteritis, kidney infection) and chronic (i.e. diabetes, asthma, angina, hypertension).

The 'wasting' of financial resources on avoidable patient admission continues to be a major problem, as highlighted by the Victorian statistics for 2002–03, which show the number rising again to 170 000 (32.86 per 1000), while the national total was 625 000. More than 100 000 of these admissions in Victoria were related to the mismanagement of chronic diseases, particularly heart disease and diabetes (Nader 2004).

As new initiatives were being introduced in Victoria, and nationwide, to improve the coordination and communication between health-care service providers, a study of ACSC was viewed as an opportunity to monitor the impact of these reforms (Ansari 2002). According to Victorian government data for 2000–01 and 2005–06, the rate of preventable admissions rose from 30.96 per 1000 in 2000–01 to 41.52 to per 1000 in 2005–06. This meant that in 2005–06 there were 215 784 preventable admissions, involving an average of 4.84 bed days per admission (Ansari 2005).

The data for 2005–06 show that diabetes complications had the highest rate of hospital admission, accounting for 50.56 per cent of the top ten ACSC admissions. ACSCs for chronic disease and for dental conditions were the four leading causes of the top five ACSC admissions, accounting for more than two-thirds of the 215 784 ACSC admissions in 2005–06. For rural areas, the admission rate for all ACSCs increased from 36.37 per 1000 persons in 2000–01 to 44.52 per 1000 persons in 2005–06. During the same period, the admission rate in metropolitan areas for all ASCSs increased from 28.82 per 1000 persons to 40.35 per 1000 persons. Large variations were found across the Primary Care Partnerships, which are designated primary care catchment areas, ranging from 33.83 admissions per 1000 persons in the Eastern Metropolitan region to 46.04 admissions per 1000 persons in the Hume region (Ansari 2005).

timely data and for small areas of particular interest to that jurisdiction, have also begun to develop and implement their own computer-assisted telephone interview (CATI) surveys to capture a range of population health issues. Special topics and populations investigated include gambling and domestic violence (South Australia), community well-being (Tasmania) and children's health (New South Wales).

All these different collections result in a number of deficiencies from an overall system perspective. The differing survey questions and data definitions mean comparability across the country is difficult to achieve. As surveys are costly, they often do not capture a sufficient sample size to allow for estimation at the local level, and they might not be repeated, so time trends are difficult to come by. Australian governments have agreed on a number of national health priorities, which are largely all chronic diseases—heart disease, cancer, mental health, diabetes, asthma, arthritis and injury. The inconsistency of information across states and territories means that coordinated public health strategies are difficult to achieve. Improvements have occurred in data collection since the first national audit of data collections on chronic disease

Table 10.1 Comparison of topics: NHS and NATSIHS and statewide population health (CATI) surveys, c. 2004

Topic area and topics	NHS 2004–05	NATSIHS 2004–05	NSW 2004	Vic. 2004	Qld 2004	SA 2004	WA 2004	ACT 2005	ACT, NT, Qld, Tas. 2004#
Health risk factors									
Adult immunisation	X	X	X	–	2003	–	X	–	–
Alcohol consumption—frequency and no. of drinks	X	X	X	X	2006	X	X	X	X
Breastfeeding	X	X	X	–	2003	X	X	X	–
Child immunisation	X	X	X	–	–	X	–	X	–
Cultural identification—family removal, stressors	–	X	–	–	–	–	–	–	–
Dietary behaviours—daily vegetable and fruit consumption and type of milk consumed	X	X	X	X	2005	X	X	X	X
Exercise	X	X	X	X	X	X	X	X	X
Height, weight, body mass	X	X	X	X	X	X	X	X	X
Smoking—prevalence and in the home	X	X	X	X	X	X	X	X	X
Substance use	–	X	–	–	–	–	X	–	–
Psychological distress (Kessler 10/Kessler 5**)	X	X (K5)	X	X	*	X	X	X	X
Health status indicators									
General health status (self-assessed)	X	X	X	X	X	X	X	X	X
Arthritis—ever told	X	X	–	X	–	X	X	X	–
Asthma—ever told	X	X	X	X	X	X	X	X	–
Cancer incidence—ever told	X[5]	X[5]	–	X	X	–	X	–	–
Cancer screening—actions taken	X	X	X	–	2003, 2005	X	X	X	–
Heart and circulatory conditions—ever told	X	X	–	X	–	X	X	X	–
Heart and circulatory conditions—used meds	X	X	–	–	–	–	–	–	–
High blood pressure—ever told	X	X	2005	X	2006	X	X	X	–
High blood pressure—last measured and/or actions to manage	–	–	2005	X	2006	X	X	X	–
High cholesterol—ever told	X	X	2005	–	2006	X	X	X	–
High cholesterol—last measured and/or medication to manage	–	–	2005	X	2006	X	X	X	–
Diabetes/high sugar levels—ever told	X	X	X	X	X	X	X	X	X
Diabetes—diagnosed during pregnancy	X	–	X	X	X	X	X	X	–
Diabetes—type	X	–	X	X	X	X	X	X	–
Diabetes—age at diagnosis	X	X	X	X	–	–	–	X	–
Diabetes—actions to manage	X	X	X	X	–	–	–	X	–
Kidney disease and dialysis**	–	X	–	X	–	–	–	–	–
Osteoporosis—ever told	X	X	–	X	–	X	X	X	–
Long-term conditions (other)—depression/anxiety—ever told/diagnosed	X	–	–	X	–	X	X	X	–

Notes: * = see last column: risk factors only ACT, NT, Qld, Tas; ** = NATSIHS only; # = DoHA-funded SNAPS risk factor survey 'Filling the Gaps', conducted in Qld, ACT, NT and Tas in 2004.

Source: PHIDU (2008:20).

and associated risk factors conducted in 2002: the ABS NHS has been conducted triennially since 2001, including a six-yearly Indigenous specific survey; statewide CATIs are well established; and data linkage systems have been developed, with further improvements to follow. However, remaining data deficiencies include the lack of a national monitoring system on chronic disease, risk factors and determinants; data gaps in nutrition, physical activity and biomedical measurements; and limited coverage of the state CATIs due to changes in telecommunications and limited access to phone numbers (Gruszin & Szuster 2010) .

From data sources to surveillance information

The information and monitoring system for all risk factors and diseases should be built on the same principles that underlie all surveillance systems, as shown in Table 10.2. While in Australia, and even worldwide, a number of communicable diseases are routinely the subject of surveillance, at present surveillance of non-communicable and chronic diseases is confined either to extremely uncommon disorders that may be identified through registers or specialised data collections (such as the occurrence of CJD) or to very common events identifiable through routine practices common to whole populations (such as births).

Each of these systems has been set up for a specific purpose, but they are very different from one another, and bear little or no relationship to each other. However, as a body of information they provide considerable data about a wide variety of health- and disease-related events. Collectively, they are powerful tools for assessing the health of Australians.

Surveillance systems have a number of features in common—most of which have been considered in many countries worldwide, including Australia. They are summarised in Table 10.2.

Monitoring the health system

Given the complexity of factors that interact in dynamic ways and thereby influence the health of the community in a continuous fashion, health information models are useful to help identify how

Table 10.2 Shared constituents of surveillance systems

Constituent	Segment
Purpose of	• Events considered to be of health importance are notified or monitored in a theoretically systematic way.
Legal basis	• Some notifications are required by local or national law. • Disease-specific circumstances and specific international and multinational requirements also exist. • Other disease-specific surveillance systems are voluntary.
Reporting mechanism	• People who may notify cases of disease to relevant authorities include medical practitioners, other health-care workers, laboratory staff, self-referrers, school health or occupational health staff, and sometimes members of the general public. • State and territory requirements are published on their websites.
Reporting time	• Notifiable diseases have specific notification timelines, set down in legislation (see state health frame department websites). Other registries are less specific.
Data collection	• All datasets include basic demographic and epidemiological information, allowing analysis of person/place/time and, to some extent, environment. • Note that the biggest datasets have the least complex information.

Table 10.2 Shared constituents of surveillance systems *(continued)*

Constituent	Segment
Data transfer	• Data used for health surveillance are usually collected according to jurisdictional constituencies (e.g. area health authorities, state and national health authorities). In Victoria, for example, notification and hospital usage data are centralised at the Department of Human Services.
	• Sometimes by law, notifications must be made by telephone very quickly. At other times, notifications are mailed. Laboratories are developing the capacity to transfer notification data electronically. Other routine data (such as hospital separation data) may be provided only periodically.
Securing and maintaining privacy and security of data	• All notification systems have security measures built into them—for example, access to raw datasets is extremely limited, requiring access to restricted rooms and password-protected disc partitions, to comply with privacy legislation.
	• Most data collections are stored in national and state jurisdictional and reference laboratory data warehouses.
	• Hard (paper) copies of notifications are kept in secure, locked rooms. Historical data is archived in secure warehouses.
	• For most conditions, full identifying details (including name, address and date of birth) are submitted, but for exceptionally sensitive conditions, such as sexually transmitted infections, only sufficient details to be sure that the case has not been notified before are provided (including name-codes, age and residential postcode).
Analysis	• Communicable disease surveillance data, cancer data, screening registry data and databases of a voluntary nature (such as CJD) are analysed continually (for example, infectious disease data is analysed on a daily basis).
	• Databases generated by statutory notification systems are summarised in quarterly reports to the Commonwealth, and yearly as the various annual reports by epidemiologists.
	• Other surveillance systems report at least annually.
	• Reports are published regularly on easily accessible departmental websites.
Interpretation	• The epidemiologist performing the surveillance report analysis usually interprets the data for the reader. If the report consists of no more than summary data, the reader will need to find previous reports to understand trends, and population data for understanding attack rates, and so on.
	• Sometimes access to other data, such as the demographic structure of the population, is also important for interpreting disease trends.
Dissemination	• Surveillance data is disseminated in annual reports, both in hard copy and on the internet.
	• Access to them is normally universal and simple.
Use	• The data is used both by the departments that produce them and by planning departments for a number of purposes. These include: – identifying and managing disease outbreaks – developing policy – planning primary and secondary care health services – planning of services for specific identified groups (for example, women's health, adolescent health).

Source: Government of Victoria (2001, 2005a).

indicators can be constructed to monitor the various factors that influence health status outcomes. Given the substantial quantum of resources invested in the health system, it is also important to monitor how well the system is performing, particularly in relation to achieving health outcomes. By developing a more comprehensive approach to health information collection, it will be possible to assess health outcomes in relation to exposures (the DoH), as well as to the adequacy of the health system (health system performance).

Such a framework is useful for mapping what information is available and what gaps and duplications exist—and therefore where there is insufficient investment in information collection. However, information systems generally tend to improve with the increased use of the information. The challenge is thus not only to achieve a more coherent information infrastructure by shifting current investments to fill the gaps, but also to ensure adequate analysis and dissemination of the information to the users, particularly decision-makers.

For the purposes of prevention, however, it is necessary to go beyond monitoring the health-care system. Monitoring systems that create health (that is, those associated with social DoH) is important. This can draw upon the same health system performance model, but give more emphasis to the DoH and data collected from outside the health system. The DoH classification shown in Table 10.3 was developed by the Public Health Determinants Classification Project.

Box 10.3 illustrates the range of objective and subjective indicators that might be used to monitor community violence.

While indicators may be developed for monitoring complex but specific health and social issues, the overall prevention effort may be served better by having a small set of indicators that point to the need for action on the 'upstream' factors that affect a range of health problems. Leading health indicators (such as those listed in Box 10.4) are based on a cross-sectional view of the world, rather than a life-course or longitudinal view, and thus do not measure accumulation and interaction of risks, cumulative exposure or the effects of the latency of adult onset. Also, when the focus is on an individual risk factor/s, the impact of that person's socio-economic status—which is related to almost all health behaviour determinants—disappears. Such indicators also lack equity and gender analysis, and seem to be selected for their importance as public health issues and thus their ability to motivate action (Lin et al. 2003).

Coordination of health information

In the early 1970s, the National Committee on Health and Vital Statistics began a gradual process to align the collections for state health authorities, with a particular focus on hospital morbidity data. In 1987, with the establishment of the Australian Institute of Health and Welfare (AIHW), a national repository of hospital morbidity records was created. Since the signing of the National Health Information Agreement (NHIA) in 1993 and under the auspices of the relevant AHMAC committee, currently the National Health Information and Performance Principal Committee (NHIPPC), Australian jurisdictions have worked to achieve agreement on national data definitions and minimum datasets (collections of similar or related data).

Within the last 20 years, Australia has been able to build on the considerable investment in information made by different jurisdictions to consolidate a process of continuous alignment and coordination of health information. Supporting the legislative bases for national collection is the NHIA—an agreement between the state and territory health authorities, the ABS, AIHW, DoHA, Department of Veterans' Affairs and Australian Commission on Safety and Quality in Health Care.

Table 10.3 Determinants of Health (DoH) classification work in progress: Overview

Behavioural DoH	Biological DoH	(Physical) environmental DoH	Socio-economic DoH
1 Risk and/or protective behaviours 2 Responses to health problems	1 Genetic 2 Body structure 3 Body functioning	1 Water quality 2 Air quality 3 Climate and geography 4 Built environment 5 Food safety 6 Land and soil quality	1 Social 2 Economic

Behavioural DoH	Biological DoH	(Physical) environmental DoH	Socio-economic DoH
1 Risk and/or protective behaviours • Alcohol use • Breastfeeding • Diet • Dietary supplement use • Hygiene • Illicit drug use • Immunisation • Oral health behaviours • Pharmaceutical use • Physical activity • Protective clothing use • Screening behaviours • Seat belt use • Sexual activity • Sun exposure protective behaviours • Tobacco use **2 Responses to health problems** • Care-seeking • Compliance with medical treatment • Health-care service use behaviours • Pain behaviours • Response to illness	**1 Genetic** • Single-gene • Chromosomal • Multifactorial • Mitochondrial DNA-linked **2 Body structure** • Height • Weight • Waist:hip ratio • Bone density **3 Body functioning** • Blood pressure • Nutritional status • Biochemical function • Sensory function • Movement and balance • Strength and robustness • Fitness	**1 Water quality** • Drinking water quality • Recreational water quality • Recycled water quality **2 Air quality** • Ambient air quality • Indoor air quality **3 (Effects of) climate and geography** • Solar radiation • Temperature • Rainfall • Fire • Severe weather events • Salinity • Sea level rise **4 Built environment** • Transport (e.g. road traffic accidents) • Public open space • Noise • Biological hazards • Material hazards (e.g. asbestos, lead) • Housing quality • Chemical hazards • Radiological hazards • Electromagnetic hazards **5 Food safety** • Contamination • Quality **6 Land and soil quality** • Contamination • Pesticides	**1 Social** • Attitudes (who holds them)§ • Community involvement, civic engagement, bridging social capitalþ • Culture • Ethnicity • Gender • Health cognition • Language • Religious belief or spirituality • Safety and security • Socal class/caste • Social and support networksþ incl. support and relationships (who provides them)§ • Trustþ **2 Economic** • Education • Employment statusß • Financial resources • Housing availability • Industryß • Literacy and health literacy • Living standard • Occupationß • Services, systems and policies (incl. health services, systems and policies)§

DoH symbols § ß þ denote existing classifications—see notes below.

Notes: Symbols denoting existing classifications: ICD § ICF (capitals indicate whole ICF chapters: e.g. attitudes), ß ILO classifications; þ AIHW AusWelfare framework.

Source: NSW Health (2010).

Box 10.3 Useful indicators for planning community violence-prevention programs

Social indicators could include:
- assault/rape
- burglary
- hospital admissions for assault
- vandalism.

But also:
- how 'safe' people feel about walking, using public transport, going shopping
- how readily the community welcomes strangers, asylum seekers; efforts towards Aboriginal reconciliation; violence-related education in schools, colleges, TAFEs, University of the Third Age, etc.

Box 10.4 Leading health indicators

The list below was developed by the US Institutes of Medicine for *Healthy People 2010*.
- Physical activity
- Overweight and obesity
- Tobacco use
- Substance abuse
- Responsible sexual behaviour
- Mental health
- Injury and violence
- Environmental quality
- Immunisation
- Access to health care

Source: Lin et al. (2003: 105).

Box 10.5 National public health information infrastructure

The **Australian Institute for Health and Welfare** (AIHW) is part of the Commonwealth Health portfolio and works in partnership with the Australian Bureau of Statistics, the Departments of Family and Community Services and Veterans' Affairs to collect health- and welfare-related information and statistics on the Australian population. The AIHW also coordinates the collection and production of information and statistics, and provides assistance to other persons and bodies collecting such information. The *Australian Institute of Health and Welfare Act 1987* also requires the AIHW to publish methodological and substantive reports, conduct and promote research into the health of Australians, and make this health- and welfare-related information available to researchers (Attorney-General's Department 2004).

The AIHW produces the biennial reports *Australia's Health* and *Australia's Welfare* in alternate years. *Australia's Health* is a national report card, which is an authoritative source of information on the patterns of health and illness over the life-course, determinants of health and major causes of disease, the protection and promotion of good health, the supply and financing of health services and the health workforce, and health research undertaken (AIHW 2012). The AIHW also produces disease-monitoring systems, data definitions and classifications and minimum datasets, and manages the metadata repository METeOR (AIHW 2012).

In addition, the AIHW produces reports on the health of particular population groups, including the Aboriginal and Torres Strait Islander (ATSI) population, children's welfare and health services, and aged care; and also on specific health topics, such as cancer, cardiovascular disease, dental health, drug statistics, injury prevention, mental health, mortality surveillance and road injury statistics (see the AIHW website for more details, <www.aihw.gov.au>).

The **National Health Information Agreement** (NHIA), which came into operation in 1993, was established to coordinate the development, collection and dissemination of health information in Australia, and helps to improve access to uniform health information by community groups, health professionals, and government and non-government organisations. It operates under the auspices of the Standing Council on Health (the group of Australian government, state and territory Health ministers) and AHMAC. The National Health Information Standards and Statistics Committee—a standing committee of NHIPPC—has the role of overseeing the development of data standards for inclusion in the National health data dictionary (AIHW 2010).

The **National Advisory Group on Aboriginal and Torres Strait Islander Health Information and Data** (NAGATSIHID) is responsible for:

- coordinating health information in relation to Aboriginal and Torres Strait Islander health and health

service delivery and advising on the improvement of the quality and availability of data
- continuing the implementation of the National Indigenous Health Information Plan
- advising AIHW and ABS on priorities in its workplan
- providing advice on indicators and targets for Aboriginal and Torres Strait Islander Health.

NAGATSIHID membership consists of representatives of the ABS, the AIHW, DoHA; the National Aboriginal Community Controlled Health Organisation; individuals and groups expert in Aboriginal and Torres Strait Islander health and welfare; and an epidemiologist with expertise in Indigenous health issues.

Gaps and problems

Although Australia has a strong public health information base relative to many countries, a criticism of the system is that there is much information on health status, but the collection of information on health risks is dependent on the political interests involved in its capture. Also, there is little information available on public health activities and inputs. Thus, the collection of data and information is not always governed by what is expedient for the delivery of public health, but rather by what is politically expedient (which, consequently, determines what receives funding).

All the data collected in these surveys by various groups and organisations contribute to a significant information base for public health action. Yet there are common criticisms that the effort made to collect

data does not always result in information being used for policy and program development and evaluation. Some of the most common criticisms from decision-makers are that the data collections do not provide data that are sufficiently timely, or that relate to particular communities of interest. This demonstrates how difficult it can be to coordinate the information needs of state, federal, local and independent public health interests. A lack of trend data (that is, identifiable patterns over time in relation to specific variables) and comparative data is also seen as a weakness in the health information system. In relation to the major health problems that confront Australia, health information gaps include psychosocial factors, social and environmental determinants of health, public health activities (outputs and expenditures) and trend data on behavioural risk factors.

Box 10.6 Evolving Priorities of the National Public Health Information Development Plan

The *National Public Health Information Development Plan 1999* responded to the growing need for

comprehensive and consistent public health information in Australia that could only be met by establishing greater cooperation and coordination between governments at the national, state/territory and local levels and their respective agencies. The current plan, the *National Public Health Information Development Plan 2005*, has an expanded scope: to address priority public health concerns within the health-care system and tackle emerging national priorities for public health action.

The recommendations of the earlier plan were concerned with strengthening the informational foundations for public health policy and programs, including improving the scope and coverage of public health information in such areas as health determinants, Indigenous peoples, socio-economic disadvantage, intersectoral information and data on the physical environment, health-promotive environments, geographical classifications, financial and economic assessment of public health programs, and defining national public health indicators. The current plan for priority work now includes information frameworks and standards for surveillance of chronic diseases, and associated determinants as a core set of national environmental health indicators for refining public health performance information, as standard geographical boundaries and standardised questions on socio-economic status.

The original plan aimed to improve the use and delivery of public health information, including analysis and presentation of information and information delivery and access. The revised plan included specific aims to further improve data on Indigenous status and on public health expenditure, to develop consistent collection of data on antibiotic-resistant infections and birth anomalies, to update information on burden of disease, to collect and analyse data on avoidable hospital admissions, to progress a national biomedical measurement survey, and to pilot a near-real-time collection of syndromic surveillance data from emergency departments.

A goal of the original plan was developing public health information capacity, such as record linkage and sentinel surveillance networks and communicable disease surveillance. The current plan includes specific goals, such as publishing a guide to the use of population health data for primary health-care agencies, to promote the use of public health information in all spheres of government and community activity, and to convene periodic national and international forums on public health surveillance.

Source: AIHW (1999, 2005b).

Public health research and development: Enriching the picture

Data and statistics form one aspect of the information base for public health action. Knowledge derived from research is another critical resource for public health practitioners. As Figure 10.2 shows, surveillance and research both contribute to the evidence base that ultimately forms the basis for public health action.

Organising the research effort

Research can happen in many ways. Curiosity about how the world works often drives the investigator. The need to solve practical problems may be another impetus for research. Public health research that has made a major contribution to health improvement has often begun with observations about patterns of health and illness in a community or population. The researcher has then looked for theories and collected data to explain why those patterns exist, and how they might be altered. An example is the program to develop and evaluate a program for Aboriginal parents aimed to restore identification with culture and promote parental confidence, knowledge and child-rearing skills by supporting parents in promoting their children's behavioural and social competence and readiness for school learning. The NHMRC identified this area of research as a priority and an unmet need, and so funded this program through its strategic awards. The types of research funded by NHMRC (listed in Box 10.7) are largely investigator driven and located in the field of biomedical and clinical

Figure 10.2 Framework for evidence and action in public health action

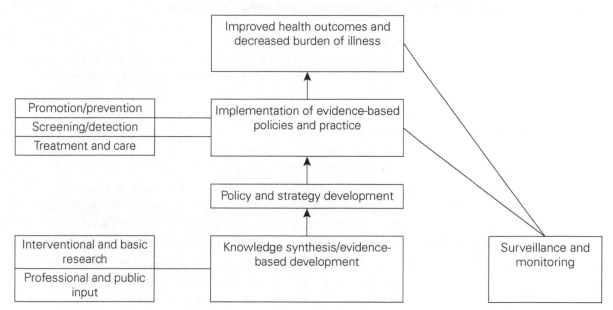

research; however, the inclusion of grant types (such as the strategic awards mentioned above, as well as capacity-building grants and partnership projects) strengthens public health research.

Given the continued and rapid expansion of scientific knowledge, research is now seldom a lone endeavour of one curious mind. Funding is required and researchers often work in multi-disciplinary teams. In Australia, government is the major funder of health and medical research, largely through the NHMRC, although public health research is also supported by the Australian Research Council. A rigorous process of peer reviewing of proposals ensures that the research projects that receive funding are of the highest possible quality. Although research is generally funded on the basis of scientific significance, meritorious methodology and the track record of research teams, from time to time the government may also set research priorities. In 2010, the National Research Priorities were designated as an environmentally sustainable Australia, promoting and maintaining good health, frontier technologies for building and transforming

Australian industries, and safeguarding Australia (ARC 2010).

There are also charitable organisations that support public health research. Bodies such as the Cancer Councils, Heart Foundation, Stroke Foundations and Asthma Foundations often receive bequests from people who hope that prevention and cure can be found for the diseases from which they suffered. These organisations typically follow a similar selection process for allocation of research funds, whereby research proposals are submitted on a set date, and are reviewed by peers.

A common criticism of this approach of organising research funding is that it is dominated by medical interests, and tends to favour biomedical research because the peer review process focuses on the track record of researchers and on traditional scientific methodology. Public health research, often being interdisciplinary, is less well understood by researchers with biomedical backgrounds and is methodologically more complex. In order to focus attention on research evidence needed in relation to global priority public health issues, the Cochrane

---

Box 10.7 Types of grant relevant to public health provided by NHMRC

Project	People
Research Fellowships	Support appointments for high-performing researchers, generally in the top 10 per cent of their field and who are viewed as 'pushing the boundaries' of research.
Translating Research into Practice Fellowships	Support future leaders in translating important research findings into clinical practice; support professionals in researching approaches to applying evidence to improve care; and develop the range of skills needed for leadership in research translation.
Career Development Fellowships (formerly Career Development Awards)	Available to researchers in the early stages of their careers to develop research leadership skills and their capacity for original self-directed and independent research in a program or as part of a research team.
Centre of Excellence Scheme	Provides support for teams of researchers to pursue collaborative research.
Early Career Fellowships	Provide opportunities for researchers to work on research projects with nominated advisers, to undertake research that is both of major importance in its field and of benefit to Australian health.
Program Grant–Teams	Provides support for teams of high-calibre researchers to pursue broadly based collaborative research activities.
Project Grant	Supports investigator-initiated research projects.
Scholarships	Support graduates early in their career, usually achieved by funding scholars to attain a PhD by full-time research.
New Investigator Project Grant	Provides an avenue for less-experienced researchers to access funding.
Partnerships for Better Health (Partnership Projects and Partnership Centres)	Provides funding and support to create new opportunities for researchers and policy-makers to not only work together to define research questions and undertake research, but also to interpret and implement the findings.
Global Alliance for Chronic Diseases Grants	Support international collaborations in research, focusing on chronic non-communicable diseases, in particular cardiovascular diseases (mainly heart disease and stroke), chronic respiratory conditions, type 2 diabetes, and several cancers, focusing in particular on the needs of low- and middle-income countries and on low-income populations in more developed countries.
Cancer Australia Priority-driven Collaborative Cancer Research Scheme	Funds cancer research in identified priority areas to help reduce the impact of cancer in the community and improve outcomes for people affected by cancer.
Targeted Call for Research	A one-time solicitation for grant applications addressing a defined research topic, to stimulate or greatly advance research in a particular area that will benefit the health of Australians.

Source: NHMRC (2012a).

Collaboration identifed reviews needed of public health topics (see Box 10.8).

Consumer health organisations also have argued that their perspectives are frequently missing from funded research—either because issues of interest to consumers are not explored, or because consumer experiences are not taken into account. The Cochrane Consumer and Communication Review Group aims to address the need for improved communication and participation by consumers and carers through producing evidence to support interventions that affect consumers' interactions with health-care professionals, services and researchers. Priority themes include evidence

for modes of consumer participation, participation and communication about use of medicines, complex health needs and the science of evidence-based health care, and the communication and information needs of specific groups, such as people with multiple sclerosis and potential candidates for vaccinations in low- and middle-income countries (La Trobe University 2012).

In the United States, a new patient-centred organisation was established in 2010 to conduct research with the intention of giving patients a better understanding of the prevention, treatment and care options available, and the science that supports those options. In keeping with the aims of

---

Box 10.8 Top 15 priority review topics

1 Community-building interventions (designed to build a sense of community, connectedness, cultural revival, social capital) to improve physical, social and mental health

2 Healthy cities, municipalities or spaces projects in reducing cardiovascular disease risk factors

3 Interventions to build capacity among health-care professionals to promote health and/or interventions to build organisational capacity to promote health

4 Physical exercise to improve mental health outcomes for adults (this topic has been turned into an intervention for reviewing effectiveness, and specified to adults to avoid overlap with existing reviews focusing on children and young people)

5 Interventions using marketing strategies to promote healthy behaviours in young people (focusing on tobacco, alcohol and/or food)

6 Pre-natal and early infancy psychosocial interventions for the prevention of mental disorders

7 Interventions using the WHO Health-Promoting School framework in improving health and academic achievements among students in schools

8 Interventions that use a combination of environmental, social and educational strategies to prevent

infectious diseases, such as malaria, dengue fever and diarrhoea

9 Interventions addressing gender disparities in family food distribution to improve child nutrition

10 Interventions to decrease/minimise adverse health effects of urban sprawl and/or interventions to increase the number of footpaths and walking trails for the public

11 Interventions for healthier food choices: 'Sales promotion strategies of supermarkets to increase healthier food purchase'; 'Pricing policies to increase healthy food choices'

12 Transport schemes to increase use of maternal and newborn health services (with a skilled attendant), and to increase community support and action for maternal and newborn health populations

13 Interventions to improve the nutrition of refugee populations and displaced populations

14 Interventions that aim to reduce health-risk behaviours through enhancing protective environments for adolescents

15 Interventions focusing on adolescent girls in order to improve the nutritional status of women of child-bearing age prior to their first pregnancy.

Source: Doyle et al. (2005: 195).

---

the organisation, the process for selecting specific topics to study includes patient input. Similarly, priorities for research are identified by drawing upon public comment obtained through various methods of patient input, including the organisation's first national patient and stakeholder dialogue. The five national research priorities in 2012 are:

1 assessing prevention, diagnosis and treatment options
2 improving health-care systems
3 communicating and disseminating information and decision-making

4 addressing disparities between populations
5 accelerating patient-centred outcomes research.

Growth of public health research funding

The late 1980s heralded significant changes in how government and Australians in general regarded health, and this resulted in an expansion of funding for public health research. The Kerr White Report recommended the establishment of a separate Public Health Research and Development Committee (PHRDC) within the NHMRC and, for the first time, public health researchers took their

---

Box 10.9 Applied public health research to improve Aboriginal medical services and health

The Audit and Best Practice for Chronic Disease (ABCD) project is an example of how public health research, aimed at improving health services and population health, can be applied successfully. Initiated in 2002, the project began as a collaboration between the Menzies School of Health Research, the Northern Territory Department of Health and Community Services, the Cooperative Research Centre for Aboriginal Health and a range of government and Aboriginal community-controlled health centres in the Top End of the Northern Territory. The approach and methods of the project built on the beneficial experiences of early coordinated care trials, which provided measurable benefits to clients and enabled the establishment of Aboriginal Health Management Boards.

The focus of ABCD is the use of continuous quality improvement (CQI) processes to improve health outcomes by assisting health services to improve their delivery systems of best practice care. Health centre staff were engaged to identify strengths and weaknesses in their organisational systems, set goals for improvement, develop strategies to achieve these goals and assess the effectiveness of these strategies

in improving chronic illness care. Participatory action research in the twelve health centres that initially took part in the project was key to showing the impacts of the approach on systems to support chronic illness care, on processes of care and on some immediate outcomes of care.

An extension phase was supported between 2005 and 2009. It sought to examine what was required to expand the ABCD CQI model to other places (remote communities, regional towns and urban settings across Australia) and to other areas of primary health care (such as maternal and child health). By the end of 2009, over 130 Indigenous primary health care services across Australia had adopted the tools and processes developed through ABCD. Factors had been identified that were necessary for scaling up the use of CQI processes and that were required to incorporate CQI into routine clinical practice across diverse settings. Since then, the National Centre for Quality Improvement One21seventy was initiated as a provider of training and implementation support to services that use ABCD CQI tools and processes. ABCD is an example of action research that has achieved not only improvements in how well Aboriginal Medical Services manage chronic disease but also improvements in health.

Source: Bailie et al. (2007).

---

place alongside medical researchers. The heyday of the 1980s also included health services research grants from the Commonwealth's Research and Development Grant Advisory Committee program, targeted efforts within a number of national public health strategies (such as HIV/AIDS and drugs), and the then new National Occupational Health and Safety Commission.

Investment in health and medical research grew steadily throughout the 1990s following the Wills Review (Commonwealth of Australia 1998). However, concerns remained about the need for increased investments in research that addresses policy priorities and the shortage of public health and health services researchers. In response to concerns about the lack of a critical mass of researchers in any one institution, the NHMRC also supported research networks (such as for injury prevention) and developed public health research capacity-building schemes as a way of building teams and new researchers. The NHMRC introduced Partnership Project Grants in 2009, in order to provide funding and support to create new opportunities for researchers and policy-makers to work together to define research questions and undertake research, and also to interpret and implement the findings. Grants are provided to researchers investigating a specific research question to influence health and well-being through changes in the delivery, organisation, funding and access to health services. In 2010, $784.9 million was distributed by the NHMRC across its funding schemes. Then, in 2011, the Commonwealth government increased NHMRC funding by 4.3 per cent and committed $700 million to building and upgrading health and medical research and training facilities.

In addition to the NHMRC, Australian governments have periodically supported the establishment of specialised research centres. The national centres in HIV epidemiology and social research, and in alcohol and drugs, work closely to support the development, implementation and evaluation of the respective national health programs. The Victorian government and the Victorian Health Promotion Foundation (VicHealth) have supported the establishment of specialist research units in areas such as mothers' and children's health, adolescent health, tobacco control, accident research and mental well-being. New South Wales Health has provided Capacity-Building Infrastructure Grants to support research units and networks focused on areas such as rural health, health informatics, infectious diseases and health services development. Building links between researchers and practitioners to improve knowledge translation and exchange has been a growing concern for research funders. (An example of action research funded by government and other agencies that connects researchers and practitioners appears in Box 10.10.) The New South Wales Sax Institute is one example of an organisation that links researchers and decision-makers. It conducts public health research as well as health services research. The Victorian Health Department has established the Centre of Excellence in Intervention and Prevention Science (CEIPS), which is focused entirely on health-promotion research (Box 10.11).

Research publications

With the expansion of research funding, the *Australia New Zealand Journal of Public Health*, initially published by the Public Health Association in the 1970s as *Community Health Studies*, began to experience an increased volume of quality submissions and a backlog of articles awaiting publication in the 1990s. Given the multi-disciplinary mix, however, public health researchers engaged in lively debates—about quantitative versus qualitative methods, priorities for particular topics and support for particular disciplines. The researchers' interests ranged from health inequalities to climate change, from cancer and heart disease to child health and women's health. Some saw sufficient differences to try to differentiate public health research from health services research.

Since the 1990s, there has been an increase in the number of public health journals in Australia, as

Box 10.10 New public health research centres: NSW Sax Institute and Centre of Excellence in Intervention and Prevention Science (CEIPS)

The Sax Institute, funded by New South Wales Health, builds partnerships between researchers and health policy and service delivery agencies, to support policy- and practice-focused research, with the aim of improving the quality and performance of health services and programs. The institute is a coalition of university and research groups undertaking public health as well as health services research in New South Wales.

Highlights during 2010–11 included:

- participation in the third conference of the Coalition for Research to Improve Aboriginal Health
- the launch of the Centre for Informing Policy on Health with Evidence for Research which will enable policy agencies and researchers to work together to develop and test new tools, skills and systems that will contribute to an increased use of research evidence in policy
- managing the 45 and Up Study, Australia's largest study into ageing, a general population cohort study designed to investigate healthy ageing
- developing the Secure Unified Research Environment project, a secure remote-access data analysis facility designed specifically for research using linked health data.

The Centre of Excellence in Intervention and Prevention Science has a greater focus on health promotion, and was established in 2011 by the Victorian Health Department as an independent public health research organisation to work with government, universities and other agencies on prevention policy and practice. Through collaborative research, the centre aims to advance the science of systems thinking and its application to population health improvement, and also to support working relationships between agencies undertaking research, policy and practice.

Recent projects include:

- working with the Institute for Research and Innovation in Social Services Scotland on the Creating a Culture of Innovation Project, which provided two organisations with tools to generate new thinking on problems and opportunities with a variety of stakeholders and encouraged them to consider developing an innovation process
- reviewing public health practitioner competency frameworks in light of developments in public health and the state Public Health and Well-Being plan
- overseeing the evaluation of the Prevention Community Model, the state's prevention system, which adopts the WHO building blocks approach, investing in workforce, new partnerships, new leadership and governance, and a new capacity to integrate research, policy and practice in relation to the determinants of health: communities, worksites and schools, the food system, the tobacco-delivery system and other determinants
- reviewing the literature on using systems thinking to develop leadership for prevention.

Sources: Sax Institute (2012); CEIPS (2012).

well as in the inclusion of public health content in journals about medicine and other aspects of health care. Table 10.4 lists some journals that are used frequently by public health practitioners.

In recent years, more attention has also been given to 'best practice' as a decision-making criteria. The rise of the evidence-based medicine (EBM) movement has challenged all decision-makers—be they in the clinical, community or government policy setting—to adopt an evidence-based approach. Systematic reviews to determine 'what works' are now expected to form part of a rigorous decision-making process. Accessing and assessing the relevance of research is now more important than ever for public health

Table 10.4 Useful public health journals

Australian	International	
Australian Health Consumer	American Journal of Epidemiology	International Journal of Public Health
Australian Health Review	American Journal of Public Health	
Australian Journal of Primary Health	BMC Health Services Research	Journal of Epidemiology and Community Health
Australian Journal of Rural Health	BMC Public Health	
Australian and New Zealand Journal of Public Health	British Medical Journal	Journal of Health Policy, Politics and Law
Health Issues	Critical Public Health	
Health Promotion Journal of Australia	Global Health Promotion	Journal of Health Service Research and Policy
Medical Journal of Australia	Health Affairs	
	Health Education Research	Journal of Public Health Policy
	Health Policy	Lancet
	Health Policy and Planning	Millbank Quarterly
	Health Promotion International	Public Health
	International Journal of Epidemiology	Public Health Reports
	International Journal of Health Services	Social Science and Medicine
		WHO Bulletin

practitioners. Fortunately, there is a growing body of literature as well as an increasing number of systematic reviews to draw upon.

With the rapid diffusion of the internet, increasing numbers of people are turning to the World Wide Web for health information. Unfortunately, there is limited quality assurance with regard to health information found on the web, although more professional journals are providing open access. The Cochrane Collaboration has placed strong emphasis on making systematic reviews readily accessible through an electronic library on the World Wide Web and in easily understood forms. Several governments are also creating portals or sites where the information is quality-assured.

While the World Wide Web may offer a vast range of information, there are some important studies and reports commonly referred to as 'grey literature' which may not be so readily accessible. Governments often commission policy research papers and program evaluations that provide a useful synthesis of the research literature and original data collections. Accessing these materials may require contacting government authorities or undertaking some good detective work.

Connecting research with action: 'Beyond the sound of one hand clapping'

Lomas (1997) has described researchers and practitioners as living in two different worlds, and has challenged them both to move 'beyond the sound of one hand clapping'. In Australia, despite the increase in research funding and publications, some have questioned how well research has been translated into practice. By the mid-1990s, the PHRDC was asking itself how to place more emphasis on the 'D' of R&D (research and development). Then the NHMRC took the decision to 'mainstream' public health—to amalgamate the PHRDC with the Medical Research Committee—thus removing the exclusive and autonomous voice of public health within the NHMRC, but also placing public health experts in a more powerful position to influence general health research priorities. Various opinions on the benefit of this move were expressed, ranging from those who felt public health researchers would benefit from having a greater profile among powerful medical research interests, to those who feared public health would be seen as a mere subset of medicine, to those who took a broader view, arguing that all of humanity would benefit from the integrated approach that public health would offer mainstream medical research in looking at health issues.

Since then, through multiple reviews, governments have given greater attention to 'priority-driven' research, meaning that research should serve the needs of policy and practice. The notion is that research and action should be intimately linked—research should be applied through commercialisation as it should respond to solving the immediate problems in the world of policy and practice. Public health researchers were asked, through this process, to demonstrate what difference their work had made, as well as what should be future priorities. Following the most recent review (NHMRC 2009b), recommendations were accepted in relation to the following actions:

- new infrastructure to support a strategic and collaborative approach for identifying priorities for public health research, particularly in relation to the government's preventative health strategy and including large-scale and long-term studies
- the establishment of National Centres of Excellence in public health research
- the development of evidence-based guidelines in relation to national health priority areas
- identifying gaps in research and minimising duplication
- 'out-of-rounds' grants in response to immediate public health needs
- increased senior public health research-funded positions
- revised selection process and criteria for grant applications, consistent with behavioural and environmental determinants of health and the multi-disciplinary nature of public health research
- definition and monitoring of research outcomes (NHMRC 2009c).

This concern about linking research and practice is not confined to the NHMRC or Australia. In the United States, major health-care providers (such as Kaiser Permanente and the Veterans Affairs health-care system) have embedded the research function within their organisations, rather than hiving off research projects to universities. Both are able to point to substantial improvements in health services as a result of their research (Lomas 2003). The Canadian government has opted for a network of funding partners in forming the Canadian Health Services Research Foundation in 1997, so that there is a coordinated approach both to funding research and to supporting the synthesis and dissemination of research results (Investment Review of Health and Medical Research Committee 2004). The US Institute of Medicine proposes 'learning collaboratives' as a means of undertaking demonstration projects and transferring their lessons to other organisations (Institute of Medicine 2003b).

In Australia, some public health research centres have taken on the need to translate research into practice as their core business (Lumley, Brown & Gunn 2003). At a policy level, the Cooperative Research Centres Program exists to link researchers

with industry so that questions of practical significance become the focus for research efforts, and so the results of research are translated into commercial benefits for industry. Public health research is less amenable to commercialisation, but the CRCATSIH does exist. Translational research is also seen as core business for the Parenting Research Centre; the Institute for Safety, Compensation, Recovery and Rehabilitation Research (ISCRR); the Sax Institute; and the Centre for Military Health. In 2012, the NHMRC established a translational research faculty in light of its importance.

In considering the challenge of research dissemination in the Indigenous context, the CRCAH nominated the approaches summarised in Table 10.5. These lessons about targeted communication are relevant to and adaptable for all instances and issues.

For public health action to be effective, the knowledge base from research is only one aspect of what is required. There remains a need to understand

---

Box 10.12 The CRC for Aboriginal and Torres Strait Islander Health (CRCATSIH)

The CRCATSIH research program has the broad aim of improving Indigenous health outcomes. The 2012–14 research agenda is defined around three programs:

- **Program 1—Healthy Start, Healthy Life:** research focused on reducing the chronic illness risk across the life-course, and improving early intervention and chronic illness management.
- **Program 2—Healthy Communities and Settings:** research focused on the capacity of local communities and organisations to develop interventions that address the determinants of health across a range of local sectors and settings.
- **Program 3—Enabling Policy and Systems:** research enabling the reform of policy and programs, workforce development and whole-of-government approaches to Aboriginal and Torres Strait Islander health.

CRCATSIH is managed by the Lowitja Institute. This is an innovative research organisation whose board has a majority of Aboriginal members and brings together Aboriginal groups, academic institutions and government agencies to facilitate collaborative, evidence-based research into Aboriginal and Torres Strait Islander health. The CRCATSIH has twelve core partners, representing researchers, practitioners and policy-makers—the Australian Institute of Aboriginal and Torres Strait Islander Studies; the Central Australian Aboriginal Congress; Charles Darwin, Flinders, La Trobe, Queensland and Melbourne Universities; the Danila Dilba Health Service; the Commonwealth Department of Health and Ageing; the Northern Territory Department of Health and Community Services; the Menzies School of Health Research; and the Queensland Institute of Medical Research.

Source: Lowitja Institute (2012).

Table 10.5 Research dissemination in an Indigenous context

Audience	Media	Actions
Remote Aboriginal community organisations	Storytelling Visual Broadcast	Involve community members in research team
Other Indigenous community	Word of mouth Newsletters Displays	Target key community organisations Use community information officers
Health policy-makers and managers	Summary reports Networking	Formal launches Mailouts Workshops
Health-care providers	Manuals Journals	Training and training materials
Research community	Conferences Publications	Networking meetings
Wider community opinion leaders	Newsletters Media interviews	Awareness-raising via a range of media

Source: Chong, Cruse & Duffy (2002).

the perceptions, preferences and particular circumstances of each community or population group for whom public health action is required. There are times when such information is not available and will need to be collected through various means. There are other times when such information needs to be discussed and interpreted with the affected community to ensure there is a shared understanding of the issue and the appropriateness of action to be taken. Action research (or participatory research) is an approach that has been adopted in a number of public health action areas. Action research is based on a partnership between the researcher and the researched (be they individuals, communities or organisations). The research typically starts with a reflection on the adequacy of current activities. The research questions are then developed in order to help improve the current action. The research findings are then directed back to practitioners, who may modify current practices and develop new activities. The research cycle then starts again with reflection on the impact of the modified action, and so it goes on. What drives participatory action

research is the need to know in order to bring about the desired change (Wadsworth 1997).

An idealised model for translating data and research into evidence-based policy and practice is offered in Figure 10.2 (above). The challenge for public health research, however, extends beyond intervention effectiveness. Public health research questions are often multi-sectoral in nature, and have strong policy dimensions. If public health research is to serve public health action, the findings need to be translated into policy and practice across relevant sectors. This is likely to require:

- more research on the context for implementation, including different community settings and population groups
- mechanisms to bring researchers and decision-makers together—to agree on shared research questions and to consider the implications of research findings for action
- investment in research dissemination efforts, ranging from broad-based publication to

workforce training (Lomas 1997; Birch 1997; Oldenburg et al. 1997).

The VicHealth Knowledge Policy signals a strengthened focus by the organisation on knowledge and its uses for health promotion. Its objectives relate not only to knowledge arising from research but also to the synthesis and production of a broader range of knowledge types, and the translation of health-promotion knowledge into health-promotion practice as well as evaluation of health-promotion practice. According to the VicHealth Strategic Framework, a key role for the organisation is to support strategies that mediate the transfer of knowledge from the knowledge pool into the decision-making processes that structure health care and the determinants of health.

The Institute for Safety, Compensation and Recovery Research (ISCRR) is another example of an organisation that operates a different model for translating research. ISCRR is a joint venture established in 2009 between Worksafe Victoria, the Transport Accident Commission and Monash University. It brings together policy-makers and researchers in fields related to safety, compensation and recovery from injury and illness in occupational settings to identify priority research questions, develop appropriate methodologies for investigating them and implement the best approaches to translating research for relevant sectors.

Conclusion: From discovery to delivery

Data constitute the basic pieces of information that point to the need for action. Research points to what kinds of public health action would work. Investments in these 'discovery' activities are central to the capacity of public health systems to be prepared to tackle new, emerging issues. However, good information and good research are useful for public health 'delivery' only when they are linked to decision-makers and practitioners.

Problems arise, however, with existing data systems. There are numerous sets of data, yet often the information needed for public health action (that is, about specific risk factors, localities and population sub-groups) is difficult to find. These gaps are filled with one-off, cross-sectional surveys, which do not allow for ongoing monitoring of health issues. Investment in surveillance systems is thus needed, in order to obtain consistent and continuous data over time. From such an information infrastructure, indicator systems can be built to track specific health concerns and their determinants.

The rise of the EBM movement has challenged public health researchers and practitioners alike, in demanding better research and research-informed practice. In transferring the framework for evaluating clinical evidence to public health, however, some immediate problems arise (NPHP 2000b). First, many public health interventions cannot be randomised, often for ethical reasons. Second, since many public health interventions are implemented in a community setting, the social and cultural contexts become important, and these are often not well documented in the published literature. Third, the question of applicability is central to evaluating evidence for public health—that is, intervention effectiveness may be found in one population or community, but the experience may not be transferable to another group or place. Finally, there are many interventions that have not been evaluated, as they have been designed and implemented in response to local need, rather than from a research perspective. From this viewpoint, it is important to recognise that evidence from the scientific literature is one part of the knowledge base for public health, but there are other types of expertise to be drawn upon for designing public health interventions.

11

Human and financial resources:
Essential foundations for action

Challenge

Since the disintegration of the Soviet Union in 1991, the public health system in that region has collapsed because of a lack of human and financial resources. The transition from a socialist to a market-based economy has been accompanied by a severe economic crisis as state-owned industries have been sold or closed down, thus creating mass unemployment. An estimated 40 000 of these former state enterprises are now in the hands of criminals, resulting in widespread tax evasion. This denies governments the billions of dollars needed to run hospitals, pay school teachers and provide for public health needs. The result has been the return of epidemics of diseases (such as diphtheria, polio and syphilis) and exponential growth in AIDS, TB, alcoholism, drug use and suicide. Between 1991 and 1996, there was a 126 per cent increase in premature deaths among men. This has caused a decline in male life expectancy from 65 years in 1970 to 59 years in 2000. The Russian population also began to decline in 1992. By 1999 only 1.2 million babies were born, while 2.1 million people died.

Nowhere is the public health crisis highlighted more than in Russian prisons. An escalating crime rate has caused acute overcrowding, creating conditions for the emergence of new strains of multi-drug-resistant TB among one in five prisoners. The prison population was estimated at 1 million in 2003. During the Soviet era, all citizens were compelled to have an annual x-ray. Any infected individuals were sent to sanatoria for months. Now there is no centralised public health system to impose screening and treatment, so TB control measures have disintegrated. The lack of

236

finances has led to the deterioration of TB-related equipment and facilities, while the lack of protective clothing (even basic protective masks) has caused large numbers of doctors and nurses to resign rather than endanger their own health. Against this background has been widespread misuse of antibiotics.

Each year, about 50 000 infected prisoners have carried these multi-drug-resistant strains of TB into the general population. The lack of a TB control system now has international implications, as these new drug-resistant strains of TB have been spread into Scandinavia and Northern Europe by Russian émigrés.

While the World Health Organization (WHO) and other international organisations, such as Médecins Sans Frontières and the Red Cross, are now contributing medical and financial support, a significant part of the problem is getting people to continue their treatments. As patients are now charged for some drugs and services that previously were free, this means many patients are discharged before the completion of treatment. Many people also cannot afford to seek medical treatment when symptoms first arise, leading to further infections. Health workers and incentive programs to encourage continuation of treatment programs are needed as part of a coordinated plan. The use of such services and approaches to treatment programs has no history in Russia because of the Soviet era's use of coercion (Garrett 2001: 113–20; 151–2; 171–84; Filipov 2003).

How can we be sure that the general situation described for Russia is not emerging in Australia?

Introduction

To deliver public health services to meet community needs and expectations, the right mix of resources and an appropriate level of investment must be available. Beyond tackling the prevailing issues—be they a food-borne disease outbreak or an increase in skin cancer—the public health system must have the skills, resources and organisational arrangements in place to respond to changing health priorities in the community and unexpected health issues.

The delivery of public health services depends on having people and money. The organisations that deliver public health services, and the basis of their authority and their knowledge base have been described in the previous chapters in this part of the book. This chapter will describe the most basic resources needed for action in Australia: the public health workforce and financing of public health activities. Investment and maintenance are required to build public health infrastructure, just as they are needed to build other forms of infrastructure (such as bridges, laboratories or trained specialists). The chapter concludes with a discussion about who is responsible for infrastructure development, thus highlighting the complexity of a health system operating within a federalist governmental system.

Human resources: Is everyone a public health worker?

Public health activities are undertaken by a range of people. There are public health professionals who specialise in particular activities, such as surveillance, policy analysis or health education. Many health-care professionals, such as general practitioners and community health nurses, also incorporate public health activities into their daily routines. Managers of health services provide leadership and organisational support for public health activities. Other professionals, such as engineers and architects, contribute to public health when they design environments for living, working and health care. Journalists play important public health roles in presenting human stories in the media that open up to debate such sensitive public health issues as suicide, road safety or sexuality. Community members also contribute to public health when they identify issues that affect health, such as unsafe environments, or when they mobilise action that leads to improvements in the health of their communities. People are thus a most important resource for public health.

Roles and functions of the public health workforce

This complex array of players makes it difficult to clearly define the public health workforce. For the purpose of examining public health infrastructure, however, the human resources for public health will be defined as those who are involved in carrying out core public health functions. This definition is still broad and includes a multi-disciplinary

workforce that is employed in a variety of health and government organisations, but focuses on those people whose work wholly concerns public health and who identify as public health workers. Madden and Salmon (1999: 20) have identified three types of public health worker, as outlined in Box 11.2.

The major Australian employers of public health workers are also diverse: Commonwealth and state or territory departments of health, regional and area public health services, universities, hospitals and statutory organisations such as the Australian Institute of Health and Welfare and Australian National Preventive Health Agency (ANPHA). Diversity is also reflected in other employers, such as non-government organisations that address specific diseases—for example, the National Heart Foundation, Diabetes Australia and the Cancer Councils, health-promotion foundations and the many community groups who focus on the health of specific populations, such as people with disabilities, younger people and Aboriginal and Torres Strait Islander people.

Box 11.1 A day in the life of a public health worker

Environmental health officer in a disease-control unit

Consistent with your commitment to a healthy environment, your morning begins by cycling to work. Your first job is the handover from the overnight on-call medical officer to check on outstanding work, as some diseases (such as measles and Legionnaire's disease) need urgent attention. You then contact the person who is handling tracing, and decide whether any site visits need to be organised.

Site visits are usually required for outbreaks of Legionnaire's disease, blue-green algal blooms and food-borne disease. While most of your day will be concerned with following up notifications of suspected outbreaks, at various times you will need to arrange

the dissemination of information to managers and the press office. By about 4.00 p.m., you can start writing the necessary routine reports and, if time allows, read journal articles and relevant textbooks in preparation for writing an article for publication.

Amid these tasks through the whole day, you will receive phone calls from the general public about head lice, travel health queries, hazardous incident reports, potential bio-terrorist incidents and a range of other matters that will call on the many skills you have acquired in training and on the job—such as risk assessment, health education, negotiation, mediation and communication.

Maternal and child health nurse

First thing in the morning, you check the problems relating to the previous day by phoning the respective mothers and checking the 'crying baby service'.

Next, you check what baby home visits are required and collect the biscuits for the new mothers' group (with about fifteen attendees) that you will run later in the morning. After lunch, the baby clinic operates, which covers health, developmental status and vaccinations—and picks up any issues the mothers might have about their own mental and physical condition, as feelings of anxiety and sometimes depression are common in new mothers. The babies are then checked by a medical officer. You then have to organise a playgroup for disadvantaged sole-parent families. The remainder of your afternoon revolves around returning phone calls and writing reports.

Policy analyst/lobbyist for a public health NGO

Each morning, you read the daily newspapers and view any relevant TV programs to see whether a story has been published that relates to the interests of your NGO. This could be a current campaign focusing on changes that either the federal or state government is proposing to a specific policy, or it may relate to legislation that is currently being debated. You then have to decide what type of action to take. For an immediate response, you can contact the relevant journalist working for a newspaper, radio or TV program. An alternative is to try to participate in talkback radio.

As a lobbyist, you will also spend time trying to directly persuade politicians to vote on legislation in a way that favours your organisation. This means that you must stay ahead of public opinion on issues and maintain regular contact with the respective federal and state ministers and their advisers. You also need to talk with backbench politicians who are known to be interested in the issue.

By mid-morning, your attention may turn to contacting the various people involved in the current campaign to get updates about a public meeting that will be held in the near future. Next is a meeting away from the office with a community group whose members are anxious about how the proposed policy changes being considered by their local council will affect them. They are requesting that you intervene on their behalf.

During the afternoon, you have to finish a report that analyses the implications of a new piece of federal legislation for the people represented by your NGO. If time permits, you may also complete the background research for the draft of a speech that you will be presenting to the meeting mentioned above, or write an article for the opinion pages of a daily newspaper.

Box 11.2 Types of public health worker

Generalist: These public health workers are required to take a broad perspective on issues, and are usually found in positions where resources and the organisational structure demand multiple skills. They can be found in positions that range from public service management, to areas of social need (e.g. drugs and alcohol), to rural areas.

Specialist: These public health workers have knowledge or skills pertaining to a particular area or setting or a higher level of skill than generalist workers.

Examples include epidemiologists, health-promotion workers and environmental health workers.

Health workers with public health components embedded in their professional practice: These workers are employed in professional roles that can include, but are not solely concerned with, public health. An example is health professionals working in an active clinical practice role (GPs and community health nurses). They need to have an understanding of evidence-based health care and population health (which is now included in general practice training).

Box 11.3 Core knowledge and skills (competencies) necessary for public health work

- Management skills, including management of change, resource management and organisational development
- Service planning
- Inter-sectoral working
- Whole-of-government approaches
- Team-building
- Community consultation/community planning
- Communication and negotiation
- Establishment and maintenance of information technology skills to support email and internet access
- Maintenance of datasets
- Descriptive epidemiology and surveillance
- Knowledge of infectious diseases
- Evidence-based practice
- Program/service evaluation
- Intervention designs
- Health promotion

Source: Madden & Salmon (1999: 20).

Such a workforce also requires specialised knowledge and skills, or competencies, with different levels of sophistication throughout a department or organisation, reflecting the variations in public health functions, duties and responsibilities.

Workforce education and training: Getting into the team

The development of the community health program in the 1970s led to concerns about whether the health workforce was sufficiently prepared to work in a different way—to be able to address broader determinants of health and work in multi-disciplinary teams, in community settings and in partnership with a wide range of organisations. This focused attention on preparation programs for public health

professionals, such as undergraduate, postgraduate and practice-based education and training.

Since 1910, responsibility for public health education in Australia had been vested in one training institution located in Townsville, which was under Commonwealth control, known initially as the Australian Institute of Tropical Medicine. This evolved into the sole national School of Public Health, located at the University of Sydney. Until the late 1980s, postgraduate education for public health was only accessible in Sydney. Various reviews of public health workforce development needs in Australia during the 1980s and 1990s focused on the importance of providing training at the postgraduate level, particularly to redress the gaps in skills in the health workforce and develop the competencies required for the public health workforce as a whole.

Public health degree programs

In the United States and elsewhere in the world, the dominant training program for entry into the public health workforce is a Master of Public Health (MPH) degree. The Schools of Public Health are accredited on the basis of being institutions independent of medical schools, and five disciplines constitute the core training for public health professionals: public health administration; epidemiology; biostatistics; social and behavioural sciences; and environmental health. Cross-cutting skills have also been defined for specialists in these public health disciplines: analytic skills; communication skills; policy development and program planning skills; cultural skills; and public health sciences (Turnock 2012).

Developments in public health education, training and professional development in Australia accelerated in the 1980s, following the release of *Australia's Bicentennial Health Initiative: Independent Review of Research and Educational Requirements for Public Health and Tropical Health* (White 1986). In line with that report, the expansion of MPH programs in the late 1980s occurred within Faculties of Medicine, and had a strong orientation towards epidemiology and public health research. In response, non-medical institutions, such as Health Science Faculties, began to develop programs with a strong orientation towards health promotion and with a foundation in the social sciences.

Why do people choose to enrol in these MPH programs and how have the courses been useful to their work? In 2004, a survey of 655 current and past students found that the main reasons they enrolled in the Victorian MPH program were to expand their public health knowledge (34 per cent), to help obtain a change in their career (25 per cent) and to gain employment in public health (14 per cent). In general, students found that while their MPH did not equate with an increased salary, or particularly help them obtain their current positions, they did feel that their training was relevant to their jobs and prepared them for other public health positions (Steering Committee of the Victorian Consortium for Public Health 2004).

In the early 1990s, a number of undergraduate public health programs were also developed, along with doctoral-level training in public health. The expansion of workforce training at different levels raised the question of what the core skills of the public health workforce should be, and what competencies should be acquired at each level of training.

A national education framework was proposed in 2002 to define the learning outcomes from MPH programs (that is, what students and employers can expect from MPH graduates). Subsequent to the identification of core public health functions, competencies were developed as a tool for ensuring the quality of graduates of public health courses in Australia. Competencies considered essential for graduates of MPH programs, consisting of 105 elements in total, are described within areas of practice that cover health surveillance, health promotion and disease control, policy and management, and evidence-based population health practice (Box 11.4) (PHAA 2009).

Undergraduate public health education

While public health education programs traditionally have been offered at the postgraduate level to students from a variety of disciplines, undergraduate teaching that focuses on health promotion and environmental health is now becoming more widespread. This raises the question of how effective undergraduate courses are in preparing graduates for the increasing diversity of public health workforce functions.

In 2001, a survey was conducted of 88 graduates of the University of Adelaide's Bachelor of Health Sciences degree, which is a traditional generalist public health program. At the time of the survey, 59 per cent of graduates were employed in the public health workforce, with the most common activity being health research (44 per cent), health program support (10 per cent), health planning and policy (9 per cent) and health education, management and promotion (8 per cent). They rated their generic skills as being the most useful in the workplace. These included working collaboratively, reading and summarising literature, and verbal and written communication skills. Of the specific public health skills, epidemiology, understanding the Australian health system and occupational health and safety were rated as the most useful.

While the study showed that a generalist degree does provide a basis for entering the public health workforce, 85 per cent of the graduates were undertaking or had completed further study. Thus, 'it appears that graduates already in the workforce are identifying areas of further study they wish to pursue, rather than finding it necessary to obtain further qualifications to find employment' (Houghton, Braunack-Mayer & Hiller 2002: 178).

Practice-based training

In the 1990s, while the federal government provided funding incentives for tertiary education institutions to work cooperatively in consortia to offer postgraduate education programs in public health, a number of health authorities opted to support

---

Box 11.4 Foundation competencies for Master of Public Health graduates in Australia

Area of practice	Unit of competency
Health monitoring and surveillance	1 Monitor and evaluate population health data or indicators
	2 Analyse the quality of findings from a surveillance or screening program
Disease prevention and control	3 Plan a disease-prevention/control strategy
	4 Formulate and implement a response to a public health emergency
Health protection	5 Describe environmental health safety standards and related management procedures
	6 Map and analyse the environmental determinants that contribute to disease in a given community or population
	7 Design an environmental health intervention in a given community or population
Health promotion	8 Prioritise population/community health needs
	9 Plan and evaluate evidence-based health-promotion initiatives
Health policy planning and management	10 Develop an advocacy strategy regarding a population health issue to influence public policy
	11 Articulate key funding mechanisms and finance sources, and distinguish costs and benefits in relation to specific population health projects/programs
	12 Analyse a government population health policy
	13 Analyse/evaluate the management of a population-level program/project
Evidence-based professional population health practice	14 Design a systematic, appropriate and ethical population health study and synthesise and articulate findings
	15 Describe core principles of just, ethical/legal public health practice
	16 Collect, organise, critically analyse and articulate secondary information
	17 Analyse own professional strengths and personal skills to work effectively with others and in teams
	18 Enable an environment of cultural safety
	19 Undertake a stakeholder analysis

Source: ANAPHI (2009).

---

stronger practice-based training programs. A public health traineeship scheme began first in New South Wales and was later instituted in Victoria. The proposed new model for the Victorian Public Health Training Scheme allocates scholarships to trainees rather than institutions, providing incentives for courses to meet requirements set out by the scheme (CEIPS 2012). Some examples of roles graduates of the Victorian Public Health Training Scheme take up include doctoral studies and policy roles, advising in areas such as alcohol and drugs, problem gambling,

Indigenous health, lifestyle risk factors and oral health. A Master of Applied Epidemiology (MAE), initially funded by the federal government, was offered through the Australian National University but based on placements—largely in state health authorities—across the country. The graduates of these schemes have taken up management and leadership positions all over Australia, and many MAE graduates have contributed to solving public health emergencies around the world, such as the SARS crisis in 2003.

Box 11.5 Fast-tracked: On-the-job training

The New South Wales Ministry of Health initiated a public health officer training program in 1990 on the basis that a series of supervised work placements provides the best approach to bridging academic studies in public health and the development of a professional public health practitioner. Over a three-year period, trainees take at least three rotations and, depending on length of placement, up to six rotations, across health services in New South Wales (including in rural areas) and gain experience across a variety of everyday public health activities. Placements are located within the New South Wales Ministry of Health, local population health organisations and New South Wales-funded research centres. The training program is based upon eleven competency areas of public health practice:

1 professional practice
2 management
3 epidemiology and biostatistics
4 information management
5 communication
6 health policy
7 health promotion
8 health evaluation
9 communicable diseases
10 risk assessment/management
11 health economics.

From day one, trainees may find themselves involved in solving such public health puzzles as a disease outbreak and having to communicate with the public or plan emergency responses in the case of bio-terrorist attacks. Graduates of the program find themselves truly 'tested' in a range of public health situations, and able to take leadership positions upon graduation.

The blossoming of multiple approaches and programs in public health has inevitably led to debates about the nature of the public health workforce. These have been focused on the extent to which public health is a specialisation and should be credentialled, the extent to which public health is a component of all health workers' jobs and the extent to which public health requires inter-sectoral collaboration and the engagement of other non-health professions as part of the public health workforce. In the United States, Schools of Public Health and public health education programs are accredited by the Council on Education for Public Health, and exams for voluntary credentialling have been introduced. Developments are occurring globally, public health education is expanding and accreditation processes have progressed to implementation. In India, new Schools of Public Health are under development and China has reviewed its national curriculum (Lin et al. 2009). In the United States in 2010, the core competencies were reviewed by a collaboration of academic and practice organisations, to encompass the varying levels of experience of public health professionals (PHF n.d.). Specific competencies have also been developed in the United States for particular areas of public health practice, including epidemiology, informatics, global health and emergency preparedness. Canada has released competencies for the public health workforce. Under the Bologna process in Europe, schools have been developing competencies with a view to educational harmonisation and, with the establishment of the European Agency for Accreditation of Public Health Education in 2011, the pilot phase commenced for the accreditation of MPH and equivalent courses (Otok et al. 2011).

Aboriginal and Torres Strait Islander health worker training

The role of the Aboriginal health worker is thought to have first developed in the 1950s, when Aboriginal women were employed as leprosarium workers; they were then appointed as medical assistants in the 1960s. It was further developed by community- and government-controlled health services and then expanded to include health promotion and community development. There have been problems with retaining Indigenous health workers, because the workforce is confronted by a variety of problems. There has been a lack of clarity about the role of such workers, particularly as each community in which they work has a unique set of cultural traditions and values. There have been problems with the coordination and planning of health worker training, both within and between the states and territories. Health workers themselves have raised questions about the quality—and relevance—of the training, as they are mainly being employed at the lower end of the wages scale, regardless of their experience. Furthermore, 40–60 per cent of health workers in some states and territories have no formal qualifications, despite the availability of training (Curtin Indigenous Research Centre 2000). The enHealth (2004) discussion paper on Indigenous environmental health workers argued that better funding arrangements were required to meet the growing environmental health needs of Indigenous communities. Indigenous environmental health workers also need to be recognised and supported by their peers and their community, because they are often involved in very stressful and contentious issues, such as housing insecurity. In 2010, Australian Health Ministers agreed that Aboriginal health workers would become a registered profession, under the National Registration and Accreditation Scheme that covers doctors, nurses, psychologists, dentists, physiotherapists and other registered health professionals. In 2011, the framework created to guide the development of the primary health-care workforce in Aboriginal health in the Northern Territory recommended the centralisation of the deployment and management of Aboriginal health workers to enable a comprehensive and strategic approach to training (AMSANT 2011).

Vocational training

In 2004, the Australian National Training Authority added qualifications and competency standards for population health workers to its Health Training Package. The training package, which includes units from the Community Services Training Package, offers qualifications such as a Diploma in Population Health. It is designed as an entry-level qualification, or to provide an additional qualification for those workers who have an existing specialist or clinical health qualification and contribute to the implementation of population health programs or projects by applying significant judgement in carrying out the broad plans devised by population health professionals. Examples of these workers are immunisation officer, gay men's educational support officer, community health worker, health promotion coordinator and senior project officer. A Diploma in Indigenous Environmental Health is also offered. For public health workers such as peer educators, who are providing basic support, such as implementing directives from superiors, a Certificate in Population Health and in Indigenous Environmental Health is offered for more senior personnel (Community Services and Health Training Australia 2004). In 2012, qualifications are offered in population health and Indigenous environmental health at certificate and diploma levels.

Public health leadership initiatives

Public health leadership has a distinctive community relations and advocacy role, which differs significantly from other leadership roles. In response, an increasing number of leadership training initiatives have been developed internationally. A premise for these programs is that many health professionals are highly proficient in their technical areas; however, advocacy and intersectoral partnership development are not typically achieved through their core or basic training. To work confidently, Coye (1994) argues, the culture of public health professionals needs to be transformed, and leadership development initiatives can play a key role. Professionals need to rise above their suspicion of the private sector and disdain for the medical care sector, shift away from a belief and reliance on public sector entitlements, develop greater appreciation for cost-effectiveness considerations and adopt organisational discipline and accountability.

In the United States, the Centers for Disease Control has supported a national Public Health Leadership Institute (PHLI) since the early 1990s, which has now spawned not only an alumni society but leadership programs for community-based leaders (for example, in the health of minority populations and women) and for specific program areas (such as reproductive health and substance abuse). In evaluating PHLI, Woltring, Constantine and Schwarte (2003) found that it had a measurable impact on the effectiveness of participants as leaders at organisational, community and personal levels; had enhanced their professional networks; and had created a commitment to the mentoring and training of others and lifelong learning. The Public Health Leadership Program is now offered at the UNC Gillings School of Global Public Health (Box 11.6).

The WHO Regional Office for the Western Pacific Region piloted an in-service health promotion leadership development program (Prolead) in 2004–05, which involved country-based teams working on specific policy projects related to health-promotion infrastructure and financing, and was assisted by the International Network of Health Promotion Foundations. Prolead has expanded to operate globally, with health-promotion leaders working on projects such as developing health-promotion foundations in Mongolia and Malaysia, implementing healthy cities in Bangalore (India) and Hue (Vietnam), and extending health-promotion partnerships in Fiji and Oman (Lin & Fawkes 2005b). By 2012, 127 fellows had been through the program, the evaluation of which has pointed to changes at individual, network and partnership, and policy and system levels.

Workforce planning: Nurturing and investment needed

For governments to invest in workforce training—undergraduate, postgraduate or in-service education and training—it is necessary to assess how many of which types of public health worker are needed. This calculation is complex. It is necessary to know how many are currently in the field, how well their skill base matches needs, and whether there are any shortages. The public health workforce is not composed of 'public health specialists', but

---

Box 11.6 Public Health Leadership Program

The Public Health Leadership Program at the University of North Carolina offers certificate and graduate degree courses in public health leadership via both traditional and distance-learning formats, developing population-level knowledge and skills with an interdisciplinary emphasis. Students participate and learn collaboratively, building upon varied professional experience.

The leadership topics offered in the curriculum of the Public Health Leadership Certificate are based upon competencies defined by the Council on Linkages Between Academia and Public Health Practice and the National Public Health Leadership Development Network. The three core units are:
- leadership style
- project management principles and practice
- core principles of leadership.

Students also choose one of six elective topics, including:
- quality improvement
- marketing
- policy development
- community assessment
- program planning and evaluation
- interdisciplinary approaches to occupational health.

Source: Gillings School of Global Public Health (n.d.)

rather people performing a number of functions that require 'the exercise of some specific expertise not usually associated with that person's primary occupational orientation' (Rotem 1995: 24). Hence workforce planning in public health is much more challenging than planning for other health practitioners (such as doctors, nurses and clinical allied health professionals).

Decision-making about personal health care workers is, on the other hand, often based on previous demand and supply data. This means the workforce required for the provision of personal health care can be predicted more readily on the basis of data associated with administration functions, such as hospital morbidity, and the workforce involved in personal health care can be counted through other administrative by-product data, such as professional registration. With the regulation of the health workforce shifting from the state to the national level, the Australian Health Practitioner Regulation Agency collects workforce data as part of the registration process, while Health Workforce Australia (HWA) undertakes health workforce planning.

Information on the public health workforce has not been easy to obtain because it involves professionals from a variety of disciplines who do not require professional licensure. Another major challenge for public health workforce planning is that the investment in public health activities is highly dependent on policy and managerial decision-making. As financial resources, community priorities or health problems change, a shift in public health workforce demand may occur. Such changes in policy direction can create an expansion within one or more public health functions, and discontinuities or relocations in others. These changes have implications for both public health workers and the services they provide. New policy developments can lead to whole new structures within departments and organisations, such as those for HIV/AIDS services and bio-terrorism preparedness (see, for example, Chapter 3, which describes the departmental and structural changes within the Commonwealth and state Departments of Health).

The predilection for ad hoc project activities causes great variability in the public health work undertaken (Ridoutt et al. 2004). Shifts in policy create short-term shifts in the demand for labour, which often creates shortages in particular areas, such as those identified in 1999: skilled biostatisticians, and people with expertise in health services research, health economics and health policy (Ridoutt et al. 2002). With major expansion of programs under the COAG National Prevention Partnership Payment arrangements, Closing the Gap (in Aboriginal health) and Medicare Locals, there are now major demands for a health promotion workforce to work in local government, school and workplace settings, Aboriginal communities and primary care, on such issues as tobacco, alcohol, overweight and obesity, physical activity and such chronic illnesses as diabetes. A study in the United States of the public health workforce (Bell & Khodeli 2004) found shortages in nursing, epidemiology, laboratory services and environmental health that were being compounded by high turnover rates and an ageing workforce with high retirement eligibility.

The ageing of the public health workforce in Australia has yet to be considered in workforce planning, and its small size and diversity means HWA has not considered the public health workforce to be a priority within its remit. The multi-disciplinary nature of the public health workforce in Australia is reflected in the membership of the national professional association for health professionals who work in over 40 different public health-related occupations. While individual organisations have undertaken specific workforce-planning efforts, such as the Faculty of Public Health Medicine in the Royal Australian College of Physicians working on estimation of need and the Australian Health Promotion Association developing competencies and sponsoring mentoring programs, there remains a gap in knowledge about what the Australian public health workforce should look like in the future.

How to identify workforce needs

The diversity of the occupational groups that comprise the public health workforce, ranging from those people who actively identify themselves as a public health worker to those people who have a public health function as part of their job description, makes it difficult to calculate demand for public health workers.

One way to ascertain the demand for public health workers is to look at what personnel and skills employers are requesting when advertising vacancies. A study conducted for the National Public Health Partnership (NPHP) (Rotem et al. 2004) scanned advertisements that appeared during June and July 2003 in the major newspapers and on websites of government agencies, employment agencies and professional organisations in each state. Some 500 job descriptions were then analysed, with the details about the employer, location, workplace setting, discipline/domain of activity, responsibilities and specific duties, level within the organisations, and salary and conditions being entered into a database.

The study 'highlighted the great emphasis given by employers to generic professional capabilities at the personal and inter-personal levels that are commonly required [for the] management and delivery of public health programs' (Rotem et al. 2004: 16). What differentiates public health workers is the 'health oriented nature of the training, capabilities and experience. This is reflected in the wide range of domains and disciplines mentioned in job titles, roles and responsibilities and the variety of formal qualifications deemed requisite or desirable' (2004: 16–17). 'Health' degrees were required in over 50 per cent of the advertisements, while management qualifications were only required in 10 per cent. The largest group (37.4 per cent) of advertisements were positions for project and program officers, coordinators and managers. The second group (10.1 per cent) comprised service directors and managers, while the smallest numbers related to three positions for epidemiologists and one for a statistician (2004: 3).

Given the difficulty of workforce planning at the system level, Ridoutt et al. (2004: 9) have proposed the adoption of a planning model at the organisational level to identify the public health workforce, which places social and service goals at the centre rather than the staff as service providers. Such a model would contain four steps:

1 Identify/measure future goals, the activities needed to achieve them and measure progress.
2 Determine what information, priorities or program changes from within an organisation generate demand for public health services.
3 Detail the organisational competencies necessary to achieve the defined goals and to implement actions.
4 Describe the competency set that is required for the future workforce.

While such a planning model might assist with determining needs for the 'generic' public health practitioner, questions remain about how to plan for the requirements of the more specialist workers, such as epidemiologists, health economists and others with a stronger orientation towards research-based work. The challenges are twofold: first, the market—private sector organisations, such as pharmaceutical companies, might offer lucrative positions so the shortage is felt in the public sector and the public sector is unable to retain graduates; and, second, career structure—as research funding is often project-based, there are few ongoing positions for researchers and career pathways are limited.

These problems are not unique to Australia. A report in the United Kingdom (Wellcome Trust 2004) suggested that there was a need for coordinated decision-making about public health research priorities and appropriate levels of support for them, along with a program of long-term investment in the academic infrastructure for public health science. The report further suggested that partnerships between universities and government

Box 11.7 enHealth Environmental Health Officer Skills and Knowledge Matrix

In 2009, the Victorian Department of Human Services conducted the Environmental Health Officer Skills, Knowledge and Experience Workforce Project to develop a skills and knowledge matrix that could underpin a national approach to managing environmental health workforce issues. The environmental health role is a role in transition, shifting from narrow compliance-based inspection and surveillance activities to approaches based on risk-management and evidence-based decision-making.

The expanding nature and scope of environmental health are shaped by an increasing awareness of the relationships between the natural and built environments and human health. Emerging challenges associated with climate change and resource depletion are being acknowledged, and these point to a continuing expansion in both the role of and demand for environmental health officers.

Identifying the skills and knowledge to undertake environmental health roles is seen as a first step towards delivering a sustainable level of environmental workforce capability. The skills and knowledge matrix aims to provide the basis for building a shared understanding about the nature of environmental health work and the related skills and knowledge required to undertake it.

The matrix is structured in three parts, reflecting distinct types of skills and knowledge.

Part 1

Adopts the generic learning outcomes required by the Australian Qualifications Framework for degree-level graduates:

- the acquisition of a systematic and coherent body of knowledge, the underlying principles and concepts, and the associated communication and problem-solving skills

- the development of the academic skills and attributes necessary to undertake research, and to comprehend and evaluate new information, concepts and evidence from a range of sources
- the development of the ability to review, consolidate, extend and apply the knowledge and techniques learnt, including in a professional context
- a foundation for self-directed and lifelong learning
- interpersonal and teamwork skills appropriate to employment and/or further study.

Part 2

Describes underpinning skills and knowledge that support environmental health work covering:
- science
- public and environmental health concepts
- research methods
- the political, legislative and policy context
- risk assessment and risk management
- compliance and enforcement
- communication, cultural awareness and interpersonal skills
- administration and management

Part 3

Describes activity-specific skills and knowledge relating to:
- safe and suitable food
- prevention and control of notifiable and communicable conditions
- water management
- environmental management
- land-use management
- the built environment
- Indigenous environmental health
- sustainability and climate change
- emergency and incident management.

Source: enHealth (2009).

public health delivery were needed, including joint posts, greater workforce mobility, commissioning of research and evaluation in support of prevention programs, and joint training. Finally, the report suggested that more informed dialogue between public health scientists and policy-makers would improve not only the position of public health science, but contribute to evidence-based decision-making.

Funding for public health: Shaking the money tree

Government investment

Investment in public health in Australia historically came from the state governments, although some activities (such as health inspections, and maternal and child health services in Victoria) had been devolved to local governments in particular states. Although community fundraising was an important source of funding for NGOs, government dollars constituted the major portion of available resources.

With the development of community health services in the 1970s, there was an expansion of resources in community-based organisations and of the public health activities delivered through those organisations. In the 1980s, there was a growth in Commonwealth–state cost-shared funding arrangements for public health programs. Resources grew for both publicly funded and non-government organisations. For the 30 years between the mid-1960s and the mid-1990s, the absolute quantum of expenditure on public health and community health increased, but the proportion of government expenditure hovered around 5 per cent of total health expenditure (Deeble 1999a). Because of differing administrative structures across jurisdictions, expenditure for public health and community health during this period should be examined together. As can be seen from Table 11.1, the larger amount of growth was in community health funding.

Subsequently, while actual government expenditure on public health more than doubled from $915 million in 1999–00 to $2300 million in 2008–09, during this period the proportion of health expenditure allocated to public health also increased by a factor of just under one-quarter, peaking at 3.2 per cent in 2007–08, due to purchase of the Human Papilloma Virus vaccine (Table 11.2). Commencing in 1997, a new approach was introduced, so called 'broadbanding', which involved Public Health Outcome and Funding Agreements, to provide funding for public health programs from the federal government to the states and territories, allowing flexibility about which programs are funded (and how) according to local population needs and changing focus from inputs to outputs (CHERE 2007).

The three core public activities that received the largest level of expenditure from all governments in 2008–09 were:

Table 11.1 Expenditure on public health and community health, 1963–1996

	1963–64	1966–67	1975–76	1985–86	1995–96
Actual expenditure ($m)					
Public health	35	46	130	152	515
Community health	42	56	194	689	2157
As % of total recurrent health expenditure					
Public health	4.1	4.1	3.3	0.9	1.3
Community health	0.8	0.9	1.6	3.1	4.2
As % of GDP	0.2	0.3	0.4	0.3	0.5

Source: abridged from Deeble (1999a).

Table 11.2 Government expenditure on public health, 1999–2009

	1999–00	2001–02	2003–04	2006–07	2007–08	2008–09
Total public health expenditure ($ million)	915	1091	1263	1727	2180	2300
Public health as a proportion of total health expenditure (%)	2.6	2.7	2.6	2.8	3.2	2.8

Source: adapted from AIHW (2011e).

- organised immunisation (27.8 per cent)
- selected health promotion (19.1 per cent)
- screening programs (14.6 per cent).

However, the priorities were slightly different between the governments. The Commonwealth government's largest expenditure was on public health research, followed by selected health promotion and prevention of hazardous and harmful drug use, while for the state/territory governments, the largest expenditures were on organised immunisation, selected health promotion and then communicable disease control (AIHW 2011e).

As well, patterns of expenditure vary between the states and territories. Differences in absolute investments obviously vary with population size and geography. Nonetheless, significant differences exist across Australia, as can be seen from Table 11.3 (AIHW 2011).

The level of resourcing for most state-based programs has either been determined by public service positions or based on submissions from service providers. With the new Commonwealth–state cost-shared programs developed in the 1980s, a range of funding formulae have been in use. Allocation by population (as a proportion of the total Australian population) is often used to determine the funding base. However, programs targeted for particular population groups (such as women aged 50–70 for breast screening or people who are HIV positive) or for particular activities (for example, immunisation, methadone treatment or births assisted by midwives) may have their funding adjusted by the specific program criteria.

The most significant injections of additional funding for public health have occurred when governments have become concerned about public health emergencies or looming crises.

Table 11.3 Expenditure on public health activities across Australia ($ million), 2008–09

Activity	NSW	Vic.	Qld	WA	SA	Tas.	ACT	NT	Total
Communicable disease control	85.2	47.0	46.0	30.1	16.8	7.0	8.7	19.0	259.8
Selected health promotion	64.5	102.0	55.0	29.3	27.2	6.6	6.3	14.5	305.4
Organised immunisation	196.5	127.6	114.6	50.5	37.4	12.9	10.7	24.5	574.7
Environmental health	15.0	6.7	25.8	13.2	5.6	4.8	3.2	5.2	79.6
Food standards and hygiene	4.9	1.9	2.0	3.2	2.6	0.5	3.0	1.0	19.0
Screening programs	64.2	52.1	56.3	18.5	17.4	6.1	3.7	7.5	225.8
Prevention of hazardous and harmful drug use	32.8	22.6	46.7	23.7	24.4	7.3	3.8	11.0	172.4
Public health research	7.1	7.5	1.4	5.6	4.9	0.3	0.3	2.6	29.7
Total expenditure	**470.0**	**367.5**	**347.9**	**174.1**	**136.3**	**45.6**	**39.6**	**85.4**	**1666.4**

Source: AIHW (2011e).

Following SARS in 2003, there was increased funding in the 2004–05 budget: $33 million for an emergency medicine stockpile, disease surveillance and public health laboratories, health security legislation and incidence response (Lin & Robinson 2005). In 2005, COAG committed significant funding ($500 million, cost-shared, over five years) for the Australian Better Health Initiative to develop a comprehensive approach to prevention and control of chronic disease (DoHA 2006), given OECD data that showed relatively low Australian labour force productivity related to the burden of chronic illness. Since the election of the Labor government in 2007, $872 million in additional national funding has been made available for preventive health measures, such as healthy communities ($23 million), healthy children ($325.5 million), healthy workplaces ($294.6 million), and closing the life expectancy gap between Indigenous and other Australians ($334.8 million) (DoHA 2010a).

Extending sources of funding

Given the limitations of government funding, public health advocates have worked creatively on other sources of funding. 'Sin tax' has become an obvious source, insofar as a public argument can be mounted that the profits from those products that lead to ill-health—such as tobacco and alcohol—should be used for prevention programs (a strategy known as tax hypothecation). In 1987, Victoria was the first state to pass legislation to earmark money raised from tobacco taxes for health-promotion programs. Western Australia followed suit in 1991. This approach also has been adopted in a number of other countries, as Table 11.4 illustrates. Other countries have also levied health insurance funds.

The advent of tobacco tax hypothecation for health-promotion foundations has expanded resources available for research and pilot programs, and for programs outside the health sector, in part because the funds had to be used for 'sponsorship buy-out' (that is, to replace the previous tobacco sponsorship of arts and sports programs). The

Table 11.4 Health-promotion financing legislation

Country/State	Year of legislation	Share of revenue	Revenue source	Defined purpose
Thailand	2010	2% + 2%	Tobacco, alcohol	Health promotion
Tonga	2007	Appropriation		NCD health promotion
Malaysia	2006	Appropriation	National treasury	Health promotion
Austria	1998	Fiscal adjustments	Value-added tax	Health promotion
Korea	1997	$0.12/capita/annum	Health insurance	Health promotion
Switzerland	1994	× Euro/insured p/yr	Health insurance	Health promotion
Portugal	1991	1%	Tobacco tax	Cancer control
Western Australia	1990	Allocation, appropriation	Health promotion	
California, USA	1988	20%	Tobacco surtax (25 cents per pack)	Tobacco control
Victoria, Australia	1987	5%	Tobacco gross sale	Health promotion
Iceland	1984	0.2%	Tobacco gross sale	Anti-smoking
Finland	1976	0.45%	Tobacco excise tax	Health education and promotion

Sources: Vertio & Catford (1995); INHPF (2012).

Victorian model became the model for ThaiHealth, the health promotion foundation in Thailand, funded from taxes on two products—tobacco and alcohol. Similar legislation has been passed or is under development in the Republic of Korea, Malaysia, Mongolia, Tonga, Samoa, Vietnam, the Lao People's Democratic Republic and the Solomon Islands. More health promotion foundations can be expected around the world as the result of the WHO's Framework Convention on Tobacco Control.

Legislation and organisational infrastructure do not in themselves ensure the continued expansion or existence of public health programs. In the 1990s, the Victorian government imposed severe budget cuts in the health sector. With a separate fund for health promotion, the Health Department was able to 'cost-shift' and withdraw from funding health-promotion activities. The South Australian Health Department absorbed its health-promotion foundation back into the department. After a successful High Court challenge by the tobacco industry in 1996 to the constitutional basis of earmarked taxes, the federal government now collects and passes on the tax to the states, and health-promotion foundations receive their allocations as part of the regular state Budget process.

Internationally, some countries (for example, the Netherlands, France and Germany) expanded resources for public health through health insurance funds, rather than tobacco tax. The funding raised in this manner has occurred either as payments for specific procedures (such as smoking cessation advice) or as direct grants to community-based health promotion programs (Vertio & Catford 1995). In Finland, gambling monopoly profits are distributed to NGOs for health-promotion activities. How countries pursue different financing options appears to be related to:

- political economy (i.e. market, planned)
- income level of the country and resources available in its health sector (e.g. low, medium)

- current sources for health financing (e.g. tax, out-of-pocket, social security)
- emerging options arising from health sector reforms (e.g. social health insurance, sin tax, donor aid) (WHO 2003b).

Bringing the marketplace into health promotion opens up many opportunities, but for the potential of these to be realised a number of conditions need to be in place: there must be a shared understanding about the respective roles of the purchaser and provider; purchasers must have adequate skills; the funding needs to be earmarked for investment in health promotion (to prevent 'raiding' by other health sectors); an effective monitoring and regulatory process needs to be in place; and training must be provided for the new tasks and responsibilities. If this private investment is not managed correctly, it may contribute to increased health inequalities, ethical issues may be ignored and health-promotion practice may be compromised (Catford 1995).

In more recent times, there have been proposals to develop public–private partnerships as a means of expanding the resource base for public health. The WHO has entered into agreements with multinational corporations, philanthropic organisations and other multilateral agencies for product development and distribution (for example, anti-retro-viral drugs, vaccines, anti-malarial drugs), and for specific disease-control programs (such as trachoma, filariasis) (Reich 2002). Since the launch of the International Health Partnership in 2007, to bring together private sector funders as well as development assistance from bilateral and multilateral funders, 31 countries and 25 development partners have entered into partnership agreements (IHP+ 2012).

Within Australia, given the Budget cuts of the 1990s, there have been particular concerns among public health advocates that a public–private partnership is a means for government to withdraw from its responsibility for public health activities. At the same time, the need for intersectoral

---

Box 11.8 Principles for developing a public–private partnership (PPP)

Principle 1: Value for money

- Factors that add value to a PPP proposal include innovation, risk transfer, improved asset utilisation, ownership and management synergies, and improved project management.
- Value for money is to be tested by comparing the outputs and costs of PPP proposals against the most efficient and best practice public sector delivery option likely to be achieved for the relevant project.
- Agencies should be encouraged to specify deliverables in terms of service outputs rather than on the basis of inputs.

Principle 2: Transparency

- Use of PPPs should not diminish the availability of information to parliament, taxpayers and other stakeholders on the use of government resources.
- Agencies must ensure that appropriate mechanisms are in place to meet established reporting requirements.

Principle 3: Accountability

- Agencies are responsible for the delivery of their outputs; where PPPs are used to deliver those outputs, agencies are not able to transfer accountability to a private sector entity.

Source: Department of Finance and Administration (2006).

---

collaborations for health improvement also requires that partnerships are formed. The challenge is to be clear about the ethical issues, and to have a set of transparent and known business rules that can govern the partnership.

Value for money: Improved decision-making in resource allocation or better advocacy?

In the 1990s, with neo-liberal reforms and Budget cuts, the voices of medicine and social movements were overshadowed by the dominance of economics. Government rhetoric was concerned increasingly with 'value for money', and how to improve allocation of limited resources became the main concern within government departments.

In 1993, the Victorian government introduced casemix-based funding for all hospitals with over 100 beds, as the first Australian jurisdiction to do so—which meant that these hospitals received their income on the basis of the clinical profile of patients treated. As the introduction of casemix funding was accompanied by Budget cuts, hospitals had to change their internal management systems

to avoid a budget deficit (Walker et al. 1996), and earlier patient discharge from hospitals increased the workload for community health services. But the allocative decision for public health was more difficult: there are no patients to count, and it is not clear what level of effort is required to prevent disease. Such activity-based funding is now being introduced across Australia as part of new national health reforms. The implications for public health is as yet unknown.

Establishing value for money in regard to some public health activities is a complex undertaking for several reasons. The outputs of public health activities consist of information about the health status of the population at a given point in time, and changes in factors that contribute to the health problem. However, the links between the outputs of particular preventive activities and longer-term health outcomes can be difficult to assess with certainty. At the program level, program activities and their impact on factors believed to favourably/unfavourably influence health are the most measurable outputs. There are many intermediate objectives that can be quantified—such as rates of smoking, dietary intake and the prevalence of a communicable disease—but the measurement of final effects that take time to develop is more difficult.

An additional problem arises from the structure of government budgets. The program budgeting framework typically separates funding for public health, hospitals, aged care, community health and so on into separate streams that are non-transferable. In theory, public health activities (and therefore expenditure) could be producing savings for hospitals, community health services or other program areas. However, in a practical sense it is difficult for these program areas to fund public health activities.

These problems of measuring output have led to the development of a variety of resource allocation techniques, such as program budgeting marginal analysis (discussed in Chapter 7), cost-effectiveness analysis (Box 11.9) and Health Benefit Groups (Box 11.10), for measuring the output, equity and efficiency of financial allocations (Deeble 2000).

Economic evaluation is applied at the intervention level while resource allocation decisions usually are made at the system level. Program budget marginal analysis was also developed as a way to bring economic analysis into administrative decision-making, and as an approach that recognises decision-making is a social process.

Economic evaluation—particularly cost-effectiveness analysis—was thought to be valuable, although in practice it was costly to conduct and did not always feed into decision-making. The multi-layered nature of Australian government means that each level will tend to be concerned about its own financial outlays, rather than the

---

Box 11.9 Use of cost-effective analysis in health promotion

A large five-year study was funded by the National Health and Medical Research Council (NHMRC) with the aim of providing a comprehensive analysis of the comparative cost-effectiveness of preventive intervention options for addressing the non-communicable disease burden in Australia, with a specific focus on Indigenous Australians. This study, entitled ACE Prevention, was the most comprehensive evaluation of health-prevention measures ever conducted worldwide, involving input from 130 top health experts. The research team assessed 123 illness-prevention measures to identify those that would prevent the most illness and premature deaths and those that represented the best value for money. For comparison purposes, 27 treatment interventions were also assessed.

The method used in the study involved modelling each intervention to apply to the relevant people in the 2003 Australian population and measuring the costs and health outcomes for as long as they occurred. Results were expressed as a cost per disability-adjusted life year (DALY) averted. Best available evidence on effectiveness of interventions was derived from the international literature. In formulating conclusions, stakeholders from government, health, academia and service organisations provided guidance to the researchers in relation to technical results and policy considerations, such as acceptability, feasibility and equity.

The study more than doubled the published economic appraisal research on health promotion/illness prevention in Australia. The main recommendations of the final report released in 2010 include taxation of tobacco, alcohol and unhealthy food; mandatory salt limits in bread, cereals and margarine; improved efficiency of blood pressure and cholesterol-lowering drugs; gastric banding for severe obesity; an intensive sunsmart campaign; increased screening for particular conditions, including pre-diabetes; subsidised nicotine replacement therapy; increasing physical activity; preventive interventions for particular mental disorders; and investment in evaluation research.

Box 11.10 Technical approaches to allocating resources across the public health system

Health Benefit Groups (HBGs) and Healthcare Resource Groups (HRGs) were introduced in the United Kingdom during the early 1990s as a tool to support decisions about resource allocation and the contracting out of health-care services. HBGs are a way of categorising the population on the basis of their health-care needs. They include those people not at risk, those at risk, those who have symptoms, those who have a confirmed disease and those with the ongoing consequences of disease. HRGs are a group of treatments that are clinically similar, use a similar amount of resources and can include health promotion, prevention, investigation and diagnosis, clinical management and continuing care. By developing a model based on HBGs/HRGs, and incorporating the appropriate process and outcomes indicators, it is possible to establish where health resources should be invested to obtain the greatest benefit in terms of health gain and cost/DALYs (Segal & Chen 2001).

HBGs/HRGs were applied to a study (for the Commonwealth Department of Health and Ageing) that was conducted to ascertain the cost-effectiveness of the current primary health-care services being provided for Aboriginal and Torres Strait Islander people in the Northern Territory, and the impact that any changes in investment patterns might have on cost-effectiveness and health outcomes. The model was based on Northern Territory data from the Australian Bureau of Statistics' population projections, coordinated care trials, and hospital morbidity and expenditure by the Northern Territory Department of Health and Community Service and the Commonwealth government. Five scenarios were modelled:

- **base model:** assumed that several levels would be provided in line with changes in costs, population and mortality

- **current situation:** assumed no real changes
- **funding decrease:** removed the Office for Aboriginal and Torres Strait Islander Health funding and its impact
- **changing mix:** changed the funding mix across diseases
- **funding increase:** doubled funding over ten years.

The main finding of the analysis was that the current projected funding allocations for the primary health care of Aboriginal and Torres Strait Islander people in the Northern Territory would not be sufficient to fund the treatment of the growing burden of chronic disease. This funding shortfall was estimated to be $7 million over five years, rising to $10 million over ten years, and within 20 years it could be $46 million. It would also impact on other parts of the health system (such as the Pharmaceutical Benefits Scheme, Medical Benefits Scheme and renal dialysis), creating a total cost of more than $136 million over five years, $470 million over ten years, and rising to $1261 million over 20 years (Beaver & Zhao 2004).

While there would be savings for the Commonwealth government if funding remains at current levels, the study found that such an effective withdrawal of resources would lead to delays in diagnosis and treatment, increased severity of chronic conditions and increased use of hospitals. The delays in diagnosis and treatment would lead to premature deaths and increased disability, which translates to a loss of healthy life years of 2.6 years over five years, 12.6 over ten years and 12.6 over 20 years (Beaver & Zhao 2004).

As the study was done in six weeks with limited expenditure and cost data available, the authors recommended that any future decision-making about funding and purchasing could be enhanced by a research program to develop a more comprehensive model and a new classification system that allowed for a comparison across the various sectors in terms of care programs and service delivery (casemix).

overall economic returns for the health system. Just as those who manage hospital budgets typically are concerned about managing their particular budgets, each level of government is concerned about its own budgets.

At the same time, public health economists (Richardson et al. 1995) suggest that conventional economic evaluation and resource allocation frameworks are insufficient, as the objective of maximising the well-being of the community from the financial resources available is not taken into consideration sufficiently. They suggest that the criteria for evaluating health-promotion programs should be:

- **technical efficiency:** achieving a desired objective at least cost
- **allocative efficiency:** trying to maximise the population health gain from a fixed allocation of resources (Appleby & Brambleby 2001: 109)
- **equity:** maximising the welfare of patients within the budget available and giving priority to those in most need (Dixon 2001: 327)
- **dynamic efficiency:** the extent to which the health-care system as a whole, and its constituent elements, can adapt to change and innovation (Duckett 2000: 229)
- **sustainability:** the ability of the system to maintain programs and health achievements
- **budgetary discipline:** managing within a predefined budget.

To achieve this broad approach, a number of preconditions need to be in place. There must be information available about the expected benefits of any program. Purchasers of these services must be well informed. There must be an institutional means of promoting and financing experimentation. A diversity of supply must also be in place. An independent process must exist to determine social justice principles. Finally, purchasers and regulators must have transparent roles and responsibilities (Richardson et al. 1995).

In the meantime, advocacy remains the primary strategy for increasing funding for public health programs. Advocacy, however, is no longer just a matter of appealing to governments on high moral grounds. It has to incorporate a sound economic argument. In the United States, the CDC began to undertake return on investment analysis. This was seen as a necessary (although not always sufficient) part of the policy process because it was difficult to justify proposed public health programs without being able to indicate the economic benefits. At the global level, the Commission for Macroeconomics and Health has also undertaken extensive studies on specific diseases (for example, TB, leprosy, HIV) to show that a significant scaling up of public health expenditure would contribute significantly to economic development (WHO 2001b). Similarly, in the United Kingdom, a major review of the resource requirements for a high-quality National Health Service in 2022 found that while more evidence about the effectiveness of public health programs was needed (especially cost-effectiveness), a number of interventions have been shown to be cost-effective on the basis of Quality-adjusted life years gained, such as interventions at most stages of pathway of disease development and progression for type 2 diabetes (Wanless 2004). The emerging investment for health approach includes a recognition of the importance of social and economic determinants in economic evaluation (WHO 2012).

In Australia, similar work was undertaken in the early 2000s, as highlighted by the Abelson Report, *Returns on Investment in Public Health* (2003a). The Abelson Report attempted to estimate the economic benefit, since 1970, of several public health programs, including programs to reduce tobacco consumption, coronary disease and HIV/AIDS; measles and Hib immunisation programs; and road safety programs to reduce road trauma. For each program, they estimated:

- the cost
- the estimated reduction in disease cases attributable to the disease

- the benefits of disease reduction in terms of increased longevity (life), improved quality of life and reduced health-care expenditures
- the total return to society of investment in public health activities
- savings to government.

The authors found that substantial gains had been achieved across all of these conditions in terms of disease (or injury) reduction. In 1998, an estimated 17 400 premature deaths were averted because of reduced tobacco consumption, including 6900 fewer deaths from coronary heart disease, 4000 from lung cancer, 3600 from bronchitis and chronic obstructive pulmonary disease and 2900 from strokes and from other cancers. The economic benefit of these public health programs was also substantial. The benefit in 1998 alone, due to reduced tobacco consumption since 1970, was $12.3 billion. This included longevity gains valued at $9.6 billion, improved health status gains of $2.2 billion and lower health-care costs of $0.5 billion (Abelson 2003a).

In a similar vein, an Australian case study of the economic ramifications of investing in population-level health-promotion programs (such as to prevent, reduce or delay the onset of type 2 diabetes) showed that they can make a favourable impact on important economic indicators (labour force participation, productivity gains and health outlays) as well as health outcomes (Murphy 2005). How the results of such studies might be built upon for improved resourcing of public health activities remains to be seen, although such reports raise the awareness of treasury officials and other senior decision-makers about the economic, social and health benefits of public health programs (Allin et al. 2004).

Another important study for advocacy was the Aboriginal Health Expenditure Study (Deeble & Goss 1998), undertaken at a time of major political debate about whether too little money was spent on Aboriginal health. What the study was able to demonstrate was that health expenditure for Aboriginal people in Australia was focused on the expensive treatment end, and the major shortfall was at the primary care end. The case was thus made for substantial increases in primary care and preventive services in particular, with the consequent rearrangement of the health-care delivery system in the Northern Territory, where the under-expenditure was most acute. The study did lead to significant reforms—in a way that had not been possible with only 'epidemiological advocacy'.

Traditionally, the public health programs had competed via the 'epidemiological advocacy' approach, where advocates for particular diseases (or risk factor or population group) competed for resources by demonstrating that their particular issue was in greatest need of support. At the international level, DALYs were developed during the 1990s as a common metric to compare the severity of health problems—in part to get away from the tendency for every clinician to lobby for their 'favourite disease'. The use of disease burden analysis was also picked up in Australia as an initial step towards priority-setting (see Vos & Begg 1999a, 1999b). With visual presentation—particularly through maps—politicians quickly came to appreciate how complex information could be reduced to simple messages able to be communicated readily to the community. The use of DALYs has also impressed upon decision-makers the value of focusing on chronic diseases as a group of preventable conditions that share many risk factors, rather than focusing on each separate disease.

There are, however, many criticisms of the DALYs methodology for not including socio-economic and environmental factors or measuring unmet health needs in the data on which the estimates were based. DALYs have also been criticised for being inappropriately used in setting national priorities in that their application does not contribute to the most efficient use of resources (Reichenbach 2001).

Nonetheless, given that the arena in which resource allocation decisions are made is dominated by economists looking for measurable outcomes and returns, technical methodologies can play an important role in advocacy.

Investing in infrastructure and capacity development: Securing the foundation for action

Government budget decisions and economic evaluation efforts are often focused on specific health programs. Yet health issues that confront and concern communities change over time. Continued funding of vertical programs, particularly on a limited-term basis, may lead to rigidities in the public health-delivery system, whereby the human and financial resources are locked into particular health issues and are difficult to divert to meet new challenges.

Given that public health is a social enterprise, communities ultimately need to be supported to develop their capacity to tackle these changing health issues. Sustainable health gain is achieved through (Hawe et al. 1997):

- infrastructure, or the capacity to develop service in response to health needs
- ownership and partnership, or the capacity and commitment to maintain programs through mobilising needed resources
- adaptation to and management of changing issues, or problem-solving capacities that facilitate the application of lessons learnt from experience to emerging health challenges.

Capacity-building efforts therefore have to be directed at a number of levels. These can be depicted as in Figure 17.3 in Chapter 17, and include the:

- **health-care service organisation:** need for commitment (resources, policies), skills (competence), structures (networks, planning, decision-making, communication) to be in place for improving health

- **health system level:** to enable the delivery of particular services or respond to a wide range of problems (competencies, performance standards, quality improvement), solve new problems and act in the face of uncertainty (workforce development, organisational development, leadership development)
- **communities:** so that health issues are addressed and initiatives maintained, and increased skills and learnings are applied to other areas of community concern.

Public health infrastructure—at the organisational, community and health system levels—must enable public health programs to be delivered. A strong public health system is a precondition for effective public health action. Many of the elements of the infrastructure, however, remain invisible, so it is difficult to mobilise financial resources and political support for them.

In the United States, as part of the national policy defined through *Healthy People 2010* (US Department of Health and Human Services 2000), public health infrastructure objectives have been set in relation to:

- **data and information systems:** to increase access to and use of information, and to track health issues
- **skilled workforce:** to ensure workforce competency, including through continuing education
- **effective public health organisations:** to ensure comprehensive delivery, improve planning and adopt modern regulatory approaches
- **resources:** to make financial resources transparent
- **prevention research:** to increase practice-based research.

These objectives were set following the recognition of the weakness and disarray in the US public health infrastructure by the Institute of Medicine's report *The Future of Public Health* in 1988 and then by the CDC's *Public Health's Infrastructure—A Status Report* in 2001. Yet it took the terrorist attacks of September 11, 2001 and the criminal use of biological agents (for example, anthrax) before Congress reacted and allocated nearly US$3 billion over three years to rebuild the essential public health functions of the system. This was done largely through CDC-administered programs. The primary goal of these programs was to enhance their ability to respond to a bio-terrorist attack. An additional goal was to strengthen the preparedness of the system to respond to population health threats related to infectious diseases. These new programs were implemented against a background of budgetary reductions at all levels of government in the United States. This posed a major challenge for the public health system as workforce, financial and organisational capacities all had to be rebuilt. Many of these problems weaken the system's ability to respond to public health threats. Following the Global Financial Crisis in 2007, President Obama included increases in public health financing as part of his stimulus package, particularly to address prevention priorities in disadvantaged communities. These were contested by conservative Republican political interests, as the US Congress struggled to reduce budget deficits (US Government 2012).

In Australia, the development and maintenance of public health infrastructure historically has been a responsibility of the state/territory governments. The Commonwealth has invested in strategic institutional infrastructure at various points in time: the Australian Institute of Tropical Medicine (discussed earlier) and its successors, the NHMRC in 1937, the Community Health Program in 1973 and the Australian Institute of Health and Welfare in 1987. A framework (through goals and targets or performance monitoring) has yet to be developed for public health infrastructure and capacity.

The NPHP was developed in 1996 as a joint approach between the Commonwealth and the states/territories to address public health infrastructure development, along with public health action. The NPHP recognised that, in the contemporary context for public health action, government direction alone was insufficient and would not be effective. The engagement of civil society—through non-government organisations—would be needed. The public health infrastructure for the coming era would require a government–community partnership and shared investment in capacity-building.

Although the NPHP initiated an examination of a range of infrastructure issues—such as workforce, financing, information and research—there remains a challenge of how to develop and effect new paradigms for funding and programming (Lin 2002). Accepting that political and sectional interests will continue to drive resource allocation, the policy and managerial challenge is to ensure that vertical programs can be translated into an integrated public health-delivery framework at the community level, and to reorient the broader health-care delivery system towards prevention and cost-effective care. In 2006, national responsibility for health protection and health promotion (health development) was divided between two principal committees of Australian Health Ministers Advisory Committee, replacing the NPHP—the Australian Health Protection Committee and the Australian Population Health Development Principal Committee (APHDPC). The APHDPC has responsibility for strengthening infrastructure and capacity, including workforce, as well as promoting the alignment of health and related sector activities with agreed national priorities. The new ANPHA, established in 2011, now has the national leadership responsibility for health promotion, and with that the infrastructure development to strengthen health-promotion practice.

Conclusion: Nothing is possible without people or money

Public health action is not possible without an organised system, and activities happen only when the building blocks of people and money are in place. A challenge in Australia, as with many other countries, is that members of the public health workforce are often not qualified in the profession, and have moved into this area of work from diverse disciplinary backgrounds. While the advantage of this situation is that people bring with them a range of skills and perspectives, plus a commitment to public health action, there can be problems in terms of there being a full set of capabilities available and accessible across the system.

While workforce capacity is central for public health action, equally important are the available financial resources. In Australia, funding for public health has remained relatively constant for decades. Funding is also uneven across jurisdictions because of the political nature of government budget decisions. Furthermore, because political lobbying has been important to secure public health funding, the financial resources available for different programs vary greatly, and there is no easy basis for deciding what the specific financial needs are for each program area.

Public health delivery relies on other critical resources—information and research knowledge—and these also require an appropriate level of funding. Although Australia's information and research base is reasonably good, its funding base remains quite low. The challenge for a federated system is to determine how the skill base, the money and the knowledge base can be assembled together, and how national services and special facilities can be funded on a shared basis. Ultimately, investment in infrastructure and capacity-building is essential to assure the continued preparedness and sustainability of the public health system.

Part IV

Public health action:
Key interventions from
past to present

12

Surveillance and disease control:
From data to intervention

Challenge

Justin and Katie were married two days ago, enjoying a happy day of celebration with their friends and families. After a long day, their best man takes them to the airport and they set off for their honeymoon interstate.

During the night they both feel unwell, and while at first they put it down to tiredness and a little too much celebrating, by lunchtime the next day they both have nausea, vomiting and diarrhoea, and resign themselves to a day of staying within reach of the bathroom instead of going on the picnic they had planned.

The next morning, Katie's mother phones with the news that quite a lot of their wedding guests are ill, and unfortunately her grandmother and one of her young nieces have been admitted to hospital. Somebody from the Health Department wants to speak to them.

What do you think the Health Department staff might want to talk to them about? Do you think the Health Department should wait until they get back home next week? Are they being too intrusive? What specific questions might they be asking? How might they use the information?

Introduction

In Chapter 4, we noted that public health surveillance has its origins with the ancient Greeks, although the practices and definitions have changed over time. We also noted that surveillance remains the foundation for public health practice. In this chapter, we elaborate on how surveillance contributes to public health action—ranging from communicable diseases control to planning other public health interventions. The different types of surveillance systems, both in theory and in Australia, are described, and their application to communicable diseases examined. How surveillance contributes to the investigation and management of a communicable disease outbreak is then explained.

Types of surveillance: Looking and finding

Surveillance is a term that relates to a collection of systematic tasks involved in knowing about the health of a population. The key elements of surveillance activities include the means by which cases are reported to a central agency, and how the resulting data collections are used. Centers for Disease Control (CDC) and the International Union for Health Promotion and Education (IUHPE) have considered the characteristics of surveillance systems in a recent paper (IUHPE 2011). There are some interesting differences in ways in which CDC and IUHPE think about the details of surveillance systems, but this is not surprising; CDC operates the cornerstone of a national surveillance system with origins in communicable disease control, while IUHPE is an organisation that focuses on special population-based surveillance for the purpose of health promotion. However, there are a number of critical similarities in their thinking about surveillance systems, and these bodies suggest that surveillance systems include the following characteristics:

- There is a theoretical basis for the existence of the surveillance system, the importance of the disease or diseases it is surveying, and for the collection of individual conditions within it.
- The system facilitates the ongoing collection, organisation, validation and continuous analysis of data.
- The data in the system are collected in such a way that the purpose and focus of the system are not on persons but on populations, and consideration is given to the control or preventability, or use in disease prevention, of the conditions being surveyed.
- Data collection is organised, analysed and reported on in time segments; changes over time can be identified and reported on in such a way that a bureaucratic response can be achieved in a timely way. The distribution of reports is thus generated in a timely way to people who will use them in planning health-related services.
- The technical features of the system are considered to be as important as the structural features. The CDC lists these characteristics as flexibility, simplicity of use, acceptability to the user, adequate sensitivity and positive predictive value (that is, cases are easy to identify and report to the system through reliable testing, and cases identified by the system are true cases) and representation of the problem, in part or whole, in a timely way (CDC 2001; IUHPE 2011; Klaucke et al. 1988).

Surveillance is different from both 'monitoring' (which is more sporadic in nature) and 'surveying' (which is about the non-experimental one-off collection of data for a special purpose).

Surveillance may be 'passive' or 'active'. Sometimes, for special reasons, a specific situation may need a targeted kind of surveillance. Such types of surveillance may be passive, active (enhanced), sentinel, rumour or syndromic.

Passive surveillance

Passive surveillance is the term given to the routine collection of cases of various notifiable events.

Surveillance systems are typically used to count cases of communicable diseases, but also are the systems that collect, for example, data on births and deaths, and immunisation records. These data collections are often underpinned by legislation. In particular, cases of certain important communicable diseases (for example, Legionnaire's disease, meningococcal disease and measles) must be notified to state health authorities by law. Notifications may be made by a variety of health-care practitioners, usually doctors or laboratory scientists.

Although in the past notifications were made on the basis of clinical diagnosis, increasingly cases have to be verified by laboratory tests. This is important when considering trends in disease, as cases may not have been identified in the same way from one year to the next, and care must be taken when interpreting the resulting data.

Furthermore, within Australia there are differences between the states in the notification requirements for a number of diseases. These things must be considered when comparing one data collection with another—even with a national data collection.

Active surveillance

Active surveillance (sometimes called enhanced surveillance) is used in two main circumstances, both to do with exposure:

- during outbreaks of specific diseases, when possible new cases are actively sought for early confirmation—for example, during an outbreak of Legionnaire's disease
- during active case-seeking and active monitoring for potential hazards following environmental concerns—for example, actively seeking to identify thyroid cancers in people and the active monitoring of radiation levels in food following the earthquake damage to the Fukushima nuclear reactor in Japan in 2011, and the subsequent detection of radioactivity in food samples from neighbouring areas (WHO 2011).

Special types of surveillance: Many eyes open

Enhanced surveillance

Enhanced surveillance involves the expansion of case definitions and ways of identifying cases in order to be sure that all possible cases are identified. This approach is used to assess a health intervention to identify its effectiveness, as in the following examples:

- From 1999, enhanced surveillance was used before, during and after the introduction of vaccine for meningococcal serogroup C disease in the United Kingdom to identify the true incidence before the introduction of the vaccination program, and to identify incidence and vaccine failures after the introduction of the vaccine (Anon 2004b: 1–25).
- Since 2000, the incidence of acute flaccid paralysis has been used as a marker to identify and ensure thorough follow-up of potential cases of polio during the implementation process of the worldwide program to eradicate this disease (Anon 2003: 188–90).
- The 2002 European Commission Group A streptococcus enhanced surveillance program (Anon 2004a) identified a doubling of cases in the United Kingdom and the Channel Islands from 2002 to 2003.

Sentinel surveillance

Sentinel surveillance systems monitor strategic sites, which act as an early warning system to the rest of the population—often leading to prompt public health action, particularly as early warning can lead to preventive or protective public health measures. In Australia, a sentinel system for warning of a rise in influenza operates through the general practitioner system. For example, in Victoria, a number of general practitioners routinely report the number of cases of influenza-like illness in their patients, and submit specimens to the Victorian Infectious

Diseases State Reference Laboratory for influenza antigen testing. Early warning of Australian encephalitis, a mosquito-borne infection that includes birds in its life-cycle, operates in protected flocks of hens on the Murray River, which are regularly bled to look for signs of infection. In the sentinel chicken program along the Murray River, chickens are bled to watch for a rise in blood antibodies to Murray Valley encephalitis (a very rare disease in Australia), which would warn of the arrival of this virus in the bird population, heralding possible disease in humans. Sentinel surveillance can be used for rare or common diseases.

Rumour surveillance

When a health problem is very rare and covers many jurisdictions without a common reporting system, rumour surveillance is one possible way of collecting and verifying sporadic reports of possible cases. It is a special type of enhanced surveillance and, in a similar way to sentinel surveillance, acts as an early warning system for a rise in cases. For example, international rumour surveillance was used throughout 2005 to search for cases of severe acute respiratory syndrome (SARS) and avian influenza. This surveillance method involves the regular and routine screening of news media and medical chat-lines and specific internet sites for reports of cases, with telephone follow-up with local ministries of Health and embassy staff to verify new cases (Li et al. 2005; PAHO 1982).

Syndromic surveillance

In some circumstances, active case-seeking may involve the use of syndromic surveillance. This kind of surveillance involves the collection of sets of signs and symptoms linked to a set of diseases and disorders, which are not necessarily of themselves exclusively diagnostic but do reflect disease patterns that might require more detailed investigation. Although often identified through passive reporting of unusual cases by astute clinicians, once these

certain sets of signs and symptoms are identified as a problem active surveillance is undertaken.

Syndromic surveillance is particularly suited to the monitoring, on a temporary basis, of a large influx of people who are predictable in that they will have health problems but unpredictable with regard to precisely what kinds of health care they will need. Influxes of people may be predictable—such as the athletes, team managers, supporters and public who came to Melbourne for the March 2006 Commonwealth Games, and who needed provision to be made for their health needs for a month or so. Refugee populations, on the other hand, can be very large and totally unexpected, and usually need longer-term care. Both types of scenario lend themselves to syndromic surveillance, and in many ways these are an adaptation of the active surveillance methods described above.

The outbreaks of a new disease, where there are no tests because the cause is as yet unknown, are another example of syndromic surveillance. For example, in the early part of the SARS outbreak, before the SARS coronavirus was identified and tests developed, cases were included when a collection of specific symptoms (including fever, malaise and difficulty breathing) were noted by a treating doctor (Koh et al. 2003). It was this level of alertness that led to the early detection of a new SARS-like coronavirus in the United Kingdom in September 2012, with all cases being linked to recent visits to Saudi Arabia (NHS 2012) and a surveillance system for visitors to the annual Hajj pilgrimage is now being planned. In the 1980s, before the identification of HIV, the virus that causes AIDS, and the development of laboratory tests for it, AIDS was diagnosed syndromically using a combination of clinical problems. These included several rare cancers—but particularly a rare cancer called Kaposi's sarcoma—along with atypical pneumonia, diarrhoeal disease and weight loss, and various other infections referred to as 'indicator diseases' (Heymann 2004).

Common sources of surveillance information: Where to go

There are a number of different ways of collecting information about the health of populations, enabling surveillance activities to occur. These include:

- routine notifications of specific diseases—for example, Salmonella food poisoning cases (see the list of notifiable infectious diseases in Box 10.1)
- health-event diagnosis-related identification—for example, a diagnosis of breast cancer
- condition-specific data collections—for example, diabetes registers
- recording of specific interventions—for example, immunisation registers. Immunisation coverage in Australia is surveyed through the Australian Childhood Immunisation Register (Department of Human Services 2013d)
- collection of routine events—for example, birth notifications
- collection of data related to health but collected for other purposes—for example, WorkCover, Transport Accident Commission (TAC)
- collections of unusual or accidental events—for example, the Coroner's Courts, TAC data
- collection of information in periodic national surveys—for example, the national health questions in the Australian Bureau of Statistics Census
- sentinel surveillance, where particular activities are in progress to identify warning events for the health of the rest of the population, and may be used for rare or common diseases
- deliberate longitudinal surveillance of specific populations—for example, the Australian Longitudinal Study on Women's Health, which to date has been going for 20 years and is funded by the Commonwealth Department of Health and Ageing through Newcastle and Queensland Universities, and the Concord Health and

Ageing in Men Project, or CHAMP, conducted by the University of Sydney.

Each of these systems has been set up for a specific purpose, but they are very different from one another, and bear little or no relationship with each other. However, as a body of information, they provide a considerable amount of data about a wide variety of health- and disease-related events. Collectively, they are powerful tools for assessing the health of Australians.

Surveillance systems worldwide share a number of common features, which are summarised in Table 12.1.

Communicable diseases surveillance: Detective work

Surveillance systems traditionally have been used for monitoring communicable diseases. Routine surveillance over time provides an excellent backdrop against which outbreaks of notifiable diseases can be identified; however, not all diseases are notifiable. There are many groups of organisms that cause disease in humans. These consist of bacteria, viruses, single-celled parasites (such as protozoa), free-living organisms that include helminthes (parasitic intestinal worms), mycoplasma and fungi. How are outbreaks of 'old' diseases identified, and how are new diseases labelled as problematic and in need of public health intervention?

Routine surveillance of notifiable communicable disease events

In Australia, communicable diseases are divided into four groups for notification purposes; similar systems are in place in almost every country of the world. In recent years, through the efforts of the Communicable Diseases Network of Australia, Australia has integrated the diseases notifiable to the state and territory notification systems, so that the same core diseases are notified in the same way all over the country. Group 1 includes the important

Table 12.1 Some examples of public health uses of environmental surveillance

Stakeholders	Food	Soil/ground	Water	Air
Communities, general public	Food-borne disease	Need for clean land for farming and housing/ recreational activities	Contamination of groundwater; pollution of recreational waters, e.g. blue-green algae	High particulate matter warnings for asthma sufferers
Industry	Food regulations, trade	Regulation of use of additives, e.g. fertiliser in farming; disposal of contaminant by-products	Regulation of use and storage of water in industrial processes	Regulation of industrial releases
Environmental planners	Regulation of the use of natural resources	Need for uncontaminated land for farming and housing, and recreational provisions	Need for sufficient potable water for population consumption; reuse of treated grey-water for some uses	Understanding of weather patterns for environmental planning
Resource managers	Food production and sales industries	Management of farming, including the growing of cash crops vs food security needs; sustainable management of land	Water authorities' need for groundwater and catchment water free from contamination	Efficient industrial production with reductions in air contamination
Local governments	Provision of staff to carry out regulation of food sales outlets and investigate breaches/ food poisoning	Safe provision of local amenities, e.g. safe playgrounds, recreational areas	Need for clean water for local communities	Participation in health promotion/ high contamination awareness
State governments	Food regulations; interstate quarantine laws	Environmental Protection Authorities; local regulation of contamination	Environmental Protection Authorities; local regulation of contamination	Environmental Protection Authorities; local regulation of contamination
National governments	Australian New Zealand Food Authority; international quarantine laws	National responsibility for reduction of pollution, e.g. continuing radioactive contamination at Maralinga following nuclear testing in the 1950s	International agreements	Implementation of national agreements
International governing bodies	Quarantine laws; trade embargoes	Displacement of refugee populations due to widespread contamination/threat, e.g. nuclear testing at Bikini Atoll; use of landmines in theatres of war	International agreements	Kyoto Agreement signatories

Source: adapted from CSIRO (1999).

and uncommon diseases, which generally have a high rate of hospitalisation, a high case fatality rate and many important sequelae (after-effects). Group 2 includes diseases that generally are less dramatic in presentation, although they include food poisoning and other vaccine-preventable diseases. Group 3 includes all sexually transmitted infections (STIs) except HIV/AIDS (the only Group 4 notification) and hepatitis B (included in Group 2).

Some diseases—especially Group 1 communicable diseases—require immediate public health interventions when even one case occurs (even before the diagnosis is confirmed), in particular measles, meningococcal disease and Legionnaire's disease. For Group 1 diseases, public health activities revolve around four intervention strategies:

- preventing further spread through person-to-person contact, either by provision of clearance antibiotics, as in meningococcal disease, or by increasing infection-control procedures
- identifying and treating potential environmental sources, as in Legionnaire's disease

- providing protection through immunisation or gamma globulin for contacts, as in the case of measles
- instituting active monitoring, so that in the event that further cases occur, treatment and further interventions can begin early.

All Group 1 diseases are covered by protocols that govern how each is handled. Generally speaking, the treating doctor or diagnosing laboratory (although sometimes it may be a teacher or relative) contacts the Health Department's communicable diseases unit, and a conversation takes place between the treating medical staff and public health staff.

The Australian states and Commonwealth, other countries and the WHO all routinely report incident cases of a similar list of communicable diseases on a regular basis—sometimes as often as weekly. Annual summaries are also published, and can be an excellent place to look for trends in disease. For example, the *Surveillance of Notifiable Infectious Diseases in Victoria 2009* notes a steady decrease in notifications of meningococcal disease (Figure 12.1)

Figure 12.1 Notified cases of invasive meningococcal disease by year, Victoria, 1998–2009

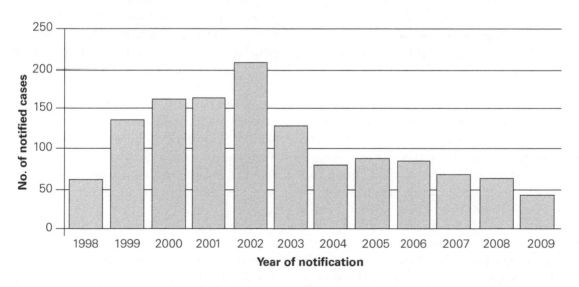

Source: Victorian Department of Health (2011).

since the introduction of routine meningococcal C vaccination in 2003. All Victorian infectious diseases annual reports from 1995 are easy to find, both in libraries and on the Department of Health website. Similarly, the New South Wales *Public Health Bulletin* reports monthly the infectious disease notifications and provides annual summaries. Queensland Health also provides regular reports, such as its Statewide Weekly Communicable Disease Surveillance Reports.

Investigation of a communicable disease outbreak or epidemic

Local outbreaks identified during the year are summarised in annual reports. For example, the New South Wales *Public Health Bulletin* provides annual summaries of disease-specific data on notifiable conditions reported by year of onset of illness, month of onset of illness, local health district, age group and sex. In 2011, there were 13 000 pertussis notifications, 3329 hepatitis C notifications and a 31 per cent increase in Salmonella case notifications compared with the annual average for the last five years (NSW Health 2012b).

During outbreaks, reports are updated on at least a daily basis, and the 'epidemic curve' (a graph of notified cases) is published on websites, or described in tabular form in medical information enews sites, such as *Promed*, in medical journals and in the media.

The definition of 'outbreak' is interesting in that it does not refer to a specific number of cases, but is considered to be more cases than one would expect through routine surveillance. Some diseases (such as the common cold, various rash-and-fever illnesses and a certain amount of diarrhoeal disease) are commonplace, and a few isolated cases do not constitute an outbreak—unless they can be shown to be due to an unusual organism, or an unusual sub-strain of a common organism. On the other hand, with a rare disease, such as Legionnaire's disease or meningococcal disease, even one case is more that we would expect and it is therefore treated as an outbreak.

There are a number of important steps involved in investigating an outbreak. First, as soon as an outbreak is suspected, a case definition must be established and enhanced surveillance put in place to identify all possible cases. A hypothesis about the possible causes of the outbreak must be formulated through careful interviewing of the case and the case's close contacts (family and closest friends with whom the case has spent time in recent days) and, depending on the possible causative organism, possible environmental causes are determined. Pre-existing appropriate clinical specimens must be identified and reserved for microbiological testing, and efforts made to collect further appropriate specimens from cases and sometimes from the environment for laboratory testing. A risk-exposure timeframe must be prepared to clarify who might have been exposed and could need health surveillance. A data-collection tool, normally in the form of a questionnaire, must be developed, tested and systematically administered to both cases and other exposed persons in order to collect high-quality data. Data must be analysed by a competent epidemiologist or statistician to establish exposures associated with a high risk of becoming ill. Lastly, a report will be written to describe the outbreak and provide scientific information for the community in general and public health practitioners for learning purposes. Table 12.2 provides an outline of the steps to be considered in investigating an outbreak.

Investigation of emerging communicable diseases

Since 1975, eighteen major communicable diseases have emerged worldwide, as outlined in Appendix I. Each of these is a very different disease and each has been identified through surveillance in different ways.

Identifying newly emerging diseases provides a number of challenges. It is notable that the presenting signs and symptoms of so many diseases are almost the same. Note in Appendix I how many diseases start with fever, chills, malaise, headache,

Table 12.2 Steps to be considered in the event of an outbreak of a communicable disease

Key question	Process of collecting existing knowledge and new information	Stakeholders	Communication strategy and outcomes
What sort of disease are we dealing with?	• List main signs and symptoms • Inquire about recent activities	• Cases and their families • Public health units	• Arrange for appropriate specimens from cases and contacts; make final microbiological diagnosis
What do the cases think caused it?	• Inquire about contacts with similar symptoms	• General practitioners	• Calculate incubation period • Identify possible causes from clinical signs and symptoms and incubation period • Identify possible intervention strategies (before confirmation of cause of disease)
How does this (probable) organism work?	• Microbiological characteristics	• Cases and their families • Public health and other laboratories • Researchers	• Identify/confirm treatment strategies • Identify protective strategies (e.g. immunisation)
Is an intermediate host or environment likely to be involved?	• Human/environmental reservoir	• Environmental health units • Engineers • Ecologists • Biologists • Media	• Decide whether reservoir intervention or monitoring is necessary
How does this organism interact with its host?	• Transmission mechanisms	• Drug companies • Social scientists • Media	• Identify behaviour-modification/ health-promotion strategies
How is the disease transmitted?	• Identify people needed for clearance antibiotics/ treatment for STIs, major bacterial infections	• Public health units • Social scientists • Media	• Contact tracing for case's friends and relatives as appropriate • Produce clear, easy-to-understand information for all contacts, at risk and otherwise, about transmission and risk of disease • In some circumstances, this may involve the media

Table 12.2 Steps to be considered in the event of an outbreak of a communicable disease (continued)

Key question	Process of collecting existing knowledge and new information	Stakeholders	Communication strategy and outcomes
Are quarantine/ isolation measures warranted?	• Identify appropriate quarantine and isolation procedures	• Cases and their families • Public health units • Quarantine and inspection officers • Hospitals • Infection-control experts • Media	• Produce clear instructions and protocols for cases, families, health-care workers and the public about precautions to be taken in the event of exposure • Nominated isolation beds known to Health Department
What options are there for preventive strategies?	• Schedule of available strategies, including vaccines, gamma globulins, antibiotics	• Public health units • Infection-control experts • Medical officers of Health • Media	• Preventive therapy options and mechanisms (immunisation, antibiotics) identified and implemented to contacts/general public
Are there likely to be environmental effects that enhance or inhibit transmission? Are there surrogate measures of disease?	• Identify environmental niche involvement (e.g. mosquito larvae in stagnant water) • If appropriate, check status of sentinel programs, including GP • Sentinel influenza program • Sentinel chickens and other animal health programs	• Cases and their families • Public health units • Infection-control experts • Environmental health units • Medical officers of health • Public health laboratories • Media	• Conduct environmental investigation as appropriate
Does the Minister for Health (or any other politician) need to know?	• For unusual outbreaks, and for new diseases, up-to-date information to political leaders is crucial	• Politicians • Public health media units	• Regular ministerial correspondence and information for the parliaments from senior managers in the outbreak team

aches and pains, a rash, sore throat, some sort of cough or breathing difficulty, nausea, vomiting and diarrhoea. In fact, most known infectious diseases and many non-infectious diseases also begin with these signs and symptoms, so Health departments must always be on the alert for a rise in cases of a non-specific illness that might herald a new disease.

Emerging diseases by definition have not previously been known and identified, and are thus not specifically notifiable. SARS is a recent example of an emerging disease, first described in February 2003. SARS had a high case fatality rate, especially in South-East Asia and Canada (see Appendix I). The main signs and symptoms of SARS are now known to be gastroenteritis, fever and shortness of breath; the disease was described as an 'atypical pneumonia' because of the type of changes seen in the chest x-rays of cases. Atypical pneumonia is characterised by fever, severe malaise, shortness of breath and sometimes a dry cough, and usually gastroenteritis symptoms. There are many causes, of which some are greatly feared—such as Legionnaire's disease, Q fever, leptospirosis and avian influenzas. Clinically,

they do not differ much from each another, making specific diagnosis impossible on symptoms alone.

Another group of emerging diseases involves animal-to-human transmission. Animal surveillance has provided some interesting examples of early warning for human disease. For example, in Queensland several examples have been reported in recent years including an outbreak of lyssavirus (one strain of which causes rabies in both animals and humans) in bats (McCall et al. 2000). Also in Queensland, a second disease originating in animals, which has recently affected humans, is Hendravirus (also called equine morbillivirus); an explanation for its emergence is that it is also associated with

---

Box 12.1 Outbreak of Legionnaire's disease—Melbourne Aquarium, April 2000

In April 2000, three cases of atypical pneumonia were admitted to different hospitals and notified to the Victorian Health Department with the same strain of *legionellosis* within a few hours of each other. It was quickly known that all the cases had recently visited the brand-new Melbourne Aquarium. Suspecting an outbreak, Health Department staff issued a press release to alert all people who might recently have visited the aquarium to watch for symptoms. Legionnaire's disease is commonly associated with human-made water environments (such as fountains, shower heads and cooling towers) so an extensive environmental investigation was begun for sources of *Legionella* bacteria, and an immediate program of disinfection commenced at the aquarium.

As all probable sources of *Legionella* were thoroughly cleaned as soon as the outbreak was identified, people were only considered to be at risk if they had visited the aquarium in the two-week period prior to the general disinfection.

More cases who had visited the aquarium were identified during the following days, and eventually

much information was collected from people who had visited the aquarium about how long they had queued, where they had queued, whether they visited with other people who had become unwell and so on. It was widely reported in the media that the cooling towers at the aquarium were contaminated with a common strain of *Legionella* bacteria, and these subsequently were removed and the air-conditioning system at the aquarium replaced with alternative air-conditioning to prevent the cooling towers ever being a possible risk again. In fact, all cases associated with the aquarium outbreak were shown to have visited before the disinfection had occurred, although the remainder of the nearly 130 cases in the outbreak continued to be diagnosed and notified from all over the world for about two more weeks.

After an extensive investigation, the important findings were not only that the disease was associated with inadequately disinfected cooling towers, but also that being a smoker increased the odds of disease fourfold compared with non-smokers, and queuing (as opposed to having pre-booked tickets) also raised the odds of disease compared with non-smokers. The combination of standing fairly still in a queue while smoking and deeply inhaling contaminated air was a risky business (Greig et al. 2004: 566–72).

bats. Surveillance has shown Hendravirus to be the cause of death in horse breeders, farmers and vets, although it remains a very rare disease in humans (Kuzmin et al. 2011; Rogers et al. 1996).

Stakeholders and disease control

A number of important groups of people need to be considered in disease control: the various key stakeholders. The stakeholders are not a ubiquitous group, and their 'need to know' about the status of a particular case, series of cases or a disease in general varies with each stage of the investigation.

In thinking about the eleven key questions in Table 12.2, it can be seen that different stakeholders will need information and support in differing degrees as an outbreak progresses. For example, the questions 'What sort of disease are we dealing with? and What do the cases think caused it?' are of immense importance to the cases and their families who are dealing with the consequences of the illness, to the public health units that must run an investigation, and to general practitioners who need to be able to provide good information to the 'worried well' seeking to protect themselves and their families, schools and other educational institutions, as well as workplaces where the cases normally spend their days.

As the outbreak develops, the question 'How does this (probable) organism work?' becomes more important to the cases and their families, to public health units, and also to the public health laboratories that are likely to experience a surge in demand for testing for a specific disease perceived as a threat. This is also the time when epidemiological researchers try to ensure that clinical investigations are carried out for all potential cases included in the outbreak so that the outbreak investigation results can be published in a timely way.

The next stage involves the question 'Is an intermediate host or environment likely to be involved?' This is of importance to environmental health units, engineers, ecologists and biologists. The media are always keen to help publicise any

> ### Box 12.2 An outbreak of *Salmonella* poisoning traced to contaminated peanuts
>
> Routine national laboratory surveillance identified less than half a dozen cases annually of *Salmonella mbandaka* before the mid-1990s; however, in 1995 there were 88 cases reported, mainly from around Sydney and Canberra.
>
> Between February and June 1996, 54 cases linked to the same strain of *S. mbandaka* serovar type 1 were identified in Victoria and South Australia, triggering an outbreak investigation. Although chicken, a common source of Salmonella poisoning, was originally thought to be responsible, laboratory testing failed to confirm this as the source of the outbreak. Further interviews with cases (people affected by salmonellosis) and controls (people of similar background who remained healthy) identified peanut butter as a possible source of infection, and opened jars were collected from affected households for testing. The same strain of *Salmonella* was identified from two of the jars, as well as another strain, *S. senftenberg*, which does not cause disease in humans (Ng, Rouch & Dedman 1996).
>
> An investigation of the peanut storage area provided some evidence for contamination by vermin, and this was assumed to have been the origin of infection. Before this outbreak, it had been thought that *Salmonellae* could not survive in peanut butter; however, subsequent research has shown that any modified peanut butter (that is, anything other than 100 per cent peanuts) is capable of being contaminated (Burnett et al. 2000: 472–7).

perceived environmental hazard—perhaps because it involves images other than 'talking heads', but also because there is always the possibility of identifying a company or person who may be at fault. Environmental hazards are interesting in that, unlike other diseases such as cancer or sexually transmitted infections, acknowledging the source of the problem does not imply a possible change of behaviour for individuals hearing the message.

Drug companies, social scientists and the media will be interested, for different reasons, in the question 'How does this organism interact with its host?' Consider how the 2003 SARS and 2004 avian influenza outbreaks generated a series of research projects aimed at delivering effective treatments and vaccines, and projects about people who live in close proximity to their livestock—all of which make excellent press. The closely related question 'How is the disease transmitted?' is of more interest to public health units.

The two related questions: 'What options are there for preventive strategies?' and 'Are quarantine/isolation measures warranted?' are key in outbreak control, but are really the province of public health unit staff, MOsH, quarantine and inspection officers, and hospitals (particularly infection-control experts). Affected individuals and their families are most interested in the question of quarantine, while the media can sometimes be seen as part of the solution if they are willing to carry Health Department messages in full without altering provided text.

'Are there likely to be environmental effects that enhance or inhibit transmission?' and 'Are there surrogate measures of disease?' are problems of interest to public health units, infection-control experts, environmental health units, MOsH, and the public health laboratories that are likely to have to undertake specialist specimen analyses.

Lastly, in an effort to keep everybody as up to date as possible, the public health units, their media teams and the minister's parliamentary secretary need to balance the question, 'Does the Minister for Health (or any other politician) need to know?' with the minister's other priorities, as well as the necessity of keeping both other health professionals concurrently up to date through professional channels and the general public informed through the media—a major juggling act by most measures.

Surveillance of environmental and occupational hazards: Where are the canaries?

Maintaining the health of the environment is just as important as maintaining that of its inhabitants, because if the world in which we live is not able to provide the basic necessities of life—food to eat, water to drink and bathe in, clean air to breathe, and safe shelter—the earth's inhabitants are more likely to become sick. Environmental disruptions are more likely to cause chronic diseases than communicable diseases, although there are some notable exceptions, such as *legionellosis*.

It is preferable to monitor environmental hazards in the community. An early practice in coal-mines, begun in Britain in 1911 and continued until 1986, was the use of canaries as a surveillance tool. Canaries were used because they were sensitive to harmful gases, such as carbon monoxide, which would not be detected by miners. When the canaries showed any sign of distress, miners were evacuated from the pits until it was safe for them to return. The canaries have been replaced by hand-held gas detectors with digital displays, which now alert miners to the presence of such potentially fatal gases (BBC News 1986). Today, when a problem afflicts the health of workers, it often serves as an early warning system of environmental disruptions that may indicate health problems within communities.

There have been numerous 'outbreaks' of diseases related to environmental and occupational hazards that had not been monitored. Box 12.3 about Love Canal tells of one famous incident. In Australia, incidents have been smaller in scale by comparison, but have also offered important lessons—such as exposure to lead in Port Pirie, South Australia, and to asbestos for the miners in Wittenoom and Baryulgil (see Box 13.2), and workers in the Latrobe Valley (State Electricity Commission) and for James Hardie Industries. These large-scale catastrophes have heightened community concerns about environmental risk factors.

Box 12.3 Love Canal

The Love Canal episode in environmental contamination also goes by the name Hooker Chemicals Love Canal. The reason? The fenced site is a hazardous waste landfill, and includes a functioning barrier drainage system with a leachate collection and treatment system. The site includes an excavated canal for a hydro-electric power scheme that was never used, installed by Mr William T. Love in the 1890s. The area was later taken over by Hooker Chemicals and Plastics for use as a dump for a number of toxic chemicals (including dioxin, pesticides and chlorobenzenes) from 1942 until 1952. Shortly afterwards, it was covered over and given to the Niagara Falls Board of Education, which later used it for development.

In the 1960s, problems began to emerge—first with smells and later, as the water table began to rise, with contaminated groundwater leaking to the surface. Investigation showed that the problems were geographically widespread and practically complex, with leachate contaminating the water supply and leaking into sewers that drained into nearby streams. An emergency was declared, and nearly 1000 families were evacuated; at the time (in 1980), 70 000 people lived within 3 miles (4.8 kilometres) of the site, 10 000 within 1 mile (1.6 kilometres). The water supply into which the leachate was leaking supplied 77 000 people with potable water.

Health studies of the exposed population are underway, and an environmental recovery plan has been instituted with a combination of short- and long-term remedial strategies. Compensation and corrective treatments have cost hundreds of millions of dollars.

A new group of people now lives at Love Canal. (US Environmental Protection Agency 2004)

In late 2003, workers who were employed in the asbestos industry in the 1950s to 1970s finally won compensation for industrially acquired asbestosis and mesothelioma, fatal diseases directly caused by exposure to asbestos fibres. A subsequent judicial inquiry found a shortfall in the established fund and a new compensation deal was not reached until 2007. In the same year, the public face of victims, Bernie Banton, died and a foundation was established in his name. A recent initiative funded by the National Health and Medical Research Council, the Australian Asbestos Network, aims to increase awareness of the ongoing risk of asbestos exposure, in particular to home renovators (Olsen et al. 2011). A further problem of concern to investigating local government health officers is the illegal dumping of asbestos by home renovators (LGA, n.d.).

Table 12.1 provides some examples of public health uses of environmental surveillance.

Designing surveillance systems: What works and what is important?

Data provided from surveillance systems are used to design public health interventions; therefore, it is critical that they include robust data collected in appropriate ways and that the people analysing the data are skilled in analysis techniques and interpretation. Surveillance data need to be collected systematically and continuously. This is an interesting difference from research data, which are normally collected for a specific purpose from a defined population; surveillance data come from whole populations rather than sections of them, and are added to over time rather than being time-limited.

Surveillance of non-communicable diseases and associated risk factors: Searching for clues

Non-communicable diseases (NCDs) now constitute the leading causes of death worldwide, and the onset of risk factors provides an important predictor for future disease both at individual and population levels. The WHO has identified five important risk factors for non-communicable disease in the top ten leading risks to health. These are raised blood pressure, raised cholesterol, tobacco use, alcohol consumption and being overweight. The disease burden caused by these leading risk factors is global. In every region of the world, including the poorest, raised blood pressure, cholesterol and tobacco use are causing serious disease and untimely deaths (WHO 2003a).

Reports by the Australian Institute of Health and Welfare (AIHW) confirm that Australia is facing an increasing economic and social burden because of chronic diseases and their associated risk factors. In 2005, chronic diseases affected 80 per cent of all Australians and they were responsible for 50 per cent of deaths and accounted for 70 per cent of total health expenditure (Walker & Colagiuri 2011: 57). Currently, non-communicable and chronic disease surveillance is confined to a few relatively uncommon disorders, which may be identified through registers and routine examinations common to whole populations. There are several difficulties in monitoring NCDs in the same way. For example, for the most part chronic diseases start gradually; there is not often an 'onset date' or 'incubation period'. However, it is also true that not all infectious and communicable diseases have a sudden onset, and some of these—in particular, hepatitis B, C and Delta and HIV infection—have to be notified even though they are generally treated as chronic diseases. Chronic non-infectious diseases might eventually be notified in the same way. Furthermore, not all non-infectious diseases are chronic—for example, incidents of heart attack, stroke and traffic accident all occur largely unexpectedly.

Unlike communicable diseases, there are no general notification forms for these disorders. While some information is available through registers of information collected for a quite different purpose (such as hospital separation data, which is collected

more for economic than health reasons), it is neither systematic in the sense that health data need to be for surveillance purposes, nor is it available on a population basis. Nonetheless, the concepts of surveillance are now beginning to be used for non-communicable and chronic diseases.

Chronic disease event monitoring and screening

Some information about chronic disease events can be extracted from hospital separation minimum datasets, such as the Victorian Admitted Episode Inpatient Dataset, surveys of GP workloads, the Pharmaceuticals Benefits Scheme, and from rebate agencies, such as Medicare, and the private health insurance funds.

For the most part, the information in these datasets is collected for financial purposes and is therefore not very reliable for the purpose of epidemiological surveillance. However, there are now some chronic conditions that are notifiable in some jurisdictions:

- Birth defects that result in death are notifiable in many places. The annual reports of the Victorian Consultative Council on Obstetric and Paediatric Mortality and Morbidity are available at <www.health.vic.gov.au/perinatal>.
- In New South Wales, abnormally raised blood lead levels became notifiable in 1997 (NSW Health 2000).
- Creutzfeldt-Jakob disease (CJD) is notifiable in many countries, including Australia. The Australian system is a registry (ANCJDR), which includes cases identified by both active and passive surveillance methods, and reports twice a year. A review of ten years of CJD notification has been conducted, showing that the ten-year incidence per million Australians ranges between 0.5 and 1.3. The registry is considered to be effective because it is simple and flexible, although it relies heavily on the competence of notifying staff (Robotin 2002: 265–72).

Another way of measuring activity related to disease is through screening registries and specialised disease registers. Some examples include:

- **BreastScreen Australia:** For Australian women breast cancer is the most prevalent cancer of all, and its incidence is rising. Breast cancer screening aims to reduce this through early detection and regular monitoring. In order to achieve this, an active system of surveying (by identifying, recruiting and screening) women between the ages of 50 and 69 is in place Australia-wide. Further information about this program is available at the BreastScreen Australia websites, <www.breastscreen.info.au> and <women.gov.au>, the National Breast Cancer Centre website, <www.nbcc.org.au>, and the HealthInsite website, <www.healthinsite.gov.au> (AIHW 2004a).
- **Cervical cancer registry:** In the same way, an active national screening program is in place to screen women for cervical cancer. Monitoring and surveillance have shown that regular population-based screening can prevent about 90 per cent of cases of the most common type of this cancer. Incidence of this cancer is now falling. Further information about this program is also available at the National Cervical Cancer Screening Program websites, <www.cervicalscreen.health.gov.au/ncsp> and <women.gov.au> (AIHW 2004a).

  Information about cancer in Australia collected via incidence data is available from the state Cancer Councils websites in New South Wales, <www.cancercouncil.com.au>, Victoria, <www.cancervic.org.au/index.htm>, and South Australia, <www.cancersa.org.au>. The Cancer Council of South Australia explicitly states that its work includes '[m]onitoring cancer and cancer risk, and undertaking applied research and evaluation to help inform services directed toward "reducing the impact of cancer"'.
- **Diabetes:** There is no centralised database containing population data about diabetes

incidence; therefore, it has to be deduced in other ways. The AIHW undertakes periodic estimates of the number of people with diagnosed diabetes in Australia. These reports are based on self-reports to the ABS through, for example, the 2007–08 National Health Survey. In 2007–08, an estimated 898 800 Australians (4.4 per cent) had been diagnosed with diabetes (excluding gestational diabetes) at some time in their lives (AIHW 2011b).

The Diabetes Australia website, <www.diabetesaustralia.com.au>, contains information and population estimates about diabetes, and a great deal of effort is made to promote a different approach to monitoring and screening for diabetic retinopathy. A great deal of information is available about this disabling by-product of diabetes, but although there is much advice about screening (for example, see Eyes on Diabetes at <www.eyesondiabetes.org.au/article/62>), no population data exist.

- **Other registries:** the Australia and New Zealand Dialysis and Transplant Registry (ANZDATA) collects a wide range of statistics that relate to the outcomes of treatment of those with end-stage renal failure. The main results are published annually. ANZDATA also provides reports on the activities of individual hospitals and treatment outcomes. (For further information, see <www.anzdata.org.au/anzdata/anzdatawelcome.htm>.) In the future, disease-specific registries could include those based on chronic diseases (for example, Alzheimer's disease and asthma), exposure to hazards in the workplace (for example, pesticides, organic chlorides and solvents) and lifestyle diseases (for example, smoking).

Monitoring behavioural risk factors

As NCDs share several risk factors, the prevention of one risk factor can help prevent several NCDs simultaneously. The WHO has developed a process that is useful for population-based assessment and surveillance. The STEPwise approach (see Figure 12.2) is a sequential process of gathering comparable and sustainable NCD risk factor information at the country level. This information can, in turn, be used to plan for and implement currently available interventions to address the disease patterns caused by these risk factors (WHO 2003a). Typically, information is obtained at two levels:

1 individuals, including such risk factors as:
   - background, that is age, sex, level of education and genetic composition
   - behavioural, such as smoking, unhealthy diet and physical inactivity
   - intermediate, for example, serum cholesterol levels, diabetes, hypertension and obesity
2 communities (or contextual factors)—for example:
   - social and economic conditions, such as poverty, employment and family composition
   - environment, such as climate and air pollution
   - culture, such as practices, norms and values
   - urbanisation, which influences housing, and access to products and services.

Health professionals in developed countries (and some transitional countries) recognise that many ill-health related behaviours can be monitored. For example, Western societies are now experiencing epidemics of obesity, considered to be extremely worrying as obesity is a marker for cardiovascular disease and cancer. Globally, the main surveillance systems for NCD risk factors are:

- the US Behavioural Risk Factor Surveillance System, which is focused on knowledge, attitudes and behaviour related to non-communicable diseases
- the Rapid Risk Factor Surveillance System from Canada

Figure 12.2 WHO STEPwise surveillance

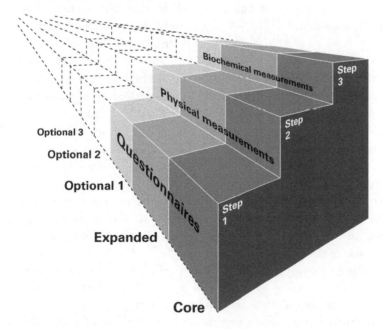

Source: Bonita et al. (2001).

- the FINBALT Health Monitor (from Finland, Estonia, Latvia and Lithuania)
- countrywide integrated NCD intervention used in the WHO (Euro) (see <www.who.dk/CINDI>)—centralised, standard-module self-reporting national surveys with objective measures and incorporation of current indicator data
- the WHO STEPwise (see Figure 12.2), which measures disease at three levels: disease events/outcomes (number of strokes, heart attacks and cancers), behavioural (such as alcohol and tobacco use, nutrition and physical activity) and physiological (biomarkers, such as cholesterol and blood sugar, blood pressure and body mass index). This is the model for developing countries, which are now instigating their own regional networks, comparable to the Countrywide Integrated Noncommunicable Diseases Intervention program, for the 29 member states of the WHO European Region and Canada or CARMEN (Conjunto de Acciones para la Reducción Multifactorial de las Enfermedades Nontransmisibles), an initiative of the Pan American Health Organization.

In Australia, the Australian National Health Survey periodically documents a range of behavioural risk factors. More recently, states and territories have developed computer-assisted telephone interview (CATI) surveys, which contain questions that can measure attitudes and behaviours associated with obesity, alcohol, tobacco and non-prescription drug use. The 2011–13 Australian National Health Survey was the largest and most comprehensive health survey undertaken in Australia and for the first time it collected physical measurements of height, weight and blood pressure for people of two years and over (ABS 2012b).

The next generation of surveillance data is likely to include more information about access to infrastructure and the underlying determinants of health and well-being. Already, the Australian Community Housing and Infrastructure Needs Survey audit includes health facilities; housing and shelter; access to public utilities, including water, gas and electricity; sewerage; and rubbish collection. There are increasing calls for monitoring health-promoting environments (such as no-hat-no-play programs in schools; smoke-free work and public places; traffic calming; and the provision of safe and adequate parks, footpaths and bicycle tracks to encourage physical activity) (AIHW 1999), along the lines proposed by Cheadle et al. (1993).

Population health monitoring

Besides behavioural risk factors, additional information about population health across Australia can be gathered systematically through the CATI surveys, and through the ABS surveys, which include a very few carefully selected and prudently written health questions. While these surveys are not of themselves surveillance systems, they are conducted regularly, providing a series of snapshots that tell a story. The difference between monitoring and surveillance lies in what is done with the information.

Through having standardised modules of questions, these surveys are capable of inquiring about shared ideas and providing comparisons across jurisdictions. Optional modules also provide the flexibility for individual jurisdictions to monitor specific concerns, such as post-traumatic stress after a disaster, as well as modify questions to local nomenclature.

Some examples of specific-interest population health surveys of an ongoing nature undertaken in Australia are:

- the CATI survey (Victoria): social networks
- the New South Wales Health Survey: child health
- the Omnibus Health Survey (South Australia): gambling, domestic violence

- CHAMP, a project to investigate the health and lives of older men (Centre for Research on Ageing, n.d.)
- Womens Health Australia: since 1995, these researchers have been following the health of more than 40 000 Australian women. While technically it is a longitudinal cohort study, in many respects the information collected acts as a surveillance system for women's health. There are many reports and publications arising from this work, accessible through the project website (Women's Health Australia 2012).
- Growing Up in Australia: the longitudinal study of Australia children, which provides similar information on the contribution of social, cultural and economic factors to well-being, and identifies policy opportunities for early intervention and prevention strategies (FaHCSIA, AIFS and ABS 2012).
- the Australian Longitudinal Study on Male Health: a study on male health and the social, economic, environmental and behavioural factors that determine the length and quality of life (DOHA 2012a).

Given the population diversity and distribution in Australia, there are major challenges involved in determining how best to reach Aboriginal and remote population groups, and how to ensure that the health needs and practices of non-English speaking people are adequately reflected in these population health surveys.

In addition to these surveys, population health monitoring can be achieved through the collection and analysis of existing statistics. Social indicator data may be extracted from sources such as the ABS and the AIHW, which are excellent sources of reliable baseline and indicator data. National programs also collect data on tobacco and alcohol use, particularly for youth. In addition, there are reported statistics on injury, violence and abuse, as well as about protective events, such as immunisation and screening data.

Surveillance of quality and safety in the health care system: Ensuring we 'do no harm'

Surveillance methods have been applied to identifying quality and safety concerns in the health-care system.

Investigation of iatrogenic illness

Iatrogenic diseases are those caused (usually inadvertently) by medical treatments. There are many types of iatrogenic illness. Examples include wound infections, such as *Staphylococcus aureus*, following surgical procedures; pain and infection caused by surgical equipment being left inside a person's body after surgery; and the effects of being given a wrong treatment or drug.

When these problems are identified, they are investigated carefully and registers of these investigations are used to improve clinical practice. For example, in Victoria the Health Services Commissioner is able to investigate cases of alleged iatrogenic disease, and make recommendations for improvements. When iatrogenic diseases are considered to be due to professional misconduct, they are investigated by the various professional boards, or even, in very serious cases, by the courts.

Adverse reactions to drugs, especially new drugs, are notified for inclusion on a special register kept by the Adverse Drug Reaction Advisory Committee (ADRAC).

Sometimes it can be difficult to identify problems because they are not particularly common, or they occur over a long time and across a wide geographical area. The thalidomide story, briefly described in Box 12.4, is an example of such a problem.

Monitoring adverse events

An important type of monitoring is that used to track adverse medical events. There is no one system that records all types of these 'medical mishaps', although some are routinely recorded.

Box 12.4 Thalidomide

Thalidomide was marketed in the 1960s as a cheap sedative and an effective treatment for tension, anxiety, insomnia and the symptoms of gastroenteritis. Because it proved safe in animal models, it was also considered to be safe to use in pregnancy. However, as the 1960s progressed, routine data collections in Germany identified an increase in the number of infants born with hypoplastic limb malformations (missing sections of limbs) and, less commonly, a number of major organ anomalies and mental retardation problems. Careful follow-up suggested that thalidomide might be the cause. Further investigation showed that the window during which it had the ability to damage the new embryo was the sixteen days between the twentieth and thirty-sixth days after fertilisation.

Active follow-up of women who had taken thalidomide as an anti-nausea drug in early pregnancy was begun. These observations were made in many Northern European countries as well as Australia. Thalidomide was withdrawn from the market, and this teratogenic (leading to foetal abnormalities) problem disappeared (Miller & Strömland 1999).

The removal of thalidomide from the drug market meant that it was not possible to use it for any reason at all. Recent reviews of thalidomide show that it can be a very useful drug in the treatment of a range of disorders, particularly in the treatment of mycoplasmas (leprosy and tuberculosis), as well as AIDS-associated wasting and a variety of immunological and skin diseases. Once again, trials of the drug are underway—with some very strict guidelines for their use (Patrias, Gordner & Groft 1997).

Box 12.5 Measurement of adverse events

As there is growing concern about the quality and safety of hospital care, several health researchers recently have used diagnosis (International Classification of Diseases, or ICD) codes to compare two different ways of identifying adverse events, using 1.65 billion routinely recorded hospital admissions. By identifying admissions where particular events had occurred subsequent to admission (modification codes), they showed that an adverse event occurred in 8.25 per cent of *all* admissions. However, fewer than two-thirds of these events were identified by ICD codes alone. The rate was much higher for people who stayed in hospital longer than one day. The rate for same-day cases primarily reflects pre-admission events that occur at home and in other health and residential facilities, but this only applies to 28 per cent of multi-day admissions. The researchers also note that:

> In contrast to purposive studies, administrative datasets provide a significantly cheaper and more timely way of monitoring rates of adverse events. When compared with 'sentinel' events' monitoring, this approach allows for identification of new kinds of events, for example, increased rates of infection of implantable devices, not anticipated in the choice of a limited set of sentinel events.

Source: Jackson et al. 2006 (quote at 2006: 24).

For example, as mentioned, adverse reactions to vaccines and new drugs are recorded through ADRAC. In Victoria, a special sentinel event monitoring system has been instituted to identify and analyse patterns of usually very uncommon adverse events in the delivery of clinical services to patients, such as an operation on the wrong part of the body, an incompatible blood transfusion, infection-control mistakes, major communication errors, and patients dying as a result of being given the wrong drugs (Victorian Department of Human Services 2004a).

The intelligent use of data linkage has provided a new way of thinking about surveillance systems. In Western Australia, the ability to provide very 'clean' and complete datasets that can be linked has the ability to enhance both standard health research and improve surveillance through the use of longitudinal data (Holman 2008). Examples of surveillance studies include birth outcomes and birth defects, the MONICA cardiac disease studies and various risk factor studies.

Conclusion: An enduring plank for public health action

The control of communicable diseases is the first major public health achievement, and surveillance is a public health practice at the core of disease control. It is also the vehicle through which new diseases are discovered and understood.

As a basis for public health action, the principles of surveillance are applicable to a wide array of public health issues. Increasingly, surveillance principles and methods are being applied to environmental health, chronic disease, and health-care safety and quality. For example, from 1 January 2004 and based on recommendations from its Scientific Advisory Committee, the UK National Disease Surveillance Centre amended surveillance system laws to make it mandatory to report to health authorities shifting patterns of illness or any unusual disease clusters that may be of public health concern. The reason for this is to be able to activate an early warning system in the event of the use of potential chemical, biological or radiological weapons (such as tularaemia and botulism) within its borders. As we have seen in this chapter, a wide range of diseases—communicable and non-communicable—exist, for which the symptoms are remarkably similar. Waiting for diagnostic confirmation is time-consuming, and can delay possible public health interventions, so this approach is likely to be very useful, providing surveillance systems with new tools for identifying outbreaks and instituting control measures in a timely manner.

13

Health protection:
From the physical environment to ecological health

Challenge

One morning on your way to work, you notice that a new planning application for a packaging plant has been posted on a large vacant site not far from a park and recreational facilities. You recall that the mayor has argued that the city needs new employment opportunities, particularly for low-skilled people. The company building the plant will be offered rate concessions and incentives, and amendments are proposed to the planning scheme to enable the plant to be built on the proposed site.

How would you respond to such a proposal? How do you balance the potential environmental health risks such as increased noise levels for nearby residents, increased traffic flows, possible air and water pollution from the industrial process and loss of visual amenity? What impact will the plant have on the health of nearby residents, particularly older people? How can the community be involved in ensuring that manufacturing practices are clean and green?

The construction of the plant will create 300 short-term jobs, and when in operation it will employ about 120 people. But the economic benefits will also spread out into the community as various businesses will be involved in the supply and transport of the raw materials and the finished products. The newly employed workers and their families will then have more disposable income, which will improve the financial position of other businesses in the city that may need to employ more part-time or casual staff.

After researching the relevant planning laws and the performance of similar plants in other locations, you decide that the environmental health risks outweigh the economic advantages. You become involved with a concerned citizens' group, whose first action is to oppose the planning permit. This involves gathering signatures from those people who oppose the plant planning permit and presenting them to the council to make sure a public meeting is convened. The group also seeks media coverage and lobbies the respective local, state and federal politicians. Supporters of the project conduct a similar campaign. What other actions can your group take? Do you explore the environmental and environmental health legislation or the idea of environmental justice?

Introduction

Chapter 1 introduced the historical connection between the health of populations and the development of cities and towns—in other words, the physical environment in which people live, work and play. The origins of both public health and the environmental movement are tied to a common genesis in terms of protecting people's health from the hazards posed by the physical environment. The foundations for public health practice today came in part as a response to the physical environmental circumstances that confronted European communities in the mid-1800s. The evolution of environmental health practice demonstrates the concept of health protection as a core public health intervention strategy.

From this time until the present day, there has been a continuous evolution of the concepts associated with public and environmental health. The long-standing understanding of the connection between 'health' and the physical environment has been shaped through broad social changes, such as the Industrial Revolution of the nineteenth century, and the continuous changes that have occurred in the urban form since then. Newer developments in understanding about human ecology and the impacts of ecosystem changes are further informing shifts in environmental and public health thinking towards a concern for human and planetary well-being in the longer term.

This chapter discusses the evolution of environmental health practice and the conceptual underpinnings associated with this practice. The chapter then reviews some of the current and emerging areas of environmental health practice, and the current issues and challenges facing public health today from an ecological perspective.

What is environmental health?

Throughout human history, societies have taken collective action to control transmissible diseases by protecting their members from exposure to hazards in the environment. Thus, health protection has always been central to the public health effort, and within that effort, environmental health is a core area of practice.

The tools of environmental health consist of a large range of legislation relating to the environment, and to protection of human health from conditions and processes in the local environment. Some of the areas regulated by law are legislation for environment protection; occupational health and safety; the storage, transport and handling of hazardous chemicals; and dangerous goods (including radioactive substances). Other tools consist of licences, registrations and permits; audits and inspections; and scientific sampling and analysis of substances, discharges, food, water and other material. Education and training constitutes an important tool—particularly in occupational health and safety, and areas involved with the supply of food and water for human consumption. So what are the origins of these environmental health tools?

Although environmental health, as a field of public health practice, has its genesis in the mid-nineteenth century, it is only comparatively recently that some attempts have been made to define it. Like 'public health', environmental health is difficult to put boundaries around, but with the publication of the *Health for All Australians Report* in 1988, environmental health hazards were identified as a risk factor to health. Within that context, environmental health can be seen as a sub-set of public health that overlaps with other areas, such as community and occupational health, and involves:

> myriad ... issues such as air quality, water quality, noise pollution, hazardous materials, the handling, use and disposal of materials such as asbestos, pesticides and industrial chemicals, ionising and non-ionising radiation, plus food safety and consumer protection (Health Targets and Implementation [Health for All] Committee 1988: 73).

This definition is rather narrow, because it is based upon a health-protection issues perspective and thus, directly or indirectly, involves the health portfolio. The scope of environmental health from a well-being perspective can be seen to include city planning, building design, transport systems, workplace facilities, and housing density and quality. At that time, it was not certain whether environmental health included issues such as deforestation or living next to high-voltage power lines (Health Targets and Implementation [Health for All] Committee 1988).

In October 1999, the Commonwealth government launched the National Environmental Health Strategy in which the definition of 'environmental' was once again considered. It was clearly articulated that environmental health was not synonymous

with the health of the environment and environmental protection, and it was not restricted to epidemic diseases of the nineteenth century, but was instead about creating and maintaining environments that promoted good public health. Environmental health was defined as those aspects of human health determined by physical, chemical, biological and social factors in the environment (Commonwealth of Australia 1999: 1, 3). From this perspective, issues such as increased air, water and soil contamination, persistent chemical pollutants and global climate change, together with the established issues of diseases associated with poverty and overcrowding were seen to be part of the environmental health milieu.

Given this new and broad perspective on environmental health, it should come as no surprise that there are many different disciplines that contribute to environmental health, including chemistry, microbiology, engineering, statistics, epidemiology, toxicology and sociology. Thus, the workforce consists of environmental health officers, researchers, academics, policy officers, urban planners, and managers employed by governments, the private sector, universities and non-government organisations. Collectively, all of these can be referred to as environmental health practitioners (Commonwealth of Australia 1999: 32). In 2007, however, the federal government redefined the definition and scope of environmental health as follows:

> Environmental health addresses all the physical, chemical, and biological factors external to a person, and all the related factors impacting behaviours. It encompasses the assessment and control of those environmental factors that can potentially affect health. It is targeted towards preventing disease and creating health-supportive environments. This definition excludes behaviour not related to environment, as well as behaviour related to the social and cultural environment, and genetics. (enHealth 2007: 4)

Clearly, the scope of environmental health was narrowed to exclude behaviour not related to environment, including behaviour relating to the social and cultural environment; this assumes that behaviours associated with each of these environments can be identified and environmental health interventions developed that target only the physical environmental factors impacting on a community.

The origin of environmental health practice: Sanitation works

Industrialisation and urbanisation in nineteenth-century England created a focus for public health action. Apart from the sudden increases in urban populations and the complete lack of infra-structure, there was direct contamination of the immediate living and working environments whereby human and other waste was allowed to accumulate in and around dwellings, streets, roads and vacant lands. Coupled with a lowering of bodily resistance to disease due to poor nutrition (starvation) associated with extreme poverty, and little personal hygiene, the result was epidemics of infectious diseases, such as cholera, typhoid and tuberculosis.

The environment was the source of nuisances and generated miasmas, which in turn caused illness and resulted in destitution and severely reduced economic consequences for the working population. The result of increased, and increasing, disease and poverty was a subsequent reduction in the labouring strength (workforce), which was perceived to be the 'wealth of the nation'. From an economic perspective, a substantially reduced labour force would be a threat to the production of goods by the factories, and the economic growth of the country.

Chapter 2 introduced Edwin Chadwick as the architect of early public health reforms. As a consequence of Chadwick's campaign, the government, after confirming Chadwick's findings through a Royal Commission on the health of towns in 1844–45, enacted the UK *Public Health Act 1848*.

Chadwick made a substantial contribution to public health, particularly in initiating the 'organised effort' as a vital ingredient of the sanitary reform movement, which had a profound impact on the environmental conditions in towns and cities. His contribution can be summarised as follows:

- Chadwick reconceptualised the connection between human illness and a community's living environment. This living environment was being polluted and contaminated, and this invariably led to the occurrence of disease. The poor lived in such environmental conditions.
- His study into the living conditions and diseases of the labouring population and the subse-quent sanitation campaign resulted in the first organised community effort to address environ-mental conditions, which was facilitated by the enactment of the *Public Health Act 1848*.
- The *Public Health Act 1848* has provided the basis for public health administration to the present day in most English-speaking countries.
- The implementation of sanitary works—for example, removing human and animal waste, providing sewers and drains, regulating food and water supplies, providing for public baths and building controls—were the right things to do, but were actually based on an erroneous idea that disease was transmitted by miasmas.

The contribution of Chadwick and those who followed him provided the basis for the environ-mental health services that are provided today in most industrialised countries.

How is environmental health practice organised?

Environmental health practice today encompasses a broad range of activities within the government sector. While different levels of government and different portfolios are involved, all their activities are designed to eliminate or reduce the risks to the public from the environment. The environmental health services and activities associated with the sanitary reforms in England in 1848, and then later in Australia, are still provided today. They generally have a legislative basis that can be traced back to the sanitary reform era. While many of these services are administered through the Health portfolio, there is a substantial number of complementary environmental health programs and initiatives provided by other government departments, notably the various state and national environment protection authorities, and Departments of Natural Resources, Conservation and Agriculture.

Appendix J provides a snapshot of the environmental health roles played by the state and territory government Health Departments, and the types and scope of environmental health services provided. As can be seen, jurisdictions define and organise environmental health in different ways. Some jurisdictions specifically refer to the administration of legislation and services as a main role and an aim in itself, while others define the role in terms of a broader management of environmental issues impacting on the health of the population.

Nonetheless, across the jurisdictions there are a number of common environmental health functions undertaken by government. These include the regulation of food safety, radiation safety, wastewater management, and poisons and pesticides regulation. Cross-cutting areas of environmental health—such as environmental health risk identification and assessment—are also included. This reflects the specialist capacity of the state portfolios and their ability to develop, interpret and use data and intelligence-gathering systems. Part of this intelligence-gathering and interpretation function is to communicate findings to other parts of the service system by way of policy and guidelines—such as to local government, which has a generalist and applied environmental health function.

Appendix J also shows that a defining feature of some environmental health issues is the involvement of several jurisdictions and portfolios in the policy-making and regulation of that issue. Food safety policy and regulation are environmental health issues that are common to all jurisdictions, including the Commonwealth jurisdiction. At this level, it involves Food Standards Australia & New Zealand (FSANZ), formerly the Australia New Zealand Food Authority (ANZFA); the Department of Agriculture, Fisheries and Forestry; the Australian Quarantine Inspection Service; and the Department of Health and Ageing. At the state level, the various Departments of Health, local government authorities and state government authorities are involved. In New South Wales, this involves all local governments, the New South Wales Department of Health and regional public health units, and Safe Food Production New South Wales, whereas in Victoria it involves the Department of Human Services, all 79 local government authorities, the Victorian Meat Authority and Dairy Food Safety Victoria.

In contrast, some environmental health issues—like radiation safety—are regulated within one portfolio by the state and Commonwealth governments. Thus, the environmental health policy and regulatory services associated with any given environmental health issue may vary significantly from issue to issue. Services may be delivered by Commonwealth, state or territory governments, and by local governments.

The snapshot of the environmental health roles played by the state and territory governments in Appendix J shows the role of agencies outside the Health portfolio, such as Departments of Environment or environment protection authorities, and the types and scope of environmental health services provided. Once again, there are common services—for example, air (including noise), land and water pollution control; and some services based on ecologically sustainable development and environmental reporting.

Local government, as has been implied, provides a set of environmental health regulatory services that have been delegated from the state governments, depending on the local government administration framework within each state. As local government and its environmental health workforce are generalists, it follows that the delegation of legislative responsibilities by parliament will reflect this generalist flavour. Consequently, substantial areas of food safety regulation are delegated, but radiation safety—because of its highly specialised knowledge and technology—is regulated through specialist state government health department units.

Table 13.1 indicates some of the core environmental health functions undertaken by local government. Although state governments delegate various responsibilities and functions to local government, there are variations in the services provided, reflecting the differences in content of the legislation and regulatory frameworks and strategies. As would be expected there are variations in environmental health services between the states and territories.

In addition to the environmental health services that are required under legislation, other programs and services are provided by local government. Mosquito monitoring and breeding control programs are found in many states. These programs are designed to control and contain arthropod-borne diseases, such as Ross River (RR) virus, Murray Valley encephalitis (MVE) and dengue fever. Many councils have also developed and implemented a range of health-promotion activities oriented to environmental health. Examples of such projects range from the development of shade policy, the erection of shades and tree planting in open public areas, and sun protection education for outdoor workers, to the safe use of recycled water in home gardens. Emerging issues that will need to be addressed in similar ways include open fires and wood smoke, and indoor air quality.

Core environmental health practice domains: What we have come to expect

Food safety

Food safety is one environmental health function performed by all states and territories, although the regulatory activity might be carried out by either state or local government. Ensuring that the food we eat is safe is a critical environmental health activity. The incidence of food-borne illness is increasing both at the national and international levels with, according to ANZFA (now FSANZ), 11 500 cases of food-borne illness being reported

Table 13.1 Environmental health functions carried out by local governments

Function/service provided	NSW	NT	Qld	SA	Tas.	Vic.	WA
Management/provision of water supplies	yes	no	yes	no	yes	no	no
Management of waste and sanitation	yes	no	yes	no	yes	no	yes
Food safety regulation	yes	no	yes	yes	yes	yes	yes
Regulation of conduct of specific businesses to prevent risk (skin penetration, hairdressing, recreational water standards, e.g. swimming pools)	yes	no	yes	yes	yes	yes	yes
Regulation of lodging houses and public buildings	no	no	no	no	no	yes	yes
Prevention and control of infectious diseases—immunisation	yes	no	yes	yes	yes	yes	yes

Note: The ACT government performs the functions of both state and local government.

Sources: Department of Human Services (2012a); ACT Government (2010); Productivity Commission (2012); NPHP (2002b).

daily in Australia—that is, over 4 million reports annually.

In a 1999 ANZFA report, it was estimated that food-borne illnesses cost Australia $2.6 billion each year, and that Australians have a one in five chance of contracting food poisoning in any twelve-month period. Australia is currently enhancing its surveillance of food-borne illnesses. This will provide better data on changes in the incidence of food-borne illness in Australia and the most likely causes (ANZFA 2002).

In 2009, there were 163 outbreaks of food-borne or enteric illness, with 2679 people affected, 342 people hospitalised and eight deaths (OzFoodNet 2010). With economic and social costs exceeding $2.6 billion annually, this is one reason for recent moves by both the Commonwealth and state governments to review food safety legislation.

Other reasons advanced for the increase in food-borne illnesses are:

* intensive farming methods
* demographic changes (ageing population, community-based care)
* new and emerging pathogens
* changes in consumer eating and shopping habits
* more frequent reportage of food poisoning and easier detection
* awareness of consumers (via media)
* compensation orientation by consumers.

These reasons provided the impetus for developing national food safety standards.

Apart from the microbiological risks, there are other issues in food safety, including food additives and labelling of food. The addition of chemicals has been conducted for many years for the purposes of preserving food so that its shelf or storage life is extended (for example, sulphur dioxide in sausage meat); improving taste, texture or colour (for example, flavour enhancers like monosodium glutamate); or maintaining quality (for example, anti-caking agents to prevent clumping of dry ingredients). There has been criticism of some food additives, such as some artificial sweeteners, being approved by FSANZ on the basis that the current scientific evidence is limited and does not provide certainty that they are safe. Food allergens are also important for increasing numbers of consumers, and the following have been declared under the Food Standards Code by FSANZ, thus requiring labels on pre-packed foods to state their presence:

* crustaceans and their products
* peanuts and their products
* soybeans and their products
* tree nuts and their products
* sesame seeds and their products
* fish and fish products
* egg and egg products
* gluten and cereals containing gluten (wheat, rye, oats, barley and spelt)
* added sulphites that are concentrations of 10 milligrams/kilogram or more (FSANZ 2012).

The mandatory fortification of foods has generated some argument among experts. The addition of folate to a large range of breakfast cereals to reduce birth defects seems to have been supported generally. The Public Health Association of Australia perceived folate-fortified foods as an extra source of folate for women periconceptionally. However, if based on a voluntary fortification system, there was doubt that this approach would ensure an adequate folate supply to women at risk. The other ethical dilemma is with mandatory fortification, as it raises concerns that everyone in the population becomes exposed to increased levels of folate and so there is a potential risk of harm to many to benefit the needs of a few (PHAA 2004). Further complexity comes from the issues pertaining to health claims and labelling of food. Currently the legislation in Australia prohibits health claims on food labels, although this is under review, with the exception of food fortified with folate. There is concern that 'health' claims can be misleading, confusing or too simplistic, and while the claims may assist sales of the product they do not necessarily recognise that there may be a variety of factors associated with diet-related illnesses or deficiencies.

In most states, responsibility for implementing or enforcing much of the food safety legislation is delegated to local government. Victoria is acknowledged as having a decentralised model whereby each local government is the registering authority for food premises and has the responsibility for enforcing the provisions of the *Food Act 1984*. Western Australia, Tasmania and Queensland also require the registration of food businesses.

In the past, the administration of food safety standards was primarily the responsibility of each state and territory. However, following the Australian Health Ministers Advisory Council in 1996, the Commonwealth and state governments agreed to move towards nationally consistent food safety legislation. The result was a draft Model Food Act and Food Safety Standards which now provide the legislative framework for the new national food system. The draft Model Food Act contains core and non-core provisions to provide flexibility for state and territory parliaments to develop arrangements best suited to their respective jurisdictions. This will also mean there may be variation in some requirements.

The development and gazetting of the National Food Safety Standards of the Australia New Zealand Food Standards Code is one outcome of this process, and each state and territory government has undertaken to adopt these standards into its legislation. Collectively, the new Food Safety Standards are intended to provide a more effective regulatory system for ensuring the safety of food in Australia and therefore reducing the incidence of food-borne illness. This is to be achieved by placing more responsibility on the food business to ensure it handles food safely into every step of its operation— from the time the business receives food into its premises until the final product is purchased or served to the customer (ANZFA 2002). This is an important shift in regulatory policy. The government policy and the legislation make it clear that the responsibility for safe food rests with the owner of the food business. Further, owners are now being required to demonstrate that risks to food safety in their business are being managed. Demonstration of risk management may involve food safety programs based on hazard analysis critical control point (HACCP) systems. HACCP systems are required in the dairy and meat industries and for any foods for export.

Apart from requirements for the safe handling of food, the standards also include requirements for design of food businesses and for the training of food handlers. In addition to the development of food safety standards, there has been the development and implementation of a national food safety protocol, including the recall of food.

Local government plays a major role in implementation of these standards and this legislation. There are two major regulatory strategies used by councils to manage legislative compliance by business:

- **Registration management strategies:** these consist of a range of business services relating to the establishment of new food premises, the transfer of registration when businesses are bought and sold, and the annual renewal of registrations for food businesses. In South Australia and New South Wales a notification system rather than a registration system will be utilised.
- **Food safety monitoring strategies:** these consist of a range of business and community services aimed at ensuring that businesses are operating in compliance with the legislation, and that the community is protected from the sale of unsafe food. Business services include inspections of premises and community services are concerned with food sampling and analysis; investigation of food safety and food-borne illness complaints; and facilitation of food recalls.

These same standards are implemented by industry-specific regulators for seafood, dairy and meat. Historically, the dairy and meat industries have been regulated by a specific authority on the basis that these industries are based within the primary producer sector. This then requires a regulatory framework for the whole system of production, if quality and safety are to be managed effectively from paddock to plate. These particular industries are also economically important because often they are engaged in the export of food, and thus need to comply with international regulatory and agreement requirements. One of the features of food safety in Australia is that, historically, the concern has been with local domestic supply and the safety of that supply; however, in recent times Australia has been a signatory to international agreements, as part of global trade arrangements that require agreed food safety standards to be put in place for exported food. One challenge is to ensure that standards are consistent and are administered in a consistent fashion. Other challenges include how government—the signatory to international agreements—must work with industry to ensure compliance with international food safety standards, as failure will result in both international public health (global) and economic (local) consequences.

Thus, there has been an important change in food safety administration in Australia, as policy and standards development now involves all three levels of government and has moved from local to global in scope. The Commonwealth and state governments are involved through extra-constitutional agreements, which have led to the development of national approaches and standards, while local government and specialist regulatory agencies are important implementers of legislation and standards.

Occupational health and safety (OHS)

Another traditional area of concern is protecting workers from hazards in the work environment. Occupational health has its roots in the sanitary reforms of the Industrial Revolution in nineteenth-century Europe and, like the broader area of environmental health, found its impetus in governments developing legislation such as the English *Factory Acts* of 1833 and 1847. The 1833 *Factory Act* was intended specifically to address child labour, so it contained provisions that prohibited the employment of children under the age of nine years, restricted children aged between nine and thirteen from working more than nine hours daily, and required all children to receive two hours of schooling daily (United Kingdom Public Record Office n.d.).

From these beginnings, occupational health has expanded to include the protection and promotion of health and safety at work through preventing and controlling hazards in the work environment and by promoting health and the work capacity of working people. Occupational health is seen as a community asset, and it makes a positive contribution to productivity, product quality, work motivation and job satisfaction (WHO Collaborating Centres for Occupational Health 1995: 2).

During the financial year 2009–10, around 640 700 people (5.3 per cent of the 11 million Australian labour force) experienced a work-related injury or disease, 303 000 workers were compensated for work-related injuries, and it was estimated that 2000 work-related deaths would result. Safe Work Australia estimated that the total cost of workplace injury and illness to the Australian economy for the 2008–09 financial year was $60.6 billion, representing 4.8 per cent of Australia's GDP. (Safe Work Australia 2011: 4; 2012: 2). Although the original focus of OHS was on injuries and injury-related deaths in the workplace, recent research indicates that broader health and disease issues have also become significant. Globally, work-related injuries and diseases are responsible for the deaths of an estimated 2 million people annually, emanating from 270 million occupational accidents and 160 million occupational diseases. Worldwide, 246 million girls and boys are

Box 13.1 Investigation of a food poisoning incident

The reporting of a food poisoning (gastro-intestinal illness) incident to health authorities is a fairly common event. Incidents of gastro-intestinal illness are notifiable under legislation to the responsible Department of Health. These reports may or may not be related, but each report is investigated on the basis that it might be part of a cluster of related incidents. Most health authorities have an investigation protocol for these incidents, and the following outlines the common steps taken in these investigations after receipt of a notification.

Interview of person(s) affected: Direct contact is made with the affected person for the purposes of obtaining further information about the person and the circumstances relating to the incident. Typically, the information to be obtained includes personal details; a description of the clinical symptoms; current occupation; travel history; and food history.

Risk assessment of the incident: Essentially, an analysis is undertaken of the data obtained to determine whether further investigation is warranted. Risks are associated with the occupation of the person affected (food handler, health-care worker, child-care worker); the possible sources of contamination, such as food, water, environment, occupation and contacts with other cases of illness; and travel and resultant exposure.

Implementation of management strategies: Depending upon the outcomes from the risk assessment, a range of management strategies will be developed. It is important to identify and contain any sources of contamination, and prevent any further cases of illness. For example, if the affected person was a food handler, then that person would be excluded from working until such time as they are cleared by a medical practitioner. Other strategies include analysing any implicated foods or water, inspecting food premises, checking for further cases and investigating these, and providing educational material to affected persons and families.

Completion of the investigation: Finalisation of the investigation requires the recording of the actions and results of investigations and any other pertinent information. This is an important step in developing further intelligence on the source and transmission of illness through food and water.

Source: adapted from Victorian Department of Human Services (1999).

---

involved in child labour, with 176 million of these children being exposed to conditions that endanger their physical, mental or moral well-being (WHO 2011e). In 1994 the WHO approved a *Global Strategy on Occupational Health for All* (WHO 1995), which had eight priority areas:

- strengthening of international and national policies for health at work
- promotion of a healthy work environment, healthy work practices and health at work
- strengthening of occupational health services
- establishment of appropriate support services for occupational health

- development of occupational health standards based on scientific risk assessment
- development of human resources
- establishment of registration and data systems and information support
- strengthening of research.

Following this, the WHO developed a Global Plan of Action 2008–2017 with the following objectives:

- to strengthen the governance and leadership function of national health systems to respond to the specific health needs of working populations

- to establish basic levels of health protection at all workplaces to decrease inequalities in workers' health between and within countries, and strengthen the promotion of health at work
- to ensure access for all workers to preventive health services and link occupational health to primary health care
- to improve the knowledge base for action on protecting and promoting the health of workers, and establish linkages between health and work

- to stimulate incorporation of actions on workers' health into other policies, such as sustainable development, poverty reduction, trade liberalisation, environmental protection and employment. (WHO 2012)

In response to Australian circumstances, Safe Work Australia has developed its draft Australian Work Health and Safety Strategy 2012–2022. This strategy has identifed the need for a nationally

---

Box 13.2 Industrial hazards: Asbestos exposure at Wittenoom and Baryulgil

Workplace exposure to asbestos fibres can occur during mining and manufacturing and when working with the end-products. When inhaled, the fibres cause various diseases, such as mesothelioma, asbestosis, lung cancer and asbestos-related pleural disease. There is no safe level of exposure to asbestos, and its deadly effects may not emerge until 40 years later. While the use of asbestos was effectively banned in Australia at the end of 2003 (Jackson 2004), its commercial and industrial use was widespread until the 1980s. Claims for compensation have since been lodged by former miners, government employees and manufacturing and construction workers against the miners and manufacturers of asbestos products CSR and James Hardie Industries. Since 1945, an estimated 7000 Australians have died from mesothelioma, and this number is expected to increase to 18000 by 2020 (Parliamentary Library 2004).

The most unhygienic and hazardous workplaces were the asbestos mines at Wittenoom in Western Australia and Baryulgil in north-central New South Wales. These two mines are an example of what can happen in vulnerable populations (recent immigrants and a small Aboriginal community respectively), with poor bargaining or political power, little contact with trade unions, and no previous mining experience or

knowledge of expected standards for working conditions. Both were isolated communities. Both mines were owned by major Australian companies but, as they were unprofitable operations, little interest was taken in them. The working conditions were like something one would expect in a developing country with a poor regulatory framework, even though the link between asbestos and lung cancer had been made in the mid-1950s.

Wittenoom, Western Australia
During the life of the mining operation, 20000 people lived at Wittenoom and were therefore exposed to potentially lethal levels of blue asbestos. The population was composed largely of recently arrived immigrants. The mine and mill were owned by CSR and operated by the subsidiary, Australian Blue Asbestos (ABA). The working conditions underground were appalling, as the men had to crawl around in hot and unventilated conditions digging out blue asbestos. Conditions at the mill, where the ore was ground down and the fibre extracted, were so horrific that floodlights were needed even in the middle of the day (Asbestos Diseases Society of Australia 2004). Tailings from the mine were also used in the town for road surfacing and land dressing at the racecourse, the local school, parking areas, around homes and on the golf course, exposing the families of miners to the risks as well. This practice continued in Wittenoom even after the mine was closed in 1966, due to its becoming economically unviable (McCulloch 1986).

While the responsibility for monitoring and inspecting the working conditions at the mine was shared between the West Australian Departments of Mines and Public Health, its isolation made such regulation very difficult. As a result, ABA made no effort to reduce the dust in the mine and mill, even though the technology was available to do so. By 1955, medical research had shown that cancer of the lung could be caused by exposure to asbestos. By 1958, six cases of asbestosis had been recorded at Wittenoom, but the true extent of the problem was masked by the high labour turnover. The first case of mesothelioma caused by asbestos was diagnosed in Australia in 1961. Since then, the number of cases of asbestosis and mesothelioma has risen steadily, resulting in increased public awareness in Western Australia and internationally in the United States and United Kingdom. The victims have found a voice through the Asbestos Diseases Society, established in 1978, which has exerted pressure on the Western Australian government to make legislative changes to enable claims to be brought forward (Asbestos Diseases Society of Australia 2004).

Baryulgil, New South Wales

Baryulgil is a small isolated Aboriginal community 80 kilometres from Grafton in north-central New South Wales. Mining of white asbestos was begun there in 1943 by a subsidiary of CSR, which was then taken over by a wholly owned subsidiary of the James Hardie Group. The mine was worked as an open-cut quarry—following blasting, a cloud of fibre drifted over the whole quarry and nearby mess areas, and the prevailing winds blew it over the town. Tailings were used on roads and in and around homes. The predominantly Aboriginal miners worked in filthy conditions, and there was a complete absence of concern by managers about hygiene. The shoeless men worked in two teams, shovelling fibre by hand into hessian bags that were often recycled from other mines (and so had blue and brown asbestos fibre in them). No industrial work clothes or boots were issued until 1974. Because of the general poverty of the community, many of these bags were taken home and used in a variety of ways. Workers' skin would be white by the end of a shift due to the dust. The New South Wales Mines Inspectorate staff—chronically overworked, but at times barely competent—made little attempt to regulate activities at the mine. The mine closed in 1979 on economic grounds (McCulloch 1986).

As there was little or no trade union presence at the mine during its working life, the workers were paid the minimum rate. The provision of housing was poor, forcing the workers to build their own housing from available materials. This included the hessian bags used to carry the asbestos fibres. Infant mortality rates were high and no medical care was provided. Major health studies were conducted in 1977, 1981 and 1982 by the New South Wales Health Commission, but conclusive evidence of widespread asbestos-related diseases was not found. As Aboriginal people in New South Wales had such poor health and low life expectancy, it was 'very unlikely that work carried out on a segment of that population could show a marked variation in mortality and morbidity' (McCulloch 1986).

In 1984, the Aboriginal Legal Service presented a submission to the Minister for Aboriginal Affairs (Clyde Holding) asking for an inquiry into the Baryulgil mine. It recommended the establishment of an Aboriginal Medical Service, that the residents of Baryulgil should be persuaded to move to another site, and that the mine site be rehabilitated (Standing Committee on Aboriginal Affairs 1984). Despite this, it has taken community members several decades to get recognition for their suffering. In early March 2005, the New South Wales Dust and Diseases Board, whose statutory function is to administer workers' compensation, sent the 'Lung Bus' to Baryulgil to assess the community's claims. But for the majority of former workers, this was too late, as many had already died (Hassan 2005).

coordinated approach to health and safety. In its first five years, it will focus on the following work-related disease priorities:

- mental disorders
- cancers (including skin cancer)
- asthma
- contact dermatitis
- noise-induced hearing loss.

The industry groupings identifed as priorities are agriculture, transport, manufacturing, construction and health (Safe Work Australia 2011).

Occupational health and safety is another environmental health function common to states and territories. Each state and territory has an *Occupational Health and Safety Act*, which sets legislative duties and obligations for workplace health and safety. The administration of OHS legislation is similar to that for food safety standards: each state and territory has sovereignty in relation to workplace safety and thus enforces state and territory legislation. Broadly speaking, OHS legislation is intended to protect all persons in the workplace, including employees and contractors. Though generally not well known, this legislation is also intended to protect visitors to the workplace, the general public, volunteers, emergency service personnel, consultants, government officials and couriers.

In 1984, the National Occupational Health and Safety Commission (NOHSC) was created to provide a national perspective and forum on occupational health and safety for state and territory governments, employer organisations and trade unions. As part of its role, the NOHSC developed national approaches, standards and codes of practice for adoption into legislation by the state and territory governments. In 2008, the Intergovernmental Agreement for Regulatory and Operational Reform in Occupational Health and Safety was signed by all states and territories and the funding provided by states, territories and the Commonwealth was used in part to establish Safe Work Australia. Like FSANZ

and arrangements for food safety standards, Safe Work Australia is a national policy body and not a regulator of work health (Safe Work Australia 2011: 11, 12). The Commonwealth government, as an employer, also adopts and administers occupational health legislation.

At the operational or enforcement end of OHS, a visit to any of the state government websites provides an insight into the level of activity associated with workplace safety regulation. In New South Wales, the responsible government agency is WorkCover NSW, which has the largest OHS inspectorate in Australia. The broad mission of WorkCover NSW is to increase the competitiveness of the New South Wales economy through productive, healthy and safe workplaces (NSW Workcover 2012a). In addition to workplace safety, WorkCover NSW has responsibility for managing the welfare of injured workers, including workers' compensation. From 2005 to 2010, there was a decrease in successful prosecutions from 699 to 103 convictions for breaches of the *Work Health and Safety Act 2011* (NSW Workcover 2012b). In 2008, the total amount for fines arising from prosecutions was $4.1 million, and $529 000 was received from infringement notices (NSW Workcover 2012b: 66).

Like food safety and other environmental health areas, over time OHS has evolved in terms of its complexity and the scope of issues to be managed and regulated by government. The government approach to regulation of OHS has slowly evolved from prescriptive legislation to performance-based legislation. This approach—again similar to food safety regulation—is based on individual industries taking responsibility for OHS, and developing systems and strategies that can be audited for compliance. Government influences this performance orientation by developing national guides and codes for adoption by industry, education and training standards, data collection and management, and research coordination and evaluation (NOHSC 2004).

The development of the Intergovernmental Agreement highlights the perceived need for a national approach and consistency between states and territories, because occupational health and safety is an important regulatory and economic issue. What is different about OHS is that the control of policy and regulation is a state or territory function, its implementation is not delegated to local government, and employers and trade unions formally participate in the policy development and regulation processes.

Vector-borne disease

As noted earlier, control of transmissible diseases was also one of the earliest public health concerns. Adopting the classic epidemiological triad model, environmental health action has focused on controlling the 'agent', or the vectors that may be responsible for carrying and transmitting the diseases.

Vector-borne diseases are those diseases mechanically carried by crawling and flying insects through contamination of body parts (feet, proboscis or gut) to humans. Plague is a classic vector-borne disease, whereby the causative organism (the bacterium *Yersinia pestis*) is carried by fleas that bite and infect humans. Malaria is also a well-known vector-borne disease, together with dengue fever and the arboviral (arthropod-borne) diseases.

Of particular public health importance in Australia are the arboviral diseases—MVE, Kunjin, Japanese encephalitis, Ross River (RR) virus and Barmah Forest (BF) virus. These diseases are spread through the bites of infected mosquitoes, most commonly *Culex annulirostris*. Of these, MVE causes the most severe disease and there was a national outbreak of the disease in 1974. In south-eastern Australia, this involved around 58 cases, thirteen of whom died (Spencer et al. 2001).

RR and BF virus are responsible for an illness known as epidemic polyarthritis and, like MVE, the virus is transmitted by mosquitoes. Unlike MVE, notifications for both these viruses are high in number; however, the fatality rate is much lower than for MVE. Both RR and BF virus illnesses are debilitating, and people suffering with the illness commonly have symptoms of joint pain and swelling, skin rashes, headaches, fever and fatigue. The illness can last for several months.

Environmental conditions are a critical precondition for the virus activity and mosquito breeding. Conditions must be warm for the virus to be active, and the environment wet enough for breeding of mosquitoes. In the north of Australia, environmental conditions are such that viruses can be active all year whenever heavy rainfall or unusually high tides occur. The notification tables for RR and BF indicate that notifications are highest in Western Australia, Queensland and New South Wales.

How are arboviral diseases controlled? There are three categories of action that are needed in controlling these diseases (Spencer et al. 2001):

- **Monitoring virus activity through surveillance of human cases of disease and sometimes activity in sentinel animals, and monitoring mosquitoes and weather conditions:** Part of these monitoring activities is the assessment of data from the various surveillance mechanisms to ascertain activity, such as the identification and reporting of human cases of the disease, mosquito trapping to determine species and predicting weather patterns that have been associated with the previous outbreaks of disease.
- **Implementation of mosquito-control programs:** Generally, this involves identification of mosquito larvae and adults, the elimination of mosquito breeding areas, and control of mosquito larvae with control programs. These programs are implemented by local councils and public health units.
- **Advice to the general public on removing mosquito breeding sites and protecting against mosquito bites:** Advising the public to take personal precautions against mosquito bites when there is increased mosquito activity

is an important control step. This also includes advising tourists and other visitors to the area.

Arbovirus diseases are a classic environmental health issue where there is a direct relationship between human health, disease and the environment (and more specifically climate change). In 1999, the former Director-General of the WHO stated that health scientists had estimated that there would be increases in the size of populations at risk of arbo-borne and other diseases from increases in global temperatures (Brundtland 1999). As the breeding environments for mosquitoes increase with changing climatic conditions, it is reasonable to expect increases in arbovirus diseases. The WHO expects that an additional 2 billion people will be exposed to dengue fever transmission by the 2080s (WHO 2009: 10).

The transmission of disease from animal to humans—that is, a disease that is infectious to both humans and animals—is referred to as zoonosis. These types of disease are not new; plague, hydatid disease, psittacosis and arboviral diseases are examples—and, in the case of plague, have been around for some time. However, in recent years there has been increased concern about emerging infectious diseases as a number of these diseases are zoonotic. SARS, avian influenza and bovine spongiform encephalopathy (mad cow disease) are some examples. The concern is that some human activities seem to increase the chances of zoonoses—activities such as the globalisation of trade in domestic animals, and increasing greenhouse emissions.

Wastewater management

With the advent of sanitary reform in nineteenth-century Europe, one of the major activities undertaken in cities was the collection, removal and disposal of human waste (nightsoil) and wastewater generated from sanitary and industrial activities, an important environmental health practice that has continued to the present day. Over time, the

Box 13.3 Why you have always disliked cockroaches

Did you know that there are 428 species of cockroach in Australia? While most of these live in the wild and fulfil a role as recyclers of decaying and dead organic matter, several species like living in houses and apartments and in restaurants and other workplaces. The most common is the German cockroach, which grows to about 15 millimetres long and can be found hiding in the cracks, crevices and cupboards in kitchens, bathrooms and living areas. The American cockroach is larger, growing to around 40 millimetres in length, and can be found in gardens, around garbage, sewers and manholes. When established in homes, they like to live behind cupboards, in the gaps between walls, under floors and in roofs.

As both species of cockroach freely move from sewers (cockroaches can pass through the S-bends of pipes), to food and food preparation utensils, they are potential vectors of disease if they harbour pathogenic organisms such as bacteria (for example, *Salmonella enteritidis*), fungi, moulds or intestinal parasites. Susceptible individuals can become allergic to cockroaches and their faeces. This allergy can lead to the development of the symptoms of asthma, particularly when there are infestations in bedrooms.

Cockroach infestations are usually controlled by the spraying of insecticides into their hiding places and breeding areas in homes, drains and garden areas. As the use of such insecticides has the potential to cause health risks to some individuals, gels have been developed that rely on the feeding and foraging habits of cockroaches. These gels use less insecticide and are combined with food, attractants and water to target only cockroaches. This means that other pests, such as ants and bedbugs, which were previously killed by sprays, are not being controlled.

Source: Miller & Peters (2004: 208–11).

development of sewerage systems included not only the collection but the treatment of these wastes prior to their disposal as wastewater. This became a critical factor in the context of urban growth, increasing industrialisation and environmental protection.

It is often assumed that all dwellings in Australia discharge waste through a public sewerage system. However, one emerging issue from an environmental health perspective is the use and management of septic tank systems. Septic tanks are used when a public sewer is not available. They involve the collection of human waste and wastewater at the dwelling and the dispersion of the treated wastewater within the boundaries of the property. Although the wastewater or effluent is treated, it still contains bacteria and chemicals that will contaminate the environment and pose human health risks.

In New South Wales, there were an estimated 250 000 septic tank systems in the late 1990s, and it has been calculated that such systems provided for 12 per cent of Australia's population (Whitehead & Geary 2000). A survey of local councils undertaken by the Environment Protection Authority and the Australian Institute of Environmental Health estimated that Victoria had approximately 238 000 domestic on-site systems. Of these, 82.5 per cent were conventional septic tanks (EPA and AIEH 2001).

Public health disease risks arise when effluent or wastewater contaminates drinking water or waters used for recreational purposes, or if there is direct human contact with effluent. Micro-organisms in the wastewater have the potential to cause diseases, including gastroenteritis, shigellosis, giardiasis, cryptosporidiosis and hepatitis. Apart from bacteria and viruses, wastewater also contains large amounts of chemicals like nitrates and phosphorus. From the environmental perspective, discharged wastewater will contaminate the environment. It is the type, concentration and location of the discharge that

determines the degree of impact on human health and the health of the environment.

In the United States, contaminated drinking water is a prominent public health risk. According to the American Public Health Association, up to 900 000 people fall ill and 900 die annually from water-borne diseases. In 1993, there was an outbreak of cryptosporidiosis that caused an estimated 403 000 cases of illness, 440 hospitalisations and 50 deaths. In a review of the reported cases of water-borne disease outbreaks in the United States between 1991 and 1998, it was found that chemical contaminants were responsible for 18 per cent of all outbreaks. Of the outbreaks associated with untreated well water, sewage contamination was identified in 26 per cent of the cases (American Public Health Association 2000). Faecal coliforms (an indicator of human sewage contamination) were found in 82 per cent of the outbreaks that were tested using water samples (Craun et al. 2002). Faecal wastes are the main source of contamination of recreational water. Research has shown that 41 per cent of water-borne disease outbreaks relate directly to overflow or seepage of sewage from septic tanks and cesspools (Reneau, Hayedorn & Degen 1989).

In Australia, the impact of failing septic tank systems has been highlighted by occurrences of algal blooms from nutrient contamination in many rivers and lakes, an outbreak of hepatitis in Wallis Lake in New South Wales (1996), and *Cryptosporidium* and *Giardia* outbreaks in Sydney's water supplies (Whitehead & Geary 2000). It was found that 444 of the hepatitis cases were due to the consumption of oysters grown commercially in Wallis Lake that had become contaminated with human waste from effluent discharges into the lake and its waterways.

A study by the Rural Water Corporation of Victoria revealed the impact of septic tank effluent on groundwater in the Murray River basin at Benalla, with nitrate-nitrogen levels higher than the WHO standards, as well as bacterial contamination. In the Piccadilly Valley, South Australia, there were found to be increasing levels of nitrate in over 50 per cent of groundwater bores between 1979 and 1994. In addition, 19 per cent of bores were found to test positive for faecal indicator bacteria attributed to leaking septic tanks (Whitehead & Geary 2000).

In a further study, a review was undertaken of alternative domestic wastewater-management options for the Mount Lofty Ranges watershed. The review was prompted by the pollution of water supply reservoirs by nutrients from failing septic tanks and urban runoff, and recommended the introduction of new guidelines for septic tank management (Geary 1988).

Even though it is recognised that all effluent—treated or otherwise—poses significant environmental health problems, the continuous expansion of Australia's urban areas without the concurrent infrastructure development (including the provision of sewerage and drains) will increase the risks of contamination of the water catchments and groundwater from which reticulated drinking water supplies are sourced.

In twenty-first-century Australia, the major issue is how we reuse treated wastewater. As Australia is the driest continent, and we have the highest per capita use of fresh water in the world, there is an urgent need to conserve water through its reuse, whether it is for agricultural, domestic or industrial purposes. Although there are sound environmental reasons for reuse, there are also concerns regarding the potential for disease if reuse is not properly managed by the user.

Chemical contamination

In Australia, chemicals such as pesticides and herbicides are used in both rural and urban environments, and in commercial and domestic settings. Their use has increased significantly since the 1950s. World attention was first drawn to the persistence of pesticides, such as DDT and organochlorines, in the environment by Rachel Carson in her 1962 book *Silent Spring* (Carson 1965). Carson revealed how

pesticides caused the thinning of bird's egg shells, resulting in lower survival rates and hence a 'silent spring' (Short 1994).

People can be exposed to pesticides through their skin (dermal absorption), residues in fruit and vegetables, drinking water, breast milk, and inhalation within homes, workplaces and agricultural areas. While exposure to some pesticides can poison an individual very quickly, many have slow impacts over a long period of time. Some effects (such as cancer, kidney or liver damage) are specific, while chemical sensitivities, nerve damage and deterioration in health and quality of life are less precise. Such exposures are frequently the result of the misuse and abuse of pesticides, which can occur because of poor training, lax safety standards, the failure to abide by directions on pesticide container labels, and not wearing appropriate protective clothing. It can result in workers, and the wider population, being directly exposed to chemical spray drift and toxic fumes (Short 1994). But exposure can also result from everyday products, such as paints, glues, furniture, carpets and clothes.

In Australia, the sale and use of chemicals is regulated by a variety of government departments and authorities. The Office of Chemical Safety, which is part of the Therapeutic Goods Administration group, 'undertakes risk assessment and provides advice on potential public health risks posed by chemicals used in the community' (<www.tga.gov.au/chemicals/ocs>) to chemical regulators, the Australian Pesticides and Veterinary Medicines Authority (<www.apvma.gov.au>) and the National Industrial Chemicals Notification and Assessment Scheme (<www.nicnas.gov.au>). NICNAS also monitors Australia's obligations under international agreements.

But regulations relating to chemicals are significantly different because of the approaches adopted by enforcement jurisdictions across Australia, particularly those relating to agricultural and veterinary chemicals. These differences have led to concerns about inconsistencies, complexity and

Box 13.4 Herbicide exposure of Aboriginal workers in the Kimberley

Between 1975 and 1985, the Western Australian Agriculture Protection Board sprayed the chemical herbicides 2,4D and 2,4,5T (which are the same ingredients that are found in the defoliant Agent Orange, which was used in Vietnam) on imported weeds that were alleged to be preventing cattle from getting access to the Fitzroy and Ord Rivers in the Kimberley. As employment opportunities were limited, Aboriginal men and women were pleased to take the jobs, although they were largely unskilled and had very limited understanding of herbicides. The workers were told the spray was harmless, so minimal safety training was provided and protective clothing generally was not worn. Many of the drums were not labelled, although at that time labelling of containers was the main source of information regarding the safe use of herbicides. The label should have alerted the user that it is was a poison with low toxicity to humans and stock, and to keep clear of spray drift (Harper 2002, 2004).

As many of the former workers became sick during spraying (with headaches, nausea, vomiting, fatigue, rashes and bleeding), and continued to suffer chronic illness, they sought for 20 years to get these problems investigated. Their illnesses were ignored by medical professionals, and thus the former workers became dissatisfied with the health-care system. Instead, they sought political intervention, which resulted in the West Australian Minister for Agriculture appointing Dr Andrew Harper to conduct the Kimberley Chemical Use Review in 2001. This review found that 321 people had been employed in the spraying, of whom 34 were deceased. The review team then interviewed 124 former workers, and documented their health problems and work experiences. They found a lack of compliance with the health and safety instructions on the manufacturers' labels, and that hygiene in the camps was left to the workers, who used the rivers for washing and drinking water. The equipment used was faulty, drums of herbicide leaked and many workers were continuously wet from the spray (Harper 2002).

The review made several recommendations based on a causal link between the workplace exposure to herbicides and current chronic illness. One of these was that compensation should be offered to those workers who had experienced loss or disability (Harper 2002). An expert medical panel has subsequently been asked to evaluate Dr Harper's findings, as it is highly likely that there will never be sufficient scientific and statistical evidence—particularly given the time period—to prove the cause–effect association resulting from exposure to herbicides (Armstrong 2003). But perhaps more importantly, the review has highlighted an 'environmental justice' issue, and a failure of the health-care system in Western Australia.

---

fragmentation (Productivity Commission 2008 pp. xxxvi and 219).

In February 2004, flooding on Tasmania's Georges River led to the death of 90 per cent of the intertidal oyster crop in Georges Bay. The oyster farmers commissioned a report by Dr Marcus Scammell, which linked the mortalities to the aerial spraying of pesticides and herbicides over private forestry plantations up-stream. The Tasmanian government admitted that it did not know what chemicals were being used and the volume being discharged into waterways, and subsequently ordered the testing of local water supplies for chemical residues. The Australian Medical Association called for a ban on aerial spraying until its safety was proven (Scammell 2004; Nettleford 2004). This incident highlighted a breakdown in environmental protection and was consistent with the conclusion of the Productivity Commission's study into chemicals and plastic regulation: 'The Commission finds that the current institutional and regulatory arrangements are broadly *effective* in managing the risks to health and safety, but are less effective in managing risks to the environment and national security.' (Productivity Commission 2008 p. xxv).

The storage of chemicals in urban areas also poses a risk to public health. This was highlighted by the Coode Island explosion and chemical fire that occurred in Melbourne in August 1991. Clouds of toxic smoke and fumes threatened nearby suburbs before being dispersed by high winds. In February 2001, half a million litres of toxic waste chemicals blew up at the Waste Control Pty Ltd plant in Bellevue, east of Perth. The company had previously been fined for contravening several hazardous waste regulations. Spot fires were started and a plume of toxic smoke and ash spread across a wide area of Perth (Skinner 2001). As the company could not provide a comprehensive list of the chemicals stored, the subsequent Western Australian government inquiry recommended the establishment of the Bellevue Health Surveillance Register to monitor the health of the exposed community (Green Dragon Consultants 2003).

In 2006 the Council of Australian Governments identified chemicals and plastics as a public policy priority and steps were taken to develop both a streamlined and harmonised national system of regulation. One of the recommendations made by the Productivity Commission was that the Australian Pesticides and Veterinary Medicines Authority should regulate the use of agricultural and veterinary chemical products after these chemicals had been sold (Productivity Commission 2008 p. XLVII). In September 2012 the Department of Agriculture, Fisheries and Forestry released a revised draft of the Agricultural and Veterinary Chemicals Legislation Amendment Bill 2012 together with explanatory documents and details of proposed regulations (APVMA 2013). Steps towards tightening the regulation of chemicals—and their subsequent risk to health, environment, and national security—have taken considerable time; however, it appears that a national framework is under development which could provide for a more consistent regulatory approach nationally.

Radiation safety

Radiation safety is a specialised area of environmental and public health and, like other environmental issues, is regulated by the states and territories through their respective Departments of Health. Within the Commonwealth jurisdiction, there was legislation regulating radiation safety before the establishment of the Australian Radiation Protection and Nuclear Safety Agency (ARPANSA) in 1998.

What are the dangers of radiation? Ionising radiation is high-frequency radiation—an example being x-rays. When absorbed into the body, this radiation causes chemical reactions that can alter the normal functions of the body, and high doses will cause cell death, organ damage and ultimately death (ARPANSA 2001: 22). Thus, there is a need to control the use of this type of radiation.

Radiation safety encompasses the use of radiation equipment, radioactive substances and electronic products that emit non-ionising radiation. Ionising radiation refers to the use of medical appliances and the safety issues resulting from exposure to this radiation by both employees and patients. The total number of diagnostic and therapeutic services involving radiation performed during 1999–2000 was almost 9.1 million, equating to $728 million in Medicare payments (ARPANSA 2001). A further use of ionising radiation is the use of x-ray technologies in the examination of imported goods in shipping containers by the Australian Customs Service.

Operators and their radiation equipment and apparatus are required to be licensed by the appropriate jurisdiction. Licensed operators are radiologists, general medical practitioners, nuclear medicine specialists, chiropractors, researchers and borehole loggers (mining industry). Registered apparatus include x-ray equipment, gauges, lasers and mineral analysers. The total number of licences and registrations in Australia exceeds 41 000, with between 30 000 and 35 000 people making use of radiation in their employment (ARPANSA 2001: 13–14).

Naturally occurring radioactive materials, manufactured radioactive material and radioactive waste, including global fallout from nuclear testing and visits by nuclear-powered warships, are subject to monitoring by ARPANSA. Analyses of food and water are also conducted, with 283 food samples and 900 water samples being analysed in 2002–01 (ARPANSA 2001).

Regulation of ionising radiation and associated environmental health risks has been managed fairly consistently by the respective Departments of Health through a legislative regime of registration, licensing and monitoring within a framework of national standards.

There have been rapid developments in new applications of radioactive substances and radiation equipment, particularly in medical diagnosis. Commensurate with this increase, there has been an apparent increase in per capita radiation dose from ionising radiation. From the public perspective, the area of ionising radiation has become more significant over time, with its increasing use in cancer treatment and increased occupational exposure (ARPANSA 2001).

Non-ionising radiation includes the radiation from powerlines, mobile telephones, microwave ovens, video display terminals, laser pointers and barcode scanners. Ultraviolet radiation is also a non-ionising radiation. Each of these areas has had a range of issues that have been the subject of public debate and concern, most notably mobile telephones and solaria. Unlike ionising radiation, there appears to be a marked absence of a systematic and consistent approach to regulation by jurisdictions. All states and territories have the power to regulate in this area, but only the Commonwealth, Western Australia and Tasmania regulate the use of non-ionising radiation apparatus, such as lasers and some radio-frequency devices (ARPANSA 2001).

Radiation safety in both the ionising and non-ionising radiation areas is rapidly expanding, and there are many environmental health issues associated with this expansion—particularly in the use of new technologies. In the case of ionising radiation safety, there has been a history and well-established regulatory framework in place in all jurisdictions in Australia. In the case of non-ionising radiation, the public has unrestricted and unprotected access to non-ionising radiation apparatus like mobile telephones, lasers and solaria.

Current environmental health policy frameworks: Shared principles for practitioners

The National Environmental Health Strategy (NEHS), launched in 1999 by the Commonwealth government, clearly espoused the perspective that people are entitled to an environment that promotes good health. Thus, environmental health is recognised as an entitlement, although the total absence of risk is not possible (Commonwealth of Australia 1999: 9). This strategy was the first national approach to the management of environmental health issues in Australia.

As part of this strategy, the Australian Charter for Environmental Health was developed, containing nine guiding principles in relation to developing and implementing environmental health strategies (see Box 13.5).

Box 13.5 Australian Charter for Environmental Health (guiding principles)

- Protection of human health
- Interrelationship between economics, health and environment
- Sustainable development
- Local and global interface
- Partnership
- Risk-based management
- Evidence-based decisions
- Efficiency
- Equity

Source: adapted from Commonwealth of Australia (1999).

The objectives of the strategy reflect these principles, particularly the need to ensure that environmental health is integrated within broader environmental, economic and social policy development. The strategy is particularly concerned with the loss of the ability to predict and reduce environmental health threats from fragmentation of management across jurisdictions and organisations. Subsequently, a number of objectives have been identified to improve environmental health management in Australia (Commonwealth of Australia 1999):

- improving collaboration through increasing support for partnerships, engaging stakeholders as partners, and increasing participation in decision-making
- improving management practices through a national approach to risk assessment and risk management, and developing national standards and guidelines, a mechanism for setting priorities in environmental health, and better coordination
- improving decision-making ability through strengthening the evidence base, providing a sound economic basis and developing a comprehensive information system
- improving communication through raising the awareness of environmental health issues, consultation on environmental health policy, education opportunities and risk communication
- increasing the capacity of the environmental health workforce through improved research and development, improved workforce development and training, and planning to meet future needs
- promoting healthy environments through recognising the central role of sustainable development and the interrelationship of health and environment, and facilitating community participation in decision-making on environmental health issues.

These objectives were ambitious, and underpinned a desire to organise the effort within

environmental health, in much the same way as has occurred in other areas such as occupational health and safety. The National Environmental Health Strategy 2007–2012 saw a shift in priorities to more emphasis on building environmental health infrastructure, including building capacity to respond to disasters. The priorities of the strategy are to:

- enhance the nation's ability to respond to environmental health challenges from disasters
- anticipate and plan for the most critical public health issues arising from climate change
- provide standards, guidelines, regulations, legislation, indicators and risk-assessment tools
- ensure environmental standards developed in other sectors
- effectively protect human health, and increase the capacity and capability of the environmental health workforce, especially in Aboriginal and Torres Strait Islander communities
- improve environmental health conditions in Aboriginal and Torres Strait Islander communities. (enHealth 2007: 5)

Clearly, the challenges of environmental health are extending beyond purely the local to become global in scope, and the strategy provides the fundamentals that need to be in place so that Australia has the infrastructure to manage environmental health.

Environmental health justice: All is not equal in the environment

One important issue raised within the 1999 NEHS is environmental health justice. The 1999 NEHS and the charter acknowledged that all Australians are entitled to live in a safe and healthy environment and that, although environmental health is inherently equitable, parts of the Australian population are disadvantaged through increased exposure to environmental hazards and risks, and decreased access to environmental health services

(Commonwealth of Australia 1999). Disadvantaged communities include people living in remote areas, isolated Indigenous communities and communities located near to industry where environmental health risks are usually identifiable—such as noise or air pollution—or where environmental health risks are unknown due to a lack of research. From the environmental health policy planning perspective, it is important to ensure that no population group or community suffers from disproportionate environmental risks, and that appropriate services—including health information resources—are accessible for these communities.

Indigenous environmental health

Living in our well-serviced cities and towns today, it is tempting to think of the environmental sanitation and sanitary reforms as issues of the past—in fact, of over 150 years ago. It is also tempting to consider that such issues, if they exist today, are issues in poor nations ravaged by warfare. Yet in Australia there remains another sanitary reform to be won, and this is in relation to the health of Indigenous Australians. While the causes of poor health in Aboriginal and Torres Strait Islander communities are complex, poor environmental health standards are a significant contributor to the 20-year gap in life expectancy between Indigenous and non-Indigenous Australians. These environmental health issues include:

> safe water and food, proper sewage and refuse disposal, adequate living space and sanitary facilities, provision of power and vector control ... Unfortunately, [I]ndigenous communities throughout Australia are too often deprived of the good environmental health standards considered normal in the greater Australian community. (National Environmental Health Forum 2000: 9)

Current priorities in Indigenous environmental health in Australia are concerned with the building of capacity and coordination. Capacity-building of the Indigenous environmental health workforce involves the development of models of essential and desirable criteria for Indigenous environmental health workers (IEHWs); ensuring representation of IEHWs on forums such as enHealth so that advice on IEHWs issues is provided directly to enHealth; recognising training issues; and the development of community education material that supports the role of the IEHW. Other priorities are concerned with ensuring that legislation that impacts on environmental health standards is binding on the Crown. For example, governments are required to comply with legislation such as that for the development of nationally consistent standards for remote Indigenous housing and infrastructure; the upgrading of Indigenous food stores to comply with the National Food Safety Standards; and the development of mechanisms to facilitate national partnerships to improve environmental health (National Environmental Health Forum 2000). Improving Aboriginal and Torres Strait Islander environmental health continues to be an issue, and was an important objective of the 2007–2012 NEHS.

Do these issues sound familiar? The very same issues that Chadwick and other public health pioneers struggled with in the mid-1800s are still present in Australian society, and have been for many years. And as with those pioneers, there are battles to be won for resources and political commitment to bring the much-needed social and environmental changes that will improve the health status of Indigenous Australians.

Monitoring environmental health: Watching out for the future

The components of 'the environment' incorporate everything around us considered to be vital prerequisites for life to exist, including the ground and soil, air, water (rainwater as well as river and lake systems and the sea) and food. The recent drought in south-west Western Australia and south-east South Australia, Victoria and Tasmania, together with climate change and a growing population, has resulted in increased pressure on traditional water supplies. Water security has become an important issue, and is demanding the development of alternatives other than building more dams, or imposing water restrictions. The Australian government has developed its Water for the Future strategy, in which it is recognised that water security will demand the integration of four key priorities:

• taking action on climate change
• using water wisely
• securing water supplies, and
• supporting healthy rivers. (Department of Sustainability, Environment, Water, Population and Communities 2012)

Likewise, food security has become a priority of the government as it is anticipated that global population growth, climate change, finite natural resources, obesity and chronic disease due to poor nutrition will shape the scope and nature of our food supply. Globally, 'one billion people suffer chronic hunger and the United Nations estimates that food production will need to increase by about 70 per cent from 2005–07 average levels to feed the projected world population of 9.3 billion by 2050' (Department of Agriculture, Fisheries and Forestry 2011: vi).

The environment also includes the less favourably viewed elements, such as chemicals, radiation, organisms that are pathogenic to humans and animals, and destructive physical forces with which we all periodically come into contact in our daily lives. We have complex ways of using and interacting with our environment. Some of them pose both immediate and longer-term threats to our own well-being. With increasing knowledge of the links between environmental influences on human health, and the impacts of human activities on the environment, increased attention has been paid to developing environmental monitoring systems, including benchmarks and status reporting, such as state of the environment (SOE) reporting by government (Australian and New Zealand Environment and Conservation Council 2000) to provide information for evidence-based environmental decision-making. Largely, these efforts seem to have relied on two sets of indicators. The first set comprises environmental indicators, which provide a measure of the health of (primarily) the natural environment. The second set consists of environmental health indicators, which provide a measure of hazards to human health within (primarily) the built environment.

Hazards to the natural environment

One of the first indicators ever used, and it *was* an environmental indicator, was smoke; to this day, we have the saying 'where there's smoke, there's fire'. According to the CSIRO (1999), environmental indicators serve management processes, and although they may vary in complexity, they usually require the integration of a range of factors, of which the physical environment is only one part. It is now realised that robust decisions require attention to social, economic and environmental factors (CSIRO 1999). Indicators actually are a communication tool between the environment and people, and are used in making decisions about managing the environment.

The recognition of just how complex our environment is resulted in the release of the report *Australia: State of the Environment 1996* (State of the Environment Advisory Council 1996), which revealed how little reliable data—and therefore understanding—of the Australian environment existed. The result was a set of a total of 454 environmental indicators that were developed specifically for the use of government in monitoring and reporting on the SOE. The *Environment Protection and Biodiversity Conservation Act 1999* requires the preparation and tabling of a national SOE report in parliament every five years. Australia also has an obligation to report on its environmental performance and progress towards sustainable development to the Organisation for Economic Cooperation and Development and United Nations Commission on Sustainable Development (Department of Sustainability, Environment, Water, Population and Communities 2012).

A core sub-set of 75 indicators were approved in 1999 by the Australian and New Zealand Environment and Conservation Council in relation to land and atmosphere; biodiversity; inland waters and marine estuaries and the sea; human settlements, including local and community uses; and natural and cultural heritage (Department of Environment and Heritage 2004). Environmental indicators for the atmosphere include indicators of an enhanced greenhouse effect—for example, annual greenhouse gas emissions. Outdoor air quality indicators include air quality standards for lead, sulphur dioxide and nitrogen dioxide concentrations. Environmental indicators for land include the total area affected by salinity; changes in land use and erosion; introduced organisms and animals, such as exotic plants and animals; and exceeding minimum residue levels (metals and micronutrients) in land and food. The State of the Environment report based on these indicators becomes an important process for undertaking a national assessment of, and reporting on, Australia's environment, with the overall aim of providing information for decision-making—as can be seen from the 2011 SOE, which was developed to:

- provide relevant, credible and useful information on environmental issues to decision-makers and the public
- increase awareness of environmental issues among decision-makers and the public
- support evidence-based environmental management decisions that lead to more sustainable use and effective conservation of our environmental resources
- identify ways in which the environmental evidence base could be strengthened (State of the Environment 2011 Committee 2011: 3).

The drivers on the Australian environment and its future condition identified in the 2011 SOE report are climate variability and change, population growth and economic growth (State of the Environment 2011 Committee 2011: 11), which show that the range of highly complex interdependent factors that impact on the natural environment and the implications of addressing these factors are highly complex.

Hazards to human health

According to the WHO, environmental health comprises those aspects of human health—including quality of life—that are determined by physical, chemical, biological, social and psycho-social factors in the environment. It also refers to the theory and practice of assessing, correcting, controlling and preventing those factors in the environment that can potentially adversely affect the health of present and future generations. Within this definition there are familiar themes relating to interaction between people and the environment. Unlike environmental indicators, environmental health indicators target hazards arising from the built environment.

The US National Centre for Environmental Health has developed a useful set of core environmental public health indicators. These are designed to identify problems in a number of topic areas:

- ambient outdoor and indoor air quality
- environmental and drinking water
- toxic and waste hazards, including environmental lead and pesticides, sunlight and ultraviolet light
- noise pollution
- disasters
- sentinel events.

However, these are conceived as hazards (indicators that include potential exposure to contaminants or hazardous situations, such as air pollution, motor vehicle emissions, tobacco smoke in homes with children, pesticide exposure, chemical contamination, residence in flood area, and contaminated fish and shellfish); exposures (bio-markers of exposure, such as children's blood lead levels); health effects (exposures that lead to adverse health events, such as lead poisoning in children); melanoma; contaminated food (especially freshwater food and seafood); noise-induced hearing loss; and cold- and hot-weather-attributed death. Attached to these hazard indicators are a set of intervention indicators—a set of official policies and programs designed to address these hazards, such as emergency preparedness programs, smoke-free environments and alternative fuels for motor vehicles (National Center for Environmental Health 2002).

Climate change: complexity and uncertainty

In 1990, the Intergovernmental Panel on Climate Change stated in its report on climate change that emissions from human activity were responsible for global warming. Since then, there has been substantial investigation into the health impacts associated with climate change. Generally the effects of climate change will be seen by rising temperatures, changes in rainfall patterns, a rise in sea level and more intense weather events, and these will lead to direct risks to human health. These direct risks are associated with:

- more frequent and intense heatwaves, resulting in more heart attacks, strokes, accidents, heat exhaustion and death
- more frequent or intense extreme weather events (particularly storms, floods and cyclones) resulting in more injuries, deaths and post-traumatic stress
- more fires, increasing the number of cases of smoke-induced asthma attacks, burns and death (Hughes & McMichael 2011: 7).

Hughes and McMichael (2011: 7) refer to flow-on effects from these increased risks, which would include—in terms of particular environmental health interest—an increase in air pollutants; changes in rainfall patterns and temperatures, which would increase the spread and activity of disease-transmitting mosquitoes and increase the risk of food-borne infections; impacts on food security; and increased pressure on health systems and services. Although it is difficult to predict health outcomes from global warming, the NHMRC (2011) suggests that the future climate-change health implications for Australia are likely to include:

- **Heat-related deaths:** If we don't adapt, heat-related deaths could more than double to 2500 a year by 2020. In the short term, warmer winters will mean fewer annual 'winter deaths' but, in the medium to long term, these would be greatly outnumbered by the additional heat-related deaths.
- **Flood-related deaths and injuries:** Increasingly frequent and extreme weather events (such as floods, droughts, hurricanes and tornadoes) are projected. Extreme rainfall is expected to increase in many parts of Australia, leading to a 240 per cent rise in flood-related deaths and injuries in some regions.
- **Mosquito-borne diseases:** Rises in temperature and rainfall may cause the southwards expansion of tropical mosquito-borne diseases, such as malaria, dengue fever, Australian encephalitis, Japanese encephalitis and epidemic polyarthritis.
- **Water-borne diseases:** As temperatures rise, the quality and quantity of drinking water could fall in some areas because of drought. As water quality falls, health disorders related to water contamination by bacteria, viruses, protozoa and parasites will rise. This contamination will also occur at the other weather extreme, as heavy rainfall and runoff cause microbial and toxic agents to overflow from agricultural fields and human septic systems.
- **Food-borne diseases:** Food-borne disease is caused by a number of different viruses, bacteria

and parasites. Because bacteria replicate more quickly at higher ambient temperatures, it is likely that the rates of food-borne diseases, such as gastroenteritis and hepatitis, will increase as average temperatures rise.

Despite these broad assessments, or predictions, it is acknowledged that trying to make judgements about risks to human health from the interacting variations in climate and the environmental changes that occur as a consequence of these variations is difficult both because of the degree of uncertainty (Western Australia Department of Health 2008: 59) and because of the significant gaps in our knowledge of potential health risks (Hughes & McMichael (2011: 3).

The reduction of carbon dioxide emissions (mitigation) has been a topic of debate both internationally and nationally, particularly around the carbon tax, and it is considered to be a critical strategy in protecting human health. However, there is also a need to implement adaptive strategies to minimise health risks that have become unavoidable from climate change (Hughes & McMichael 2011: 33, 38). One specific adaptive strategy has been planning for hotter temperatures. In New South Wales, South Australia, Western Australia and Victoria, heatwave planning has been undertaken at the state, local and institutional levels, in recognition that there are population groups that are at higher risk of illness from increased temperatures.

Climate change and its impact on public health represent a challenge because of the gaps in evidence and because it consists of a range of complex interacting variables that will be different for each geographical location. Clearly, it will impact on and change the traditional areas of environmental health practice, such as food safety and vector control, and introduce new challenges to the organised effort.

Conclusion: Our environment, our health, our future

The history of environmental health—particularly since the Industrial Revolution—has been a story of grappling with environmental threats to human health. Initially, the thinking was around protecting human health from the hazardous environment. Over time, there has been a shift to a realisation that our strategies should instead be about protecting and conserving the environment from the incursions and impacts of human development, particularly urbanisation and economic activity. There has been a growing recognition that the health of the environment is at risk, and that human health very much depends upon the sustainability of environmental systems (Brown et al. 2001).

According to Brown et al. (2001), environmental health practice in the twenty-first century will be about addressing the human health outcomes of human–environmental relationships, principally through:

- **environmental security for human biology:** preserving the physical conditions for life
- **environmental security for human population:** protecting communities from local and global environmental risks to health
- **physical security for workplace and human settlements:** managing place-based economic, social and environmental risks
- **long-term security for global self-supporting systems:** re-establishing human–environment sustainability.

This has implications for the environmental health workforce in that there will be a greater need for specialisation across a broad range of activities—from Indigenous environmental health and the challenges of removing the barriers to environmental health justice to the challenges of biosecurity and sustainability.

Ecologically sustainable development (ESD) is one model that has been discussed, and that is used as a planning approach in some local environmental health-planning processes and public management (for example, triple bottom-line reporting). The essential elements of ESD are a need to consider the wider economic, social and environmental implications of our decisions and activities, which have implications for the international community and the biosphere, and a need to take a long-term rather than short-term view when making those decisions (Commonwealth of Australia 1992a: 6). In 2012, the United Nations Secretary General's High-Level Panel on Global Sustainability affirmed that sustainable development was 'about recognising, understanding, and acting on interconnections—above all those between economy, society, and the natural environment' (United Nations Secretary-General's High-Level Panel on Global Sustainability 2012: 6).

The ongoing challenge is for all governments to think in terms of the global community and the global environment, and to ensure that local actions are taken to give substance to that thinking—the global organised effort.

14

Preventive services:
Linking public health and personal health care

Challenge

On the first Thursday of every month, you meet with a group of parents whose children attend the local primary school. At one particular meeting, a debate begins about a vaccine that is now available for children under ten years of age. One mother declares that as there are potential side-effects and risks, she will not be allowing her child to be vaccinated. This is countered by someone else who says that she has a social responsibility to have her child vaccinated because vaccination is a social good that not only helps prevent her child from getting the disease, but helps to limit its spread to the wider population. Therefore, the potential benefits outweigh the possible risks.

One of the fathers present is concerned that, as his family GP no longer bulk-bills, there will be a high cost to the consumer, particularly for his family with three children aged under ten. This prompts another person to suggest that the vaccine should be provided free by the Commonwealth government and organised through local schools. This will ensure that everyone is covered and that no one has to miss out because of their economic circumstances.

How should a new vaccine be made available? Is prevention a matter of individual choice, or does your social responsibility override such a decision? Should the government pay the cost of vaccinating whole sections of a population if it is known that the disease will only affect a small number of children each year?

Introduction

Public health services are delivered through a range of settings and by a variety of providers, including government public health workers and private sector public health consultants. This chapter is concerned with those services that are delivered to individuals in clinical settings but, when brought together to cover defined population groups, constitute a public health approach. What underlies the public health nature of individually delivered clinical services is the organised effort. When services are provided on an opportunistic basis, rather than an organised or targeted one, the health benefit for the public is not necessarily achieved. However, with an increasing orientation by health-care organisations to primary health-care services, there is an increasing emphasis on population approaches to service delivery.

This chapter describes the interface between public health and clinical care, offering a conceptual framework and a historical perspective. The chapter then offers a review of various fields where organised approaches to personal health care have led to public health achievements. The discussion starts with the traditional clinical public health services—those that have focused on infectious disease control—and then moves on to the screening services that assist with early detection. A review follows of more recent developments in public health efforts provided through the primary care setting, and the chapter concludes with details of current developments in general practice and public health.

How public health and clinical care interface: Friends or foes?

As discussed in Chapter 1, the term 'public health' has been used historically in two senses. In the first sense, it was a way of differentiating between public and private health services, with the former being resourced from the public purse and delivered either directly by government or not-for-profit

agencies. The second sense is associated with community health, or the health states of populations as distinct from personal or individual health services of clinical medicine (Turshen 1989; Peterson & Lupton 1996).

Lasker (1997), in attempting to define medicine and public health, took the two vantage points of 'health' and 'disease', whereby healers were provided to care for individuals who were sick (medical sector), and to prevent disease from occurring and promote healthful conditions in the community at large (public health). Although the strategies of public health and the medical sector are quite different, there have been close links between them at times. For example, during the mid-nineteenth century, when infectious diseases were rampant, effective strategies had to include the community-focused preventive activities of sanitary reform and medical care. Leaders in the two sectors have also overlapped, and history recounts the numerous contributions made by medical practitioners to public health—particularly when neither the medical nor public health sector could address the problem alone, such as in the case of infectious diseases (Lasker 1997).

When communicable disease was replaced as the leading cause of death by cardiovascular disease and cancer in the mid-twentieth century, the medical sector sought to tackle the issue by focusing on the biological mechanisms of these diseases within the body, and developing procedures and drugs for diagnosis and treatment. The public health sector, on the other hand, worked to identify the environmental, social and behavioural risk factors, and developed population-based interventions to reduce or prevent those risks (Lasker 1997).

Preventive medicine is therefore concerned with the reduction of the number of sick individuals who form a clearly definable minority of the population (Rose 1992). This notion of 'vulnerable' or 'high-risk' population groups provides common ground between preventive medicine and public health, and the need for a complementary set of management strategies. Within this population group are individuals who may have a high risk of disease, or may be suffering from the disease. From the public health perspective, it is important to understand the environmental, social and behavioural factors impacting on a population group that lead to disease, and to devise means by which these factors can be detected and managed. Thus, in the case of breast cancer, the promotion of screening and early diagnosis and treatment can be seen as a combined public health and preventive medicine approach. Other public health strategies include education on risk factors and behaviour modification, and support for seeking and following medical advice.

The continuum of public health and clinical interventions is complementary, and although the public health approach is generally applied at a population or community level, individuals related by health, disease, location or other circumstance constitute a community of interest. According to Rose (1992: 10–11), there is also a continuum relating to clinical or medical activities:

Preventive medicine should be concerned with the whole spectrum of disease and ill health, both because all levels are important to the people concerned and because the mild can be the father of the severe. The visible tip of the iceberg of disease can neither be understood nor properly controlled if it is thought to constitute the entire problem.

Starfield (1996) has also examined the complementarity between public health and medicine through various types of health service intervention and the target groups for these interventions. Table 14.1 provides examples of different types of preventive intervention and the target group for each intervention, and shows that both fields contribute to different levels of prevention, either singly or together. In Table 14.2, Starfield makes generalised observations concerning the locus of responsibility—public health or clinical medical care—for these types of intervention, and illustrates how public health and medical care work in partnership.

Table 14.1 Examples of interventions by type of function and target group

Target	Type of function*		
	Primary	**Secondary**	**Tertiary**
Generalised populations	• Environmental planning	• Environmental monitoring and product control	• Public advocacy • Community mobilisation
Individuals	• Health education campaigns • Immunisations	• PKU screening • Breast cancer screening	• Information systems:** data standardisation, collection, analysis and dissemination
Selective	• Genetic engineering***	• Blood lead screening	• Outreach/access, e.g. home visiting
Indicated	• Communicable disease control • Prophylactic antibiotics • Practice guidelines	• Frequent follow-up for disease recurrence	• Address problems: quality assessment of clinical services

* Primary: intervention to prevent a problem from occurring; secondary: intervention at a stage before a problem is manifested; tertiary: remediation to reverse the manifestation of a problem.

** Activities involve monitoring health statistics and surveys of health status, access and people's experiences with services.

*** Should such an effort ever be considered ethical or practical.

Source: adapted from Starfield (1996: 136–7).

Table 14.2 Locus of responsibility for interventions by type of function and target group

Target	Type of function*		
	Primary	Secondary	Tertiary
Generalised populations	Public health	Public health	Public health
Individuals	Public health/clinical medical care	Public health/clinical medical care	Public health/clinical medical care
Selective	?	Public health/clinical medical care	Public health/clinical medical care
Indicated	Public health/clinical medical care	Public health/clinical medical care	Clinical medical care

* Primary: intervention to prevent a problem from occurring; secondary: intervention at a stage before a problem is manifested; tertiary: remediation to reverse the manifestation of a problem.

Source: adapted from Starfield (1996: 136–7).

From a policy perspective, there are constraints to integrating the clinical and public health responses in Australia, and in many other countries. Many clinical services are provided by the private sector, whereas most public health activities are provided by the public sector. The issues of professional autonomy, perceived interference with the doctor–patient relationship and compulsory reporting, and service competition are a few of the barriers to integration. The organised public health effort is concerned with overcoming these constraints and coordinating all the relevant players in order to ensure that the interventions achieve health improvements at the population level.

The following sections describe and analyse traditional and contemporary clinical public health interventions, including those used for specific diseases and population groups. Included are illustrative examples that have been the subject of organised public health interventions.

Organised clinical services for infectious disease control: Maintaining early achievements

The prevention of infectious diseases was one of the earliest public health concerns, and clinical services were an integral part of the strategy of containment.

Although most deaths in Australia occur through cancer and cardiovascular disease, infectious diseases still remain a threat within the Australian community. In the developing world, communicable diseases remain major killers, and this partly reflects an insufficiently organised approach to disease prevention and control.

However, a low incidence of an infectious disease always has the potential to become an epidemic if there is a breakdown in any area or areas of surveillance, response or treatment. Clinical services provided by institutions (such as hospitals, clinics and community health centres) are an important way to deliver public health services. The ways in which clinical services for infectious diseases are organised provide lessons for how public health objectives can be achieved across other conditions. The degree of organisation— whether they are provided for the whole or specific parts of the population—is also a central aspect of when a clinical service is a public health service.

The following topics illustrate how public health clinical programs have been developed in relation to infectious disease control across populations.

Immunisation

Immunisation is a good example of the use of a clinical intervention at the individual level that is also used as a public health strategy to prevent disease within a population group or community.

As outlined in Chapter 2, the first government- and community-organised public health interventions were initiated in the mid-nineteenth century during the sanitary movement. Environmental hygiene initiatives were undertaken as the primary means of controlling and reducing the transmission of disease within rapidly expanding urban communities. These measures had a great impact on 'filth' diseases, such as typhoid and cholera, and diseases associated with poor living conditions, such as tuberculosis. Environmental sanitation had little impact on the incidence of diseases such as smallpox. It was only with the development of vaccines that it became possible to target and prevent specific infectious diseases through immunisation.

The man credited with discovering vaccination was an English doctor named Edward Jenner. In 1796, he took the fluid from the sores of milkmaids recovering from cowpox (a milder disease than smallpox), and put this on the cuts of an eight-year old boy, James Phipps. Phipps subsequently developed cowpox blisters, but when Jenner exposed him to smallpox eight weeks later he did not develop any symptoms of smallpox. As it was not understood then that infectious diseases were caused by micro-organisms, there was no satisfactory explanation for this important discovery. Jenner called his procedure 'vaccination', from the Latin *vacca* for cow (Rosen 1958).

By 1880, Louis Pasteur had discovered that infectious diseases were caused by micro-organisms. Pasteur developed cultures of bacteria in his laboratory, and discovered that older bacteria lost the capacity to kill experimental animals. He injected this weakened or attenuated bacteria into animals and found that it could render animals immune to fresh, virulent bacteria of the same type. The experiments were so successful that he later used the same method to develop a vaccine against rabies (Rosen 1958).

The development and administration of vaccines is an important element of the organised public health effort. Appendix K provides an indication of the timeframes over which vaccines have been introduced in Australia. Note that there has been much activity in vaccine development and usage in recent years, indicating a renewed emphasis on immunisation.

Traditionally and globally, immunisation coverage is often one of the major indicators of the overall health of a nation, and a key population health initiative. However, in 1995 only 53 per cent of children in Australia were fully immunised, a rate that was considerably lower than for other Organisation for Economic Co-operation and Development countries. From the public health and government standpoint, this was unacceptable, as such low rates of immunisation exposed Australian communities to a range of vaccine-preventable diseases, such as whooping cough, poliomyelitis and rubella. The achievement of community protection from vaccine-preventable diseases is based on the notion of 'herd immunity'. This is a concept whereby there is indirect protection from infection of susceptible members (those that are not immunised) of a community or population, which is brought about by the presence of immune individuals (those who have been immunised). To attain herd immunity, between 85 and 90 per cent of the population (depending on the disease) needs to be immunised, or to have had developed antibodies against the specific disease or diseases. How, then, could the Australian community be protected against vaccine-preventable diseases? What would be the features of this public health organised effort?

Despite the accessibility of general practice, local government and community health services for immunisation services, the public health objective was not being realised. The Immunise Australia Program was developed to organise the public health effort for immunisation. In 1997, the Commonwealth government approved a Seven-Point Plan, with an important component being the development and funding of policy initiatives targeting parents and GPs.

The first policy initiative was the linking of welfare benefits (the then Maternity Allowance, Childcare Assistance and the Childcare Rebate) to children's immunisation status (notwithstanding medical contra-indications or conscientious objections). The Maternity Immunisation Allowance, a non-income tested payment, provided a bonus to parents for ensuring that their child's immunisation coverage was complete. In 2012, the first payment of $129 was made if a child was fully immunised between eighteen months and two years and the second—also $129—if a child was fully immunised between four and five years of age (Department of Human Services 2012b).

The second initiative was the introduction of financial incentives for GPs to monitor, promote and provide immunisation services in accordance with the immunisation schedule to children under the age of seven years. Under the General Practitioner Immunisation Incentive (GP II), two payments are made, one on the completion of each schedule, and one paid quarterly to practices that reach immunisation levels of 90 per cent or greater coverage for children under seven years old. The introduction of this initiative was a cornerstone of the organised public health immunisation strategy because GPs have significant levels of contact with children, and each of these contacts provides an opportunity to assess and monitor each child's immunisation status (Department of Human Services 2012c). Local council and community health service providers also receive incentives, although at much lower rates than those offered to GPs.

Supporting the medical practitioners was the enhanced role of the Divisions of General Practice (recently replaced by Medicare Locals), funded by the government to work closely with other immunisation providers, develop educational and training materials, and identify and target groups with low immunisation levels. Additionally, a national database, the Australian Childhood Immunisation Register (ACIR), was developed to record details of vaccinations given to children under the age of seven. The ACIR is administered by Medicare Australia (then the Health Insurance Commission) and is updated from the Medicare records of all children younger than seven years of age. The data held on the ACIR is used to determine entitlements to Commonwealth benefits, and is accessible to professionals to monitor coverage levels, service delivery and disease outbreaks.

Other strategies under the immunisation program have been immunisation days, which have involved social marketing activities to increase coverage rates in geographical areas of low coverage, and education and research focusing on epidemiological and sociological aspects of immunisation and vaccine-preventable disease. Legislation has also been used to require parents to provide their child's immunisation history when they enrol at school. These legislative requirements are now in place in New South Wales, Victoria, Tasmania and the Australian Capital Territory.

The Immunise Australia Program has led to a dramatic turnaround in the levels of childhood immunisation. The proportion of fully immunised children at twelve months had increased from 75 per cent in 1997 to 91.4 per cent by the end of 2009 and at 24 months, from 64 per cent to 92 per cent (DoHA 2011b: 135). The vaccination coverage rate (the number of children fully immunised by age group as appropriate in relation to the total number of children by age group in a postcode area) is an important indicator of the effectiveness of immunisation programs. The National Immunisation Program Schedule in Table 14.3 outlines the age at which vaccines are to be administered.

Australian data in 2011 indicated a high level of coverage for children at two years of age, with coverage rates above 90 per cent for all vaccines in all state and territories, in line with NHMRC targets. The second target of near-universal immunisation coverage at school entry has not been achieved as yet. Schools provide a high-risk setting for disease

Table 14.3 National Immunisation Program Schedule as at May 2012

Child programs

Birth
- Hepatitis B (hepB)

Two months
- Hepatitis B (hepB)
- Diphtheria, tetanus and whooping cough (acellular pertussis) (DTPa)
- Haemophilus influenzae type b (Hib)
- Polio (inactivated poliomyelitis) (IPV)
- Pneumococcal conjugate (13vPCV)
- Rotavirus

Four months
- Hepatitis B (hepB)
- Diphtheria, tetanus and whooping cough (acellular pertussis (DTPa)
- Haemophilus influenzae type b (Hib)
- Polio (inactivated poliomyelitis IPV)
- Pneumococcal conjugate (13vPCV)
- Rotavirus

Six months
- Hepatitis B (hepB)
- Diphtheria, tetanus and whooping cough (acellular pertussis) (DTPa)
- Haemophilus influenzae type b (Hib)
- Polio (inactivated poliomyelitis) (IPV)
- Pneumococcal conjugate (13vPCV)
- Rotavirus

Twelve months
- Haemophilus influenzae type b (Hib)
- Measles, mumps and rubella (MMR)
- Meningococcal C (MenCCV)

Eighteen months
- Chickenpox (varicella) (VZV)

Four years
- Diphtheria, tetanus and whooping cough (acellular pertussis) (DTPa)
- Polio (inactivated poliomyelitis) (IPV)
- Measles, mumps and rubella (MMR)

School programs

Ten to thirteen years
- Hepatitis B (hep B)
- Chickenpox (varicella) (VZV)

Twelve to thirteen years
- Human Papillomavirus (HPV)

Ten to seventeen years
- Diphtheria, tetanus and whooping cough (acellular pertussis) (DTPa)

Immunisation for special groups

Six months and over: at-risk individuals
- Influenza (people with medical conditions placing them at risk of serious complications of influenza)

12 months: at-risk individuals
- Pneumococcal conjugate (13vPCV)
- Hepatitis B (hepB)

Twelve to 24 months
- Hepatitis A (Aboriginal and Torres Strait Islander children in high-risk areas)
- Pneumococcal (23vPPV) (18–24 months) or Pneumococcal (13vPCV) (12–18 months from 1 October 2012) (Aboriginal and Torres Strait Islander children in high-risk areas)
- Hepatitis A (Aboriginal and Torres Strait Islander children in high risk areas)

Four years: at-risk individuals
- Pneumococcal polysaccharide (23vPPV)

Fifteen years and over
- Influenza (Aboriginal and Torres Strait Islander people)
- Pneumococcal polysaccharide (23vPPV) (Aboriginal and Torres Strait Islander people medically at risk)

Fifty years and over
- Pneumococcal polysaccharide (23vPPV) (Aboriginal and Torres Strait Islander people)

Pregnant women
- Influenza

Sixty-five years and over
- Influenza (flu)
- Pneumococcal polysaccharide (23vPPV)

Source: DoHA (2012i).

transmission, and there has been an increased effort in improving vaccination coverage rates amongst school children—for example, the New South Wales Adolescent Vaccination Program. In New South Wales, the coverage rate in 2004 for diphtheria, tetanus and acellular pertussis ranged from 48 to 63 per cent (Ward et al. 2010: 240) and in 2010 it was 70 per cent (Hull et al. 2011: 190). Similar initiatives to increase school vaccination coverage rates are being taken in other states, such as Victoria, where it is estimated that the adolescent vaccine coverage rate is 75 per cent (Victorian Department of Health 2012b: 1).

In terms of adolescent immunisation, it appears that there are similar barriers to those for immunising young children, such as a lack of parental knowledge and concerns about side-effects. In addition, however, there are some uniquely adolescent issues, including:

> rapidly changing emotional, cognitive, and physical development, and lower rates of contact with the healthcare system … Knowledge of vaccine-preventable diseases and mistaken concerns about immunization side effects become important not only for the parent but also for the adolescent. (Kaplan 2009, p. 525)

Addressing these issues will be a critical factor in achieving optimal universal immunisation coverage for adolescents.

The turnaround in immunisation coverage rates has come about through using a public health approach that has involved developing policy, coordinating professional practice, securing the cooperation of the appropriate jurisdictions, developing and making accessible a comprehensive and integrated database, conducting research into scientific and social aspects of the issue, and using social marketing activities to educate and involve the broader community. The progress to date of using a public health approach provides some optimism that immunisation coverage rates will continue to increase.

Tuberculosis control

As with the recent successes with immunisation coverage, tuberculosis (TB) control in Australia is another success story for the organised public health effort, and contrasts sharply with the global situation.

Tuberculosis is an infectious disease caused by the bacterium *Mycobacterium tuberculosis*, with most infections occurring in the lungs. Pulmonary TB is easily treatable, and is almost 100 per cent curable if treatment is undertaken and completed.

Internationally, tuberculosis remains a major global health problem and cause of human suffering, with the World Health Organization (WHO) estimating that there are 9 million new cases of tuberculosis, and 2 million deaths, annually. Most of the cases occur in Africa (30 per cent) and Asia (55 per cent), with India and China accounting for 35 per cent of all cases globally. Complicating the picture is the fact that 13 per cent of tuberculosis cases occur among people living with HIV and there are around 0.4 to 0.5 million cases of multi-drug-resistant TB (WHO 2011d: 1), thus making treatment more complex and demanding. Nonetheless, the incidence of TB is in decline (WHO 2011d: iv), and this is associated with the WHO Global Plan to Stop Tuberculosis launched in 2006 together with the current Global Plan to Stop TB 2011–2015.

The Australian population has been spared many of the problems experienced elsewhere with tuberculosis. The annual incidence rate is stable at five to six cases per 100 000 people (Lumb et al. 2011: 154), which is among the lowest in the world. Indigenous Australians continue to have higher rates (6.6 per 100 000) of TB than the non-Indigenous Australian population, although rates are falling and drug resistance is associated mainly with people born in countries located in the Western Pacific and South-East Asian regions (Barry, Konstantinos and the National Tuberculosis Advisory Committee 2009: 134).

A total of 1135 cases of tuberculosis were notified in Australia in 2007, representing a crude rate of 5.4 cases per 100 000 people, continuing a stable trend over 25 years. The distribution of cases by state of residence is shown in Table 14.4, which indicates the range of notification rates for all Australian-born people from 0.5 per 100 000 in Western Australia to over 15 per 100 000 in the Northern Territory. This higher rate reflects a notification rate for the Northern Territory Aboriginal population of 32.2 per 100 000.

So why has Australia been successful in controlling tuberculosis? Unlike other countries, Australia avoided the resurgence of tuberculosis in the late twentieth century that saw the declaration of a global emergency on tuberculosis by the WHO. Essentially, improved living standards, national TB campaigns after World War II, free specialised TB services and, more recently, pre-migration screening, have all contributed to the control of TB in Australia (Ralph & Kelly 2009: 578). The global emergency arose because of a number of factors, including the HIV pandemic and the collapse of primary health-care services following political upheaval in some countries. However, the high incidence of disease in developing countries is in part due to a lack of basic infrastructure, such as fresh food and safe water supplies, and the absence or scarcity of primary health-care services.

The public health campaigns of the 1950s in developed countries consisted of a management approach referred to as vertical or specialised control programs. Each of these programs had its own direct line of command structure, staffed with specialists from the central level through to the local level, where the control services were delivered. The elements of the service included mass case-finding through the screening of the population using mobile x-ray units and bacteriological diagnosis (skin testing); Bacillus Calmette-Guerin (BCG) immunisation; and specialised case management through specialised hospitals and clinics whereby patients were segregated while undergoing drug treatments. All of these were independent of the general health infrastructure and other vertical control programs, such as those for leprosy. Specialisation of control programs was seen as an appropriate way by which to control TB (and other diseases). This was a successful approach in developed countries as it accelerated the decline in the risk of infection (Raviglione & Pio 2002).

Table 14.4 **Notifications of tuberculosis and notification rate per 100 000 population in all Australian-born cases, Australia, 2007, by state or territory and Indigenous status**

State or territory	Indigenous Australians		Non-Indigenous Australians		Total Australian-born	
	Notifications	Rate	Notifications	Rate	Notifications	Rate
ACT	0	0	2	0.9	2	0.8
NSW	3	1.9	52	1.2	55	1.2
NT	21	32.2	2	2.4	23	15.5
Qld	7	4.7	12	0.4	19	0.6
South Australia	3	10.5	9	0.8	12	1.1
Tasmania	0	0	3	0.8	3	0.8
Victoria	1	2.9	30	0.9	31	0.9
Western Australia	0	0	6	0.5	6	0.5
Australia	35	6.6	116	0.9	151	1.0

Source: Barry et al. (2009: 308).

As a pupil attending primary school in the early 1960s, the author remembers lining up with the other pupils and undergoing tuberculin skin testing and, a week later, lining up again to have the skin test 'read' and receiving the BCG immunisation. At the same time, while accompanying my parents shopping, it was not unusual to see the mobile chest x-ray unit parked on the street and signs on the street encouraging people to have a chest x-ray.

Years later, while completing my nursing training, I worked in the Tuberculosis Chalet on the hospital grounds and saw at first-hand patients undergoing treatment for tuberculosis, and heard the orchestra of early-morning coughing and expectorating. Some time later, when working in a local government Environmental Health Department, I remember reading the regulations and seeing the signs saying that it was an offence to spit on the pavement due to the risk of the spread of TB.

The same approach was taken by the WHO in developing countries; however, there was not the same expected decline in TB that had been experienced in developed countries. The major reasons were that the vertical control program approach was beyond the resources of developing countries—particularly the cost of the drugs used in the treatment of active TB. Importantly, the vertical program approach and its specialised structure could not provide services to the whole population (Raviglione & Pio 2002).

The WHO (2005a) then developed the directly observed treatment—short course (DOTS) strategy, which consisted of five steps required for the control of TB:

1 a sustained political commitment
2 access to quality-assured TB sputum microscopy
3 standardised short-course chemotherapy for all cases of TB under proper case-management conditions
4 an uninterrupted supply of quality-assured drugs
5 a recording and reporting system enabling outcome assessment.

The shorter-term aim of the Global Plan to Stop TB 2011–2015 is to halve TB prevalence and death rates by 2015, with the longer-term goal being the elimination of TB by 2050. Subsequently, the DOTS strategy has been expanded to include the management of drug-resistant TB and TB/HIV, and further laboratory strengthening as one part of the plan. The second part of the plan is focused on research and development on new diagnostics, drugs and vaccines (WHO 2011d: vi, vii). The WHO acknowledges that these measures are required at the TB prevention program level; however, the prevention of TB on a global basis requires political commitment, a nationwide public health effort, and social mobilisation to address the underlying determinants of TB, which include: access to general health care; improved nutrition, living and working conditions; reduced exposure to HIV infection; and reduced levels of smoking, alcohol abuse and drug abuse (WHO 2011d: 2).

The implication for Australia, given that a large proportion of TB cases are associated with people from overseas, is that surveillance assumes an even greater importance to ensure control of TB.

The lessons from TB control at the global level are that any organised approach must be considered in the context of the local social and economic circumstances, and an understanding that these will determine fundamental disease-control strategies. From the Australian perspective, the global incidence of TB coupled with international travel, immigration and the entry of refugees and asylum seekers means that there is a need for vigilance and no room for complacency.

Sexually transmitted infections

The control of sexually transmitted infections (STIs) or diseases was one of the earliest global public health efforts. Although much attention has focused on the dramatic impact of the Black Death (plague) that killed millions, there were epidemics of other diseases, such as leprosy, smallpox and venereal syphilis. Syphilis was introduced into Europe at the end of the fifteenth century (Gordon 1976). Numerous famous historical figures have been documented as suffering, or suspected to have suffered, from the disease—Beethoven, Schubert, Abraham Lincoln, Vincent van Gogh, Friedrich Nietzsche, Oscar Wilde, Karen Blixen, James Joyce and Adolf Hitler to name a few (Hayden 2003).

STIs are primarily passed from person to person by sexual contact. Some STIs—such as chlamydia, gonorrhoea, human papilloma virus (HPV), hepatitis B, HIV and genital herpes—often cause infections that exhibit no obvious symptoms (are asymptomatic), thus the person suffering with the infection may not be aware that they are infected. However, there are serious complications associated with some STIs that remain untreated, including pelvic inflammatory disease and infertility in women. Sometimes complications can be fatal for individuals. The morbidity associated with STIs has a profoundly adverse effect on the quality of life and economic productivity of many women and men, their families and, consequently, entire communities. The WHO estimates that annually there are more than 448 million new cases of curable STIs in men and women aged between 15 and 49 years (WHO 2011a), and millions of viral STIs along with many millions of incurable viral STIs—including HIV, herpes and HPV. It is expected that populations at risk of STIs will grow substantially, given social, demographic and migratory trends (WHO 2007b: 3).

In 2010, the most frequently reported notifiable condition in Australia was chlamydia (74 305 diagnoses) with a population rate of 319 diagnoses per 100 000, and this level has been increasing for the last ten years. Similarly, the number of diagnoses of gonorrhoea and syphilis increased by 25 per cent and 60 per cent respectively from 2009 to 2010, with substantially higher rates of diagnosis of chlamydia and gonorrhoea recorded in the Aboriginal and Torres Strait Islander population compared with the non-Indigenous population. At the end of 2010, there were 30 486 cases of HIV infection diagnosed, and it was estimated that 21 391 people were living with HIV infection (The Kirby Institute 2011: 7–8).

Individual treatment for STIs is necessary but insufficient for control of disease transmission. Early approaches to the control of STIs included contact tracing of symptomatic patients, the use of specialised clinics and treatment with low-cost antibiotics (UNAIDS 1998). In the United States, the requirement for a pre-marriage blood test was imposed as a screening measure. In Australia, the approach to the control of STIs has revolved around mandatory notification of the disease and the surveillance of these notifications, tracing of contacts and the use of specialised clinical services. These services have been state or territory based. Historically, risk factors for STIs have centred on age (younger than 20), partnership status (in some cultures), new sexual partners, multiple partners, partners with multiple partners, having a partner who often travels, history of an STI or reproductive tract infection, and having a partner with symptoms of an STI or current symptoms or signs. It is recognised that the successful prevention of STI/HIV needs to go beyond information and awareness-raising, and also beyond individual behaviours, to the contextual factors that make people vulnerable to STI/HIV infection, and that influence or determine behaviour (EngenderHealth 2004).

These factors include social determinants like social norms, gender inequalities and poverty. Economic and political forces make people vulnerable to infection, and these too must be considered risk factors for STIs (UNAIDS 1998). Factors that affect social vulnerability include gender inequities, economic power, youth, cultural constructs and government policies. Women in particular may be vulnerable to infection because of gender inequities and a lack of power within sexual relationships, and this makes it difficult—if not impossible—for them to negotiate safer sex with partners. Lack of economic power can lead to vulnerability as some women are forced to enter into sex work or to form temporary partnerships to barter sex for economic survival.

Simply advising of the risk behaviours is generally not enough because a person must know which practices can put them at risk, and have a belief that they are 'at risk'. Interventions must then be based on people knowing what they have to do to protect themselves, feeling that they have the ability to effect change, and having the skills and resources to do so. Importantly, people must have willing partners and a supportive environment underpinning these interventions.

A public health approach to addressing STIs requires an organised effort across the scope of determinants that influence individuals and at-risk populations, together with clinical service and policy strategies that integrate the efforts of general health services, and specialised screening and support services. The WHO public health package for STI prevention and control (see Box 14.2) clearly identifies the range of interventions that are required for a 'public health approach'. Importantly, comprehensive case management is a significant part of the approach.

An example of this approach can be seen in Australia through the Second National Sexually Transmissable Infections Strategy 2010–2013, one of five national strategies to reduce the transmission of STIs and blood-borne viruses. The guiding principles of the approach are based on the framework of the Ottawa Charter, and encompass:

- the active participation of affected communities and individuals to increase their influence over the determinants of their health

---

Box 14.2 WHO public health approach to prevention and control of STIs— the key elements

- Promotion of safer sexual behaviour
- Promotion of early health care-seeking behaviour
- Introduction of prevention and care activities across all primary health-care programs, including sexual and reproductive health and HIV programs
- A comprehensive approach to case management that encompasses:
  - identification of the sexually transmitted infections syndrome
  - appropriate antimicrobial treatment for the syndrome
  - education and counselling on ways to avoid or reduce risk of infection with sexually transmitted pathogens, including HIV
- Promotion of the correct and consistent use of condoms
- Partner notification

Source: WHO (2007b: 10–11).

- the formulation and application of law and public policy that support healthy behaviours and respect human rights
- the adoption of harm reduction principles to underpin measures to prevent transmission of HIV and viral hepatitis
- recognition of the rights of people with HIV, STIs and viral hepatitis to participate in the community without experience of stigma or discrimination, and having the same rights to comprehensive and appropriate health care as do other members of the community
- effective partnerships between governments, affected communities, researchers and health professionals, characterised by consultation, cooperative effort, respectful discussion and action to achieve the goal of the strategy. (DoHA 2010c: 11–12)

Within both the public health and case-management spheres, there is an emphasis on developing the capacity of primary health care facilities for STI prevention and care. A public health approach to managing the prevention of STIs is about focusing on developing and integrating systems and services, including development of capacity for STI case management in primary care and strengthening of STI services in other reproductive health services; epidemiological surveillance of STIs; control of epidemics; and the provision of affordable, accessible and acceptable care for STI patients and HIV-infected people.

Organised approach to screening

Early detection of precursors to diseases is a central plank of the secondary prevention strategy. Screening is most commonly seen as the standard tool for early detection, and has been defined in a number of ways. The US Department of Labor Occupational Safety and Health Administration defines screening as: 'a method for detecting disease or body dysfunction before an individual would normally seek medical care' (2012). The aim of screening programs is to pick up very early cancers in healthy individuals who do not have symptoms (Cancer Council Australia 2012b).

> The World Health Organization (WHO) defines screening as the presumptive identification of unrecognised disease or defects by means of tests, examinations or other procedures that can be applied rapidly. Screening is intended for all people, in an identified target population, who do not have symptoms of the disease or condition being screened for. (AHMAC 2008: 1)

The consistent theme of these definitions is the administering of these activities before people have symptoms of ill-health.

At the individual level, the purpose of screening is to refer people for early diagnosis and treatment and, where possible, to provide preventive measures. Early identification is important when dealing with conditions that are more difficult to treat when fully developed. In the case of communicable diseases, it is particularly important in the prevention of disease transmission in the broader community. The public health application of screening is aimed at detection and early prevention. Clinical screening can be distinguished from public health applications, as it is concerned with diagnostic application and assisting treatment decisions and interventions at the individual level, and includes such activities as assessment of activities of daily living, diagnostic imaging/radiology, disease/disability-specific screening/diagnosis, general laboratory tests, general physical examinations, genetic testing and screening, paediatric evaluation and physical fitness assessment.

Health checks by GPs are seen as a screening test for both clinical and public health purposes. Screening programs for HIV, high cholesterol, high blood pressure, genetic abnormalities and other risk factors, if offered as a diagnostic procedure or as an opportunistic preventive measure, do not constitute a public health service. Such screening activities can be considered of public health benefit when they are targeted at the appropriate population and can cover sufficiently large portions of that population.

Sometimes, advocates for prevention suggest that it is desirable for all screening procedures to be organised at the population level. This is not necessarily appropriate either, as a great deal of resources may be invested but with very little return in terms of health improvement at the population level. From a public health perspective, screening programs should not be commenced without careful consideration of a range of factors. Suitable criteria for screening include:

- Is the disease or condition suitable? It should have a long detectable pre-clinical phase, the prevalence should not be rare (or have high incidence), and it should be a significant cause of morbidity or mortality.

- Is there a suitable test? It must be valid and reliable.
- Will early treatment be advantageous?
- Is an organised program feasible and desirable? Is it cost-effective, and will benefits outweigh costs (economic, social, psychological)? Is it acceptable to the population?

Whether a program should be directed to a single risk factor/disease or multiple risk factors and diseases is another issue. The distinguishing feature about public health screening programs is that they are organised efforts, as seen from the above framework, rather than opportunistic clinical services.

A number of screening programs in Australia are discussed below. They demonstrate that screening for disease has become almost commonplace in Australia, and screening technologies are constantly being developed for early detection and treatment. Critical success factors for any screening activity include:

- funding and resources required to establish the service and, importantly, to maintain the service

---

Box 14.3 Population-based screening framework

The Australian Health Ministers' Advisory Council (AHMAC) has adopted a population-based screening framework in which a screening program must:
- respond to a recognised need
- have a clear definition of the objectives of the program and the expected health benefits
- have scientific evidence of screening program effectiveness
- identify the target population that stands to benefit from screening
- clearly define the screening pathway and interval
- ensure availability of the organisation, infrastructure, facilities and workforce needed to deliver the screening program
- have measures available that have been demonstrated to be cost-effective to encourage high coverage
- have adequate facilities available for having tests and interpreting them
- have an organised quality control program across the screening pathway to minimise potential risks of screening
- have a referral system for management of any abnormalities found, and for providing information about normal screening tests

- have adequate facilities for follow-up assessment, diagnosis, management and treatment
- have evidence-based guidelines and policies for assessment, diagnosis and support for people with a positive test result
- have adequate resources available to set up and maintain a database of health information collected for the program
- integrate education, testing, clinical services and program management
- have a database capable of providing a population register for people who are screened that can issue invitations for initial screening, recall individuals for repeat screening, follow those with identified abnormalities, correlate with morbidity and mortality results, and monitor and evaluate the program and its impact
- plan evaluation from the outset and ensure that program data are maintained so that evaluation and monitoring of the program can be performed regularly
- be cost-effective
- ensure informed choice, confidentiality and respect for autonomy
- promote equity and access to screening for the entire target population
- ensure the overall benefits of screening outweigh the harm.

Source: AHMAC (2008: 11).

- a high level of participation by the community to ensure that a reduction in mortality is achieved and the service is cost-effective
- screening activities, including interpretation and diagnosis, communication and referral, and information management of high quality
- a skilled professional workforce and management
- a high standard of integration of services.

Maternal and child health

Maternal and child health (MCH) screening and monitoring services are historically government-funded. MCH is a universal service that has linked two population groups: mothers and mothers-to-be; and children. This service has been provided in Australia since about the early 1900s, when there were concerns about the high maternal and infant mortality rates (Lawson & Bauman 2001). An organised approach to antenatal and postnatal care for mothers and screening of infants was central to the improvement of maternal and child health.

Figure 14.1 shows the steadily decreasing infant mortality rate (IMR) in Australia since 1901 until 2001, which reflects the relative impact of immunisation and antibiotics. Although the rates for the total population and Indigenous groups have decreased steadily since 1972–73, it is quite clear that the Indigenous population's IMR is almost 2.5 times greater than that of the total population.

Australia's IMR has declined steadily over time. This decline was evident over the whole of the twentieth century: for every 1000 babies born in Australia in 1904, nearly 82 died before their first birthday; by 2010, the rate was just over four deaths per 1000 live births. The decline in infant mortality was due largely to improvements in prenatal and postnatal care, birth conditions and sanitation, as

Figure 14.1 Australian infant mortality rates, 1901–2010

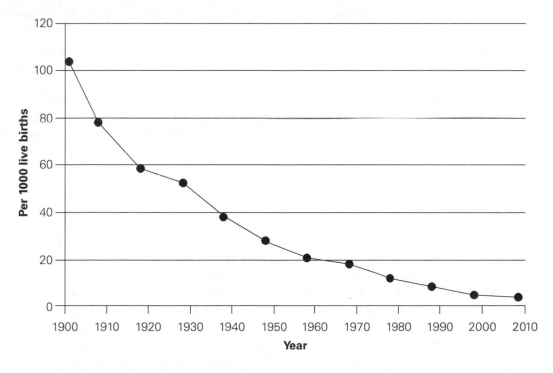

Source: Australian Bureau of Statistics (2010, 2012c).

well as drug development, mass vaccination and lower rates of infectious diseases (ABS 2012c).

Organised MCH services commenced in Paris around 1880, when it was recognised that knowledge about infant nutrition, hygiene and infant care were common needs for new mothers (White 1994). The organisation of MCH services soon became generalised in Western countries, and services were aimed at improving the survival and fitness of infants. As a result, governments funded and further organised MCH services largely because they were consistent with governments' nationalist ideals: the concern with the need to produce a healthy and strong population so as to improve national efficiency, productivity and an ability to fight and win wars.

Maternal and child health services were based on clinics in which nurses monitored infant health and provided advice to mothers. Monitoring consisted of vision screening; physical examination; measurement of weight and height; activities to check posture and coordination; games to check hand and eye coordination; assessment of hearing, speech and communication; observation of concentration and cooperation; and assessment of social development and play skills. Emphasis was also placed on infant nutrition and hygiene. Today, with the declining birth and infant mortality rates, and a reduction in the incidence of childhood infectious disease, maternal and child health services also emphasise quality of life, parenting skills and health promotion. Services tend to provide information, advice and referral for parents regarding child health, child development, breastfeeding, child and infant nutrition, maternal health, parenting, accident and injury prevention, home safety, immunisation, and local support services and resources. A major emphasis is placed on the physical development of the child, with regular screening activities to detect early signs of physical and sensory impairment, and the monitoring of the child's progress.

An important aspect from the population health perspective has been the development of service linkages. All births are notified by the hospital or birthing centre to the maternal and child health nurse, and arrangements are then made for home visits by the nurse and regular attendance at the nearest centre. Further service linkages come from referrals arising from screening activities to a range of primary service and secondary service providers. The activities of screening, referral and early intervention are well integrated within this primary health-care service.

Maternal and child health is a long-standing public health clinical service that has continued to evolve from a focus on the survival of children to a focus that encompasses the child and their family, backed by a network of services. The service continues to be based on fundamental screening and monitoring of the health of the child measured against the expected development milestones of a healthy child. Importantly, it is organised such that it is a universal service in Australia.

Antenatal screening

A systematic approach to antenatal care has been historically important in the reduction of maternal mortality rates, through early detection and improved management of high-risk conditions. While such an approach remains important in developing countries with high maternal mortality rates, antenatal care is now seen in Australia as a program of care for all pregnant women, regardless of their level of risk. Programs are usually made up of three quite distinct elements: the provision of information about pregnancy and childbirth generally, and about arrangements for the birth of individual babies; antenatal classes; and screening of pregnant mothers. Historically, falling perinatal mortality rates have been associated with increasing numbers of antenatal visits.

Antenatal screening is concerned with regular check-ups in the first and second trimesters of pregnancy, with the aim of monitoring the well-being of the mother and child during pregnancy. Typically, foetuses are screened for Down syndrome, Edward syndrome and open neural tube defects. The medical practitioner records the physical signs, and may order tests as required and act upon any symptoms of illness or abnormality detected from this process. The tests and examinations range from measurement of blood pressure and determination of blood type to sophisticated ultrasound screening and the use of a range of other screenings, including amniocentesis and chorionic villus sampling.

From a public health perspective, there are questions about which screening tests should be available to which women, especially as more older women (who are at higher risk) are having babies. There are public health questions about over-use of expensive technologies as well as insufficiently targeted use of beneficial technologies. Ultrasound is the most widely used of the screening tests, with a routine ultrasound at eighteen weeks being almost universal in Australia. However, baseline screening tests are determined by individual practitioners and care institutions. A study by O'Leary et al. (2006: 432) into the variations in prenatal screening concluded that in Australia, antenatal screening was uncoordinated, and operated with variable policy and practice and also occasionally with indeterminate quality. The use of routine ultrasound is somewhat controversial. For example, O'Leary et al. (2006: 431) argue that as a primary screening for foetal chromosomal abnormalities, ultrasound is no longer viewed as adequate.

Coupled with concerns relating to inconsistent baseline screening, there appears to be inadequate counselling of women about the nature of a screening test and possible adverse consequences of routine scanning, and the difficult decisions they may have to face from having an ultrasound. Antenatal screening of women and foetuses is an issue that has generated considerable interest and concern among consumers, clinicians and health administrators. Major concerns consistently raised relate to the increasing range of screening tests offered to women and the frequency with which they are performed, the concomitant growth in expenditure on screening and a lack of evidence about the efficacy of many

of the tests now performed (Senate Community Affairs References Committee 1999; O'Leary et al. 2006; Hunt & Lumley 2002).

The Royal Australian and New Zealand College of Obstetricians and Gynaecologists (RANZCOG 2009) recommends the following in relation to antenatal screening in the absence of pregnancy complications:

- full blood examination
- rubella antibody status
- syphilis serology
- HIV
- hepatitis B and C
- cervical cytology
- obstetric ultrasound scan (18–20 weeks)
- Down syndrome
- gestational diabetes.

A public health approach to antenatal screening would point to the need to address these concerns and examine the AHMAC Population Based Screening Framework, particularly in areas of establishing an evidence base, agreement on screening criteria and cost-effectiveness. The Western Australian Department of Health has developed a best practice model for prenatal screening choices, which includes a number of the elements of the AHMAC Framework. This model aims to inform the delivery of prenatal screening services by describing service provider roles and responsibilities, and defining best practice across the screening process (Western Australia Department of Health 2010: 7). Importantly, the model emphasises the need to provide information to support decision-making by women and identifies post-test counselling and support as a part of best practice.

Women's cancer screening services (breast and cervical)
With non-communicable diseases (NCDs) a leading cause of death, there has been much interest in finding strategies for the early detection of cancers.

The incidence of breast and cervical cancers in women has prompted the development of nation-wide screening activities. Both illustrate the shift from a clinical diagnostic service to a public health effort.

The focus of both services can be seen by examining their aims. BreastScreen Australia aims to maximise the early detection of breast cancer in well women without symptoms who are aged 50 to 69 years through an organised approach using screening mammography (DoHA 2012b). The aim of the National Cervical Screening Program (and the National Cervical Screening Program Renewal, which is examining the science and tech-nologies used in the program, as well as access to the program) is to reduce the incidence of and death from cervical cancer through an organised approach to cervical screening—that is, Pap smears every two years (DoHA 2012f).

There have been concerns about the high rates of mortality from cervical and breast cancers, particularly when screening and early detection are possible. Cervical cancer is one of the most prevent-able and curable of all cancers, and is the thirteenth most common cancer affecting Australian women. It is estimated that up to 90 per cent of the most common type of cervical cancer (squamous cell carcinoma) may be prevented if cell changes are detected and treated early. In 2007, there were seven new cases of diagnosed cervical cancer per 100 000 women and two deaths per 100 000 women. This was an historic low, and since the introduction of the program in 1991 both incidence and mortality have been halved. However, both cervical cancer inci-dence and mortality were higher in Aboriginal and Torres Strait Islander women, with the incidence more than twice, and mortality five times, that of non-Indigenous women (AIHW 2011a: vi).

In 1988, the AHMAC Cervical Cancer Screening Evaluation Steering Committee recommended the establishment of an organised approach to screening to provide better protection against cervical cancer. In 1991, the Organised Approach to Preventing Cancer of the Cervix was established as a joint initiative of the Commonwealth, state and terri-tory governments, and in 1995 it was renamed the National Cervical Screening Program (DoHA 2012f).

One of the concerns leading to the 'organised approach' to cervical screening was the over-use of Pap smears by some groups and their under-use by other at-risk groups. The basis of the 'organised approach' was an agreement on screening intervals (based on cost-effectiveness), a registry and recall system, education and outreach to at-risk groups, and a cytology service. The National Cervical Screening Program broadly targeted all women aged from eighteen to 70, with an emphasis on the 35–70 age group. There was an extensive use of media, including television and women's magazine adver-tising and a public relations program. A component of the campaign was a targeted strategy for women from diverse cultural and linguistic backgrounds aimed at informing them about the importance of cervical screening.

Service providers were also the subject of the campaign, not only to inform providers about the National Cervical Screening Program, but to reinforce the important role they have in encour-aging women to be screened. In 2001, a Cervical Screening Incentives Program was launched by the Commonwealth government. Eligible general practitioners received a service incentive payment for screening women aged 20–69 who had not had a cervical smear in the last four years. In 2002, a further payment was made to practices that reached their target levels of cervical screening (Wooldridge 2001).

Data collection, analysis and feedback were important components of the campaign, and cervical cytology registries were developed to provide feedback to GPs, nurse practitioners and women's health centres. Feedback included advice on the technical adequacy of the smear, offering a reminder service for women who were overdue for a routine Pap smear, helping ensure that women with significant screen-detected abnormalities were appropriately followed up, and providing assistance to pathology laboratories with internal quality control (DoHA 2004f).

In the period 2008–09, more than 3.6 million women participated in the program—that is, 59 per cent of eligible women. Participation was highest in urban areas and lowest in more remote areas; however, rates of participation were higher with increasing socio-economic status, with a rate of 53 per cent of participating women residing in areas of lowest socio-economic status compared with a rate of 64 per cent of women in areas of highest socio-economic status. Participation level by Aboriginal and Torres Strait Islander women is not known, but there is evidence that this group is under-screened (AIHW 2012: vi).

Breast cancer is also a major health issue for women aged 34 to 75 years, causing more deaths of Australian women than any other form of cancer. In 2007, a total of 2680 Australian women died from breast cancer, and it is predicted that one in eleven Australian women will develop the disease. Age is the biggest risk factor in developing breast cancer, with the incidence rate significantly increasing in women over 50 years (DoHA 2009: 18; DoHA 2012b). In June 1990, the Ministers for Health in all states and territories joined the Commonwealth in agreeing to jointly fund a national mammography screening program. BreastScreen Australia was established in 1991, and is now recognised as one of the most comprehensive population-based screening programs in the world. BreastScreen Australia is targeted specifically at women without symptoms aged 50–69, and operates in over 500 locations nationwide, via fixed, relocatable and mobile screening units. The program's aim is to achieve a participation rate of 70 per cent among women aged 50–69 years. The participation rate for BreastScreen Australia is 54.9 per cent of the target population, with 1273 403 women being screened in period 2007–08 (DoHA 2012b).

In the context of the national program, 'screening' refers to population-based screening for breast cancer of apparently well women in the target age group. Screening mammography is carried out in an organised and systematic manner to detect unsuspected cancer so that early treatment can reduce illness and death from breast cancer. This population-based approach is distinctly different from the use of mammography to investigate symptoms in an individual woman, which is a diagnostic procedure.

Both the cervical and breast screening campaigns have the hallmarks of the public health approach in that there are policy elements that provide for a national or population focus, appropriate funding to underpin the campaign from all governments, identification of at-risk groups and a recognition that a multiplicity of strategies need to be utilised for these groups, acknowledgement of the service providers' role, and the need for a data-collection and feedback system—the organised approach.

Other cancer screening

The success of cancer screening programs has resulted in the government providing funding to explore other cancer screening programs, such as for bowel (colorectal) cancer, which is the second most common cancer affecting both men and women in Australia. In 2007, there were 14 234 new cases of bowel cancer reported (7804 men and 6430 women) and 4047 deaths. The incidence rate of bowel cancer rises steadily with advancing age, and most cases occur after the age of 50 years (Cancer Council Australia 2012).

With clinical evidence showing that screening via faecal occult blood testing (FOBT) can reduce mortality by 15–33 per cent, the Commonwealth government provided funding to undertake a pilot screening program that was found to be cost-effective, and had a participation rate of over 45 per cent of the target population group. As the pilot screening program showed that it was acceptable, feasible and cost-effective, it has paved the way for a national screening program (DoHA 2005d). The National Bowel Cancer Screening Program commenced in

January 2011, and free bowel cancer testing kits were mailed to the target group of Australians who turned 50, 55 or 65 years of age as identified from Medicare records. As part of the 2012–13 Budget, the federal government announced that the program would be expanded to include Australians turning 60 years of age from 2013 and those turning 70 years of age from 2015 (DoHA 2012e).

The screening program, using the FOBT kit, has been found to detect almost triple the number of Stage A cancers (40 per cent) compared with those diagnosed through symptoms (14 per cent), thus having the potential to reduce mortality in the target groups. According to the Cancer Council of Australia, these findings, together with an independent cost-effectiveness analysis estimating that the program would save up to 500 lives each year, are consistent with international evidence showing that bowel cancer screening on a population basis significantly reduces mortality and morbidity (Cancer Council Australia 2012a).

Over the last few years, there has been much debate on taking a population-based screening approach to prostate cancer using digital rectal examination and levels of prostate-specific antigen (PSA). According to Cancer Council Australia and AHMAC (2010), almost 3000 Australian men die from prostate cancer annually and, as with many cancers, it is expected that the number of cases will continue to grow as the Australian population ages. Over 80 per cent of new prostate cancer cases occur in men aged over 60, and 97 per cent of prostate cancer deaths will occur in this age group. In a joint position statement, Cancer Council Australia and AHMAC (2010) stated that the current evidence indicates that the PSA test is not suitable for population screening, as the harms outweigh the benefits. In terms of diagnosis, the issue is that many prostate cancers grow slowly without requiring treatment or intervention, and thus a normal life can be led, whereas other men will experience life-threatening prostate cancer where the cancer grows and spreads rapidly and there is no

test that adequately differentiates between these cancers (Cancer Council Australia & AHMAC 2010). Chapman, Barratt & Stockler (2010: 9) quote the following scenario that may occur if men undergo a treatment based on PSA screening for which the evidence is unclear but the risks of the surgery are well established:

> A 2003 review of the issue in the *Lancet* concluded that if one million men over 50 were screened, about 110 000 with raised PSAs will face anxiety of possible cancer, about 90 000 will undergo biopsy, and 20 000 will be diagnosed with cancer. If 10 000 of these men underwent surgery, about 10 would die of the operation, 300 will develop severe urinary incontinence and even in the best hands 4000 will become impotent. And then came the crunch: The number of men whose prostate cancer would have impinged on their lives is unknown.

Health screening for migrants and refugees

Screening can be used as a tool to identify prevention opportunities for the individuals screened, but it can be also used as a tool to 'protect' people in the Australian community from exposure to infectious diseases.

The history of public health provides us with many examples of the relationship between the movement of people and public health issues. Colonial expansion, gold rushes, disease, famine, persecution and wars result in the movement of people and the spread of disease. The traditional response by governments to these disease threats has been the introduction of quarantine controls for both people and goods.

There are a number of public health implications for those people on the move and the populations that come into contact with them. In the early settlement of Australia, the long voyage from England to Australia served as a 'quarantine period'. The barrier of geography and isolation has long since been overcome, with the ease of international travel today. This, together with an explosion in global trade, allows diseases in one country to be quickly transferred into another, thus exposing the host population to current epidemics, such as avian influenza and SARS. The capacity for people to move easily and quickly around the world means that isolated or contained communicable diseases can very quickly become outbreaks, thus raising the public health issues associated with traveller's health, the health of co-travellers, the health of contact populations and, ultimately, the health of the host population.

Migrants and refugees pose potential public health risks to the Australian (host) population, and subsequently the systematic management of this risk has become the responsibility of the Commonwealth Departments of Immigration and Citizenship and Health and Ageing. Government strategy is that all refugees applying for a permanent visa must have a pre-departure health assessment, which includes a chest x-ray and HIV test. Specific diseases that are screened for are tuberculosis, hepatitis B and HIV (DIAC 2012).

Screening programs for refugees (persons who have had to flee their home and country, are living outside their country of nationality and are unable to return for fear of persecution) were developed in the 1970s to monitor Indo-Chinese people arriving by boat in Australia. This coincided with the ending of Australia's restrictive immigration policies and a government commitment to accept refugees from South-East Asia. Reid, Goldstein and Keo (1986) found that the advocates for refugee screening justified this screening on the basis of the protection of the Australian public from refugees with disease, and reassurance for the Australian public that they were not being 'invaded' by 'bugs'. A further justification for conducting screening is its value as a personal medical service, rather than a public health service, whereby diseases such as diabetes and heart disease can be detected and treated, providing individual benefits. The critics of this view are concerned

with the added stress on refugees, the protection of refugee rights and the validity of public health arguments for maintaining or expanding screening. Reid and Trompf (1990) conclude that there is some validity for all arguments, but there is also a need for compulsory screening for those diseases that are missed at overseas screening, and that pose a significant threat to public health—namely tuberculosis, syphilis and hepatitis B. Immunisation is also regarded as important.

In contrast to the refugee screening for South-East Asian refugees, the government conducted Operation Safe Haven, when from May to June 1999, a total of 3920 ethnic Albanians from Kosovo arrived in Australia. The arrival of a large number of refugees in a short timeframe was unprecedented in Australia, and there were no pre-existing Australian guidelines for the establishment of health surveillance in a rapid-response setting. A health surveillance system was established and critical health data were collected to assess health status, plan care, monitor for potential outbreaks of communicable diseases, track service use and meet international reporting requirements (Bennett et al. 2000).

The primary aims were to:

- determine the health status of incoming evacuees to plan for appropriate care
- ensure timely ascertainment of active cases of tuberculosis
- monitor for potential outbreaks of communicable diseases.

The secondary aims were to:

- document health status over the duration of stay, including communicable disease incidence, prevalence of chronic disease, mortality and births
- record preventive health care activities, such as immunisation
- collate health status data for repatriation

- provide data to assist in monitoring costs of health services for the evacuees.

Screening was in accordance with a protocol specifically developed for the Kosovar evacuees by the National Centre for Disease Control, including specific screening for tuberculosis (Bennett et al. 2000). As seen from the primary and secondary aims, there was an emphasis on personal medical care. It would appear that refugee screening will continue to encompass a range of public health and clinical services, although emphasis may change to reflect the current political environment.

In 2010–11 Australia granted 13 799 visas to refugees or people in the special humanitarian program and granted them access to a wide range of services, including health services (DIAC 2012). However, refugees who enter Australia without authority are detained in immigration detention centres while their reasons for being in Australia are investigated. Newly arrived refugees undergo a protocol-based health assessment, which is concerned with conditions of public health importance and identifies the minimal health requirements (including vaccinations) necessary to protect both the health of other detainees and the Australian community. King and Vodicka (2001), in a study of 7000 detainees screened by the New South Wales Refugee Health Service between 1 January 2000 and 30 June 2001, concluded that:

> the health-screening program at the immigration reception and processing centres detects significant numbers of conditions of public health importance, enabling treatment and surveillance to the benefit of the people detained and the Australian community (King & Vodicka 2001: 604).

A similar conclusion was reached by Martin and Mak (2006: 610) in their review of infectious disease screening of refugees in Western Australia in 2003 and 2004; the authors comment:

Our study demonstrates the need to monitor the prevalence of diseases of public and personal health significance in refugees entering Australia to provide cost-effective services that protect the health of both individual refugees and the wider community.

Outside of the infectious disease issues, there are a number of refugee health needs associated with specific sub-groups within the refugee community, including nutritional problems relating to vitamin A, vitamin D and/or iron deficiency, and untreated health conditions and injuries exacerbated through poor living conditions and a lack of access to treatment. The most frequently treated physical conditions are dental caries, digestive complaints, respiratory problems, skin lesions, dermatophytosis, otitis externa and infections of the upper respiratory tract. In addition to these physical conditions, mental health is also a priority issue for refugees; this stems not only from the the pre-arrival experience itself, but it is believed that the detention and settling in period may have an even greater negative impact on mental health (Bowers & Cheng 2010).

Migrant and refugee screening is an element of an overall immigration policy administered by a non-Health portfolio of the Commonwealth government. The area of immigration and refugee policy is controversial, but there is merit in a systematic screening process for the benefit of both the Australian population and the newly arrived immigrants and refugees.

New developments in primary care and public health: Moving to shared ownership

The ageing of the population, increasing prevalence of chronic diseases and workforce shortages have led to concerns that greater partnerships are required between clinical care and public health in prevention. In recent years, there have been increasing efforts to develop primary care services based on population health approaches. These have included the development of both basic criteria for these services and the institutional arrangements by which they can be delivered to the community.

Divisions of General Practice and Medicare Locals: An organisational approach to institute public health in primary care?

While new Commonwealth–state cost-shared programs were being introduced in the 1980s and delivered largely through state-based service-delivery systems, a different policy discourse emerged about the role of GPs in the provision of public health services. A number of disparate factors contributed to this development, including the following:

- As GPs were paid by the Commonwealth government, it was possible for states to cost-shift—that is, close down immunisation and maternal and child health services on the basis that families would go to their GPs for that service.
- Many GPs thought the state governments and the public sector were competing for work, and therefore lobbied to be recognised and included in public health programs.
- Commonwealth reforms of general practice moved towards developing population-based divisions, hence providing a framework for public health activities to link with individual clinical care.
- Many national public health strategies suggested that educating GPs was a key intervention for improving health in the community.
- The Royal Australian College of General Practitioners began to promote putting prevention into clinical practice, and developed guidelines to assist GPs in this area.

In 1991, the Commonwealth government announced a number of reforms to general practice, including funding arrangements. These reforms were concerned with the supply and distribution of medical practitioners, accreditation of general practices, funding of complementary fee-for-service reimbursement, and the amalgamation of solo and small-group practices into larger entities. It was seen as important that local GPs were able to work together more closely, and have an input into health-care planning for their respective communities. This led to the establishment of Divisions of General Practice.

Although the prevention agenda was not prominent at the outset, Divisions of General Practice became increasingly important as a vehicle for linking public health activities and primary medical care. In the mid-1990s, the Commonwealth began to develop payment incentives for GPs to offer immunisation services. In 1998, a Joint Advisory Group on Population Health, formed between the National Public Health Partnership and the GP Partnership Advisory Group (a policy advisory group to the minister), proposed the SNAP (smoking, nutrition, alcohol and physical activity) framework to guide GPs in primary prevention for chronic diseases. In the late 1990s, other new payment schemes were introduced (called 'Enhanced Primary Care') to improve such things as the continuity of care and health checks for older people.

In August 2011, the then Prime Minister, Julia Gillard, announced a National Health Reform Agreement between state and territory government and the federal government, the aims of which are 'to deliver better access to services, improved local accountability and transparency, greater responsiveness to local communities and provide a stronger financial basis for our health system into the future through increased Commonwealth funding' (DoHA 2013a). A key element of the reform agenda was the establishment of a new primary health care organisation, Medicare Locals, replacing the Divisions of General Practice and having the role of coordinating primary health care delivery and addressing local health care needs and service gaps. There are five objectives of Medicare Locals:

- **Objective 1:** Improving the patient journey through developing integrated and coordinated services.
- **Objective 2:** Providing support to clinicians and service providers to improve patient care.
- **Objective 3:** Identifying the health needs of local areas and development of locally focused and responsive services.
- **Objective 4:** Facilitating the implementation and successful performance of primary health care initiatives and programs.
- **Objective 5:** Being efficient and accountable with strong governance and effective management.

The public health role is enunciated in Objective 3, particularly in relation to maintaining a population health database, providing input into population health profiles and undertaking population health needs assessment and planning (General Practice Victoria 2011). Given that the government has already signalled that community health promotion and population health programs should include preventive health as an area for exploration (Commonwealth of Australia 2010), the advent of Medicare Locals may see the development and integration of public health, primary care and preventive services at a regional level throughout Australia.

The public health community was divided over the initiatives associated with the development of Divisions of General Practice, and it is early days in regard to Medicare Locals. Certainly the resources budgeted for the new Medicare Locals and the stated aim of integrating primary and population health planning and service coordination as key roles are consistent with public health principles. There is some concern with regard to ensuring that appropriate governance structures are established within each Medicare Local, that accountability is to the local community and that the organisations are not dominated by professional elites.

Screening for NCD risk factors

NCDs now constitute the leading causes of death in the developing world, and the onset of risk factors is an important predictor for future disease—both at an individual and a population level. The WHO has identified five important risk factors for non-communicable disease: raised blood pressure, raised cholesterol, tobacco use, alcohol consumption and being overweight. The disease burden caused by these leading risk factors is global. In every region of the world, including the poorest, raised blood pressure, high cholesterol levels and tobacco use are causing serious disease and untimely deaths (WHO 2003a). The top four risk factors for chronic disease in Australia are the same as for high-income countries overall: tobacco smoking, high blood pressure, overweight and obesity, and physical inactivity (AIHW 2012, citing WHO 2009).

A report of the Australian Institute of Health and Welfare confirms that Australia is facing an increased economic and social burden because of chronic diseases and their associated risk factors. Fourteen chronic diseases and conditions accounted for an estimated 32 per cent of the total disability-adjusted life years lost in Australia in 2003, indicating that the total disease burden could be reduced by about one-third if these risk factors could be eliminated (AIHW 2012).

In Australia, it has been recognised that effective public health interventions into these key risk factors would result in significant health gains. The comprehensive model of chronic disease prevention and control (see Figure 8.3 in Chapter 8) outlines how and where GPs can make a contribution to the public health organised effort. This was further reinforced by the Australian Better Health Initiative in 2006.

The model clearly indicates that GPs can adopt a range of interventions to help people manage health risk factors and to promote healthy behaviours. In the 'at-risk' population groups, interventions include screening and early detection, and the collection and forwarding of this information—which can then be used to develop the evidence base for interventions across the population. The role continues into the disease management areas, where GPs can plan and integrate their efforts with others to enable those who have specific diseases to improve and maintain well-being.

The SNAP framework is a tangible entry point to bring prevention into clinical practice. The concept is to use general practitioners as the largest, most accessible single entry point for the community into the health-care system, and to support them to provide illness care together with preventive care and chronic illness management, thereby contributing to population health outcomes

(General Practice Partnership Advisory Council 2002). Table 14.5 outlines the specific activities that GPs are advised to undertake for the SNAP.

The SNAP framework is indicative of public health thinking, as it clearly identifies the integrated levels of activity; these have been described as GP–patient consultation, GP practice, and Divisions of General Practice and community, at the state and Commonwealth levels. It is also recognised that, in order for these activities to be effective, there is a need for systems to support changed ways of working for GPs. These support system elements include organisational structures and roles, financing systems, workforce planning, education and

Table 14.5 Recommendations by the Royal Australian College of General Practitioners on preventive activities for general practice in relation to SNAP

Risk factor	Recommendations
Smoking	• Start screening of all people aged 10 years or over. • Take every opportunity to ask about the smoking of cigarettes, pipes or cigars. • Include smoking status as part of routine history-taking. Consider implementing systems changes at the practice or clinic. • Patients who smoke (regardless of the amount they smoke) should be offered brief advice to stop smoking. • Patients not interested in quitting smoking should be offered brief advice on the risks of smoking and encouraged to consider quitting.
Nutrition	• Patients should be encouraged and supported to follow Australian dietary recommendations. • Patients should be advised to eat at least seven portions of fruit or vegetables per day.
Alcohol	• Start screening from 14–15 years on quantity and frequency of alcohol use, using Alcohol Use Disorders Identification Test. • Individuals in high-risk groups should be screened at each presentation. • Brief interventions to reduce alcohol consumption should be offered to all patients drinking at potentially risky or high-risk levels.
Physical activity	• Patients should be asked about their daily physical activity and assessed to determine whether they walk or participate in leisure-time physical activity of sufficient intensity and duration for health benefits. • Patients may be referred to cardiac rehabilitation or physical activity programs, or classes run by local community organisations. • Patients who are insufficiently active and have a chronic medical condition with complex care needs may benefit from an EPC multidisciplinary care plan.

Source: Adapted from Royal Australian College of General Practitioners (2004).

training, information management and technology, communication, community awareness and patient education, partnership and referral mechanisms, and research and evaluation (General Practice Partnership Advisory Council 2002).

The framework is also an example of overcoming the patient–doctor relationship as a constraint to public health action, and using it as a basis for the organised effort that underscores public health approaches.

Consumer self-help groups and chronic disease self-management

With the rise of chronic diseases, people have to learn to live with symptoms that persist and affect their various roles in life (such as social, family and work). Doctors are able to prescribe medications that provide symptomatic relief or help manage the disease, but the role of consumers has become particularly important.

Self-help groups are not new. They have been established in Australia since the 1930s, but until recently have not become organised to the point where it is now recognised that they constitute a social movement. Self-help groups have formed and individuals have joined such groups because they are affected by a condition or life circumstance (for example, alcoholism and Alcoholics Anonymous). According to the Collective of Self-Help Groups, what makes self-help groups different from welfare or charity organisations is that the people being assisted are the same ones who control the activities and priorities of the group:

> Self help is about people coming together with others who are affected by a particular issue (experience, disadvantage, discrimination, etc.) to support each other and to work together to change the disadvantage affecting them. The activities that groups are involved with include community education, information, mutual support, research, services and advocacy.

> Self help groups are not charity, or simply community based groups run by volunteers and that are made up of, and controlled by, the people affected. Importantly members work to change their own situation and the support is mutual. (Nash 1999)

Over time, self-help groups have become more focused on understanding and changing the situations in which their members find themselves. Such situations are usually associated with disadvantage and discrimination, and are often expressed through their needs not being met, community attitudes causing discrimination, or a lack of power over decisions or resources needed to live full lives (Nash 1999). Many self-help groups have been formed because of a specific health or illness, such as asthma and arthritis, and advocacy for equitable distribution of resources is an important activity of the group.

Governments—notably the Whitlam government in 1972—have tried to harness community self-help into a more organised effort through funding support for community groups. However, as funding is provided with certain conditions and requires financial accountability, this has tended to cause a tension in regard to the independence of the group. Further, the removal of funding at a later time, or the inconsistency of funding associated with changing governments and policies, has also exposed groups if they have developed their activities on the basis of a certain level of funding.

The way in which self-help groups work is also quite different from that of service providers and welfare-style organisations. Self-help groups take an individual approach to dealing with an issue so individuals can gain power over their lives—they do not develop structures, such as 'programs', or provide a service delivered by a 'professional'. Thus, the organiser of the effort is not government but rather the individuals forming the group, who are empowered through a community development model. The public health approach in these circumstances is to accommodate and support the notion of self-help within the public health policy process, and involve self-help groups in policy development and system reforms.

More recently, the notion of self-help has become incorporated into the health-care system in the form of chronic disease self-management. Chronic disease now accounts for three-quarters of all health expenditure, and self-management for people with chronic disease is now seen to be a necessary part of treatment. Lorig and Holman (2000) define self-management as a term used to describe patient education, patient behaviours and health-promotion programs. The patient's role is to monitor symptoms, report them accurately and otherwise manage the disease on a day-to-day basis. The role of the health carer is as a partner in care, consultant, interpreter of symptoms and resource person. Within the confines of the chronic disease self-management model, the public health approach is not just to teach individual patients to care for themselves better, but to create support

structures among patients using lay educators and peer support approaches.

The Lorig and Holman (2000) model, developed at Stanford University and now extended to numerous countries, shows that self-management and peer support are based on the social and psychological needs of patients, which arise from the disease—such as learning to cope with new social and family roles, limitations in functional ability, and living with pain, rather than on the specifics of an illness. Evaluation of self-management also points to a reduction in doctor visits and hospital admissions, as well as improvements in life satisfaction. On the basis of this, a public health approach to chronic disease self-management is to organise a scaled-up effort to ensure access by all who would benefit.

The Commonwealth government's National Chronic Disease Self-Management Initiative in 2000 was based on a recognition of the value of chronic disease self-management when organised

---

Box 14.4 Quality use of medicine

In Australia, the most common health-related activity is taking medicines. But many medicines are being over-used, and there are an estimated 80 000 annual hospital admissions associated with medication-related problems, which include antibiotic resistance and medication misadventure by older people (DoHA 2002b). There is also concern about the increasing government expenditure on the PBS. To address these issues, Quality Use of Medicine (QUM) initiatives have been developed. The National Prescribing Service (NPS) (established in 1998) defines QUM as being 'about ensuring that all Australians have access to high quality, safe and effective medicines. It also relies on rational use of those medicines' (National Prescribing Service 2005). Thus, QUM is essentially about changing the way in which medicines are used both at the practitioner and community level; this

should be done by using an approach that encompasses individual and community development, and public health perspectives in policy planning, implementation and evaluation (DoHA 2002a: 9).

This is reflected in the NPS, which is funded by the Commonwealth government and is a partnership of government, the pharmaceutical industry, health professionals and consumers. The NPS supports QUM by providing support to health professionals through the development of tools for managing information about medicines and telephone advisory and information services. The NPS supports consumers by working with the Consumers' Health Forum of Australia to provide the public with resources and information, conducting national awareness campaigns and community-based programs for specific population groups, and providing a telephone information service through the 'Medicines Line' (National Prescribing Service 2005).

at a population level. The objectives of the initiative were to improve the health-related quality of life for people with chronic disease, and to encourage people with chronic disease to use the health-care system more effectively through a partnership model, rather than to decrease the incidence of chronic diseases. The current Sharing Health Care Initiative continues with the aims of self-management and building an evidence base on the efficacy of chronic disease interventions to support self-management available to people with chronic diseases, and to their carers and families (DoHA 2012l).

The significance of the self-management approach is that all parties take responsibility for actively managing the chronic disease, which becomes an integrating or coordinating mechanism for the efforts of all those parties concerned. The person with the chronic disease is therefore empowered to manage their disease with support from professionals and voluntary carers.

Conclusion

Clinical preventive services for early detection and prevention have made a significant contribution to improving population health, whether in the control of infectious diseases or risk factors for chronic diseases. A preventive service offered on an opportunistic basis—that is, as a patient walks into the clinic—does not produce a health benefit at the population level. Clinical services become central to the public health effort when at-risk populations are provided with these services in an organised fashion that ensures sufficient coverage of the population group at risk or of concern.

With demographic and epidemiological transition, an organised partnership between public health and primary health care becomes an urgent priority for the public health system. While the specific health concerns will undoubtedly change over time, the principles of how to organise a preventive effort across the clinical and community setting remain the same.

15

Health promotion:
From lifestyles to societal determinants of health

Challenge

Recently, many voices in your community have been calling for 'something to be done' about the increasing proportion of children and teenagers who are overweight or obese. Teachers, parents, doctors—and children too—all have something to say about the scale and causes of the problem, how it affects young people (as well as the broader community) and its longer-term impacts.

You are a staff member of a rural primary health care service that is also a partner in a local network of health-care services. As you, and some of your colleagues, think that the data about weight trends are too ominous to ignore, there is agreement that a local strategy needs to be devised to bring down the rate of increase of obesity in young people.

Focus groups have explored the perceptions of different groups of people living in the town and surrounding areas. They show a general belief that the problem has many dimensions—poorly maintained sports facilities that are uninviting as venues for sports activities; parents who work at times when young people want to have adventures in parks and natural settings but are encouraged to 'stay safe' inside, playing computer-based games; vending machines in workplaces and schools that supply cheap, carbonated drinks to children and workers; lack of time for parents to prepare and cook meals when juggling full-time work and the demands of family life; and the preference of children for takeaway foods as their snack of choice.

While some community members appreciate the interest expressed by health workers to stimulate action on the rising incidence of residents who are overweight or obese, others point out that there are many other problems and issues that need attention, from road maintenance to petrol prices to ensuring all children have access to computers in classrooms. These community members also think that bringing attention to individuals who are overweight or obese will cause more harm than good, as it could stigmatise them, or encourage them to form more unhealthy habits in defiance, or more generally make them feel badly about themselves.

As a health professional with a commitment to wellness in your community, what would you do? What do you see as the problem and its causes? Would the Ottawa Charter for Health Promotion be useful to you in taking action? How would the role of others in the community differ from your role in responding to this issue? What ethical issues might you face in responding to the problem?

Introduction

Canadian Minister of National Health and Welfare Marc Lalonde is widely credited with using the term and concept of health promotion for the first time in 1974. In his landmark report, *A New Perspective on the Health of Canadians*, Lalonde (1974) proposed that health care was only one of four main factors (human biology, health care, lifestyle and environment) responsible for patterns of health in a population. Changes across all of these were required to improve health status. He recognised that although much more evidence was required to establish scientific proof of cause-and-effect relationships between these factors and health, the magnitude of health problems in Canada demanded that 'action has to be taken on them even if all the scientific evidence is not in' (Lalonde 1974). Lalonde presented this wider view of health and its improvement as a basis for government policy, embedding a philosophy of social justice and political accountability for population health outcomes.

Since the early 1970s, the term and concept of health promotion has been applied to frame international policies and programs geared to improving health. An 'organised effort' aptly describes the multi-strategy, multi-level approach required in contemporary health promotion which, taken as a whole, has been shown to be more powerful and effective in improving population health than the use of specific interventions.

As discussed in Chapter 6, health promotion continues to evolve as a concept and area of public health practice, but remains concerned with collective and individual actions designed to enhance quality of life, reduce the burden of illness and prolong life expectancy. In broad terms, effective health promotion leads to actions that create living and working conditions conducive to health and well-being in populations and support people to adopt and maintain healthy lifestyles. Over the last three decades in particular, the theoretical foundations and practice of health promotion have matured through an accumulation of experience and research, combined with lively, ongoing debates in the field and literature about principles, values, methods and effectiveness.

The basic concept of health promotion is depicted and explained in the Ottawa Charter for Health Promotion, which was formulated in 1986 at the first of a series of international WHO meetings (WHO 1986). The charter has been applied to policy, planning, projects and research in many different national and organisational contexts. Demonstrating what some regard as its visionary quality, the charter continues to serve as the internationally recognised frame of reference, or foundation 'blueprint', for health promotion. The charter defines health promotion as the process of enabling individuals and communities to increase control over the determinants of health and thereby improve their health.

This chapter reviews the evolution of health promotion and shows how health promotion has been applied in contemporary settings and systems. Case studies of health promotion are used to illustrate approaches to planning, implementing and evaluating health-promotion programs. They are also used to highlight current issues in health promotion, such as how to ensure effectiveness of health-promotion programs.

Evolution of health promotion: Learning from doing

Contemporary accounts of public health distinguish three major phases in the evolution of health promotion—disease prevention, lifestyle or behaviour change, and social-environmental change—by the different emphasis given to particular health determinants and intervention aims. Interactions between program evaluation, research, health-promotion practice and debates among public and professional groups have driven the general development of the field. Some specific drivers of this maturation process are:

- **international research**, which is producing evidence about relationships between health and its determinants and about the efficacy of interventions to bring about change in individuals, communities, organisations and public policy and practice
- **professional groups**, such as the International Union of Health Promotion and Education, and government technical agencies, such as the Centers for Disease Control and Prevention, which are making notable contributions to compiling evidence of health promotion effectiveness
- the **World Health Organization**, which has sponsored invitational conferences on health

promotion since 1986. These have examined and debated concepts, theories and practice and renewed strategic directions for health promotion. They have been held in Ottawa, Canada (1986); Adelaide, Australia (1988); Sundsvall, Sweden (1991); Jakarta, Indonesia (1997); Mexico City, Mexico (2000); Bangkok, Thailand (2005) (WHO 2005b); Nairobi, Kenya (2009); and Helsinki, Finland (2013).

The changing role of health education in health promotion

As discussed in earlier chapters, health education has endured as a valuable public health strategy for centuries—informing people about isolation measures during the plague, encouraging families through household visits to use soap to prevent disease transmission in nineteenth-century England, and in recent decades educating the public through campaigns about the dangers of smoking or fast driving and the benefits of participating in vaccination programs or of breastfeeding infants. Health education is part of action on many current issues to bring about changes in health behaviour, including the nurturing of infants and children, dental care, food choices, physical activity, sexual behaviour, social participation, and the use of alcohol, tobacco and illicit drugs.

In the 1970s and early 1980s, behaviour was emphasised as a major determinant of health, and this led to health-education programs for individuals and groups, and also social marketing strategies, becoming popular ways to influence population health. Health-education programs typically were delivered face to face, through settings that had a health or educational role, such as health services (for example, general practices, hospitals, pharmacies, maternal and child health, or MCH, services), schools and community groups (for example, those with a health focus, such as self-help groups for people with chronic diseases). Social marketing strategies applied techniques developed in the retail sector in order to 'sell' a message about behaviours, products or services to choose. Posters, pamphlets and other information materials were combined with the placement of television advertisements to reach mass audiences.

Two examples of this are advertisements advocating active lifestyles in community settings—for example, the Life. Be In It campaign—or raising awareness about HIV—for example, the Grim Reaper campaign (see Box 15.1).

Health-education programs are often based on simple assumptions about what determines health patterns in a population and what is required to improve and sustain health, relying on people being both ready to accept information and able to apply it in their own circumstances. Definitions of health

---

Box 15.1 Early Australian campaigns leading people through stages of change

Life. Be In It

'Norm' was a cartoon character developed for the 'Life. Be In It' campaign launched in 1975 by the Victorian government and later adopted by the Commonwealth government and implemented in other states. Norm—overweight and sedentary—was invented at a time of increasing prevalence of cardiovascular disease to raise awareness in the population about the benefits of moderate, regular exercise and to motivate individuals to initiate changes in their daily lives. The first advertisements used negative motivators to raise awareness among segments of the population who were not even contemplating a change in their exercise patterns (like Norm) or just moving towards a change. Later advertisements highlighted positive rewards for becoming more active. Norm was portrayed as a role model for how people could commit to increasing activity in their daily lives—walking or flying kites—and initiate change. Community level programs offering opportunities for people to 'come an' try' new activities complemented the advertisements.

Grim Reaper

In 1987, an advertisement was developed by the Australian government to challenge a commonly held view in the community that the main population group at risk of acquiring HIV infection comprised men who have sex with men. A powerful image of the Grim Reaper—the harbinger of death—was used to grab the audience's attention. The Reaper was shown poised in a dark bowling alley, scythe in hand, ready to strike down startled citizens of all ages. The voiceover warned, 'at first only gays and IV drug users were being killed by AIDS, but now we know every one of us could be devastated by it'. The campaign was regarded by many people to have not only missed an opportunity to inform the general public, but to have increased the stigmatisation of people infected with HIV and gay men. Among the most important responses to the campaign was that group affected by HIV/AIDS led community-level education.

National campaigns following in the early 1990s were based more explicitly on theories about how to change behaviour (social learning theory and social marketing approaches), and included the National Heart Foundation's 'Exercise: make it part of your day' and 'Exercise: take another step' campaigns. Evaluation suggested that, rather than increasing physical activity participation rates, these campaigns may have reinforced regular physical activity habits among the population groups who were already active.

To bring about change in behaviours across the population, more emphasis is now given to incorporating health education into an ecological approach—that is, transforming relevant environments—social, built and natural—so that they encourage positive health behaviours.

Sources: Owen et al. (1995); Recreation Australia Limited (2001).

---

education from this period emphasised behaviour change related to personal health practices as the goal of health education, while later definitions suggested that health education could inform and activate people to change their environments, as well as personal health practices.

Since the early 1980s, the locations and modes of delivery for health education programs and social marketing strategies have progressively expanded. Common locations now include workplaces; sports, leisure, entertainment and recreation facilities; educational institutions; shopping centres; libraries and other public spaces. Forms of media used to deliver health messages have changed alongside innovations in technology, such as the internet, DVDs and mobile phone and tablet applications ('apps'). This has dramatically increased the potential for information and messages about health to permeate routine domestic life, use of personal communications devices and people's experience of public spaces. However, while availability of information has increased, assuring its quality and reliability—especially in cyberspace—is a rising and complex problem.

Health education is a useful aspect of broader strategies operating at the level of individuals or groups, but experience across the world has shown that for a number of reasons it is inefficient and insufficient as the major strategy for improving population health. Delivering health-education programs to the whole population across all possible health topics and on an issue-by-issue basis is clearly neither feasible as an organised approach, nor sustainable. People whose lives have led them to have poor literacy and low levels of power to make and exercise personal decisions are unlikely to benefit from health-education programs that rely on written forms of communication to bring about behaviour change. Indeed, the issues that those organising programs might regard as important might have low priority among those groups they seek to influence. Health education can achieve some objectives related to increasing knowledge,

but leave future populations exposed to the major structural forces (such as persistent unemployment, social dislocation, housing or food insecurity or an increasing social divide between the rich and poor) that are at the heart of, and sustain, health problems.

The widening perspective on how to improve population health

From the early 1980s, as evidence about strategies to improve health accumulated, stronger recognition was given to two themes: first, the need to change social and economic structures that influence population health; and second, the need to involve community members in framing what needs to be changed and the processes of change.

Working synergistically with health education, structural changes (to public policy and institutional practices, for instance) can alter social and physical environments and shape behaviours in ways that support health (Waas 2003). This notion is reflected in the Ottawa Charter and also in Green and Kreuter's (1991) frequently cited definition of health promotion—'any combination of health education and related organisational, political and economic interventions designed to facilitate behavioural and environmental changes conducive to health.' (p. 161)

The involvement of community members in achieving change is integral to improving health: from framing and prioritising health issues or problems (for themselves or their communities), to identifying which factors are involved in creating and sustaining the issue or problem, to participating in activities to change these factors, such as lobbying local members of parliament for legislative reforms. The rationale for personal and community education that emphasises participation can be traced to the work of Paolo Friere (1973), who asserted that education should be a force that enables and liberates people. While active participation is seen as desirable, the 'politics of participation' (Dwyer 1989) must be recognised: who decides who participates, how they participate and what control they have over decisions and actions? This thinking underpinned the greater emphasis on a different form of education: education for raising consciousness about oppression, to stimulate community mobilisation for social change, and about the importance of empowerment. Notions of power and control characterise mature definitions of health education, which in turn have seeded contemporary definitions of health promotion. For example, empowerment concepts stand out in the Ottawa Charter for Health Promotion's definition in the way it refers to people 'increasing control' over the determinants of health in order for their health to be improved (WHO 1986).

Widening the perspective on what factors need to be targeted for change and what methods are useful to achieve change has become an important theme in the evolution of health-promotion practice.

Evolving approaches to health promotion: From disease prevention to social-environmental change

While the development of the germ theory provided a strong basis for interventions that could help populations stay healthy by preventing disease—thorough identifying and dealing with the germ—it also brought on a narrowing of the role of public health because people looked for the 'germ behind every disease'.

In the latter part of the twentieth century, a broader approach to prevention was called for as epidemiological evidence revealed the increasing prevalence of cardiovascular disease, cancers and other non-communicable diseases (NCDs). The public health field was called on to rethink what actions were needed to reverse this epidemic. From the 1980s, epidemiological evidence accumulated that suggested causal links between prevalent NCDs (such as cardiovascular disease and some cancers) and personal health habits (smoking, food intake, physical activity and stress management). This gave

impetus to many programs that sought to change health behaviours associated with NCDs. Existing theories, such as the health belief theory of reasoned action and stages of change (trans-theoretical) models, were applied to motivate and support individuals to effect behaviour change.

However, whether our concern is with cardiovascular diseases, cancers or other conditions, population-level shifts in health will not be realised by designing interventions that primarily aim to change the behaviours and lifestyles of individuals. A critique of this approach has been pursued along several lines:

- First, the focus on individuals will be ineffective in covering the large numbers of people who already have risks for diseases plus the number of people who continue to enter into the 'at-risk' population (Syme 1986). As well as being ineffective, such approaches are not cost-effective, and raise significant ethical questions.

- Second, as described in Chapter 5, patterns of health behaviour, morbidity and mortality tend to be distributed along a socio-economic gradient, leading to worse health among disadvantaged groups. This has been demonstrated for many conditions, including mental health problems such as affective disorders, anxiety disorders and suicide attempts and suicide (Taylor et al. 2005). Yet positive health behaviour change has a propensity to occur more readily in educated population groups, especially where such changes are reliant on using specific resources. As a consequence, health inequalities can be exacerbated by health-promotion campaigns even though they might be considered successful among some sections of the population.

- Finally, a focus on health behaviour as the responsibility of individuals not only ignores the broader societal determinants but suggests an attitude of 'blaming the victim'. From the community perspective, the demands of daily life and the material resource limitations may

---

Box 15.2 Behaviour change theories

The theory of reasoned action (Ajzen & Fishbein 1980) has been used in research since its inception in 1967 to explain and anticipate behaviour. In essence, it states that a person's behaviour is determined primarily by their intention to perform it. Intention is based on a person's attitude to carrying out a behaviour. This attitude is also based on the person's belief about the consequences of carrying out the behaviour. Hence, consequences are a key feature of the reasoning underlying behaviour. The process of changing behaviour is explored by other theoretical models, such as the trans-theoretical model and social cognitive theory. Both of these have been useful in planning interventions. Prochaska and DiClemente's stages of change model (1984) is another common name for the well-tested trans-theoretical model. It proposes that behaviour change proceeds according to five stages:

1 pre-contemplation (when the person is not considering change)
2 contemplation (when the person moves towards change)
3 determination (when the person makes a commitment to change)

4 action (when the person initiates change)
5 maintenance (when the changed behaviour is maintained).

It also identifies ten processes of change: consciousness-raising; counter-conditioning; dramatic relief; environmental re-evaluation; helping relationships; reinforcement management; self-liberation; self-re-evaluation; social liberation; and stimulus control. Such a model is useful because it conceptualises behaviour change as a process—not an event—that occurs in a social context, and it indicates critical points where an intervention (such as a smoking cessation program or media advertising campaign) is likely to be most beneficial.

This model has been used as a basis for many health-education programs conducted in communities and health services. It underpins the Commonwealth government's preventative health program, 'Lifescripts', launched in 2005. Lifescripts provides written 'prescriptions' that general practitioners are encouraged to use in the context of motivational interviewing to prepare patients for behaviour change. It covers advice about quitting smoking, increasing physical activity, eating a healthier diet, maintaining healthy weight, reducing alcohol consumption or a combination of these (DoHA 2005e).

---

constrain the possibility to 'go jogging, stop smoking or eat brown bread' (McCormack 1994), or adopt other behaviours espoused as having positive impacts on health. To make demands of individuals to adopt such behaviours presupposes that they are fully responsible for their circumstances of poverty.

Health promotion has been reconceptualised as a social change strategy, as evidence from social epidemiology points not only to the role of a socio-economic gradient in health in modifying levels of risk (Langenberg et al. 2005) but also to the importance of social support and control (Berkman & Glass 2000). These findings indicate that interventions at the organisational and community levels are likely to be particularly influential in promoting health and preventing disease. Interventions based on a social change approach will focus on altering social structures, emphasise change in policy or environments (rather than behaviours) and shift the level of interventions 'upstream' towards the fundamental *social* determinants of health.

Health promotion at the organisational level
Health-promotion practitioners working in the social change tradition are interested in changing

organisations and ways in which organisations relate to each other so that they can make explicit contributions to protecting and promoting the health of workers, managers and their associated families and communities. Organisations are systems that embody and transmit values and norms and are influential social environments for much of the population. By changing values and norms that work against health (for example, the exclusion of employees from decision-making processes about work routines, or bullying and sexual harassment) and encouraging values and norms that support health (for example, using breaks for physical activity or relaxation, or providing leave to fulfil caring responsibilities), members of organisations will behave differently with each other and organisations will pursue their goals using different methods.

The manner in which organisations relate to each other also creates community norms, so intersectoral action for health involves social change strategies at both the organisational and community levels. The extent to which a local government works cooperatively and in common purpose with other local governments, community health services, citizen groups, local businesses and government sectors (such as housing, education and social security), for example, will affect the achievement of sustainable health initiatives and changes in a local community.

Approaches to changing organisations include organisational development, organisational learning or developing the 'learning organisation', action research and project management (Iles & Sutherland 2001). While different in their approaches, they are all concerned with influencing organisational values, norms and behaviour.

Health promotion at the community level

At the community level, three main approaches to health promotion based on a community organisation model have been widely used (Glanz, Lewis & Rimer 1997; Bracht 1990; Baum 1998):

- locality development
- social action
- social planning.

The locality development approach is concerned with building the capacity of a community to make

---

Box 15.3 Organisational change that enhances health

Though still developing, the theoretical foundations of organisational development suggest that action in a range of domains, and on a variety of levels, is needed for an organisation to change. These ideas are encapsulated in the 'Seven 7s' model—shared values, structure, strategy, systems, style, skills, staff (Iles & Sutherland 2001)—and a four-stage model for organisational change—awareness-raising, adoption, implementation and institutionalisation (Goodman, Steckler & Kegler 1997).

The value of using a multi-level, staged approach to bring about change is illustrated by two examples:

first, the 'MindMatters' mental health-promotion program, developed in the late 1990s as a whole-school approach to mental health promotion and suicide prevention in Australian secondary schools (Hunter Institute of Mental Health 2005); and second, the Australian Football League's (AFL) 'Respect and Responsibility' program, which addresses the issue of violence against women.

MindMatters

An evaluation of MindMatters in 2005 used case studies of fifteen schools, a professional development questionnaire and key informant interviews to explain what organisational and other changes resulted. Key organisational changes included the following:

- **School structures, services and systems:** the introduction of a pastoral care session; inclusion of MindMatters in schools' charters as an element of learning; introduction of 'release cards' so students can leave class to access counselling without the associated stigma and loss of privacy; timetable changes to provide more time for student-led activities and breaks; restructuring of schools to increase cohesion and support; creation of flexible learning options for at-risk students; the introduction of a restorative justice approach to conflict resolution; more teachers for students with difficulties; the introduction or redevelopment of peer support programs and school transition processes.

- **School policies and procedures relevant to social and emotional well-being:** critical incident policies and plans, including responses to social and emotional issues; bullying and harassment policies; more consistent behaviour-management policies; drug and alcohol policies; and uniform policies.

- **Curriculum or classroom content:** resources introduced in a broad range of class levels to increase learning about grief and loss, mental illness, resilience; reworking of curriculum in a range of subjects (for example, maths, science, English, religious education and physical education) so as to incorporate MindMatters issues and materials in an integrated way.

- **Partnerships or external relationships:** few changes were made in this area, although some schools continued existing relationships, such as with community-based youth services.

All students, but especially students with particular needs, experienced increased support for their well-being. The program led to improvements in communication and articulation of emotions, help-seeking (including reports of and responses to bullying) and attachment to school. Teachers increased their awareness of mental health generally, and were better able to identify and respond to students at risk. They were also more personally and professionally satisfied. Schools developed a shared understanding of and ability to talk about mental health and a stronger commitment to student well-being as central to their role, demonstrated in a more coordinated whole-of-school approach to well-being. Overall, staging the introduction and implementation of MindMatters and working on multiple levels were found to be important to improve the effectiveness of schools' efforts to promote mental health among students, teachers and the school community.

Source: Goodman, Steckler & Kegler (1997); Hunter Institute of Mental Health (2005); Iles & Sutherland (2001).

Respect and Responsibility

In 2005, the AFL launched its Respect and Responsibility policy. It signalled a shift within the league to actively address violence against women; to work towards environments that are safe, supportive and inclusive for women and girls across the football industry, as well as the broader community; and to build broad understanding that violence against women and behaviour that results in harm to women or is degrading are never acceptable. The policy is relevant to the high-profile, elite level of the sport as well as the wider football community. Initiatives and programs seek to promote equal and respectful relationships between men and women. They are based on the principles of 'respect', 'responsibility' and 'participation' as the basis for club cultures. Player-education programs increase understanding of how sexual assault, violence, harassment and abuse can impact on women and girls. Issues covered include the meaning of consent, situations that have the potential to go wrong and ways to build and maintain healthy and respectful social relationships with women. The reach of the program is extending to community clubs from 2012.

Source: Australian Football League (2012).

collaborative and informed decisions; the emphasis is on consensus development, participation and self-help. The social action model, by contrast, is concerned with shifting power relationships and resources through confrontation and direct action; the focus is on changing institutional structures and redressing social injustice through agitation. Social planning involves a problem-solving process with a focus on particular social or health problems in the community (such as environmental pollution, insecure food supply and inadequate support for people with mental health concerns); a range of analytical tools are used to characterise the problem and strategies are then devised and deployed to address it. In reality, these approaches are not necessarily adopted in a mutually exclusive manner. Labonte (in Baum 1998) suggests there is an 'empowerment continuum' that health organisations could adopt in their practice, as shown in Figure 15.1.

From a health-promotion perspective, the central concern with community organisation is the activation of the community to act for change in the first place. Instead of triggering individual-level behavioural change, the task for public health practitioners is to assist a community to become aware of a problem, to agree on that problem as a priority for action, to institute steps to address the problem, and to establish structures and mobilise commitment to implement and maintain program solutions (Bracht 1990). The stimulus for communities to respond to health issues has been depicted by Bastian (1998) in the following way:

- groups that form around local geographical interests, generally in response to a single issue of local public concern (for example, toxic chemicals in children's playgrounds, traffic management signalling)
- groups that form among people sharing the same health condition or experience (for example, people with chronic illnesses such as cancers or diabetes)
- groups that are forged among people with a shared experience of being harmed by a product (for example, tobacco), or by people advocating a particular treatment or practice (for example, complementary therapies)
- groups that protest particular practices or developments on an ideological basis (for example, assisted reproduction)
- population groups with a shared identity who come together to represent their concerns and interests (for example, refugees, women, parents of children with developmental disabilities)
- generic groups and coalitions that are formed to advocate on behalf of the whole population (for example, in relation to protecting universal health coverage or cost of essential drugs).

For a community organisation model to be effective in promoting health, some essential

Figure 15.1 The community development empowerment continuum

Personal empowerment	Small group development	Community organisation	Coalition advocacy	Social and political action
Developmental casework, increasing self-esteem	Improving social support, strengthening personal identity	Raising awareness, developing local action	Lobbying for policy change	Links with broader social and political movements

Source: adapted from Labonte (1990); Laverack (2009).

Box 15.4 Control of an epidemic through a community engagement approach: HIV/AIDS

Following the outbreak of the human immuno-deficiency virus (HIV) infection in the early 1980s, a rapid increase in the incidence of the disease occurred in many countries over several years. Australia was one of the first countries in the Asia-Pacific region to be affected by the virus. By the mid-1980s, the incidence of HIV infection in Australia began to fall (Butler 2003). Australia's estimated annual number of people newly diagnosed with HIV has declined from a peak of around 2300 in 1987 to a current and relatively stable number of around 1100 cases per year (McDonald 2011). By December, 1996, an estimated 16150 Australians had been diagnosed with HIV and 5250 had died of AIDS. Approximately 80 per cent of infections were due to sexual contact between men (NPHP 1998c). In a small number of cases, the virus was contracted through blood products, the sharing of infected needles or medical equipment (NHMRC 1997a).

Australia's response has had three main components, built on the platform of partnership between the health system, government and affected communities: (1) recognition of the social context and impact of HIV/AIDS; (2) cooperative partnerships between all levels of government, community organisations, health professionals, clinical and social researchers and people living with HIV/AIDS; and (3) non-partisan political support by the Commonwealth government, which has facilitated appropriate parliamentary mechanisms, such as multi-party liaison groups and a consultative approach to policy development (Feacham 1995; NPHP 1998c). The main public health responses have been securing the blood supply, introducing needle and syringe programs for injecting drug users, and educating the population about the virus and the consequences of infection. Education campaigns have targeted both high-risk groups (for example, MSM, and injecting drug users) as well as the general population. While there is no cure or effective vaccine for HIV, there have been increases in both treatment efficacy and options since the introduction of triple therapies, including a protease inhibitor in 1996. Cooperative partnerships have facilitated the control of the spread of HIV, and have minimised the social and personal impacts of the disease. In particular, people living with HIV/AIDS have been involved in decision-making and policy formulation.

Evaluations of the effectiveness, efficiency and appropriateness of the second and third national HIV/AIDS strategies have found that they have been effective in working towards their stated goals. Feacham's review of the second strategy states that Australia has been successful in containing epidemics among intravenous drug users (IDUs), sex workers and heterosexuals (Feacham 1995; ANCARD 1999a). National-level strategies have been instrumental to Australia's response to the HIV/AIDS epidemic. However, past success in containing the epidemic must also be attributed to the high level of community participation and the leading role of community groups. Efforts to promote safer sex among homosexual and bisexual men are the result of community action, and the decline in the rate of HIV transmission through sex between men began before the government-funded programs began in the mid-1980s. Community development and peer-education programs have been used extensively in the gay men's community. Effective community-based organisations have been set up to advocate for the needs of the gay men's community and sex workers, and access to services and information about legal, welfare, medical and political matters has increased. Sex worker organisations have lobbied for better laws to protect their workers against the risk of HIV infection, among a number of issues (NHMRC 1997a).

There has been a recent resurgence in HIV infection among MSM, and smaller epidemics among Australians travelling and working in countries with high HIV prevalence (DoHA 2011a). These trends indicate that we cannot be complacent and instead need to revitalise a national concerted effort featuring strong leadership and sustained community-driven approaches to preventing HIV transmission.

Source: McMichael & Lin (2004).

elements must be in place. The community needs to have the necessary skills and leadership, the process needs to start from 'where people are' (that is, people's current concerns, understandings, goals and skills) and to foster community participation, and critical consciousness must be created among members of a community (Minkler & Cox 1980). Trust—its establishment and maintenance—is an often-overlooked ingredient of social processes like community organisation, and is a critical factor influencing the quality and effectiveness of relationships between professionals engaged in health promotion and communities (Tyler 2001).

Obesity

The need for engagement by community members to address a health issue is evident in Obesity Prevention and Lifestyles (OPAL)—a whole-of-community approach to reducing obesity levels that was initiated in fifteen South Australian communities in 2009. It focuses on supporting children (through families and communities) to be and remain healthy, and has expanded to include communities in other states and territories. OPAL applies a model developed and tested in France, which was successful in preventing increases in obesity among children. The French study of two towns (Fleurbaix and Laventie) found that children in the town with the program had changed their eating and physical activity choices and developed better nutritional knowledge. The critical success factor in the program was found to be the broad community engagement in action that went well beyond schools to families, general practitioners, pharmacists, shop-owners, community-based sports and cultural associations, and local government.

In contrast to interventions based on individual behaviour change, there is less documented experience with those focused on organisational change and community organisation for health promotion. This is in part because both the research and evaluation for such programs, and the systems that they seek to transform, are more complex. Indeed, designing such interventions is also complex, requiring consultation with and acceptance by members of the organisation or community, development of appropriate support and policy among decision-makers, and provision of appropriate incentives to bring about and maintain changes at the levels of individuals and social systems (organisations and communities).

Multi-strategy health promotion

The evolution of health-promotion practice is demonstrated in the use of multi-strategy approaches to increase health-promoting behaviours, such as regular physical activity, and to prevent diseases such as those associated with tobacco use. In Australia in the 1980s, public anti-smoking campaigns sought to advise people about how to quit smoking—or to not start—rather than directly tackling the availability of and exposure to tobacco products in society. Over the last two decades, education programs have been continuously available to individuals who desire to quit smoking, but major efforts have been stepped up to deal with complex social, economic and legal questions of the regulation and marketing of tobacco products (see Box 15.5).

A risk to governments from using an approach that controls or prevents access to products or services is that they may be accused of supporting a 'nanny state'. This term is thought to have arisen in the United Kingdom in the 1960s, and refers to child-care workers for families whose role it is to take responsibility for making decisions for young children. A government accused of supporting a 'nanny state' is viewed as being authoritarian and overstepping its role, unduly interfering with decisions that should be a matter for individuals—especially those related to food, alcohol and tobacco.

In summary, it is now recognised that successful health-promotion practice relies less on encouraging changes in individuals' behaviour in order to produce improvements in population health and gives more emphasis to changing underlying factors

---

Box 15.5 Reduction of tobacco consumption in Australia: Beyond an educational challenge

In Australia, tobacco is the largest single preventable cause of death and disease (Scollo & Winstanley 2008), and is estimated to be responsible for over 15000 deaths annually (Begg et al. 2007). Tobacco is estimated to be responsible for nine out of ten drug-caused deaths—fourteen times more than alcohol and seventeen times more than illicit drugs. The risk of death from tobacco consumption is greater than that for any other addiction, exposure or injury. Since the early 1970s, tobacco consumption has fallen considerably. At a national level, the proportion of adult male smokers fell from 75 per cent in post-World War II Australia (1945) to 45 per cent in 1974 and then to 27 per cent in 1995. The proportion of adult female smokers declined from 33 per cent in 1976 to 29 per cent in 1986 and to 23 per cent in 1995 (Abelson & Taylor 2003; NHMRC 1997a). The proportion of adults who smoke on a daily basis is currently 17.5 per cent (AIHW 2012).

While it is difficult to quantify the relative contributions of Australian public health programs to reduced tobacco consumption, the decline in tobacco consumption has been attributed predominantly to mass media-led campaigns, provision of information on the potential health effects of tobacco consumption and strategies for quitting, regulations that restrict where and to whom tobacco products are promoted and sold and where they are consumed (such as work-places), and the introduction of taxes that increase the price of cigarettes (Pierce, Macaskill & Hill, 1990; Tan, Wakefield & Freeman, 2000; Abelson & Taylor 2003; Scollo 2012).

Most recently, the 1997 National Tobacco Campaign has achieved excellent results. The key strategy areas of this campaign have been strengthening community action; promoting cessation of tobacco use; reducing the availability and supply of tobacco; reducing tobacco promotion; regulating tobacco; and reducing exposure to environmental tobacco smoke (QUIT 2003). This combination of diverse strategies for tobacco control in Australia recognises the complex causes of the problem and the range of effective methods for preventing uptake and reducing smoking prevalence.

A social gradient exists in relation to tobacco consumption and the effects of smoking on health status. Since 2004, campaigns have targeted various population groups with messages to not take up, or to quit, smoking. These have included youth, Aboriginal and Torres Strait Islander populations, selected culturally and linguistically diverse groups, pregnant women and prisoners. Legislation has played a major role in reducing demand by affecting tobacco product availability and marketing. Arising from globally significant landmark legislation in 2012, tobacco companies are required to only package their product in plain (olive green) wrapping bearing graphic health warnings and no trademarks.

Despite the successes in tobacco control over 30 years, smoking remains the largest preventable cause of death in Australia. The highest rates of consumption exist within Aboriginal and Torres Strait Islander populations and among people from lower socio-economic groups. Nevertheless, reduced tobacco consumption has led to many significant health benefits, particularly reductions in premature deaths from lung cancer, chronic obstructive pulmonary disease and coronary heart disease (Abelson & Taylor 2003; NHMRC 1997a).

Sources: McMichael & Lin (2004); Scollo & Winstanley (2008).

(that is, social, technological, economic, environmental and political factors) that shape health behaviours and population health patterns. Health promotion has evolved to represent a process of personal, organisational and political development towards health (Kickbusch 1997). Indeed, as the globalisation of economic models and communications intensifies, debates about shifting power and control are particularly pertinent to those working to promote health. The human rights agenda and social justice concepts of equity have brought fresh awareness about the need for health-promotion activities to consider the politics of health and be based on engaging with—and benefiting—groups experiencing long-term social, economic and health disadvantages. In this context, working at the level of individuals, groups, organisations and even communities may be successful in achieving local-level change, but ultimately such a strategy faces limitations in terms of improving population health.

Integrated health promotion

The popular model of integrated health promotion introduced in Chapter 6, which has been implemented since the mid-1980s, is 'healthy settings'. Its conceptual origins can be traced to the WHO Health for All strategy (WHO 1980, 1981) and the Ottawa Charter for Health Promotion: 'Health is created and lived by people within the settings of their everyday life, where they learn, work, play and love.' (WHO 1986) Healthy settings was consolidated as a popular approach for integrated health promotion action in the 1990s, building on the successful take-up of the Healthy Cities Project example. The concept has been interpreted in policy frameworks, pilot projects and networks for a variety of settings all over the world, in both urban and rural environments, and in developed and developing countries.

Principles

Principles of health promotion, originally outlined in the Ottawa Charter and backed up by a growing body of international experience, have been adopted and adapted to guide quality practice in a variety of contexts. Government and institutional policy documents now commonly

---

Box 15.6 Guiding principles for integrated health promotion

Address: the broader determinants of health, recognising that health is influenced by more than genetics, individual lifestyle behaviour choices and provision of health care, and that political, social, economic and environmental factors are critical.

Base: activities on the best available data and evidence, both with respect to why there is a need for action in a particular area and what is most likely to effect sustainable change.

Act: to reduce social inequities and injustice, helping to ensure every individual, family and community group may benefit from living, learning and working in a health-promoting environment.

Emphasise: active consumer and community participation in processes that enable and encourage people to have a say about what influences their health and well-being, and what would make a difference.

Empower: individuals and, through information, skill development, support, advocacy and structural change strategies, to have an understanding of what promotes health, well-being and illness, and to be able to mobilise the resources necessary to take control of their own lives.

Consider: explicit difference in gender and culture, recognising that gender and culture lie at the heart of the way in which health beliefs and behaviours are developed and transmitted.

Work: in collaboration, understanding that while programs may be initiated by the health sector, partnerships must actively be sought across a broad range of sectors, including those organisations that may not have an explicit health focus. This focus aims to build in communities the capacity of a wide range of sectors to deliver quality integrated health-promotion programs, and to reduce the duplication and fragmentation of health-promotion efforts.

Source: Victorian Department of Human Services (2003).

set out guiding principles to influence the practice of health promotion. These reinforce the need for multi-level and multi-strategy approaches that engage relevant settings (Victorian Department of Human Services 2003). A nine-year investment in integrated health promotion by the Australian government occurred under the National Partnership Agreement on Preventive Health in 2009–10. It seeks to establish the foundations for healthy behaviours through eleven initiatives, including Healthy Children, Healthy Workers and Healthy Communities. In Victoria, the Department of Health is using these funds to establish the Prevention Community Model in twelve local community areas to improve health and reduce health disparities through these initiatives.

Application: Healthy settings

Healthy settings principles, and the strategies of health promotion outlined in Chapter 6, have been applied in many contexts (for example, hospitals and health services, schools, communities and workplaces) to bring about changes in relation to:

- population group issues across the lifespan (maternal and child health, adolescence, ageing)
- risk factors (tobacco use, poor nutrition, lack of immunisation, illicit drug use)
- protective factors (social connectedness, community resilience, safe neighbourhoods)
- conditions and diseases (non-communicable—some cancers, heart disease, asthma, injury, road injuries—and communicable—HIV, sexually transmitted infections).

A healthy setting has been defined as: '[t]he place or social context in which people engage in daily activities in which environmental, organisational and personal factors interact to affect health and wellbeing' (WHO 1998). Settings have been classed as 'elemental', referring to specific types of organisations and facilities (schools and universities, marketplaces, hospitals and health-care facilities, prisons and workplaces), and 'contextual', referring to settings defined geographically (cities, communities, villages, towns and islands).

The potential for settings to positively influence health goes well beyond offering a convenient location and 'audience' for health education (Rowling 2005). A setting is 'where people actively use and shape the environment and thus create or solve problems relating to health. Settings can normally be identified as having physical boundaries, a range of people with defined roles, and an organisational structure.' (WHO 1986) The healthy settings approach has been part of a move to using a salutogenic approach—that is, improving population health and well-being, rather than treating or ameliorating disease (Kickbusch 1996).

The healthy settings approach aims to change the many social and physical aspects of organisations and environments so that they function in support of health: values and culture; norms for decision-making; organisational policies; physical work conditions; facilities for employees and others accessing the setting; and programs and activities undertaken within the setting (Fawkes 1997). In schools and workplaces, for example, a strategy might aim to improve factors that impinge on mental and physical health, such as changing the number and flexibility of working hours across a week, increasing opportunities to engage in regular physical activity, expanding healthy food choices in canteens, updating furniture to meet ergonomic standards, increasing availability of health-related information, changing organisational decision-making to be more inclusive of staff values and views, or creating links into the community to work in partnership to address local health-related issues (such as public transport access).

The rationale for a healthy settings strategy brings together some key ideas in health promotion (Dooris 2004):

- Health is largely 'produced' outside of illness [healthcare] services.

Box 15.7 Road injury prevention: Success through an integrated approach

Until recently, road transport injury was the most common form of death caused by injury. Measurable impacts have been made over time on this major public health issue, using a range of road injury-prevention interventions. Deaths on Australian roads are estimated to have fallen by 80 per cent since 1970 (National Preventative Health Taskforce 2008), when 3708 people died on the roads. In 2011, a total of 1291 people died (including drivers, passengers, pedestrians, motorcyclists and pedal cyclists) (Bureau of Infrastructure, Transport and Regional Economics 2012). The road fatalities per registered road vehicle also fell steadily (NPHP 1998a; Abelson 2003a: 99). This decline has been achieved despite the fact that the amount of road travel has almost doubled since 1970 (NHMRC 1997a).

This trend reflects the general improvements in roads, vehicles, driver skills and road safety education. In 1970, public safety programs began with the mandatory fitting of safety belts in all new vehicles (Abelson 2003). The progressive introduction of enforcements of seatbelt use, random breath testing and speed limit enforcement have played major roles in increasing road safety, along with education programs designed to promote safe driving (NPHP 1998a). Effective improvements to the road system have included construction of high-standard roads, skid-resistant footpaths, road delineation, staggered T-intersections, roundabouts, traffic signal installations, removal of roadside hazards, audio tactile edge lines and other 'blackspot' treatments. Safety features in vehicles have also improved significantly, beginning with the introduction of compulsory seatbelt installation and now including anti-burst door latches and hinges, energy-absorbing steering columns, minimum head restraint heights and minimum side door strength (NHMRC 1997a).

Overall trends in Australia suggest that road safety programs focusing on behaviour change (education, speed reduction, drink-driving reduction) are responsible for a significant component of the fall in road crashes since 1970. This improvement has been achieved despite inherent barriers: Australia is a large country that is heavily reliant upon road transport; there is an extensive road system supported by relatively few taxpayers; and there is a culture that condones the consumption of alcohol. A frontier for further reducing fatalities and injuries from road crashes is to better understand the circumstances of crashes. Statistics on single-driver crashes are thought to potentially mask road crashes that might more accurately be classified as road traffic suicides. Available data, though scarce, indicate that this phenomenon is more common among males aged 25–34 and where particular risk factors are present: the person has previously made suicide attempts, experienced mental illness, and consumed alcohol or other drugs (Routley et al. 2003). Linking strategies for reducing road crashes and alcohol consumption might be of particular importance in the next phase of public health action on this issue—for example, changing cultural attitudes to drinking; regulating the licensing, location and opening hours of outlets; and changing alcohol service practices in pubs and other venues.

Source: McMichael & Lin (2004).

- Effective health improvement and public health development require investment in the social systems in which people actually live their lives (such as homes, workplaces, local communities).
- The settings approach represents a tangible and logical way of investing for health at a local level—with health being seen as both an asset for and a result of the development and effective functioning and productivity of organisations.

While the theory of healthy settings is appealing, in practice the concept can be quite difficult to implement and evaluate. Swerissen et al. (2001) suggest that to investigate what works and what does not, there needs to be a blending of evaluation designs that are qualitative (case studies, action research, formative methodologies and longitudinal designs) and quantitative (quasi-experimental designs). When real-life constraints associated with implementing and evaluating whole-system changes pose political, technical and resource barriers (such as organisation-wide support for change or costs), there is a risk that the focus of

work might be narrowed to smaller-scale, single issue-focused projects that are simpler to evaluate (Lin & Fawkes 2003).

Figure 15.2 and Box 15.8 portray the characteristics of common settings to which the principles of health promotion have been applied (cities and schools) and illustrate the influence of the Ottawa Charter in conceptualising change across multiple dimensions.

As well as looking at individual settings, work over the last decade has explored the potential

Figure 15.2 Dimensions of a health-promoting school

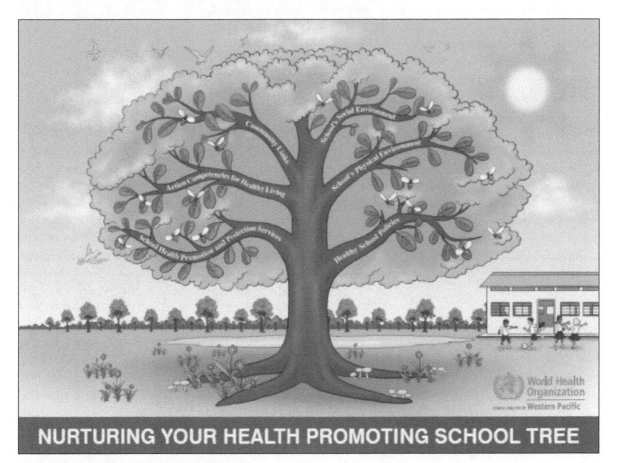

Branches of the health-promoting school tree:
- school health promotion and protection services
- action competencies for healthy living
- community links
- the school's social environment
- the school's physical environment
- healthy school policies

Box 15.8 Healthy Cities

In 1986, the WHO Healthy Cities Project launched an integrated way of developing the health-promoting potential of urban settlements. It has been adapted for use in a diverse range of settlements—communities, towns, villages and islands. Core principles are that a city should strive to provide (Tsouros 1994):

- a clean, safe physical environment of high quality (including housing quality)
- an ecosystem that is stable now and sustainable in the long term
- a strong, mutually supportive and non-exploitative community
- a high degree of participation and control by the public over decisions affecting their lives
- the meeting of basic needs (food, water, shelter, income, safety and work) to all people
- access to a wide variety of experiences and resources, for a wide variety of interaction
- a diverse, vital and innovative city economy
- the encouragement of connectedness with the past, and heritage of city dwellers and others
- a form that is compatible with, and enhances, the preceding characteristics
- an optimum level of appropriate public health and sick care services accessible to all
- high health status (high levels of positive health and low levels of disease).

Enabling networking between cities is a key strategy of the Healthy Cities movement, and facilitates both political and technical cooperation. The Alliance for Healthy Cities, launched in 2003 in the Western Pacific region, is an international network that has taken on the roles of supporting the exchange of information and experience, advocacy and international cooperation. Members include Australian cities and communities in Casey and Corio (cities in Victoria), the Illawarra and Kiama (NSW), the Gold Coast and Logan City (Queensland), Marion (South Australia) and Townsville (Queensland).

benefits of a more 'fully developed scenario' for healthy settings in which synergies are created when the same type of healthy settings work together in sub-national, national, sub-regional and international networks (such as networks for health-promoting schools or health-promoting hospitals—see Box 15.9) and unlike settings working together at the local level—such as schools, workplaces and health-care organisations (Dooris 2004). This approach is potentially valuable because it offers the means for health policies to be aligned, skills and resources to be pooled, and actions—such as advocacy—to be better focused and coordinated.

Refocusing health-promotion practice: Consolidating lessons learned

Recognising context

It is certain that the character of health promotion will transform over the next decades under the influence of social, technological, economic, environmental and political change. Based on previous experience, we can speculate that globalisation in various forms will transform the nature of health-promotion interventions (such as health education, advocacy and social marketing) and practice issues (such as ethics and professional standards). Of all the drivers of change, technological innovations are likely to play an important role in reshaping the values, beliefs, attitudes, knowledge and skills of populations that are relevant to health. Personal mobile communications devices, which allow communication 'anytime, anywhere', as well as home computers, are already influencing how many people perceive and respond to health matters, and how and when they acquire and use health knowledge. Furthermore, technology might play an interesting role in changing relationships between communities and professionals promoting health, as access to information becomes more accessible and contested. Approaches to health

---

Box 15.9 International cooperation to promote environmental health: Healthy hospitals networks

The European Health Promoting Hospitals Project was initiated by WHO as a multi-country pilot in the late 1980s to demonstrate the application of the healthy settings approach in health-care organisations and systems. Building on the experience of six pilot countries, WHO established an international network of health-promoting hospitals and health services (HPHs) in Europe to promote wider cooperation and sustain development of this field of health-promotion policy, practice and research. The network expanded beyond Europe and became independent, retaining close links with WHO through a Memorandum of Understanding. It extends its global reach through national and sub-national networks in a number of regions, and partners with international and inter-governmental organisations on issues of mutual concern.

While a range of issues—such as tobacco and alcohol—have been sustained as priority themes for taskforces and working groups in the network to tackle collaboratively, new issues have come on to the agenda that reflect current or emerging social challenges. These include health care and ageing, the health of migrants and refugees, physical activity and the environment.

The growing importance of reducing the harmful impact of hospitals and health services on the environment led to the creation of a specialised taskforce of the International HPH Network in 2010. Later, a 'networking of networks' formed to diffuse the concept across regions through a partnership between the taskforce and a stream of the Health Care Without Harm movement—the Global Green and Healthy Hospitals Network. Nine goals of this alliance were developed to provide direction to participating institutions:

• leadership—to prioritise environmental health
• chemicals—to substitute harmful chemicals with safer alternatives
• waste—to reduce, treat and safely dispose of health-care waste
• energy—to implement energy efficiency and clean, renewable energy generation
• water—to reduce hospital water consumption and supply potable water
• transportation—to improve transportation strategies for patients and staff
• food—to purchase and service sustainably grown, healthy food
• buildings—to support green and healthy hospital design and construction
• purchasing—to buy safer and more sustainable products and materials.

In a period of only a few months, the impact of 'networking networks' resulted in over 3500 hospitals and health systems from six continents signing commitments to action to reduce their ecological footprint, and by so doing improving environmental health.

Source: International Network of Health Promoting Hospitals and Health Services <hphnet.org>; Global Green and Healthy Hospitals Network at <http://greenhospitals.net>.

---

promotion, such as healthy settings, will need to respond as factors one might plan to change in local settings come under the control of non-local agents. For example, what flexibility will workplaces or schools have in determining which foods and beverages are sold if food services are contracted to multinational food companies?

Change is also likely in terms of how health promotion is understood and the issues it faces. The re-emergence of communicable diseases might change the focus of health promotion, with a possible blurring of boundaries between health protection and health promotion, and a weakening of the close identification of health promotion with lifestyle and behavioural risk factors associated with NCDs.

Appropriate planning and evaluation

Whatever the issues of the future, behavioural, organisational and environmental assessments provide the starting points in health-promotion planning. They help to clarify the nature of an issue, how it might be framed to secure support, the factors needing to be altered, the capacities of people and organisations that need to be developed, and which interventions to use. They also indicate what will need to be evaluated and by whom.

The assessment of this context, then, needs to be coupled with an examination of the evidence about intervention effectiveness for different population groups, in a range of settings and for relevant health issues (see Table 15.1). Ultimately, how a health-promotion program is planned depends on whether its orientation is to improve health or prevent a specific disease. Looking ahead, an approach that places emphasis on how to create health, as represented in the salutogenic model (Antonovsky 1996), may become more important. Such an approach would build on but avoid the pitfalls of working only with quantitative indicators of diseases and risk factors as the basis for health promotion (Tannahill 2002). It would recognise the links between behaviours and social context, and ensure that interventions encompass both individuals and their environments, as well as incorporate their subjective outlooks and understandings of health.

Recognising that the evidence base for complex interventions is still limited, a panel of representatives from global health organisations identified priority areas for the conduct of systematic reviews in public health (discussed in Chapter 10). In so doing, the panel called attention to areas in which public policy and health-promotion action are needed, but for which an evidence base has not been adequately established. These priority systematic reviews will contribute to strengthening program planning evaluation in the future.

Health-promotion planning in the future is likely to aim explicitly at strengthening community assets important for health action—such as the levels of 'connectedness' between community members or means for communication (Hawe et al. 1997). It is also more likely to aim to bring about participation, ownership and even control among groups affected by an issue and able to contribute to action. An evidence base for intervention that contributes to 'empowerment' is emerging to underpin this work (Wallerstein 2006).

A successful health-promotion program will produce measurable changes to health status and quality of life (morbidity, mortality, disability and dysfunction), but these might not occur until months or even decades after program interventions have occurred. It will be important to track the intermediate outcomes (such 'proxy' measures as changes in the wider environment) to ensure that health-promotion efforts are on track and can be expected to lead eventually to changes in health status and social outcomes.

Table 15.1 The health-promotion effectiveness equation

Effectiveness	=	Evidence	+ Infrastructure	+ Action
Efficiency		Policy, planning and financing framework		Appropriate targeting
		+ organisational structures and resources		+ sufficient coverage
		+ workforce and community capacity		+ skilled actions
		+ monitoring and evaluation		+ community ownership

Source: adapted from Lin & Fawkes (2005b).

The Nutbeam model (see Figure 6.4) suggests that changes in three main domains will be important:

1 health literacy (health-related knowledge, attitudes, behavioural intentions, interpersonal skills)
2 social mobilisation (community participation, community empowerment, social norms, public opinion)
3 healthy public policy and organisational practices (policy statements, legislation, regulation, resources allocation, organisational practices).

If these changes are observable, then the achievement of intermediate health outcomes (related to determinants of health) may be expected some time later, including healthy lifestyles (tobacco use, physical activity and food choices), healthy environments (safe physical environments and supportive economic and social conditions) and effective health services (provision of preventive services, and access to and appropriateness of health services).

As depicted in Chapter 6 (Figure 6.5), the pathway from using evidence (of what works in specific contexts), to designing and effectively implementating programs, to producing outcomes is complex and can take considerable time to be realised (Lin & Fawkes 2003). To achieve program effectiveness, the ultimate challenge is to translate theory into practice. Key elements for achieving effectiveness, regardless of the health challenges, are outlined in Table 15.2 (Lin & Fawkes 2003).

Box 15.10 The Walking School Bus™: A neighbourhood journey to better health

The Walking School Bus™ program is operating in many parts of Australia and internationally. It is based on a simple concept. According to a roster, volunteer parents or carers (a minimum of two adults are needed) escort children along a set route through a neighbourhood to and from school, with children joining in or being dropped off at designated 'bus stops' along the way. One adult is the 'driver' and joins up with another adult along the way who is the 'conductor'.

The Walking School Bus™ program has short, medium and long-term effects on a range of factors. The 'bus' provides a pollution-free alternative to using a car, reducing congestion around neighbourhoods and schools, increasing road safety and improving local amenity. Children, as well as the 'bus' drivers and conductors, get regular exercise, which can boost fitness, moderate weight, support effective learning in classrooms and establish a healthy pattern of activity that might be carried into adulthood. Children meet other children from a range of age groups with whom they might not ordinarily socialise, expanding their local circle of friends and building their sense of self and their neighbourhood and social skills. Parents meet other parents and also benefit socially. Parents share the task of transporting children to and from school, providing them with more time during the week to use for other activities on the days when the 'bus' operates. Children learn road sense and safety in traffic. Children and their parents or carers are more visible on neighbourhood streets, contributing to the social milieu and conviviality of a community.

The popularity of the Walking School Bus™ program stems primarily from its practical approach to transporting children to and from school. The program's effectiveness, however, can be measured in terms not only of its actions (the program and how it operates), but its impacts and longer-term effects. These are also desirable from a population health point of view and include contributions to prevention of disease, community health and wellbeing and environmental sustainability.

Source: VicHealth, <www.vichealth.vic.gov.au>.

Table 15.2 The health-promotion effectiveness checklist

Framework	Checklist to ensure effectiveness/avoid implementation failure
Evidence	• Literature search and systematic review conducted • Program evaluations reviewed
Infrastructure	• Policy authority in place • Funding secure and adequate • Organisational commitment assured • Workforce developed and adequate • Stakeholders engaged • Information system in place for monitoring and evaluation
Action	• Target groups identified, quantified and reachable • Population coverage specified and achievable • Community commitment gained • Implementation protocol in place • Feedback reporting mechanism in place

Source: Lin & Fawkes (2003).

Affirming principles

At the Fourth International Conference on Health Promotion, held in Jakarta, Indonesia in 1997, more than ten years after the Ottawa Charter was designed, participants reviewed the experiences of health promotion across both developed and developing countries and concluded that:

• 'Comprehensive approaches to health development are the most effective. Those that use combinations of the five strategies are more effective than single-track approaches.'
• 'Particular settings offer practical opportunities for the implementation of comprehensive strategies. These include mega-cities, cities, municipalities, local communities, islands, markets, schools, workplaces and health-care facilities.'
• 'Participation is essential to initiate and sustain efforts. People have to be at the centre of health promotion action and decision-making processes for them to be effective.'
• 'Health learning fosters participation. Access to education and information is essential to achieving effective participation and the empowerment of people and communities.'

Participants recognised that poverty continues to be among the greatest threats to health, and transnational factors (such as population mobility and international trade) influence the spread of non-communicable diseases and new and re-emerging infectious diseases.

The priority strategies nominated in the Jakarta Declaration are likely to remain highly relevant into the future:

• Decision-makers must be firmly committed to social responsibility.
• Increased investment is needed for health development.
• It is vital to consolidate and expand partnerships for health.
• It is essential to increase community capacity and empower the individual.
• Infrastructure for health promotion must be secured.

This shift in thinking about where the determinants of health are located in societies was reinforced by the WHO Commission on the Social Determinants of Health (CSDH 2008a). Evidence and case stories were presented from a number of countries on the links between poverty, inequality and health, and an agenda for global action on social determinants of health was articulated by the Commission.

Subsequent global health promotion conferences have drawn a high-level focus to debates on areas that have been difficult to progress, while renewing thinking about concepts and strategies. The conferences have emphasised the importance of globalisation as a major consideration for health promotion and health inequalities (global conference held in Bangkok in 2005); what capacity and resources are required to achieve the practical realisation of health-promotion aspirations and goals (Nairobi in 2009); and how to achieve intersectoral action on social determinants of health and cross-government, healthy public policy through a Health In All Policies approach (Helsinki in 2013).

Conclusion: Individual plus societal change

Like many other countries, Australia has been successful in using the health-promotion strategy defined by the Ottawa Charter to improve the health of the population, reduce premature deaths from some causes, reduce morbidity and risk-behaviour prevalence, improve health literacy and skills, and change the policies and environments that determine people's access to healthy choices (NHMRC 1997a).

The 'good news stories' presented in this chapter offer important insights into successful health promotion. Typically, they show good use of theory and evidence to design their approach. Using a combination of methods, they engage the relevant levels of society (from individuals to social and economic environments) and sectors (for example, health services, schools and urban planning) to bring about changes that will improve population health outcomes. Brief case studies in this chapter related to HIV, tobacco and road trauma provide a glimpse of health-promotion practice that has been effective in making a difference to health at the population level.

As the evidence base for health promotion expands, the case for investing in health promotion to improve public health will be strengthened and the role of health promotion in an organised approach to public health will be consolidated further (see Table 15.3). Current emphases on

Table 15.3 Evolution of strategies to improve health

	Health information	Health education	Health promotion
Approach	Information	• Information, communication, education	• Ottawa Charter: enable, mediate, advocate

Special characteristics	One-way	• Teacher–learner interaction
		• Participation
			• Participation
			  – multi-sector
			  – multi-level
			  – multi-strategy

Focus of change	Knowledge	• Beliefs, values, attitudes, knowledge and skills pertinent to risk factors, protective factors, behaviours	• Structural and personal • Determinants of health • Community
Presumed result	? Retained	• Sustained	• Governance, community, organisational and personal capacities increased

evidence-based policy and practice will see an acceleration of 'evidence' impacting on methods, high-level support for health promotion, and levels and sustainability of investments. Such investments are needed to further develop health-promotion theory (concerning change in behaviour, organisations and societal factors) and practice.

The successes in Australian public health should not, however, obscure the significant issues that require further action. Reducing inequalities in health status between the most and least socio-economically disadvantaged populations remains fundamentally important as a measure to improve health, and will require innovative approaches—such as social entrepreneurship—that are not well captured in the 'scientific literature'. Improving the quality of interventions and sustaining infrastructure support and capacity (NHMRC 1997a) will be critical, enduring tasks.

16

Health maintenance and improvement for vulnerable populations:
From needs to rights

Challenge

Roxbury is an urban secondary school with a vibrant mix of students from a range of ethnic and cultural backgrounds. Within the past five years, Roxbury has received a large number of students who arrived in Australia as refugees. Several of the teachers have become concerned about the health and welfare of the students in this group. Some have noticed that these students often come to school without lunch or do not have any money to purchase food at lunchtime. Additionally, there has been concern about inappropriate behaviour in the classroom when some of the boys have attempted to solve conflict through loud arguments and, in some cases, threatening behaviours. Finally, some of the teachers have heard that there are cases of active TB among some of the newly arrived refugee communities.

The school has asked the Diversity Unit in the state Health Department to advise it on how to approach these problems. The school has won several awards for its policies on inclusion and diversity, but the teachers now feel a little overwhelmed about not being able to cope with these new students, and they are also grappling with their own fears about being exposed to communicable diseases. Some parents in the school community have also expressed concerns, asking that students with infectious diseases be excluded and that those with aggressive behaviours be expelled. Although the teachers have usually adopted a supportive approach to all students, they are feeling under increasing pressure from the larger community to act in its interests.

In thinking about the 'problem', what different public health strategies could you draw on to begin to elaborate on possible 'causes'? In what ways might public health thinking inform a range of possible approaches to begin investigating the nature of this problem? What types of public health knowledge would you draw upon to begin to formulate possible approaches to resolving this problem?[1]

Introduction

Public health practitioners naturally tend to have an orientation towards prevention in their work. However, prevention and restoration of health is not always possible. Shifting concepts of health and well-being have placed greater emphasis on the importance of quality of life and the mainten-ance of social functioning for people who are ill, have chronic conditions or disabilities or terminal illnesses, or whose health is compromised because of social disadvantage. Additionally, as seen in previous chapters, risk factors and ill-health are not randomly distributed but are clustered in popula-tion groups, so that some people are more likely to be in need of support and care than others. Given that all members of society are entitled to the best possible levels of health and quality of life, regardless of whether they are well, distressed, sick or disabled, it is particularly important that consideration be given to how health care and social support can be organised for those who are experiencing, or are particularly vulnerable to, poor health.

Every society has strategies to ensure that its vulnerable members are looked after. However, there is considerable diversity in the criteria that different societies use to determine vulnerability. This, in turn, impacts on how societies respond to vulnerable members and where the responsibility for this response is located. In some societies, the family is seen to be solely responsible for its more vulner-able members, such as those who are aged, sick

and/or disabled. In Australia, vulnerable members traditionally have been the responsibility of the state in partnership with charity organisations.

While public health approaches to advancing the health of vulnerable populations in Australia have varied over the years, an area of tension has centred around the different responses to the locus of responsibility. Societal values and norms are influential in shaping the nature of public health responses. Social values in turn relate to whether the cause of vulnerability is seen to be 'fate' or bad luck, genetics, social inequalities stemming from state policy, or the ways in which responsibility is exercised by individuals. There has also been varia-tion in the extent to which responses to people with certain vulnerabilities punish rather than support them. In short, public health responses to vulner-able populations in Australia have been shaped by the politics of cause and responsibility.

This chapter begins by discussing briefly how the notion of vulnerability is conceptualised. Five case studies are provided that focus on different groups—people with mental illness, people from refugee backgrounds, people living with hepatitis C, people with chronic and terminal illness, and people who are in prison—to illustrate different forms of vulnerability and the variations in the ways the public health system in Australia has responded.

The first case study shows how 'stigma' and 'shame' have played a large role in shaping societal responses to mental ill health, and how public health responses have shifted away from a clinical

---

1   This chapter has been written with a major contribution from Sandy Gifford

perspective. The second case study discusses how the state, by viewing 'offshore' refugees as 'deserving', has taken a major role in providing integrated approaches to public health within the resettlement context. We show how vulnerabilities are shaped by factors that are influential prior to and after displacement. The third case study considers the ways in which stigma has shaped responses to prevention and treatment for people who contract a disease as a result of 'illegal' behaviours, such as when hepatitis C is transmitted through illicit drug use. We highlight the ways in which vulnerabilities associated with hepatitis C stem both from the impact of this illness on physical and mental health and the ways in which the association with injecting drug use has acted to stigmatise people with this condition. This has resulted in a range of discriminations that both act to isolate people socially and create barriers to prevention and treatment. Public health responses have had to focus particularly on reducing stigma and combining treatment and care with harm-minimisation approaches to prevention. The fourth case study looks at how people with chronic and terminal illness can benefit from a comprehensive health-promotion approach to their health maintenance. Finally, in considering people who are in prison, we show how vulnerabilities are related to social inequalities and a lack of power to exercise prevention and care, and how the movement towards a harm-minimisation and rights-based approach within prisons is a critical part of an effective public health approach.

Overall, these case examples illustrate that Australian public health responses to vulnerable populations have been positive; however, they have varied over time in terms of their effectiveness, and reflect the prevailing social values and political climate of the time.

What makes a group of people vulnerable?

Although the Australian public health system is a story of success benefiting the majority of the population, the approaches adopted have not always met the needs of particular communities. Consider the following.

Indigenous Australians (Trewin and Madden 2005):

- have life expectancy at birth approximately seventeen years lower than that of the non-Indigenous population
- have higher rates of mental ill-health compared with the non-Indigenous population
- have higher rates of chronic illness, including diabetes, heart disease, hypertension, kidney disease, and eye and ear problems compared to the non-Indigenous population
- are half as likely to have a non-school qualification than the non-Indigenous population and are under-represented in the higher education sector.

People from culturally and linguistically diverse backgrounds and experience in general have:

- lower utilisation of breast and cervical cancer screening programs (DoHA 2009; Cancer Council Australia and Federation of Ethnic Communities' Councils of Australia 2010)
- lower utilisation of mental health services (Victorian Department of Human Services 2006)
- poor dental health and immunisation status among newly arrived refugee communities (Briggs & Skull 2003).

People with developmental and acquired disabilities may:

- lack access to appropriate institutional care for people with mental disabilities
- lack access to home support
- have inappropriate institutional care for young people with severe disabilities
- lack provision for mobility, toileting and self-care in public facilities and spaces.

People incarcerated in Australian prisons:

- lack access to harm-minimisation programs for hepatitis C and STIs
- have higher rates of mental ill-health.

People living in rural and remote locations, when compared with metropolitan populations, have:

- poorer access to healthy food
- higher rates of obesity
- higher rates of suicide among men—especially young men (Caldwell et al. 2004)
- poorer access to all types of health services, including emergency and specialist services.

People residing in Australia who have not been granted permanent residency have:

- no access to Medicare if they are on certain visa types
- limited or no access to housing, social and economic support.

Frail and elderly people:

- may lack access to appropriate residential care or services to enable them to live independently in their own homes
- often use medications inappropriately
- are at risk of injury from falls and other accidents
- may have poor food intake, causing nutrient deficiencies.

Clearly, public health practitioners face particular challenges in meeting the health and welfare needs of vulnerable segments of the Australian community.

The notion of vulnerability is contentious. The term 'vulnerable' stems from the Latin word *vulneratus*, 'to be exposed to the chance of being attacked or harmed'. In a public health context, 'vulnerability' refers to individuals or populations being at risk of ill-health or other harms, such as injury. Linked closely to definitions of vulnerability are concepts of 'risk'. While everyone in a community is potentially vulnerable or at risk of ill-health or injury at some time, those at the bottom of the social hierarchy—however that social hierarchy is structured—are most at risk. This is because those who are socially disadvantaged have the least social capital and economic resources (Aday 1994), and consequently have the weakest ability to protect themselves. Thus, within public health, vulnerability can be conceptualised as a set of circumstances or conditions that place people at a disadvantage in terms of being able to access social and economic goods in a society and make decisions that are in their own interest. Put another way, vulnerability can be thought of in terms of an individual's or group's exposure to a range of psycho-social environmental factors that raise the chances of ill-health (Siegrist 2004). Thus, vulnerability is essentially a product of inequalities in society, and the outcomes—ill-health and injury—are the result of social inequalities.

When taking a public health approach to redressing vulnerabilities, it is important to consider how the criteria for defining the root causes of vulnerability are defined. Here, there is considerable debate about who has the power to define the circumstances or conditions that lead to inequality: lay people or experts (Milburn 1996; Stead et al. 2001). There is strong evidence to suggest that lay perceptions of social inequalities—for example, perceived social status—impact on subjective and objective health outcomes. People whose subjective perceptions are that they are on the bottom of a social hierarchy have been found to suffer from poorer health outcomes (Adler et al. 2000). Another common issue is that there are differences between lay and expert knowledge in perceptions of what constitutes vulnerability and disadvantage. For example, disadvantaged neighbourhoods, considered by epidemiologists to lower the health of individuals who reside there, may not always be perceived as a risk to their health by those individuals. Indeed, some studies show that residents of some disadvantaged neighbourhoods in the United Kingdom consider their neighbourhood to be a positive place to live (Bennett et al. 1999). There can also be differences between what epidemiologists and lay people consider to be risk factors for a particular illness. For example, epidemiologists working on issues of diabetes among Aboriginal communities in Victoria have identified that high consumption rates of foods high in fat and sugar make people vulnerable to adult onset diabetes. However, Aboriginal people have identified these foods as having significant social meanings, and as desirable because they are inexpensive and readily available (Thompson & Gifford 2000). Lay understandings of diabetes and its risk factors can stand in contrast to expert definitions of risk. What is important here is that it is essential to take into account lay views of risk and protection when defining vulnerabilities (Popay et al. 2003).

A second issue at stake, especially for public health, is whether the focus on vulnerability should be on health inequalities or social inequalities. Approaches that focus first on health inequalities as the cause of vulnerability will favour strategies for improving the 'health' outcomes first, while a focus on social inequalities will favour policies that influence the social conditions that give rise to ill-health. In the case of refugee health, which is described in more detail in this chapter, there is a tension between public health professionals who argue that people's physical health needs should be given priority (immunisations, screening for communicable diseases, dental health) and those working from a more holistic model of health, who argue that ensuring the well-being of refugees in terms of safety, security, housing and capacity-building will enable new arrivals to take control over their own health needs. Currently, public health responses to vulnerable populations can be divided into these two broad approaches, with the first focusing on improving health outcomes and the second focusing on improving social inequalities. In reality, a combination of approaches is required; however, it is important to note the growth of evidence that vulnerability is primarily associated with the social causes of ill-health (Marmot & Wilkinson 1999), including the impact on health outcomes of social class (Scambler & Higgs 2001), structural violence (Farmer 1996), social exclusion and stigma (Link & Phelan 2001) and discrimination.

A third important issue at stake when considering public health definitions and responses is to ask whether the response to vulnerability is a 'need' or a 'right'. Defining vulnerability as a 'need' implies the adoption of a welfare-based approach. Critics of a needs-based approach have argued that such policies promote dependency, whereas a rights-based approach leads to emancipation and individual and collective action (Fraser 1989). Responses based on a rights-based model would focus on entitlements instead of needs. For example, in conceptualising poverty as a health issue, instead of thinking about addressing poverty in terms of 'needs', a rights-based approach would argue that all people are entitled to certain social goods, and that the right for food and to live a life free of poverty is a basic human right (Sen 1997, 2001). Again, the critical aspect is the question of who gets to define 'needs'.

Fourth, vulnerability can be defined in terms of structural factors that act as barriers to the availability of, or access to, public goods and services. For some populations, services and programs may not be available for a range of reasons, including a simple lack of services in a particular geographical area. However, even in the case where goods and services are available, a range of other barriers can exist that prevent people from accessing services (Gatrell et al. 2001). These include economic barriers, a lack of knowledge about goods and services, or inappropriateness of services for specific groups (defined, for example, by age, gender, ethnicity, language spoken, location in relation to services, and availability to access services, based on hours of provision).

Fifth, social stigma and discrimination can increase the vulnerability of individuals and groups. Stigma is a marker of disgrace that socially devalues a person in the eyes of their family, friends and the wider society. It reduces one's social standing and most often is managed by negative social sanctions. Stigma often stems from conditions (for example, leprosy) or behaviours (injecting drug use or sex outside of marriage) which may be seen to be socially undesirable. While stigma can be thought of as a social label, in effect it translates into discrimination. Discrimination is the action that results from stigma, and this places stigmatised individuals or communities at risk of poorer health outcomes (Link & Phelan 2001; Alonzo & Reynolds 1995; Ren, Amick & Williams 1999). Increasingly, public health has identified stigma as a root cause of ill-health, and approaches to addressing stigma include public awareness-raising, education and legislative change.

Finally, it is important to discuss vulnerabilities that stem from particular behaviours that are harmful, illegal and difficult to change. Behaviours such as injecting drugs produce vulnerability because they can directly harm health, and the often illicit nature of these behaviours places individuals at risk of criminal or social sanctions. These factors in turn act as barriers to health care and support. Many of these behaviours are difficult to change, and place individuals in ongoing situations of risk. In these contexts, harm-minimisation approaches coupled with peer education, care and support have been the key to assisting vulnerable communities maintain an adequate level of health while still engaging in the behaviours that compromise their health (Louie et al. 1998; Aitken, Kerger & Crofts 2002).

However vulnerability is defined, it is now well accepted that the health and well-being of vulnerable populations is worse compared with the 'non-vulnerable', and that public health approaches offer particularly effective strategies for reducing vulnerability and improving health and well-being. The following sections illustrate different public health responses to vulnerable populations in Australia. Each of the case studies chosen highlights the tensions between different ways of thinking about vulnerability, but also the strengths of an integrated and holistic public health approach. This integrated approach is a common theme shared by contemporary public health approaches to vulnerability, in Australia. As the case studies illustrate, all approaches combine protection, prevention and care; seek to integrate a range of responses and strategies from community-based primary care to self-help; and aim to involve affected communities in partnerships with professionals and governments to reduce vulnerability and improve health.

Addressing vulnerability and mental health: Historical shifts

Historically, responding to the needs of certain vulnerable population groups has been the responsibility of the state, through direct institutional service provision and through funding of not-for-profit organisations for community-based support services. These groups include people who have a mental illness or intellectual disability, children who are orphans or people who are frail and aged.

Mental illness in its many different forms puts both affected individuals and their families at a disadvantage in a range of ways. In many cultures, including mainstream Australian culture, mental illness is highly stigmatised, and many societal responses have been to contain mentally ill people and render them 'invisible' to the rest of society. In the past, those with severe mental illnesses were hospitalised or cared for by charities, and those with mild health conditions were either cared for within the family setting or became indigent. All too often, the result of these strategies was to make the already vulnerable even more at risk.

Although the earliest Australian asylums were meant to be places of refuge, 'providing cleanliness, kindness, nutrition, medical attention, recreation, and good record keeping', they largely evolved into 'bins' into which deviants were 'dumped and forgotten about' (Barrand 1997). Since the 1960s, there have been numerous inquiries into how to address problems of overcrowding and abuse in institutions. Out of these, the concept of community-based psychiatric care was introduced, along with efforts to remove patients with psychiatric illness from institutions and settle them into the community.

In the 1970s, the movement towards deinstitutionalisation picked up pace, driven partly by public health concerns about the medicalised approach to psychiatric care and partly by state interests to share costs and save money (Palmer & Short 2000). The result of this deinstitutionalisation was to again render many already vulnerable people even more vulnerable—at risk of homelessness, substance abuse and extreme poverty. Many health professionals became concerned about patients with long-standing or chronic problems being discharged into communities that were unprepared to look after them or ill-disposed towards them. The demand for care fell not only to community-based, not-for-profit organisations, but also to families and other carers.

Since the 1970s, people with mental illnesses and their carers have advocated for better health and social services, and this movement stemmed largely from a partnership between consumers and mentally ill people who experienced little or no access to support and care. In 1991, after a number of years of consultation, the Australian Health Ministers' Conference adopted the Statement of Rights and Responsibilities, which tried to promote 'social justice, equity, access, and a compassionate society with mental health as its primary goal' (Barrand 1997: 139). It attempted to balance consumers' right to respect with their responsibility to respect others. Along with the UN Principles for the Protection of Persons with Mental Illness and for the Improvement of Mental Health Care (see <www.unhchr.ch/html/menu3/b/68.htm>), these principles were subsequently incorporated into the National Mental Health Policy of 1992 (see

<www.health.gov.au/internet/wcms/Publishing. nsf/Content/mental-pubs/$FILE/nmhp92.pdf>). The subsequent National Mental Health Strategy of 1993 called for a range of improvements to mental health services, including integration with mainstream health services and a stronger focus on community-based care. Equally importantly, the strategy included additional goals of advancing the human rights of those with mental illnesses, removing the stigma of mental illness and promoting the mental health of all members of the Australian population. Mechanisms to enable consumer input into policy decision-making were also incorporated into the implementation structure for the strategy (Palmer & Short 2000), and projects were funded to ensure that consumers were involved in the education and training of mental health professionals (Hazelton & Clinton 2002).

Since the promulgation of the National Mental Health Strategy (and with substantial financial investment by federal and state governments), there has been a strong shift towards developing new models and approaches to deal with mental health conditions and to promote mental health. This has seen an emphasis on de-stigmatising mental illnesses such as schizophrenia and depression through public education and media campaigns, preventing mental health problems through programs that help to build a sense of community and social support, and providing early diagnosis within the primary care setting and more comprehensive acute care and treatment services through new funding initiatives. A key thrust of the public health effort in these developments has been to ensure that a comprehensive approach is taken towards mental health in the Australia community.

Statistics associated with the prevalence and incidence of mental health conditions in Australia reinforce the importance of giving this area priority attention in public health. Mental ill-health is the largest cause of disability (Commonwealth of Australia 2009: 16–17). It is estimated that one in five people aged sixteen to 85 years in Australia will experience one of the common forms of mental illness annually. Mental health problems disproportionately affect rural and remote Australians, particularly Aboriginal people and those experiencing socio-economic disadvantage (Fuller et al. 2002). There is not only a need for better care for individuals, but also for early detection and prevention among population groups. This means that the public health system needs to have a focus on and address the sources of vulnerability. Thus, public health practice has been pressured to shift its focus upstream, and to develop strategies that combine health-promotion programs, community services and family support. Ensuring that all individuals can benefit from social participation, employment and non-discrimination may be some of the most important goals, at the societal level, for the promotion of mental health and well-being (Victorian Health Promotion Foundation 2005). This focus is reflected in the the Fourth National Mental Health Plan, which has incorporated a population health framework and recognises the importance of vulnerability and the complex interactions between a broad range of biological, social, psychological, economic and environmental factors (Commonwealth of Australia 2009: 10).

The most significant government initiative relating to disability and mental health was the announcement of a National Disability Insurance Scheme in 2012 (see <www.ndis.gov.au>). The scheme aims to provide the appropriate and necessary care and supports through a centralised funding pool, thereby assisting people with disabilities to reach their full potential.

Promoting refugee health: Towards best practice

Australia is one of a handful of countries receiving refugees for resettlement under the United Nations High Commission for Refugees humanitarian resettlement program (2005). In 2010–11, Australia granted 13799 visas to refugees or people in the special humanitarian program, which enabled them to access a wide range of services, including health services (DIAC 2012). While countries that have been the source of refugees have changed over the years, and refugee communities represent considerable cultural and ethnic diversity, all refugees who come to Australia share a set of common experiences that impact on their health and well-being over the resettlement period. They have all been forcibly displaced from their home by violence of some kind (Pedersen 2002). Many have witnessed the killing of family members; had to leave their homes with little notice; spent many years in refugee camps; had family members go missing; experienced torture; and had to deal with the loss of their community, livelihood and, in many cases, their sense of hope for the future. People with refugee experiences are made vulnerable by these experiences. However, many argue that, rather than accepting the identity of a refugee in Australia, they are ordinary people with extraordinary experiences. Most new arrivals want to get on with their lives and be 'ordinary' once again.

When arriving in Australia, individuals and their families are offered an integrated package of resettlement services, including income support, housing, English language instruction and health care (DIMIA 2005). People who suffer from the mental health effects of torture and trauma are offered counselling and support provided by torture and trauma services located in each state and territory. These services are funded by state and Commonwealth governments. Despite this program of integrated humanitarian support services, people from refugee backgrounds face many challenges during their resettlement period. Recent research indicates that factors that come into play after displacement play a critical role—and in some cases can be more important than those affecting pre-displacement— in shaping mental health and wellbeing (Porter & Haslam 2005). Establishing a sense of security, trust, and control over the future is one of the key tasks in the resettlement process, and public health approaches need to address the impact of both pre- and post-displacement factors that affect this process. Public health approaches that incorporate the broader needs of refugees within the resettlement context are widely recognised as being more effective than strategies that focus on only one aspect of the settlement challenge (Watters 2001). Indeed, Australia's integrated approach to resettlement has been recognised as one of the world's best, and Australia has authored the *UNHCR Resettlement Handbook* (UNHCR 2002). This broader approach to refugees and resettlement has shaped the ways in which public health systems are expected to respond.

Although new arrivals to Australia may have a range of physical health needs, there has been a move away from implementing screening and disease-specific treatment carried out in isolation from responses to other social needs. The value of an integrated approach to addressing the needs of a typical family newly arrived in Australia can be seen in Box 16.1.

Public health approaches in Australia have recognised the complexity of the refugee experience. The response has been shaped by a range of frameworks for recovery that take account of the psychological, social and physical factors that impact on the resettlement process (VFST 1998, 2004b).

Box 16.1 Integrated approach to meeting refugee health needs

A family of six—father, mother and four children—arrived in Australia relatively intact (although many do not). Before that, they spent four years in a refugee camp. They left behind one child who had gone missing and two children who were killed. They also left behind an elderly father and mother, a sister without a husband who has three children to support and 20 other family members who were scattered between different refugee camps, many of whom they have not heard from for five years. The father in the family has suffered from torture and the mother headed up the household for a number of years on her own when her husband was missing. The family had to flee their home with little notice, leaving behind all their belongings.

Having spent four years in a refugee camp, the children's schooling has been severely disrupted. The family suffered from poor nutrition, malaria, and a lack of immunisations and basic health care while in the refugee camp. Although both the mother and father have training in a trade or profession, neither has been able to bring with them evidence of their qualifications and neither has been employed in their profession for

years. Neither speaks English, while the children speak a number of languages, including some English. The two oldest children entered Years 9 and 10 in school; however, their numeracy and literacy skills are limited due to the disrupted schooling.

This family faces many immediate problems. In the longer term, it is likely that one of their key goals will be to reunite with family members who are still overseas and at risk by sponsoring them. Over that time, this family is likely to face many challenges and disappointments, even if they are successful in bringing family members to Australia (Rousseau et al. 2004). Finally, before coming to Australia, they underwent numerous health screening tests, which were stressful. Particularly stressful was the fear that one of the family might be HIV positive, which would mean that no members of the family would be accepted into Australia. As a result of the screening, three of the family were treated for TB before leaving for Australia, and they fear this might impact on their health and well-being in Australia. In a situation like this, where the complexity of needs of the family is high, an integrated approach that empowers them to take control over their own health and social requirements is an approach that will assist with successful settlement in both the short and longer term.

Public health responses have included advocacy on behalf of refugee communities; capacity-building with health and social services to better meet the needs of refugees; capacity-building among refugee communities themselves; intersectoral partnerships established with the aim of meeting a range of resettlement needs, by working with the education and health sectors; and community development, by creating opportunities for economic and civic participation and through recreation, sport and cultural events (Victorian Health Promotion Foundation 2003). For example, an integrated approach to refugee health in Victoria includes training and capacity-building among general practitioners to be able to treat the whole family; the introduction of a new medical benefit category to compensate general practitioners for longer consultations; the training of teachers, school health nurses and welfare officers to be able to address the needs of refugee children and their families; lobbying for better access to dental health and oral hygiene services; advocacy on behalf of refugee communities to improve access to services, including interpreter services, and to enable services to become more aware of the needs of refugee clients.

In sum, Australia's approach to the vulnerabilities of refugee communities has combined advocacy with primary care, self-help with specialist services for those suffering from the mental health effects of torture, and capacity-building among refugee communities as well as among the wider health and social sector. It is an example of a public health approach that has addressed the social factors as well as the physical factors that are the root causes of vulnerability among this population.

Vulnerability, illegal behaviour and stigmatised infections: The case of hepatitis C

Hepatitis C virus (HCV) infection is now the most commonly notified communicable disease in Australia, accounting for 90 per cent of new infections and 80 per cent of existing infections (DoHA 2010b: 3). There are an estimated 226 700 people living with HCV infection and, although the rate of newly diagnosed cases is falling, HCV infection continues to be a major public health challenge. Infection by HCV results in a chronic condition that has a major impact on population health and on the quality of life of individuals. HCV is a major cause of liver cirrhosis, and is the leading reason for liver transplants in Australia (Hepatitis Australia 2012a, 2012b). Although a small proportion of people live with the virus without chronic infection, the majority of those infected suffer from a range of symptoms, such as chronic fatigue, nausea, and aches and pains, all of which impact on an individual's quality of life. A key feature of living with HCV in Australian society is the stigma associated with the nature of its transmission: approximately 83 per cent of infections are associated with unsafe injecting drug use (Hepatitis Australia 2012a).

HCV is a blood-borne virus, and prior to 1990 a major risk factor for acquiring the infection was having a blood transfusion. However, since then, people with HCV antibodies have been excluded from donating blood and thus the main risk factor for acquiring HCV is unsafe injecting practices (Crofts, Dore & Locarnini 2001; Dore et al. 2003). At present, there is no vaccine to prevent HCV infection and there is no simple treatment that will bring about a cure once infection has occurred. HCV therefore presents the public health system with a significant challenge.

Responding to people with HCV involves tackling the stigma associated with how it may be acquired because stigma has led to a range of discriminatory practices, both overt and unintended, which have acted to marginalise people living with the virus. For example, people with HCV infection report being excluded from their families, being prevented from having close physical contact with their children (such as hugging them), and having to use separate plates, cups and cutlery to other family members. There are reported cases of people being discriminated against at work—losing their jobs or not being hired because of their HCV infection status (Platt & Gifford 2003). HCV has also been reported to be a factor in the way that people are treated in the health-care setting. People living with HCV report experiencing a range of behaviours that they regard as discriminatory, such as being scheduled as the last dental patient of the day, and judgemental treatment by doctors and nurses (Anti-Discrimination Board of New South Wales 2001; Gifford et al. 2003: Hopwood & Southgate 2001). Finally, it has been difficult for public health practitioners to find effective strategies for partnering with affected communities, as has been successful in the case of HIV/AIDS. This is partly due to the fact that, in Australia, those at risk of contracting HCV are generally more vulnerable than those at risk of HIV/AIDS. HIV continues to mostly affect men who have sex with men, whereas HCV infection is a risk for people who often are addicted to injecting drugs; are living in conditions of poverty; are already marginalised from their family and the broader society; and are living with a range of other challenges, including lack of secure housing, unemployment and ill-health. As a result of these issues, public health strategies have focused primarily on an integrated approach to prevention and care, informed by strategies to normalise the perception of and response to this condition through the removal of the attached stigma.

One of the major planks of prevention has been harm minimisation (Watson 2000) and peer education (Aitken, Kerger & Crofts 2002). Both of these public health responses have been shaped by Australia's successes in containing the HIV/AIDS epidemic, which has in turn shaped public health policy for HCV (Puplick 2001). A key feature of HIV/AIDS policy in the early 1980s was the requirement that three conditions be met: first, the affected community had to be involved in the response; second, responses needed to be informed by solid evidence; and third, responses needed to include

policies that were not only health related but included law reforms, changes to public perception and provision of social support and care. Informed by the successful policy response to HIV/AIDS, a National HCV Action Plan was adopted by the Australian Health Ministers' Advisory Council in 1994. This had two key objectives, both of which focused on 'minimisation', the basis of an integrated public health approach. The first focused on minimising the impact of HCV infection on those already infected and the second focused on minimising transmission. Harm-minimisation policies that focused on promoting blood safety (including safe injecting practices) were the key plank in preventing new infections. Improving treatment and health care for those affected was a second plank to this integrated approach. This involved professional development for general practitioners, extending access to specialist liver clinics to current injecting drug users, and capacity-building across the health sector to improve responses to people living with HCV. A third plank of this integrated approach was to invest in research, and to this end targeted NHMRC funding was allocated to increase medical and social research. A key focus of this integrated approach was to extend partnerships, through the funding of Hepatitis Councils in each state and territory, a series of public consultations and the establishment of an advisory committee comprising people from a range of backgrounds, including those living with HCV. The Third National Hepatitis C Strategy continued on from this first strategy, and was based on a range of guiding principles, including harm reduction, effective partnerships, the right to participate without stigma and discrimination, and the adoption and maintenance of protective behaviours (DoHA 2010b: 11–12).

Although Australia's public health response to HCV has not been easy, it can be regarded as a success story because, in global terms, it is the first national policy that integrates support and care for, and treatment and prevention of, HCV infection. A key challenge, however, has been the controversial nature of one of the 'risk' factors for infection: injecting drug use. Although a harm-minimisation approach has been the central plank of prevention, it remains controversial. For example, it has been difficult to establish effective policies that can be translated into safe injecting practices in community settings. Needle-exchange programs, although successful despite unreliable funding, have been criticised for being too few in number and inaccessible to many of the people who need them. Supervised injecting facilities continue to be controversial. Although there have been some successes in trial conditions, such as in Sydney, these facilities are still not being publicly funded as part of the prevention strategy in Australia. Engaging the affected community has been a further difficulty in HCV policy development, in large part due to its members' extreme disadvantage and the reluctance of governments to promote participation of community-based organisations that are working at the coalface with this vulnerable population. Thus, the case of HCV infection illustrates two important points for public health practice: an integrated public health approach can be adopted to address an urgent Australian health issue; and integrated approaches that work well for one condition—for example, HIV/AIDS—cannot be directly transferred to address a similar issue. While the two conditions have much in common, their differences are striking, and it is important that these differences inform the shaping of a unique, integrated and effective response to HCV.

Sustaining health and quality of life among people with chronic and terminal illnesses: Linking individuals and the community

Health-promoting palliative care

Organised care of people who are dying has long been provided by hospices run by religious organisations. In the 1960s, the palliative care movement began to spread in the United Kingdom, North America and Australia, and—with government support—patient-centred care that focused on good symptom control, privacy and autonomy became more widely available (Kellehear 2003).

Health-promoting palliative care (HPPC) offers an innovative approach by drawing on principles of health promotion as represented in the Ottawa Charter and applying these to the core concerns of the hospice tradition that is the basis of contemporary palliative care. It recognises the physical, psychological, social and spiritual dimensions of life-threatening illnesses, is concerned with the importance of good quality of life for what remains of life and does not deny the inevitability of death.

The essential elements of the HPPC approach are health education, death education, social support, health service reorientation towards the patient and policy development. HPPC refocuses attention particularly upon the social and spiritual dimensions of care. It also draws attention to the wider contribution that palliative care services can make to maturing understandings of death in the community through partnerships with other agencies and groups that share common concerns around living with loss, disability, ageing or life-threatening illness. A service modelled on the HPPC approach will be able to demonstrate that it (Kellehear 1999, 2005):

- extends the activities or complements existing support groups with adult learning groups
- provides death education for patients, staff (including volunteers), caregivers and community members
- provides education in social approaches to care for staff (including volunteers), caregivers and community members
- has (non-clinical) partnerships with public health agencies and associations, community groups, community health agencies, community services groups, churches and schools
- provides education resource material—both to the client and professional

- participates in research devoted to social issues in palliative care, and/or has staff reading groups or journal clubs devoted to social, cultural and spiritual research topics, and/or encourages staff toward future education in welfare studies, public health, social sciences, humanities, or legal and political studies.
- acts in advocacy roles, including making regular policy submissions to members of parliament, government committees of inquiry, Health Departments and local councils
- has a staffing profile that includes socially trained professionals, especially social workers and pastoral care workers; provides access to a health promotion and/or health educator worker; and resembles the cultural and social profile of the community it serves
- develops health-promoting settings by minimising the impact of clinical settings and creates environments that recognise and enhance individual identity, allow opportunity for community access and participation, and provide genuine opportunities for health improvements (relief of distress, such as emotional, physical, social and spiritual distress; physical mobility; and sense of wellbeing).

The HPPC concept can be extended further to the local community with the idea of 'compassionate cities', which builds on the WHO's model of healthy cities. Compassion is considered to be both an attitude and action that can be defined as sharing the suffering of another. The main aim of compassionate cities is that care for the dying, or those who are experiencing loss, has a health-promotion approach that involves palliative care services taking a leadership role in the initiation of community-wide action. The characteristics of a compassionate city are listed in Box 16.2.

Health-promoting palliative care illustrates how the principles of comprehensive care for people with HIV/AIDS can be extended more broadly. Although HIV infection and the development of AIDS are

> **Box 16.2 Characteristics of a compassionate city**
>
> - Has local health policies that recognise compassion as an ethical imperative
> - Meets the special needs of its aged population, those living with life-threatening illness, and those living with loss
> - Has a strong commitment to valuing social and cultural differences
> - Involves the grief and palliative care services in local government policy and planning
> - Offers its inhabitants access to a wide variety of supportive experiences, interactions and communication
> - Promotes and celebrates reconciliation with indigenous peoples and the memory of other important community losses
> - Provides easy access to grief and palliative care services
> - Has a recognised plan to accommodate those disadvantaged by the economy, including rural and remote populations, Indigenous people and the homeless
> - Preserves and promotes a community's spiritual traditions and storytellers
>
> *Source:* Kellehear (2005).

different from many other health problems (that is, infection is lifelong and ultimately fatal, and transmission is related to sexual behaviour—usually a domain of privacy and secrecy—such that initial reactions of society to the disease were characterised by fear, stigma and discrimination, ultimately leading to social rejection of those affected by HIV/AIDS), innovative approaches to the broad and humane care of those affected by HIV/AIDS provide an illustration of how the health needs of people who are ill can be supported through an organised approach, one that recognises the various contributions of many groups and organisations in society. Box 16.3 outlines how such an approach works.

Box 16.3 Comprehensive care for HIV/AIDS

As a first step in developing new approaches for HIV/AIDS care, it is crucial to identify the needs of those individuals who are infected and their families. Rapid appraisals of the medical, psycho-social and welfare needs of HIV/AIDS-affected individuals should be conducted with the active participation of the patients, families and communities. Based on these needs, a comprehensive HIV/AIDS care program can be developed. This should cover four areas:

- clinical management, including appropriate diagnosis using flowcharts, rational treatment and discharge planning for follow-up
- nursing care
- counselling, including helping individuals make informed decisions on HIV testing, stress and anxiety reduction, planning for the future, positive living and networking, and behavioural change
- home- and community-based care, including training family members, neighbours and community members as care providers; providing supervision/guidance by community-based workers and social workers; managing common symptoms; providing palliative care and moral support; providing support for families to maintain hygiene and nutrition; and providing linkages to social welfare systems.

HIV/AIDS patients and their families require a comprehensive continuum of services that ensures that care is provided at various levels of the health-care system. Such a continuum links facilities (including major hospitals, district hospitals and local community health centres) with families in their homes and supportive community networks. In other words, HIV/AIDS care is not only integrated into all levels of the health-care system, but also includes whole communities and families in the spectrum of care, and thus ensures the provision of care throughout the lifespan of people affected by HIV/AIDS.

Community-based care, which provides psychological, social, medical and nursing support to HIV/AIDS patients and their families, is seen by many countries as the only realistic approach to the crisis. Care for chronic conditions is given by families and members of society in the home and at the community level through hospice and other residential settings. Health-care settings support community-based care by providing diagnosis, clinical management and the treatment of acute conditions. Thus, referral networks between communities and health settings are key elements of the continuum of care.

Community-based care can further be defined as the interaction of support mechanisms of communities and governmental and non-governmental organisations to meet the physical, emotional, social and spiritual needs of persons who are sick. Community-based care should build upon or make use of the strengths of communities and families, and should take into account social and cultural norms and traditions. Community health workers, community development groups, religious groups, traditional practitioners, volunteers and social workers are involved in raising community awareness, initiating preventive activities and coordinating social support.

Home-based care refers to the provision of services by family members, neighbours or trained community members within the home to meet the physical, emotional, social and spiritual needs of people who are sick. These services can be supervised by existing support mechanisms in the community.

Source: WHO SEARO (1993).

Meeting the health needs of people with altered legal status: Prisoner health

The custodial system in Australia has no over-arching national system—it is entirely state and territory based. There are 98 custodial institutions in Australia, and in a liberal democracy the principle of imprisonment is punishment through the deprivation of liberty. However, in reality imprisonment brings with it a range of punishments that go beyond the lack of liberty. Risks to health are one of these, and in Australia there are no uniform standards for the provision of health services in prisons (Levy 2005). Prisoners lose their access to Medicare and the Pharmaceutical Benefits Scheme (PBS). Although prisoner health services are funded by state and territory governments and care is available, the fact that they lose such citizenship rights as Medicare (and voting) indicates how they are perceived by governments and society at large.

Prison populations consist predominately of people from the most economically disadvantaged and marginalised sections of societies. The majority of prison populations are young and male. Aboriginal and socially disadvantaged people are disproportionately represented (Butler 2003). Up to half of all people who enter prison have been exposed to HCV, and many have a current or past history of injecting drug use and are at risk of HIV/AIDS (Crofts, Dore & Locarnini 2001). While many prisoners may have a pre-existing chronic disease or have been involved in risk behaviours (such as injecting drugs), there are significant possibilities that they may contract a chronic, life-threatening communicable disease caused by infections from hepatitis C, TB or HIV while in prison, due to overcrowding, poor environmental conditions and other risk factors. If these communicable diseases go undetected, released prisoners can then spread them into the general population. In the United States, for example, there are at least 2 million people in prison, representing a 77 per cent increase

since 1990. In 1996, at least 41 per cent of inmates in Californian prisons had hepatitis C compared with 2 per cent of the general population (Restum 2005).

During most of the twentieth century, prison health services received very little attention from either prison managements or local health services. This situation began to change in the 1980s for two main reasons. The first was the break-up of the Soviet Union and the emergence of newly independent states in Eastern Europe, which were faced with widespread social, economic, political and environmental problems, including the development of new criminal justice systems and the reorganisation of their overcrowded prisons (see the 'Challenge' at the beginning of Chapter 11). The second was the rapid spread of the HIV/AIDS epidemic and the resurgence of communicable diseases, such as tuberculosis. This focused attention on the public health consequences of poor prison health services and the growing threat to the wider community of contracting communicable diseases. In Europe, the inability of countries to develop any clear ideas of how to implement control measures led to the initiation by the WHO, in 1995, of the Health in Prisons Project (HIPP), with the aim of bringing about improvements in all aspects of health in prisons through changes in prison health policies (Gatherer, Moller & Hayton 2005).

While the HIPP has sought to address issues such as communicable diseases, mental health, use of illicit drugs, the special needs of minority groups and how to bring prison health into a closer working relationship with the public health system (see the 'Prison Health as Part of Public Health' Declaration, Moscow 2003, at <www.hipp-europe. org/NEWS/moscow_declaration_eng04.pdf>), many problems remain. These include overcrowding and unhygienic facilities due to the failure of new prison construction to keep up with expanding prison populations, the low priority given to prisons in government spending, and ambivalent public attitudes to prisons and prison reform (Gatherer, Moller & Hayton 2005).

In Australia, interest in prisoner health emerged in 1996 when 789 prisoners in New South Wales prisons were screened. The survey found that those in the New South Wales prison population come from the poorer and more vulnerable sections of society, and that they are at a greater risk of blood-borne infectious diseases, mental health problems, sexually transmitted diseases and tobacco-related diseases (NSW Corrections Service 1997). Another survey of 914 prisoners was conducted in 2001, and it showed that there had been increases in the prevalence of hepatitis C among men (34 to 40 per cent), as well as in the proportion of men and women receiving treatment for psychiatric illness, and in the proportion of men who were current smokers and illicit drug users (Butler & Milner 2003).

In response to these surveys and the increasing prevalence of hepatitis C (which by early 2004 saw 60 per cent of women and 40 per cent of men infected), NSW Justice Health established a network of specialist clinics providing services relating to blood-borne viruses and sexually transmissible diseases in all of the state's 29 correction centres. These centres provide targeted health services that are run by public health nurses and supported by a network of visiting specialists (Pollard 2004).

Furthermore, New South Wales Justice Health established the Centre for Health Research in Criminal Justice in 2004 to undertake research and to evaluate the programs that underpinned its service delivery programs, with the priority areas being mental health; blood-borne viruses; drugs and alcohol and Indigenous health; providing support for undergraduate, graduate and postgraduate training in custodial health care; and improving public health through diminishing the harms and maximising the benefits of incarceration (Centre for Health Research in Criminal Justice 2004). Box 16.4 sets out the findings of two research projects on prisoner health, one that looked at what the priority areas of research are and the other that examined NSW prisoners' health concerns.

From a public health perspective, it is clear that there is still much work to be done to address the health disadvantage among prisoners. Just like injecting drug users who have HCV infections, the fact that prisoners have committed crimes does not make their entitlement to health and health care any less than that of others in the community. Recognising their right to health, along with their social vulnerabilities, is the starting point.

Challenges for Australian public health practice

All the above case studies highlight how a public health approach is central to informing how best to support and advance the health and well-being of vulnerable populations. They also highlight how responses to the health needs of people who experience different vulnerabilities can be tailored using a 'toolkit' of public health strategies. The strength of the public health approach is that it is multidisciplinary in theory, method and practice, and thus lends itself to addressing the broad scope of issues affecting health that arise from different forms of vulnerability. This multidisciplinarity has been at the core of creating the intersectoral partnerships required for developing and implementing policies and practices critical to all public health successes.

While the health and well-being of vulnerable populations is of concern to many key stakeholders, it is perhaps important for public health practitioners to remember that the public health system cannot and should not assume all responsibility for dealing with vulnerable populations. In Australia, action in support of the interests of vulnerable communities and individuals is shared by various government portfolios at the federal and state levels, local communities, non-government organisations, and charities and community-based organisations, as well as by families and individuals. It is important to remember that public health is not only about the prevention of disease and injury, but that it is an integrated approach to responding to the health

Box 16.4 Prisoner health: An emerging field of research in New South Wales

Research on Aboriginal prisoner health is limited. In response to this gap, the Cooperative Research Centre for Aboriginal Health, supported by the Public Health Association of Australia and the Australian Institute of Aboriginal and Torres Strait Islander Studies, instigated the Aboriginal Prisoner Health Industry Roundtable in 2007. The roundtable brought together advocates, researchers, community representatives, correction staff, community-based service providers, and health and government representatives, and achieved results in two key areas: priority areas for research and how best to undertake Aboriginal prisoner health research. The roundtable identified several priority research areas: establishing an evidence base for interventions across the prisoner life-cycle (arrest, remand, sentencing, incarceration and release stages); examining the scope of prison health services and service delivery models used in prisons, with particular consideration given to continuity of care before and after release; determining how best to deliver health services across the country and within jurisdictions; and identifying which mechanisms and strategies could reduce rates of recidivism. Issues identified by the roundtable relating to the conduct of research included cultural appropriateness; use of Indigenous research methods; recognition of circumstances and experiences of prisoners ('prisoner-centred' research) and their relationships to family, community and the broader society; and use of collaborative approaches to developing research.

The importance of having up-to-date and accurate data on which to base plans and decisions led to New South Wales Justice Health conducting a survey, for the first time, of Aboriginal health within the New South Wales custodial system in 2009. Aboriginal prisoners in Australia comprise one-quarter of the total prisoner population and have a rate of imprisonment that is fourteen times higher than for non-Aboriginal people. In New South Wales, the proportion of male inmates who are Aboriginal increased from 12 per cent of the inmate population in 1996 to 22 per cent in 2009, and for female Aboriginal inmates the increase was from 17 to 29 per cent over the same period (Indig et al. 2010b: 6). The health survey, as expected, found that there were 'higher levels of disadvantage, unstable housing, violence, alcohol and drug use, and mental health issues among Aboriginal inmates' (Indig et al. 2010a: 11). One particular finding was that, due to a range of barriers, Aboriginal inmates—especially men—were significantly less likely to have accessed prevention and treatment services outside prison than non-Aboriginal inmates (Indig et al. 2010a: 11).

Source: Davis & Brands (2008: 5).

problems and concerns of the whole population, including people who are vulnerable because of illness or social disadvantage. In this context, public health practitioners have an important duty to advocate on behalf of vulnerable groups to other government portfolios, sectors and stakeholders, and to ensure the health and well-being of vulnerable groups is given priority in public policy and partnership-based initiatives. This dynamic is a key strength of public health in Australia, and one that needs to be strengthened further to ensure public health approaches for vulnerable segments of our community are effective and sustained organised efforts.

For the public health system to make progress in responding to the interests of vulnerable populations, it is important that their interests and needs are reflected in all domains of activity, from research to policy development to program evaluation. In research, novel methodologies may be needed to sensitively and ethically gain insight into the circumstances and views of vulnerable groups—such as aged migrants, or teenagers with a mental illness—and the interplay between social and environmental factors at work in shaping their lives and experience. In policy development, new mechanisms might be necessary to engage vulnerable groups in framing and assessing key public health issues. Innovations in program-evaluation methods might need to be created so that people whose literacy skills are limited can provide input.

While the public health system steadily gains insights into how different forms of vulnerability arise and might be prevented, and what strategies are effective in responding to health needs arising from vulnerability, the public health landscape continues to change and produce new forms of vulnerability. In the coming decades, how might the interaction of social, technological, economic, environmental and political forces alter the nature of vulnerability and what can we do about it? How will the trend towards older populations change the type and scale of populations at risk? In the digital age, what health consequences might there be for population groups who cannot access a home computer or mobile communications technologies? On the other hand, will the opening up of access to the internet and other technologies produce new forms of vulnerability? Which population groups might fall into conditions of defencelessness or exploitation under the influence of globalisation of production and service industries, privatisation of energy and water sources or decoding of the human genome? What would the impacts be if policy support for the PBS were to be withdrawn?

Conclusion: Universal rights

The Universal Declaration of Human Rights 1948 (<www.universalrights.net/main/declarat.htm clearly>) identifies in Article 25 that health is a basic right of all people:

Article 25

Everyone has the right to a standard of living adequate for the health and well-being of himself [sic] and of his family, including food, clothing, and housing and medical care and necessary social services, and the right to security in the event of unemployment, sickness, disability, widowhood, old age or other lack of livelihood in circumstances beyond his control.

Australia's public health system has gone a long way towards ensuring these rights are upheld for the majority of the country's population. However, despite the adoption of the Universal Declaration more than half a century ago, Australian society continues to debate whether the condition of vulnerability should invite punishments (such as withdrawal of rights to access health care) or support (through the provision of material resources and social supports). A public health approach considers the problems facing an individual within the context of family, community and society, and looks for ethical solutions that work at these multiple levels.

While the history of implementing public health strategies for vulnerable population groups has not been without problems (indeed, state-run and top-down programs have been the sources of human rights abuses), it has been the consumers and carers, self-help groups and other social movements that have successfully used advocacy to pursue a rights-based approach. As the case examples portrayed in this chapter suggest, there are now a number of useful lessons to be drawn from the range of innovative public health strategies adopted for various vulnerable population groups and applied to other groups.

Part V

Public health challenges:
Emerging issues and responses

17

Public health governance:
Politics of participation, decision-making and accountability

Challenge

The fast-food chain McDonald's has developed a global profile and significant reach into industries and the lives of people on every continent. In 1990, the infamous McLibel trial began between McDonald's and a gardener and a postman from London (Helen Steel and Dave Morris), members of a group called London Greenpeace (Vidal 1997). The case was based on claims made in a brochure distributed by the group, such as 'McDonald's try to show in their "Nutrition Guide" that mass-produced hamburgers, chips, colas, milkshakes, etc. are a useful and nutritious part of any diet. What they don't make clear is that a diet high in fat, sugar, animal products and salt (sodium), and low in fibre, vitamins and minerals—which describes an average McDonald's meal—is linked with cancers of the breast and bowel and heart disease.' (McSpotlight 2005)

At the end of the 313-day trial (the longest trial of any kind in England), Judge Bell delivered his 762-page judgment, ruling that McDonalds 'exploit children' with their advertising, are 'misleading' with their advertising, are 'culpably responsible' for cruelty to animals, are 'antipathetic' to unionisation and pay their workers low wages. However, Steel and Morris were not able to prove all the points claimed in their brochure (for example, that McDonald's had used lethal poisons to destroy significant areas of rainforest in Central America), so the judge ruled that they had to pay £60 000 damages on the basis that they had libelled McDonald's. The defendants refused to pay and this was not pursued (BBC 2005).

Regardless of the outcome, this case illustrated with startling clarity how a globally successful organisation can have a major impact on public health—directly because their products are consumed and indirectly through the ways in which they set up and defend their means of production. The case also flags some key issues for public health in the context of globalisation: will an organised approach be able to assure the fundamental determinants of health, such as a nutritious food supply, income and human rights? What instruments will be available to regulate market forces (including product supply and marketing) in the interests of public health? What avenues should be available to consumers to assert their viewpoints and demands for change in the face of multinational industries?

Introduction

Public health actions have long been linked to government roles and activities. Historically, governments have provided funds and legislative authority, along with a range of services. Yet public health action does not rest with government alone—it relies on the mobilisation of resources (human and financial) within the community. As such, it is dependent on community interest, support and the resources available. Community values will shape government legislation. Community interest and support will also shape government interest in and commitment to allocating funds for particular health programs.

As public health action draws from public finances, and there is a finite amount of resources available, how these scarce public resources are to be used is a central concern of public health policy-making. Should funds be used for the health problems experienced by the largest number of people? Should funds be used for the most preventable health problems? Should funds be used for the most disadvantaged people? A consistent thread in public health policy and program development is the question of whether programs should be directed to particular diseases and risk factors or around geographical locations and population groups. In addition, given limited resources and the evolving list of priority health issues in the community, how can health gains and public health programs be sustainable?

Organisational arrangements for the delivery of public health programs are also a matter for debate. Is this best done by government or by non-government organisations? Should the organisation and delivery of public health activities be centralised or decentralised? How important are the roles of medical doctors and those with clinical training? What is the relationship between public health units and personal health-care service-delivery units?

In the face of multiple health needs and multiple perspectives from the participants in the public health enterprise, priority-setting is an inherent component of decision-making about which public health problems should be tackled, as is the question of who participates in those decision-making processes and how. Public health decision-making is both a technical exercise of trading off options as well as a political process. This raises the more fundamental question of governance. What should be the mechanism for decision-making? Who should be involved? What mechanisms should exist for accountability? What is the role of the community in decision-making?

This chapter is concerned with what drives decision-making and the current debates on how choices should be made in the face of competing needs and interests. It also raises questions about how the public health system should be governed in the face of competing interests and needs. The chapter starts with a brief discussion about the concept of governance, and then moves on to consider the choices involved in designing and allocating resources for public health programs, and the relationship between government and society. As the relationship between government and society evolves, so the chapter considers the changing approaches to public-sector management and their implications for public health practice. Given that public health issues have moved from being local to global, the chapter will conclude with discussions on emerging issues for global health governance.

A word on 'governance': One idea, diverse views

'Good governance' has become an important principle for governments and corporations alike in recent years. In its most general sense, governance means a system of authority and control. In the narrower sense used in everyday parlance, the term means achieving effective, efficient, transparent and accountable processes for decision-making.

It includes establishing policies and processes for decision-making and holding decision-makers responsible for their actions. Figure 17.1 depicts the typical elements of a framework for governance (Cameron 2003: 5).

Given that public health is a societal enterprise, the concept of governance includes both formal political institutions and processes and their relationship to society. For public health governance, the concern is for the totality of processes and arrangements, both formal and informal, by which power and public authority are distributed, regulated and exercised. Burris (2004) considers that task of public health governance consists largely of the 'policing of social relations, environmental conditions, and the allocation of resources essential to wellbeing'. The relationship between state and civil society is as important as how government works. This connection is at the heart of democratic governance and notions of locating the

Figure 17.1 Framework for governance

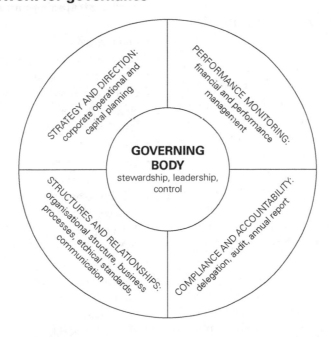

Source: adapted from Cameron (2003).

citizen—as a target and an agent—at the centre of policy-making concerns.

Maddox (2005) argues that a contemporary approach to governance in Australia will have five features if it is to be considered democratic. First, democracy rests on 'constitutional order', with government action being limited to appropriate domains. Second, there must be a 'responsible' executive that is strong enough to fulfil government functions and ensure adjustments to social demands. Third, this executive must be a constitutional opposition, to query, interrogate and help the Australian community to control government's power. Fourth, all political institutions should apply the democratic ideals (such as justice, liberty, equality and community) to their procedures and processes. Finally, the society the political structure supports should be pluralistic, participatory and thrive through group engagement. Together, these features would underpin citizen engagement and participation in policy matters, including those concerned with health.

How do governments frame public health strategies?

As discussed throughout the book, governments have been involved in public health through legislation and allocating funds for programs. Chapter 7 pointed out that government involvement in public health may be justified on economic grounds (as a public good—offering diffuse benefit, containing externalities, addressing public interest) or as part of its stewardship role (investing in society). Governments may also initiate programs on the basis of responsiveness and political pragmatism—either to perceived need or health threat, or to political lobbying.

The framing of public health policy is dependent upon the interplay between community, professional and political interests. Duckett and Willcox (2011) suggest that there have been three phases of public health policy in Australia: (1) medical

dominance via the National Health and Medical Research Council (NHMRC); (2) interest group competition; and (3) the importance of the social environment as a determinant of health and ill-health. In the first phase, decision-making was dominated by the experts—particularly the doctors—and lasted from the initial establishment of the NHMRC into the 1980s. During the 1980s, dramatic increases were seen in government funding and in the number of public health programs (see Figure 8.2). Since the 1990s, although public funding has been in decline, the number of public health strategies and programs has continued to grow. Many of these were in the form of government policy documents, prepared through a consultative process with expert and community input but without substantial funding attached.

At first glance, the programs listed in Box 17.1 would appear to be responses to a mix of diseases, population groups and risk factors, with no apparent

---

Box 17.1 Australian national public health strategies and programs

- Immunisation
- National health emergencies
- Communicable diseases
- Chemical and biological risks
- Natural disasters
- Health surveillance
- Mental health
- Suicide prevention
- Substance misuse
- Preventive health
- Healthy living
- Ageing
- Palliative care
- Chronic diseases
- Child and youth health
- Women's health
- Men's health
- Indigenous health

organising logic. How did these programs arise? Was it the result of lobbying by interest groups? Was it based on epidemiological analysis? Was it political vision? Which individuals, groups or institutions were involved? In most of these cases, some of the principles at work included:

- broad and respectable constituency for the issue (for example, clinicians, a wide range of people)
- valuing immediate results (that is, 'saving lives')
- the importance of epidemiological evidence, but only if numbers are large and distributed across different groups.

The naming and framing of issues is an important part of how issues 'get up' on the political and funding agenda (Gibson 2003). Disease outcomes are more readily understood by the community at large, and by politicians as their representatives. Risk factors are an important focus if avoiding them or minimising their effect seems to be out of the control of individuals. For instance, Australian states and territories have implemented programs in nutrition education for many years (including media campaigns, community education and school-based programs), and in more recent times have begun to promote physical activity targeted at various population groups in a range of settings (such as schools, community centres and workplaces). Although nutrition and physical activity programs have long been part of campaigns to promote healthier lifestyles and are essential components of any effort to reduce chronic diseases (such as heart disease, stroke and diabetes) and their predisposing conditions, it has been the naming of the problem as 'obesity', with summits and taskforces that began in 2003 across Australia, that has captured both the popular and the political imagination, along with heightened concern within the health care system.

At times, there is a coincidence of political policy with health policy. In 1992, a new government was elected in Victoria and a 'Heart and Cancer

Offensive' was launched. This public health initiative was concerned with the two leading causes of death in Australia. That may not have seemed unusual at first glance, but it signalled a shift in political policy (Tehan 2002). At the political level, instead of small interest groups receiving funding for various programs (for example, women's health, HIV/AIDS), the new policy focused on the health problems that faced the majority of the population, and brought the medical interests, in particular, into the policy fold. As a health policy, it was easily justified on the basis of leading causes of mortality, morbidity, hospitalisation and health-care costs.

The framing of programs around specific disease end-points and the desired health outcomes reflects the greater chance that 'vertical' programs (that is, programs directed at single diseases and risk factors, with top-down planning) will gain political attention and support. Single-issue programs, however, pose a number of problems (NPHP 2000d), including:

- cost and sustainability—there is a need to continually fund them
- administrative burden for service providers—because each program has its own reporting and funding arrangements
- failure to address comorbidities—since many risk factors and health conditions coexist but are not necessarily covered by single vertical programs
- mismatches with local priorities and poor ownership by local communities—as communities may not identify the funded program (be it a disease or a risk factor) as their most important problem.

As many public health activities are concerned with acting on underlying causes of ill-health, attention has turned toward defining the nature of intermediate outcomes (Nutbeam 1996) that would be more appropriate measures for public health programs. For example, it is now well accepted that sustainable health outcomes depend on capacity in

Box 17.2 Development of women's health policies

When two new policies on women's health—the National Women's Health Policy (NWHP) and Breast-Screen Australia—were developed during the late 1980s and early 1990s, political pragmatism resulted in one policy being privileged over the other in terms of resource allocation.

The NWHP was a governmental response to the women's health movement of the 1960s. It sought to reform the health system by getting policy-makers to recognise that women had special needs, that the focus should be on prevention and primary health care rather than curative medicine, and that there was a need to establish specific health services for women (Willis 2003). In 1987, the Hawke Labor government appointed a special adviser on women's health to coordinate the development of NWHP with the Australian Health Ministers' Advisory Council. Through informal consultations conducted Australia-wide, evidence on women's health perceptions and needs were gathered from service providers, government representatives, women's organisations and individuals. The resulting discussion paper, which was distributed throughout Australia, combined with meetings held in each state, gave more than one million women the opportunity to contribute to policy development (Women's Health Queensland Wide 2003).

The NWHP was launched in April 1989 with a goal to 'improve the health and wellbeing of all women in Australia, with a focus on those most at risk, and to encourage the health system to be responsive to the needs of women' (quoted in Women's Health Queensland Wide 2003). Seven priority issues (reproductive and sexual health; the health of ageing women; women's emotional and mental health; violence against women; occupational health and safety; the health needs of women as carers; and the health effects of sex role stereotyping) and five action areas

were identified to improve women's health by 2000 (Willis 2003).

BreastScreen Australia, on the other hand, was a programmatic response to the importance of breast cancer as a contributor to women's morbidity and mortality. Governments needed to be seen by the electorate to be actively doing something about the problem. Eleven pilot programs were established throughout Australia during 1988–89, which received support from clinicians, researchers and advocates for women's health. The subsequent policy was developed using epidemiological and clinical data (evidence) from randomised controlled trials conducted in Canada, Sweden, the United Kingdom and the United States (Willis 2003). Launched in 1991, BreastScreen Australia is a population-based national screening program that specifically targets women in the 50–69 years age group who do not have symptoms of breast cancer (DoHA 2004a). Political pragmatism dictated that more financial resources be given to BreastScreen Australia even though the scientific evidence contested the effectiveness of such a large-scale screening program. The BreastScreen policy had the potential to deliver results to the electorate.

Overall, the NWHP was a less-clearly defined policy than BreastScreen, developed using qualitative data that sought to respond to the demands of the 1960s women's health movement by giving legitimacy to its argument that health is a gender issue. Also, '[t]he political reality of a social change agenda within women's health policy, no matter how strongly argued, represents a challenge to the dominant discourses and to the accepted social order' (Willis 2003: 220). While BreastScreen Australia received a federal government allocation of $64 million for the first three years of the program (which increased to about $80 million a year once fully implemented), the NWHP only received $34 million over a four-year period from 1989 to 1993, with 94.5 per cent of those funds being allocated to improving health services for women.

the community to maintain these programs and to evolve lessons from current efforts to apply to new health challenges (Hawe et al. 1997). Community capacity is itself shaped by a complex array of factors (see Figure 17.2), many of which are outside the narrow concerns of a health-care system. Yet the goal of community-building is difficult to translate into a central aim for popular public health programs that are readily supported in the political arena. Rather, government generally names a program in terms of a health problem and then funds a purported solution for it.

Burris (2004: 354) argues for the need for governments to shift the way they think about public health strategies. He recommends a shift in the orientation from solving problems to 'influencing the generative dispositions of a system'. This means that we need to build a system capacity to understand the links between the different problems and across different communities and population groups, and to organise our decision-making processes in a way that can influence both underlying issues and the ways in which different organisations and communities respond to perceived problems. From the viewpoint of the stewardship role of government, therefore, there is an argument to be made that government should focus on investment in the capacity of the public health system, as well as building the capacity of communities to address local health problems. The effectiveness of interventions relies not only on adopting evidence-based intervention designs, but also on sufficient quantity and quality of human and financial resources to implement them. An adequate coverage of the target population is dependent on the resources available. The feasibility of implementing in accordance with intervention design specifications depends on workforce capacity (Fawkes & Lin 2002). The

Figure 17.2 Influences on community capacity

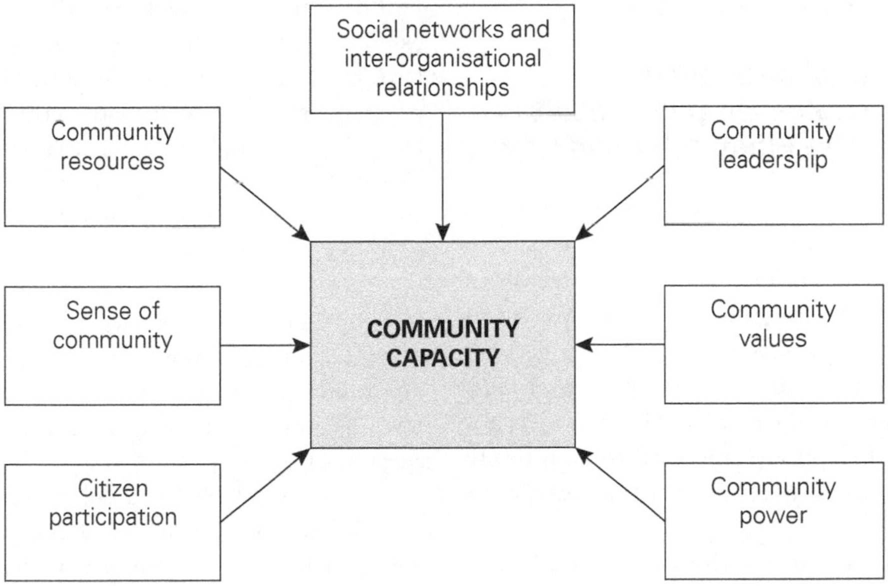

Source: adapted from Lin (2000).

Figure 17.3 A healthy and well community

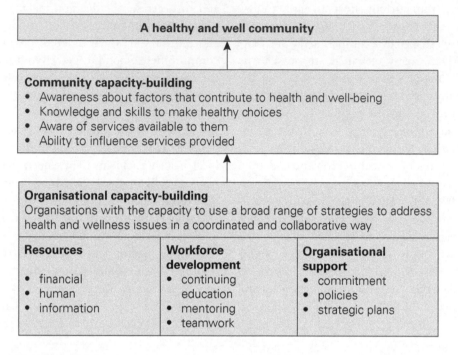

Source: adapted from Lin (2000).

relationship between system capacity and community capacity is outlined in Figure 17.3.

Organisational and resource allocation choices in public health programs: The what, who and how

As well as the prioritisation of issues or problems to tackle, the persistent tension in public health programming, as outlined above, has been about whether vertical programs (that is, programs directed at single diseases and risk factors, with top-down planning) are most effective in producing health improvements, or whether a locally integrated and responsive approach to local health needs is more effective in producing sustainable health gains.

In the latter part of the twentieth century, the question of whether public health activities and organisational units should be centralised or decentralised also came to the fore. As Australian health authorities have developed regional or area-based frameworks for health administration, there have been questions about whether public health programs should remain with central office or be located in regional offices or area health services. The argument runs in parallel with the debate about vertical programming versus integrated local practice—that is, a centralised approach can offer expert direction, give directives and mobilise resources in times of emergency, while a decentralised approach allows for greater community input, and programs and strategies more tailored towards the needs and culture of the local community.

In New South Wales, a decentralised approach was chosen when divisions of population health were formed within the Area Health Services (AHSs). This restructuring was an attempt to 'overcome the marginalisation and fragmentation that often characterise population health workers within AHSs' (Sainsbury 1999: 119), through better coordination of activities and focusing on similar goals. As each AHS contains a different mix of professional skills and services, and has to cater for the varying needs of the local population, this is reflected in the functions these divisions of population health provide (Sainsbury 1999). This approach has been continued in New South Wales in the development of Local Health Networks, which are part of the national health reforms in 2011.

In the final decade of the twentieth century, public health delivery faced a further challenge. With neo-liberal economic reforms, including reforms in public-sector management, questions arose about whether public health services should be delivered by government or outsourced (to another level of government, to community organisations, to health providers or to private-sector entities). In Victoria, a range of organisational types—such as community health centres, local government and NGOs—have always been involved in public health delivery, but compulsory competitive tendering was introduced in the 1990s. Organisations that historically have provided the services had to compete with a range of public- and private-sector organisations to continue receiving public-sector funding for their service provision. Most significant, though, was the tendering of the inspectorial services so that the powers of the state could be exercised by those winning government contracts.

Regardless of who provides the services, there remains a question of how these programs should to be coordinated. An uncoordinated approach often leads to service providers (such as GPs) and other organisations (such as schools) being bombarded with requests to undertake highly specific health-education activities. Separate and singular efforts may also lead to inconsistent, if conflicting, health messages being conveyed to the community. Furthermore, there is potential for the duplication of resources and 'reinventing the wheel'

if those who are managing programs fail to learn from each other.

Thus, planning efforts at the organisational, community and system levels will require leaders and senior managers to pay attention to collaboration and coordination mechanisms across myriad public health strategies and programs. The focus for coordination may be on (NPHP 1999): intervention type (for example, a media campaign), population

---

Box 17.3 Guidelines for consumer representatives (on committees)

- Be clear about whom you represent, to whom you are accountable and what you are expected to do.
- Before you start, obtain information about the committee's structure, scope of activity, authority, mode of operation, membership and duration; also find out about workload expectations.
- Prepare well for meetings by reviewing previous meetings' minutes, setting short-term goals, obtaining different consumer views and examining the agenda.
- During meetings, request additional agenda items, take notes of significant points and major decisions, record dissent and use the lunch break to advantage by speaking informally with other members.
- Between and after meetings, report to your organisation, keep in contact with the secretary and other committee members, seek help from the chairperson, the secretary, your organisation or other consumer representative if you are having difficulties dealing with the committee, reflect on and evaluate your work on the committee.
- Be effective by creating a positive first impression, consulting, networking, reporting regularly to your organisation, planning your tactics, and forming alliances and coalitions.

Source: Consumers' Health Forum of Australia (2001).

---

group (for example, Aboriginal communities, young people or rural communities), intervention setting (for example, general practices or schools), infrastructure (for example, data collection or research) and common or shared determinants of health (for example, tobacco or social support). The coordination may cover not only programs, but may bridge specialist expertise. In such a way, generalists may be the frontline program providers, knowing that specialist back-up is readily accessible.

Expanding participation in decision-making: Bringing 'the public' into public health

The dominance of medical professionals in health policy decision-making, including public health, was challenged by the social movements of the 1970s. The women's health movement, workers' health movement and Aboriginal health movement, in particular, advocated successfully for new forms of health care-delivery organisations. The Alma-Ata Declaration of 1978 further provided international support for consumer/community participation as an integral component of primary health care.

In the 1980s, structures for consumer participation in decision-making in the health system were designed and implemented in a number of jurisdictions. The Commonwealth government established the Consumer Health Forum (CHF), which was granted a seat at the table in all policy advisory bodies. Although some people in the health system ridiculed CHF representatives as 'professional consumers', there were strict guidelines for all CHF representatives, along with training programs and reporting mechanisms.

At the state level, Victoria already had a long tradition of community committees of management in all spheres of life. When community health centres were set up in the 1970s, such committees were established. During the 1980s, the *Health Services Act 1988* required their members to be elected, while some states also developed mechanisms for

community involvement at a broader level of oversight of the health system. In Victoria, the District Health Councils (DHCs) program was in place from 1985–93. South Australia similarly established Health and Welfare Councils in 1988.

The initial concept of DHCs was that they act as a 'local government for health'. Such a program required substantial support and training for consumers, but the powerful players in the health system (such as doctors and hospital administrators) generally saw no reason to take notice of their existence or views. Over time, the focus of DHCs evolved towards involvement in health-promotion and community-development activities, rather than calling health services to account. Although this experience illustrates the challenges for consumers to be overseers of the health system, consumer participation has been legislatively enshrined in other ways—such as in the requirement for lay representation on health professional registration boards (for doctors, nurses, psychologists and so on), and for health services (metropolitan health services in Victoria and area health services in New South Wales and South Australia) to have consumer advisory mechanisms.

The value of consumer involvement in policy deliberations did remain a central plank in public health policy-making at the national level. The National Women's Health Policy (1989) and the National Aboriginal Health Strategy (1988) were both developed within a framework of participation by community members. Subsequently, the notion of 'partnership with the affected community' was strongly incorporated into the initial national HIV strategy and, given its success, the concept has become embedded into national public health strategy development generally. In 1999–2000, the national Sharing Health Care Initiative supported twelve demonstration projects, which involved clients attending a chronic disease self-management course to learn new skills to help with the daily management of their chronic disease. Structures to support consumer participation were an integral part of the projects. In the case of two projects in Queensland and the Australian Capital Territory, it was found that consumers influenced how the courses were marketed, the establishment of self-help groups and the education of health professionals (Allwell, Spink & Robinson 2004).

At the policy level, consumer representation was also enshrined in the *National Health and Medical Research Council Act 1992* and formalised by the Statement on Consumers and Community Participation in Health and Medical Research (NHMRC & the Consumers' Health Forum of Australia 2002). Given the NHMRC's origins and its place as a symbol of medical dominance, this legislative move showed

that Australia had truly moved to a new framework for decision-making. In 2009, the Australian Research Council funded a three-year project involving the Australian Institute of Health Policy Studies, together with industry and academic partner organisations, to investigate consumer engagement in health policy.

One policy area where shifts in participation in health policy and decision-making have been evident is Aboriginal health. These are outlined in Box 17.4. Tracing changes in the type and composition of mechanisms enabling participation and influence reveals flux in the level at which

---

Box 17.4 Shifting mechanisms enabling participation by Indigenous Australians in health decision-making

1971 First Aboriginal Medical Service (AMS) initiated on a voluntary basis in Redfern, Sydney.

1973 Aboriginal Health Branch established in the Commonwealth Department of Health to provide professional advice to government.

1974 National Aboriginal and Islander Health Organisation (NAIHO) formed.

1983 Responsibility for all Commonwealth Aboriginal health programs, including the Department of Health's role in the funding of some AMSs, consolidated within the Department of Aboriginal Affairs.

1987 Joint Ministerial Forum on Indigenous Health established.
National Aboriginal Health Strategy Working Party (NAHSWP) appointed to develop a strategy on Indigenous health that would encompass issues pertaining to funding, Indigenous participation and intersectoral coordination and monitoring, and meet with the approval of all stakeholders.

1988 Royal Commission into Aboriginal Deaths in Custody initiated.

1989 NAHSWP final report, *A National Aboriginal Health Strategy* (NAHS) presented to Joint Ministerial Forum.
Aboriginal Health Development Group (AHDG) established.
AMSs protested against the limited representation of Indigenous community interests on the AHDG. A community advisory group, the Aboriginal Health Advisory Group, established in parallel with the AHDG.

1990 Aboriginal and Torres Strait Islander Commission (ATSIC) established and assumes national responsibility for Indigenous health.

1991 Final report of the Royal Commission into Aboriginal Deaths in Custody published, providing a comprehensive review of Indigenous health needs, and government strategies addressing those needs. NAHS implementation supported.

1993 The National Aboriginal Community Controlled Health Organisation replaced NAIHO as the new national AMS umbrella organisation.
The *Native Title Act* became law, recognising and protecting native title and giving Indigenous land rights statutory authority.

1995   Health Ministers agreed to a process for developing multilateral Framework Agreements with states and territories, to enable the establishment of consultative national and state/territory forums to provide policy and planning advice on Indigenous health issues.

1996   The national health advisory forum proposed in the Framework Agreements, the Aboriginal and Torres Strait Islander Health Council, established. Six states and territories sign the Framework Agreements.

1997   The Human Rights and Equal Opportunity Commission (HREOC) released *Bringing Them Home: Report of the National Inquiry into the Separation of Aboriginal and Torres Strait Islander Children from Their Families* (AHRC 1997).

1998   The Australian National Audit Office concluded its performance audit of the Department of Health and Aged Care and released its report on the Aboriginal and Torres Strait Islander Health Program.

The final two jurisdictions, Tasmania and the Northern Territory, signed Framework Agreements.

2003   The Commonwealth and state/territory governments endorsed the *National Strategic Framework for Aboriginal and Torres Strait Islander Health: Framework for Action by Governments*. It built on the 1989 *National Aboriginal Health Strategy* and addresses approaches to primary health care within contemporary policy environments.

2004   Responsibility for delivery of all Indigenous-specific programs is transferred to mainstream agencies and a 'whole-of-government' approach is adopted. The new approach is based on a process of negotiating agreements with Indigenous families and communities at the local level in accordance with concepts of mutual obligation and reciprocity for service delivery. ATSIC and its service delivery arm, Aboriginal and Torres Strait Islander Services, are abolished. The Office of Indigenous Policy Coordination is established in the Department of Immigration, Multicultural and Indigenous Affairs.

2005   ATSIC Regional Councils are officially disbanded.

2006   The Commonwealth Department of Health and Ageing released the *National Strategic Framework for Aboriginal and Torres Strait Islander Health 2003–2013: Australian Government Implementation Plan 2003–2008*.

2007   Oxfam's *Close the Gap: Solutions to the Indigenous Health Crisis Facing Australia* outlined disparities of life expectancies between Indigenous and non-Indigenous people in Australia (Oxfam 2007).

HREOC's *Social Justice Report 2006* identified two major problems with how the government has dealt with Indigenous reform: the new whole-of-government approach does not adequately include Indigenous people in decision-making; and the government has no framework or benchmarks to gauge improved access to services.

2008   Prime Minister Kevin Rudd formally apologised to members of the Stolen Generations on behalf of the government.

Statement of Intent signed between the government and Indigenous health leaders, signalling an intent to collaborate in achieving equality in life expectancy and health status between Indigenous and non-Indigenous Australians by 2030.

The Indigenous Health Equality Council is established to advise on development and monitoring of health-related goals to support the government's commitment to closing the gaps in health between Indigenous and other Australians.

2009 Australia's official support for the United Nations Declaration on the Rights of Indigenous People, adopted by the UN General Assembly in 2007, is announced.	2010 The National Congress of Australia's First Peoples is established as an incorporated body, succeeding ATSIC as an advocate for the recognition of Indigenous peoples' rights.
	Source: Australian Indigenous HealthInfoNet (2010).

community control and self-determination have been able to be exercised.

Decision-making and priority-setting: Technical or participatory process?

Although consumer participation has been accepted as an integral part of health-care decision-making, questions remain about how best to support community members to make decisions about funding, resourcing and priority-setting in public health (Australian Institute of Primary Care 2004). In the 1990s, with neo-liberal reforms and budget cuts, the voices of medicine and social movements were overshadowed by the dominance of economics. Economic evaluation tools became increasingly important in public policy, as decision-makers raised questions about returns on investment. Several countries experimented with explicit forms of priority-setting and rationing for health care.

In Oregon in the United States, the controversial Oregon Health Plan (OHP) was enacted in 1989 and implemented in 1994 to expand access to health insurance (Medicaid) for the state's uninsured population by rationing medical care services that 'would be explicitly prioritized according to their medical benefit and contribution to the population's overall health status' (Jacobs, Marmor & Oberlander 1999: 164). The prioritised list of services (based on 709 condition–treatment pairings) drew on cost-benefit analysis (value for money) and a consultative process, which capitalised on Oregon's culture of public participation and built a coalition of support for expanded access. While the actual implementation of OHP failed as a demonstration

of cost-benefit analysis to resource allocation in health care (because additional funding was provided and very few services were actually cut), it showed the importance of public participation and coalition-building in the reform process (Jacobs, Marmor & Oberlander 1999). Unlike this very technical rationing approach, the New Zealand Department of Health established the National Advisory Committee on Core Health and Disability Services in 1992 to identify the broad priority areas to be covered by publicly funded health care. This was achieved by holding public meetings and conferences between health professionals and expert lay people. A consensus (or bargaining process) resulted, which produced four principles to be used in assessing whether a service should be included or excluded from public funding. They were: What benefit does the patient gain? Is the service cost-effective? Is it fair (in terms of equity between the different regions of New Zealand and socio-economic groups)? Is it consistent with the values and priorities of the community? (Coast 1996).

In 1991, the Dutch government established the Committee on Choices in Health Care with the aim of establishing 'a broad consensus to solve the problems of scarcity, priority setting and patient selection'. The committee proposed a basic health care system of a funnel with four sieves to establish which types of care would be retained and those which fell through. They were: 'Is the intervention necessary/useful to all members of society? Does it have documented effectiveness? Is it efficient (on the basis of cost-effective analysis)? Should it be left to individual responsibility?' (Hermans & den Exter 1998). Overall, while more explicit evidence bases, processes and criteria were adopted in all countries, societal values remained an important facet of decision-making.

The 1990s also saw the rise of the evidence-based medicine movement. Begun in part as epidemiologists calling clinicians to account for the effectiveness and efficiency of medical interventions, the notion of evidence-based practice and policy has quickly filtered through to all parts of the health system. The Cochrane Collaboration is comprehensive in its coverage of health care, in reviewing and promulgating the evidence base to improve health-care practice. Recognising the potential influence of the Cochrane approach, consumers and their representatives who have become a part of the health policy landscape have also ensured that consumer issues and perspectives are incorporated into the international Cochrane network. Given the extent to which consumers have been involved in the Australian health system, it is perhaps not surprising that Australians take lead roles in the Cochrane Consumers and Communication Review Group and the Cochrane Consumer Network.

While much of the priority-setting debates have been focused on personal health care, there are similar challenges in allocating finite resources (human and financial) for interventions aimed at prevention at the population level. Two examples illustrate the complexity of bringing diverse stakeholders together for shared decision-making, and point to the importance of both a credible evidence base and a well-managed process for decision-making. In an initiative of the National Public Health Partnership, key stakeholders in food and nutrition—ranging from governments to industry to professional organisations and consumer representatives—were brought together. They were presented with epidemiological and economic data about the impact of poor diet for Australia, and possible benefits that could result from increased consumption of fruits and vegetables. Tools for priority-setting which more explicitly recognised stakeholder values and participation were shown to be useful for developing a shared understanding of the decision-making contexts for each of the stakeholders and exposing the complexity involved in choosing a preferred intervention strategy. They enabled agreement to be reached about shared intervention goals and objectives, priority target groups, criteria for choosing interventions, and ultimately a portfolio (or mix) of intervention activities (NPHP & SIGNAL 2000). In an AIHPS project on citizen engagement in chronic disease prevention and health promotion, funded by VicHealth, deliberative forums were held in rural and metropolitan Victoria to look at prevention priorities and tradeoffs between prevention and treatment. Community members first responded to hypothetical policy scenarios—designed to be controversial and encourage discussion. Next, they learned about the realities of implementing prevention policies from an experienced public health professional and

---

Box 17.5 Cochrane Collaboration

The Consumers and Communication Review Group is responsible for the preparation and maintenance of reviews on how best to communicate with people about their health and health care. The group is based in the Faculty of Health Sciences at La Trobe University in Melbourne and is funded by the Victorian Government Department of Health and the NHMRC. The group's reviews fall under six broad communication categories:

- interventions directed to the consumer
- interventions from the consumer
- interventions for communication exchange between providers and consumers
- interventions for communication between consumers
- interventions for communication to the health-care provider from another source
- service delivery interventions.

Source: Centre for Health Communication and Participation (2012).

Box 17.6 Cochrane Consumer Network (CCNet)

CCNet supports a consumer perspective on Cochrane reviews and other activities within the Cochrane Collaboration because it believes that such 'consumer participation aids the development of high-quality and relevant systematic reviews and these can actively inform evidence-based practice in health care with effective dissemination'. The Cochrane Collaboration invites consumers to work collaboratively with health-care providers and researchers in order to:

- ensure review questions are relevant to people requiring health care who are offered an intervention by their health-care provider
- identify outcomes from health-care interventions that are important for consumers—which may be different from outcomes identified by service providers
- improve access to reviews by ensuring that reviews can be read by a wide audience and that the language is sensitive to consumers
- weigh up the benefits of a health-care intervention against the potential harms—from the perspective of health-care users
- prioritise topics for new reviews.

    CCNet also provides support to consumers in several ways:

- It provides means of communication for consumers through a Facebook page and a blog, as well as regular newsletters.
- It develops training materials and workshops to facilitate effective consumer participation.

Source: Cochrane Consumer Network (2012).

discussed a number of issues. Finally, they worked within a fictional budget to make resource allocation decisions (AIHPS 2009).

For all the technical developments related to decision-making, the questions of governance—Who should participate and how should they be accountable?—have yet to be resolved. Differences in views exist. For example, Daniels and Sabin (2002) argue that continuing to try to develop the correct set of priority-setting principles with appropriate weights will not contribute much to the problem of resource allocation. They believe that there is little chance of a consensus developing on the proper balance between competing principles. Instead, they argue for an acceptable, fair process for setting limits. For them, a fair process would mean that:

- decisions, and the grounds for making them, must be public
- the grounds for decisions must be seen as relevant by fair-minded people
- the decisions must be subject to revision and appeal
- the process must be governed by some type of regulation.

Political policy, health policy or public health policy?

The issues of who participates, who decides and whose priorities dominate in decision-making are based on the notion that resources are scarce. But who decides how much of GDP should be spent on health care? Is the 17.9 per cent spent in the United States more beneficial than the 8.7 per cent spent in Australia? In a similar vein, what is the right percentage of GDP to be spent on education, the environment or defence? Harvey (1974) raises the question of whether the size of the pie really is finite, and whether resource scarcity is real and absolute.

From a public health perspective, given the importance of non-health sector influences on health outcomes, the resource allocation tradeoff between health and other sectors becomes an important policy question. This concept of allocative efficiency refers to where the investment should be made to maximise health gain. However, not every minister in a government, nor every group within the community, will make decisions that have regard to health outcomes as a key criterion. Even health professionals may have greater regard for their own interests, and so focus on the development of health services institutions, rather than public policies that promote health and well-being.

In the face of the political nature of public health policies and programs, experts have attempted to develop technical tools for priority-setting—such as the various methods of economic evaluation and burden of disease analyses. Despite the availability of these tools, decision-making remains an art form, and technical tools have yet to take the place of political processes and judgement calls. The inherently political nature of public health decisions means that policies, strategies and programs are likely to receive support when the technical solution fits the political solution.

Stakeholder analysis and the involvement of stakeholders in priority-setting and decision-making processes become central issues for public health governance. The argument in support of community involvement can be made either on equity or human rights grounds—that people, particularly those with weak voices in the community, have a right to have a say. The argument can also be supported on political and/or utilitarian

---

Box 17.7 Citizens' juries: A new approach to participation?

As many Australians seem to have a growing interest in being involved in decision-making about what health-care services are provided and where, the idea of citizens' juries is emerging. The choice of jurors is based on random selections of individuals from electoral rolls. They are asked to make decisions for the whole community, rather than for themselves. The evidence presented to these juries must be balanced, and sufficient time must be allowed for discussion and decision-making. They differ from 'health consumer advice' (usually patients with a particular interest) because the juries are composed of a cross-section of the community (such as actual and potential patients, taxpayers and people with private health insurance), and hence are more likely to bring the values and interest of the whole community into their decision-making (Mooney & Blackwell 2004).

A citizen's jury on health priorities was conducted in 2010 in the ACT at the request of the territory Health Minister, to advise her on community priorities for health services spending. The facilitator, a health economics professional, had experience in conducting juries and had undertaken research on them. Jurors were addressed by a panel of expert witnesses who provided them with factual information about the ACT health system and health challenges. Issues of interest to jurors were the health status of the ACT population, the differences in health and life expectancy of different groups and the scope of services provided by ACT Health. Following the presentations, jurors began determining their priorities in health with guidance from the facilitator about principles to apply to determine priorities.

Overall, the jury developed a broad consensus that ACT Health should focus on the health and quality of life of the population overall; prioritise equity over efficiency and have added concern for children, Aboriginal people, people living in poverty and people suffering mental illness; emphasise illness-prevention and health-promotion but avoid blaming people for their health conditions (e.g. obesity); ensure both health services and individual health professionals communicate better; rebalance spending on hospitals by increasing spending on community-based health services; cut expenses in some areas in order to spend more on critical services, explaining decisions and tradeoffs to the public clearly; and avoid introducing inequitable user fees to boost public health service provision.

Sources: ACT Health (2010); Mooney & Blackwell (2004).

grounds—that involvement will produce more acceptable, more sustainable and more implementable programs.

The contested nature of public policy and public health policy means that policy advocacy skills are crucial for public health professionals—including understanding government processes, being able to work with the media, building coalitions of groups with similar views and so on. Judgements will be required about when to engage from within the system, and when to build coalitions to lobby from outside.

Since the late twentieth century, opportunities for citizen participation in policy-making and program management have increased. To be effective, community representatives will require skills in order to ensure that the outcomes of these processes truly serve the interests of the health of the public.

Evolution of public-sector management in the 1990s and beyond: New possibilities and partnerships

Given the importance of government in the funding and provision of public health services, frameworks for public administration are important for how public health programs are delivered. The shifts that occurred in the public administration framework during the 1990s, with the introduction of new public-sector management, are particularly important. At the more fundamental level, these shifts also represent new thinking about the changing roles of state, market and civil society.

Concepts and buzzwords like 'steering not rowing', 'small government', 'contract management', 'unit-cost funding', 'purchaser–provider split' have, over the last two decades, signified a shift from the expectation that government will provide for the population to a plurality of service provision arrangements that rely on private-sector and community-based organisations. For many public health advocates, the reformist

language, the microeconomic reforms and the policy drive to improve technical efficiency have been unpalatable—as if human needs were not being valued. There is an argument to be made that, if resources are limited, it is an ethically appropriate position to take to ensure that all available resources are used to their maximum effect. The question remains, though, of who determines the priorities and resource allocation decisions.

The language of public administration has started to shift again in the early part of the twenty-first century—to such concepts as 'social inclusion', 'community strengthening', 'social capital' and 'partnerships'—and there is a continuing trend towards greater involvement by community and private-sector organisations. Government continues to adopt a role oriented towards strategic direction rather than direct service provision.

Hess and Adams (2002) suggest that public administration evolved over the twentieth century from a focus on manuals and forms in the 1930s, to planning and policy in the 1960s, then to management and contracts in the 1990s. These trends can be seen in the ways in which public health programs were managed and delivered.

Hess and Adams (2002) also suggest that the body of knowledge that has underpinned these developments has shifted from law and history, to social science, then to public-choice theory. The major tools adopted by administrators have moved from regulation, to program planning, to competition. These trends and features are shown in Table 17.1.

They further suggest that changes in the relationship between markets, states and communities at the dawn of the twenty-first century are placing new demands on governments. They predict that the policy-making world will shift away from searching for the 'right' definition of ideas and applying objective knowledge to the rational pursuit of policy objectives. Instead, the policy process will entail a fluid movement of ideas emerging and shifting as they are debated across policy networks. This fluidity will require a

Table 17.1 Evolution of public administration

	1930s	1960s	1990s	2020?
Character	Manuals and forms	Planning and policy	Management and contracts	Knowledge and energy fields
Core subject	Constitutional law	Policy analysis	Management	Brokering meaning systems
Body of knowledge	Law, history	Social science (deductive, positivist)	Public choice (inductive, empirical)	Interpretive
Unit of resourcing	Functional sphere	Programs	Individual outputs	Public service outcomes
Problematic	Administration	Poverty, employment	Legitimacy	Coherence of economic, social and human capital
Main tool types	Regulatory budgeting	Planning, management	Competition, productivity	Sustainability, deliberation
Organising focus	Bureaus	Programs	Output groups	Networks

Source: adapted from Hess & Adams (2002: 68).

constant search for new ideas and approaches, and for new intellectual foundations for public administration and policy-making.

Evaluating public policy?

As governments have begun to take a more integrated approach to health and development, a new approach known as health impact assessment (HIA) is being used to evaluate social, economic and environmental policies. HIA can be defined as 'a combination of procedures, methods and tools by which a policy, program or project may be judged as to its potential effects on the health of a population, and the distribution of those effects within the population' (European Centre for Health Policy 1999: 4). HIA has its origins in environmental impact assessment (EIA). Traditionally, EIA has only evaluated the negative physical and natural impacts of projects, so HIA has developed to give a structured consideration to the positive impacts on human health (enHealth 2001).

An HIA should take place early enough in the development of a policy or project so as to permit changes or modifications to be incorporated in the implementation process, but late enough so that a clear idea of the nature of the policy or project is available. In other words, an HIA should be able to maximise the positive benefits and minimise the negative impacts on the health of a defined population (Scott-Samuel 1998).

There are two basic categories of HIA: a tight (rapid) focus, which is retrospective, technocratic and concentrates on the quantitative aspects of public health (that is, the risks involved) and is applied as a corrective measure to existing health inequalities; and a broad (comprehensive) focus, which takes a holistic approach to health policy, places an emphasis on the social determinants of public health, welcomes input from the community and stakeholders and is applied as a forecasting device (Mahoney & Durham 2002). While there is no formally agreed manner in which to conduct an HIA, the core elements include screening, scoping, appraising or assessing, developing evidence-based recommendations, having further discussions with policy-makers, and then conducting ongoing

Box 17.8 Rapid HIA of town centre street redevelopment

As part of the strategic policy of Queensland Tropical Population Health Services to work with local government in order to facilitate the creation of healthy physical and social environments, a rapid HIA was undertaken on Townsville's Flinders Street Redevelopment concept planning documents. Staff from the state Health Promotion and Environmental Health Services worked together with Townsville City Council staff and expert advice was provided by the Centre for Health Equity Training, Research and Evaluation. The process involved cross-sectoral work as the city council staff involved were from the council street redevelopment project team as well as staff from council's Community and Environmental Services. Recommendations were developed as a result of the HIA, aimed at enhancing health outcomes for residents and visitors who accessed the city centre area.

The decision had been made to reintroduce traffic access to the town centre in order to improve access for residents and visitors to the heart of the city. This decision raised concerns about the possible negative health impacts in relation to safety and equity, access for all ages and abilities, social connectedness, and participation and identity. The redevelopment of the street was also seen as an opportunity to address some existing health needs in the local community. Interviews and workshops were conducted with key informants, including council project design staff as well as environmental health staff, and a community consultation was conducted in relation to the street redevelopment. A literature review was also conducted, and evidence in relation to addressing the social and environmental determinants of health through urban design was used to inform the findings of the HIA. The proportion of the Indigenous population was noted to be higher than the state average and, while breastfeeding rates were noted to be low statewide, local breastfeeding facilities were noted to be sub-standard. The local population was noted to be ageing, with the proportion aged over 85 years increasing at the fastest rate.

The findings of the HIA extended across three themes: safety and security; identity and sense of place; and health-promoting and sustainable environments. Recommendations to improve safety and security included the use of community streetscape design to promote access and participation for all ages, abilities and population groups via walking, cycling and public transport use; and using pedestrian friendly design, increased lighting and shade and active street fronts—such as street cafes near bus stops. A participative planning approach was recommended to address the possible health impact on identity and sense of place, engaging with key community groups and stakeholders to develop interpretive signage and public art. To address the impact on environmental determinants of health, design features were recommended, including provision of bicycle parking, alteration of the bus route so as to travel through the reopened mall, provision of pedestrian links to neighbouring destinations and railway stations, and the use of a comprehensive partnership approach to increase access to healthy food in the town centre.

Source: Population Health Queensland (2008).

monitoring and evaluation (Health Development Agency 2002).

While HIA has been part of the Australian public health agenda for several decades, it has been embedded in the EIA process rather than being used as a tool in decision-making. Following the NHMRC recommendation that an HIA be incorporated into the environmental decision-making process, the Tasmanian government passed legislation in 1996 stating that all proposed developments requiring an EIA must provide an HIA. This includes activities that exhibit characteristics such as causing possible changes in the demographic or geographical structure of a community, increasing the potential for individuals to be exposed to hazardous products and processes or contaminants, increasing traffic flows that will increase the risk of injury, and environmental changes that will impact on disease vectors and parasites. In this context, HIA is being used as a decision-support tool, as it is part of the EIA process, which means that health authorities can only provide advice to the responsible statutory body. The Tasmanian experience of HIA embedded in the EIA process has been used as the basis for the EnHealth HIA guidelines (EnHealth 2001).

Over the past few years, the application of HIA to programs and projects has moved away from its original risk assessment/health protection model to an application within the actual policy process based on the determinants of health. In Australia, a two-year research project has resulted in:

> the development of an equity focused health impact assessment framework that can be used to determine the unanticipated and systemic health inequities that may exist within the decision making process or activities of a range of organisations and sectors (Mahoney et al. 2004: 1).

An equity-focused health impact assessment (EFHIA) is concerned with equal access to services for equal need, and allows policy-makers to focus on the specific needs of the most vulnerable and disadvantaged groups within society. An EFHIA therefore seeks to identify and assess those health differences that result from factors which are both avoidable and unfair, and then suggest ways in which a policy can be amended or improved before it is implemented (Mahoney et al. 2004).

The implementation of the use of HIA in the health system in New South Wales is under development. A review completed in 2008 in the state Population Health Division and Area Health Services found that processes need to be identified that will ensure HIA is prioritised as a core business

activity. The review also recommended that HIAs need to be operationalised at the organisational level and supported with policy at the state level, as well as being aligned with WHO social determinants of health. Ongoing funding and workforce capacity-building was necessary, with consideration being given to cost-effectiveness (CHETRE 2008).

Working in partnership?

From the late 1990s onwards, the notions of partnership and collaboration became more important as communities and citizens reacted against the decade of neo-liberal reforms. These notions also sit comfortably with public health principles—that the achievement of better health requires working across sectors.

Common forms of collaboration include:

- **network**—organisational links that facilitate the exchange of information for mutual benefit
- **coordination**—organisational mechanisms or processes that require altering some common activities in order to achieve a common purpose and mutual benefit
- **cooperation**—organisational commitment to share resources for a common purpose and mutual benefit
- **collaboration**—risks and responsibilities, resources and rewards being shared by organisations, which results in enhancing the capacity of each partner to achieve defined objectives (Himmelman 1996).

Walker (2000) suggests that there is a continuum for collaboration. At the loosest level of information-sharing, networking meetings between organisations or professionals in various program areas may be a way of increasing mutual awareness and shared problem definition. Joint working parties between programs or organisations on shared concerns may be the next step in arriving at shared solutions or coordinated action. Joint planning is another step towards securing ongoing collaboration, as operational plans may be linked, resources shared and continued interaction planned. Programs and organisations may wish to proceed into formal coordination arrangements, whereby services may be provided jointly on a contractual basis and the institutional relationships defined through binding agreements.

The achievement of successful partnerships rests on some preconditions, as well as on the hard work of building and maintaining relations. Six factors have been identified as critical conditions for an effective partnership:

- **necessity**—agreement that a partnership is useful
- **opportunity**—receptivity for partnership to occur
- **capacity**—organisational ability to carry through
- **relationship**—clear definition of organisational links for achieving the purpose of the partnership
- **planned action**—agreement on clear roles and responsibilities as well as activities
- **sustained outcomes**—the existence of a system to monitor progress and achievements (Harris et al. 1995).

Recognising the importance of partnerships in health-promotion work, VicHealth has developed a resource for use by organisations entering into or working in a partnership. The partnerships analysis tool outlines three activities organisations can undertake to explore the nature of partnerships, to help embed partnerships as an ongoing way of working and to reflect on the partnerships they have established, and to monitor and maximise their effectiveness (VicHealth 2011).

Conversely, the major variables, or potential barriers, that impact on the success of building and sustaining a partnership are:

- **people in structures**—leaders who are not able to search for mutual benefit and focus on problem-solving

- **turf**—professional defensiveness and concern for administrative domains
- **structural complexity**—the number of organisations involved and asymmetry in resources and power
- **product diversity**—a large variation in the volume and range of activities or services
- **policy congruence**—divergence in basic objectives
- **planning capacity and philosophy**—disparities in skill level and timetables, and differing emphases on strategic versus operational issues (Challis et al. 1988).

Typically, intergovernmental collaboration occurs to resolve problems of blurred boundaries, to resolve policy disputes, to speed decisions or to develop consensus on new policies and programs (Gray 1989). Partnership between government and civil society—a crucial ingredient for successful public health action—is more difficult to achieve, given the power imbalances. Governments have financial resources, extensive information resources and administrative authority, and sharing these with non-government organisations is necessarily a learned behaviour.

Challenges in global health governance: Acting beyond national interests

Public health issues have moved from being local concerns in the nineteenth century to become global concerns in the twenty-first century. Public health action has evolved from being a matter for local government to requiring nationally coordinated policies and programs. Just as Australian states and territories are the members of Australian intergovernmental coordination mechanisms (such as the Australian Health Protection Committee and the Australian Population Health Development Principal Committee), governments around the world participate as member states of the WHO.

There are numerous economic and social activities spanning national boundaries that have implications for health (see Table 17.2 for examples). Such events as the destruction of the World Trade Center on September 11, 2001 and the SARS epidemic of 2003 have highlighted the interdependencies that countries have with each other, as well as the interrelationship between health and economic and social development. The United Nations held special General Assembly sessions on HIV/AIDS in 2001 and Children and the Environment in 2002, as well as a High-Level Meeting on the Prevention and Control of non-communicable diseases in 2011. In 2002, the Global Fund to Fight HIV/AIDS, Tuberculosis and Malaria was established. In 2003, the WHO revised international health regulations to address emerging and re-emerging diseases, including improving global surveillance and response to epidemics.

In the face of developments such as these, Lister, Lee and Williams (2003) suggest that the governance arrangements for global health need to be examined at:

- **the international level:** to develop a legal and regulatory framework for health as part of the UN Charter and examine the health impacts of trade, investment and migration
- **the national level:** to bring together government departments NGOs and private businesses

- **regional levels:** such as ASEAN and the European Union, to develop shared health policies.

Ingram (2003) suggests that not only would these activities involve government departments (Health Departments as well as other departments), but there is also a need to develop relations with civil society, to engage expert and stakeholder input, to develop interdisciplinary knowledge and skills, and to provide a public forum for community and business participation.

Beyond structures and participation, there remains the question of whether there are shared values that could underpin global decision-making about public health priorities. The principles used by Australian consumer representatives to lobby Australian governments have global relevance:

- **the right to satisfaction of basic needs**—food, clothing, shelter, health care and education
- **the right to safety**—protection against products, production processes and services that are hazardous to health or life
- **the right to be informed**—to be given the facts needed to make an informed choice, and

Table: 17.2 International social and economic activities and health

Domain	Specific activity	Health implications
Population movement	• Travel • People-smuggling	• Infectious diseases • Health risks to undocumented immigrants and refugees
Trade	• Promotion of 'modern lifestyle' products • Drug trafficking	• Increased tobacco use and consumption of prepared foods • Increased use of and addiction to illicit drugs
Armed conflict	• Displacement of people • Destruction of infrastructure	• Physical and mental trauma • Loss of health services; problems arising from lack of sanitation and clean water
Industrial development	• Environmental pollution • Inequitable distribution of wealth	• Poisoning and related chronic diseases • Poverty and health inequality

Source: elements drawn from Lee & McInnes (2003).

protected against dishonest or misleading advertising and labelling

- **the right to choose**—to select from a range of products and services offered at competitive prices with an assurance of satisfactory quality
- **the right to be heard**—to have consumer interests represented in the making and execution of government policy, and in the development of products and services
- **the right to redress**—to receive a fair settlement of just claims, including compensation for misrepresentation, shoddy goods or unsatisfactory services
- **the right to consumer education**—to acquire knowledge and skills needed to make informed, confident choices about goods and services, while having an awareness of basic consumer rights and responsibilities
- **the right to a healthy environment**—to live and work in an environment that is non-threatening to the well-being of present and future generations (Consumers' Health Forum of Australia 2001).

Kickbusch (2004) further suggests that public health advances at the global level will depend on recognition that health is a global public good, and that it is a key component of global security as well as a key factor of good business practice. Thus, global health governance involves not only the organisations (international, national government, non-government and private businesses) involved in the health sector, but requires all the international relations instruments available across sectors, along with a shared set of ethical principles focused on the notion of global citizenship.

Instruments for global governance range from voluntary codes to binding legislation. The International Code of Marketing of Breast-Milk Substitutes, adopted by the World Health Assembly in 1981 (see <www.who.int/nutrition/publications/code_english.pdf>) is an example of a voluntary code. Due to campaigning by the WHO, UNICEF and non-government organisations, the code was instrumental in drawing attention by governments and the public to marketing practices being used by infant formula manufacturers, and their consequent health damage in developing countries. Campaigns such as this have the potential to mobilise public opinion and action, thus creating pressure on governments to adopt regulations and on companies to adhere to them (Lutter 2012).

However, while voluntary codes have been effective in raising awareness, they are not enforceable, and therefore stronger governance instruments may be needed. The WHO Framework Convention on Tobacco Control (FCTC) is an example of an international treaty that binds governments to legislative action. The adoption of this enforceable approach was also built upon an active campaign by civil society groups in conjunction with several governments (see Box 17.9).

Conclusion: Making room for diverse voices

Government has traditionally been the key decision-maker for public health action, in framing appropriate societal responses and allocating resources. This chapter has raised the question of what the basis for decision-making should be, as well as asking who should participate in decision-making. Given the breadth of health concerns that call out for public health action, the complexity of society and the need for mobilisation of diverse resources, questions can be raised about whether traditional forms of government decision-making, with professional input, remain appropriate.

In the late twentieth century, debates arose about the appropriate role to be played by consumers and the community in health policy, and the extent to which decision-making should be centralised or decentralised. Over this time, and with the adoption of market-based reforms, public-sector management also evolved away from the top-down, command-and-control paradigm. New approaches

Box 17.9 The WHO Framework Convention on Tobacco Control (FCTC)

The WHO FCTC is an example of a global public action that has been designed to strengthen local, national and international coordination to combat the tobacco epidemic. While cigarette smoking is one of the major causes of preventable death in developed countries, the epidemic of disease is also rapidly shifting to developing and transitional market economies. The treaty was negotiated over a period of four years by WHO member states—and requires governments to implement restrictions on cigarette advertising, sponsorship and promotion; ensure that health warnings are put on packaging; establish clean indoor air controls; and legislate to stop tobacco smuggling.

The idea of an international convention for tobacco control began when Ruth Roemer (UCLA School of Public Health) and Allyn Taylor (University of Maryland School of Law) decided to apply the WHO's neglected constitutional authority to develop a treaty on any matter that affected global public health. Roemer promoted the idea at the first All-Africa Conference on Tobacco or Health (1993), and discussed it with senior staff members at WHO headquarters in Geneva and with tobacco control colleagues at the annual meeting of the American Public Health Association (APHA). One colleague, Judith Mackay, the director of the Asian Consultancy for Tobacco Control, supported their idea and was to become a key advocate for the convention.

Roemer and Taylor further promoted the idea at the Ninth World Conference on Tobacco or Health in Paris in October 1994, which saw the adoption of a resolution (drafted with the help of Mackay) urging the development of an international instrument for tobacco control. Shortly after this conference, Jean Lariviere, a Canadian delegate to the World Health Assembly, was contacted by a number of Canadians who had attended the Paris conference, expressing their support for the idea. With the backing of delegates from Mexico, Finland and Tanzania, Lariviere then drafted a resolution that was adopted—despite some objections by the WHO secretariat—by the 95th WHO executive board meeting in January 1996. The subsequent World Health Assembly voted to proceed with the development of 'an international instrument for tobacco control'.

But these initial efforts to support a global treaty lacked political support and policy direction. The turning point was the election of Gro Harlem Brundtland as the WHO director-general in 1998, because her two priorities were tobacco control and combating malaria. This meant that resources became available to turn the idea of a framework convention into a global public health movement. The tobacco industry opposed a comprehensive treaty—particularly the provisions for increased taxes on tobacco products, limitations on free trade and public smoking bans—and instead supported voluntary agreements and regulations. In 1998 and 2001, the APHA passed resolutions supporting a framework convention, while other non-government agencies offered strong support. Subsequent negotiations by WHO member states thus led to the 2003 World Health Assembly adopting the first international treaty under WHO auspices.

Source: Roemer, Taylor & Lariviere (2005).

to governance are now emerging, with greater partnership between the state, the market and civil society elements. This new framework is relevant for public health governance. Given the global scope of public health issues, the challenge for good public health governance will be to develop coordinated structures at multiple levels, and shared principles for decision-making. New forms of technology capable of mediating participation and decision-making present an interesting array of public health governance challenges that are yet to be fully explored.

18

Futures of public health:
Where to now for the organised effort?

Challenge

With energy costs rising steadily, Alison—88 years old and as hardy as they come—no longer used the air-conditioner in summer and only sparingly used the portable heater in winter. The cost of operating major appliances, lights and TV seemed to be high enough without running an electricity-hungry air-conditioner as well. There were numerous calls on her fortnightly pension, with electricity bills being only one of many. Like most of her peers, she lived on her own, took responsibility for managing her money and cut costs where she could. Her groceries were mainly 'no name' brands and she did all her own housework and tending of the garden instead of accepting home help from the local council.

Alison had heard the Weather Bureau's warning about a three-day heatwave and made sure she had plenty of food and milk in stock to avoid having to go out to shop during the intense heat. She had sweated through many city heatwaves over the decades, but felt that summers had become longer with more intense heat than when she was a child. Now, living by herself after her husband had died and her two adult children had moved away, she had worked out ways to keep cool in her inner-city weatherboard home. Despite her years of experience, Alison did not expect that her strategies to get through the high day and night temperatures would be insufficient if the heatwave continued on for over a week.

It was after being reminded by the evening news reader of the risks of heat to elderly people that Alison's neighbour knocked on her door to check on her. Receiving no response, he let himself in through the back door, only to discover Alison slumped in her chair. She stirred when she heard her name, but the neighbour was distressed to see that her eyes were sunken, she was listless and she appeared confused and disoriented. The temperature in the house was high and uncomfortable. Within a short time, thanks to the quick reactions of the neighbour, an ambulance had arrived and treatment for heat exhaustion and dehydration was underway.

This scenario flags some key issues for public health in the future, given the significance of global warming, energy scarcity and demographic changes. Will an organised approach be able to assure the fundamental determinants of health, such as safety in the face of extreme weather events? What instruments will be available to regulate market forces related to energy and other markets (such as food) in the interests of public health? Will the voices of vulnerable citizens be heard by multi-national industries in defining policies that set prices and assure access to essential services and goods?

Introduction

It is probably hard for children growing up in the first decades of the twenty-first century to imagine how their parents communicated and were entertained without the relatively recent technological innovations that are now all-pervasive, such as personal computers and the internet, DVDs, iPods, email and smartphones. Similarly, for those working in the health system in the 1950s, the rapid advances in technology and health interventions that have led to widespread changes and opportunities for health would have been unimaginable. Doctors training at that time would not have dreamt of CAT scans, MRI and laser technology, remote diagnostic technologies, interventional radiology, robotic surgery, organ transplants or even coronary bypass surgery. The elimination of dangerous diseases such as scarlet fever, polio or typhoid would have been an aspiration rather than a probability; indeed, where diagnosing these diseases would once have been commonplace, most medical personnel who trained in the latter part of the twentieth century in Australia would now not be able to recognise these diseases. Medical personnel today are regularly involved in treating older people with various conditions, such as cancers, cardiovascular diseases and other chronic diseases, which were not as familiar to their counterparts of past decades. Such

problems have long latency periods and are now revealing themselves because people are living longer. Preventing these problems was not a priority for health systems in the past because they were not as common in populations and we did not have adequate knowledge about causative factors and the role of exposure to risks early in life.

As discussed in the first chapter, George Rosen, the public health historian, notes that while health issues change (or are framed differently) over time, there are some constants about the field of public health (Rosen 1958). These relate to the way in which prevailing scientific and technical knowledge is turned into social and political action, to address whatever happens to be the health concern of the day.

Increasingly, though, the health concerns that deserve immediate interest are not only the problems facing present-day populations. Rather, they include issues whose significance only becomes clear when a long view—from a global perspective—is taken. 'Given the pace and scale of the changes unfolding in the twenty-first century, it is becoming essential to step up efforts to complement conventional techniques of risk assessment based predominantly on past observations with forward-looking approaches that give greater weight to likely future development.' (OECD 2003: 95)

While new health challenges require a changing

technical toolkit for public health action, there are also implications for the concept of governance and the role of the state in relation to public health. Conversely, changing assumptions and expectations about the role of government also lead to different strategies for tackling health challenges. Despite the changing issues, the fundamentals of public health are reaffirmed.

This chapter asks how public health practitioners can think about and track futures—the trends, scenarios and challenges, and possible ways forward. As the Challenge box at the beginning of the chapter illustrates, powerful driving forces are shaping public health in critical ways. Insights into them, and their potential ramifications, are needed to anticipate alternative futures and act in the interests of healthy futures. Are there ways in which we can anticipate and prepare for alternative futures—or even act to shape preferred futures? What is currently known about possible and plausible futures? How can we take this knowledge into account in decision-making from the local to the global level to pursue preferred futures?

Why think about futures?

Thinking about futures has probably always accompanied human existence in one way or another. It inhabits natural cycles of inquiry that can be triggered by fear (Will a pandemic such as the post-World War I 'Spanish influenza' happen again?), proactive efforts to prevent disasters (How can we avoid accidents at nuclear power plants in the event of natural disasters?) or secure achievements (How can we maintain social cohesion in this community over the next decades?). Scientists, journalists, bureaucrats, civil society leaders and community groups, academics and others have long communicated ideas about futures that reflect their role in society and the tools they have to gauge and interpret emerging phenomena.

In the public health field, quantitative and qualitative analyses of drivers of change and trends (social, technological, economic, environmental and political) are fundamental inputs to processes for designing strategies to achieve long-range public health goals. Gaining insight into how these trends interact and integrate to create different futures is also necessary—not just short-term futures that can readily be visualised, but long-term futures that are gauged in terms of trends, cycles and events over decades, even centuries. McMichael (2001) argues that this 'long view' is needed to decipher patterns in biological and ecological systems and to prioritise areas for action, and is thus critical to securing a healthy future for populations. For example, the perspective gained from analyses that span the centuries since humans gathered closely in social groups, grew their own food and herded animals has provided valuable insights for tracking down the origins of modern-day threats—SARS and avian influenza.

The long view is also needed because today's health issues do not remain within local boundaries: over time, they can amplify to become the concern of continents and regions. With the influence of globalisation (of markets, technologies, knowledge and culture), issues such as epidemics, terrorism and environmental concerns have expanded to have international as well as domestic implications (Marsh & Yencken 2004).

The current context for public health is characterised by rapid changes in almost every dimension of living and working, and in new threats and opportunities, thus motivating people to seek out ways to increase control, or at least reduce uncertainty about the future. At its simplest, thinking about futures can stem from a desire to reduce this uncertainty and aid present-day decision-making. Comparisons between 'now' and 'possible' or 'probable' or 'preferred' futures can then provide a powerful source of energy to act on preventing something from occurring or introducing steps to bring about a particular outcome. An emphasis on forecasting is not unanimously supported as the main goal of futures work; rather, 'the goal of futuring is not to predict the future but to improve it. We want to anticipate possible or likely future conditions so that we can prepare for them. We especially want to know about opportunities and risks that we should be ready for.' (Cornish 2004)

The concept of risk management—a major concern for those involved in governance—links futures work to a major concern of public health: that it is necessary to make efforts to predict, influence and minimise risks in the major systems on which society depends (energy, health, transport, environment, food, communications and so on) if population health is to be protected and improved.

The emerging dimension of systemic risks is shaped by the view to the future. A multitude of driving forces for change, trends, developments and obstacles are at work; in important ways, these will affect the nature of risks and the context in which they are managed. Thus, factors influencing the evolution of hazards and the vulnerability of systems over the next ten to fifteen years (and in some cases longer) are of great significance. But so too are factors that might modify the propagation of damage, or that affect the likely responses of institutions and the perceptions of the public (OECD 2003: 33).

Ways to think about futures: Guesswork or structured inquiries?

Structured ways of thinking about the future have been developing in the West since the mid-twentieth century through two main trajectories: industrial and military forecasting, and corporate, government and institutional strategy development (Bell 1996). The field of futures studies encapsulates a range of qualitative and quantitative analytic methods and approaches that can be used to create alternative perspectives on the future and can assist decision-making by assessing the implications of policies and actions. Highly accessible computer-based technologies—which permit access to information, ideas and people to an extent that is

unparalleled in history—have propelled futures studies in new directions in recent years. Global conversations about methods and depictions of the future are occurring, and studies can more easily engage experts, citizens and other groups from across the world. Thus, pan-national, cross-cultural and multi-generational insights can be brought into the process of thinking about the future.

Since 2000, the State of the Future Index (<www. millennium-project.org/millennium/SOFI.html>), for instance, has been produced annually by the United Nations' Millennium Project as a resource for decision-makers and educators. A 'global lookout panel' informs the process, and all continents are represented on the panel. It examines and summarises changes in a range of key variables and forecasts indicators. Progress is assessed in relation to fifteen global challenges constructed from key variables and forecasts that, when taken together, depict whether the future promises to be better or worse over the next ten years. Views from experts about the best and worst expectations and probabilities of specific developments are also obtained through a Delphi process. According to the index, the outlook for the future is getting *better* as a result of improvements over the past 20 years to the infant mortality rate and life expectancy at birth; food availability in low-income countries and the share of households with access to safe water; gross domestic product per capita; the adult literacy rate; women in parliaments; the percentage of the world's population living in countries that have free secondary school enrolment; HIV prevalence; and share of the population with access to local health care in the fifteen most populated countries. (Glenn & Gordon 2004, 2012) Despite the positive implications of these improvements for population health, there are no reasons for complacency: significant inequities are hidden in these generalisations and achievements can be eroded if political support, continued action and resources are not sustained. The index also shows complex and far-reaching challenges for public health posed by forces that are shown to have impeded improvement in relation to carbon emissions, the share of the population unemployed, loss of forestlands, the ratio of global average income of the top 5 per cent to the bottom 5 per cent, annual AIDS deaths and developing-country debt.

In the public health domain, structured inquiries about futures, beyond assessments of risks, are relatively recent inputs to policy-making and planning. These processes typically have drawn on methods that are bound to past contexts and events, such as epidemiological and economic forecasting, which are quantitative methods that are highly valued in the quest for evidence-based policy. While projects specific to public health have been few and far between, projects in fields regarded as key drivers of population health—such as the natural and built environment, social change and sustainability—represent valuable inputs to public health policy. Examples include foresight projects convened by the CSIRO on megatrends shaping life in Australia, energy futures, and environmental and economic challenges arising from our dependence on fossil fuels for transport (<www. csiro.au/Portals/Partner/Futures/Futures-Reports. aspx>). In recent years, the Prime Minister's Science, Engineering and Innovation Council's (PMSEIC's) Expert Forum on National Enabling Technologies Strategy has used foresight methods to identify challenges and opportunities arising for Australia from enabling technologies over the next five to ten years. The forum briefs policy-makers, regulators, industry and the broader community on future developments in this field of innovation, and informs other government agencies with an interest in emerging technologies about these findings. The PMSEIC has also investigated themes that have long-term importance for the country in general and public health in particular: food security and the energy–water–carbon intersection (PMSEIC 2010a, 2010b).

Inquiries into health futures need to analyse the wide range of driving forces that shape population health by altering the nature of threats and opportunities and the ways in which they are handled. Significant forces for change in public health include:

- **social factors:** social values, demography, education, housing, mobility, migration, social inequalities, education, literacy and health status
- **technological factors:** developments in information technology and telecommunications, and medical technology
- **economic factors:** demand and supply dynamics, employment, income and its distribution, inflation and consumer spending on resources for health
- **environmental factors:** ecological sustainability, resource-use patterns (such as energy) and their impacts, and transportation
- **political factors:** government stability, ideological climate and policy priorities.

Interactions between these forces will produce new opportunities for communication and action to improve population health. On the other hand, they will also 'modify usual hazards or create new hazards, change the way disasters and accidents spread and generate reactions, or amplify the vulnerability of vital systems' (OECD 2003) in societies and economies in the future.

Ways of constructing and communicating ideas about futures have expanded over the last few decades, and brought in the voices and perspectives of different groups. They have increasingly recognised the complex nature of life and change. Approaches have ranged from the superficial to deeper, multi-level approaches. 'Pop futurism' (Slaughter 1996) appraises and portrays interacting forces in forms of mass entertainment, such as fiction (George Orwell's *1984*), movies (*Mad Max*), music (David Bowie) and cartoons (*The Jetsons*). Intriguing images and concepts about the future are presented in these media, drawing on novel social and scientific innovations and forecasting changes to ways of living and environments. While very accessible, this form of futures work is often super-ficial and weakly grounded in theory and insight. It can shock people or provide interesting, fleeting ideas for conversations, such as scenarios about the long-term impacts of genetic engineering of animals or colonisation of space.

In contrast, other forms of futures studies provide deeper and more complex analyses of how forces interact to create trends, cycles and events (Inayatullah 2005; Slaughter 1996). They provide critical perspectives and delve into the dynamics of communities, organisations, cultures, indus-tries or societies to detect patterns and ways in which meaning is created, and to understand the dynamics of life and change. Depending on which methods are used, they might call on fields such as philosophy, psychology, studies of civilisations and macro-history to shed light on past patterns of thinking or behaviour and signify future conditions.

For example, the causal layered analysis (CLA) approach (Inayatullah 2002) seeks to uncover four levels of an issue or problem, and reveal new ways of thinking about or framing a problem, its contributing factors and solutions. The first level, 'litany', refers to a public description of an issue or problem (such as 'over-population'). The second level is concerned with systemic causes of an issue or problem (social, technological, economic, environ-mental and political). The third level, 'discourse' or 'world-view', considers the ideologies underpinning the causes (such as Indigenous, Western, Islamic, Confucian and feminist), and helps to reveal how a situation or problem has come to be framed in a particular way. The fourth level is that of the deep, socially constructed myths or metaphors that might be at the heart of an issue.

Applied to the issue of ageing in some Western societies, for example (Inayatullah 2003), the problem might be framed as 'older people are dependent, sick and alone' and an increasing burden on society. Systemic causes of this problem might relate to a combination of factors, such as social attitudes to getting older, media representations of the ageing

process and life in old age, access to preventive health care, taxation regimes, and government social and housing policies. The world views or ideology underpinning the ways in which the system operates and the framing of the problem might be charac-terised as 'ageing is a collective burden', while the fundamental myths or metaphors sustaining and giving meaning to the system might be related to notions that 'baby boomers are the problem—they have stolen from future generations'. Bringing about a positive change to the status of older people in future societies would then involve social processes that expose these layers of understanding and culti-vate myths and metaphors that embed more positive views of ageing and older populations.

The context, purposes and characteristics of futures work, as well as currently available tech-niques, are summarised in Table 18.1.

In public policy, approaches that apply input from recognised experts and formally collected data—quantitative and qualitative forecasts, scen-arios and expert-based statements—are commonly used, although the rationale for choosing them over other approaches is often obscured or not made explicit.

Projecting health futures: Anticipated challenges

In the health field, quantitative projections of trends are commonly used forms of futures inquiry. For example, in the planning of health services in Australia, projections about a range of issues are made as a basis for decision-making about service types and location, and resourcing matters, such as (Eager, Garrett & Lin 2001):

- incidence or prevalence of conditions
- behavioural and environmental factors that determine the health outcome
- factors that influence care-seeking behav-iour, including financial, household structure, socio-cultural, logistical and other variables

Table 18.1 The nature of futures studies

Current context (early twenty-first century)	Purposes of futures inquiry	Questions to explore the future	Characteristics	Futures techniques
• Increasing complexity • Rapid change • Increasing competitiveness • Increasing connectivity through networks • Knowledge orientation • Developing world is growing, younger and poorer • High levels of risk and uncertainty	• Raising issues of common concern that may be overlooked in the conventional short-term view • Highlighting dangers, alternatives and choices that need to be considered before they become urgent • Publicising the emerging picture of the medium-term future in order to involve the public in the decision-making process • Contributing to the body of knowledge related to foresight and the macro-processes of continuity and change that frame the future • Identifying the dynamics and policy implications of the transition to a sustainable world and placing them on the global political agenda • Facilitating the development of social innovations • Helping people to become genuinely empowered to participate in creating the future • Helping organisations to evolve in response to the changing global outlook • Providing institutional niches for innovative futures work	• What stays the same? • What are the major trends? • What are the most important change processes? • What are the most serious problems? • What are the main discontinuities? • What are the new factors 'in the pipeline'? • What are the main sources of inspiration and hope (social, technological, economic, environmental, political)?	• Trans-disciplinary • Complex • Global outlook • Normative • Scientific • Dynamic • Participatory • Decision analysis	• Trend exploration or analysis • Environmental/horizontal scanning • Cross-impact analysis • Delphi technique • Strategic conversations • Scenarios • Gaming, simulations and models, and environmental scanning • Time series forecasts • Trend impact analysis • Brainstorming

Source: adapted from Slaughter (1996).

Box 18.1 Knowledge needs in safety, compensation and recovery research over the next 25 years

The Institute of Safety, Compensation and Recovery Research (ISCRR) is a joint initiative of WorkSafe, the Transport Accident Commission and Monash University. In 2012, ISCRR designed and implemented the Futures Research Initiative to provide a rich information context and opportunity for debate among its stakeholders about knowledge needs in safety, compensation and recovery over the next 25 years. A staged approach to gathering and debating information used selected futures studies methods.

Information on national and global trends and futures writing across eleven areas of interest was gathered by a horizon-scanning project. From over a million references, the project selected fewer than 200 articles that considered trends and possible futures, and factors that shape them. The major themes considered in the articles were 'environmental crisis' and 'hi-tech new world' while the common underlying drivers were 'global cooperation' versus 'pursuit of sectoral interests' and 'proactive' versus 'reactive' approaches to the future.

These articles became the catalyst for the first stage in a stakeholder dialogue project—eleven online discussions (blogs) involving invited contributors. Outcomes of these discussions were analysed, and generated nine themes of critical significance to the future of safety, compensation and recovery:

- universal care and support for disability
- greater focus on non-financial needs, especially emotional needs, to reduce unintended harm of compensation schemes
- increased engagement with workers through the employment relationship and with clients through consumer empowerment in care systems
- broader ways of measuring success in improving the health of society—needing an evidence base
- new ways of assessing and managing risks—dealing with emerging risks
- new relationships (partnerships and collaborations): governments, NGOs, business, unions, workers and communities, including globally
- technological change paced by social change—reclaiming humanity
- diversity as the norm—equity as the challenge
- system integration.

The blog themes seeded discussions at a futures workshop convened at Parliament House involving a wide range of stakeholders. They contributed to the production of both optimistic and pessimistic scenarios for health, safety and compensation futures. The context of these scenarios was generally characterised as one of economic flux. The workshop then used a backcasting method to address the critical paths required to achieve participants' preferred scenarios in which prevention was the focus and partnership was the operating model. This process laid the groundwork for brainstorming research questions that could develop the knowledge needed to achieve a preferred future. Through a voting process, participants identified that the most critical research would focus on improving intervention policies and programs, ahead of developing new indicators of health, identifying future social issues, translating research more effectively and increasing the capacity of systems in research and program delivery.

The project concluded that, in each of these nine areas, there would be opportunities for developments at the global level and for those in Australian safety, compensation and recovery to inform and engage with each other.

Source: Fawkes et al. (2011).

- changes in technology and clinical patterns of care
- selection of provider, referral patterns and attitudinal factors affecting preferences for providers
- health expenditure and government budget outlays.

Internationally, the Global Burden of Disease study (Murray & Lopez 1996) projected trends through to 2020 in the burden attributable to a variety of diseases and conditions. These projections were based on a set of assumptions about the forces underlying disease patterns. The study anticipated some major changes in the prevalence of a variety of conditions, such as notable rises in neuropsychiatric conditions (such as depression) and conditions related to violence and war. Studies such as these shed light on emerging global agendas for health care as well as prevention and health promotion (see Table 18.2).

What the figures do not reveal is the rapid rate at which some epidemics are developing in some regions of the world—particularly HIV/AIDS and conditions arising from tobacco use. These are problems for which some countries have adopted effective containment strategies, but they remain

major challenges for other countries. The problem of newly emerging diseases (be they drug-resistant diseases or new forms of zoonosis, such as avian influenza) is not yet quantifiable, but it is already testing existing paradigms about disease prevention and control.

Changes are occurring at both the micro and macro levels—disease profiles are shifting as a result of changing risk factors within the context of large-scale changes in environment, society, economy and technology. Understanding the drivers of these changes and how to intervene to influence their positive impact on health is an essential public health activity. The addition of tools of futures inquiry to the existing public health toolkit facilitates broader and deeper analyses of what public health issues could lie ahead and what might cause or contribute to them. Work undertaken in different parts of the world has been valuable in highlighting the role of scenario development to portray integrated depictions of health futures, and raise important issues for health and associated policies at national and global levels. For example, Marten and Huynen's work (Box 18.3) has brought to the surface the question of how political will and leadership—combined with social, technological and economic means—can

Table 18.2 Disease burden measures in DALYs

Estimate 1990			Projection 2020		
Rank	Cause	% total	Rank	Cause	% total
1	Lower respiratory infections	8.2	1	Ischaemic heart disease	5.9
2	Diarrhoeal diseases	7.2	2	Unipolar major depression	5.7
3	Perinatel conditions	6.7	3	Road traffic accidents	5.1
4	Unipolar major depression	3.7	4	Cerebrovascular disease	4.4
5	Ischaemic heart disease	3.4	5	Chronic obstructive pulmonary disease	4.2
6	Cerebrovascular disease	2.8	6	Lower respiratory infections	3.1
7	Tuberculosis	2.8	7	Tuberculosis	3.0
8	Measles	2.7	8	War	3.0
9	Road traffic accidents	2.5	9	Diarrhoeal diseases	2.7
10	Congenital abnormalities	2.4	10	HIV infections	2.6

Source: Murray & Lopez (1996: 375).

Box 18.2 Health 2020: Queensland Health

In 2002, trends in health and health care were analysed to shape the Queensland government's vision for population health and the health system to the year 2020. Key trends investigated related to social, economic and environmental systems, scientific and technological knowledge and providing support for the growing and ageing population in a sustainable way.

According to the analyses, Queensland's population will increase in size, become older and be made up of more people from Asian backgrounds. Life expectancy will be 81 for men and 85 for women. Older people will account for around 17 per cent of the population. A greater proportion of the total population will be living alone, with up to a quarter of people aged 75 years and over likely to be living alone; most of them will be women. Almost one-third of children aged from birth to four years could be living in one-parent families.

Queensland's economic growth and workforce patterns will be influenced by lower birth rates and the ageing of the population. There will also be many changes to career patterns and conditions of work:

workers can expect seven career changes over a working life and more people will work in part-time or casual employment, with associated lower levels of income and job security. The widening gap between the rich and the poor will have significant implications for health.

Changes to the environment will impact on Queensland's population in the following ways. Changing weather patterns (including global warming) could set up conditions for existing communicable diseases (for example, malaria and dengue fever) to spread geographically and for new ones to emerge. Unstable weather patterns could expose more populated areas to natural disasters, such as cyclones. Ozone layer depletion might increase rates of development of skin cancer and cataracts. Diseases associated with air pollution, including respiratory problems, could increase in urban areas. Queensland's population, like the world more generally, could face a lack of safe drinking water and changes to food production patterns under the influence of global warming and unstable weather patterns.

Source: Queensland Health (2002).

Box 18.3 Potential future health strategies

Martens and Huynen (2003) propose that epidemiological health transition occurs through a sequence of stages that reflect shifts in the patterns and causes of death in countries.

Three stages of the health transition are evident in countries today. The first stage is the **Age of pestilence and famine**. It is characterised by the kind of mortality that has prevailed through most of human history. The second stage, which most developing countries are either in now or moving toward is the **Age of receding pandemics**. The prevalence of infectious diseases is reducing with a consequent fall in mortality rates. The third stage is the **Age of chronic**

diseases. Infectious diseases are eliminated, making way for chronic diseases to increase in prevalence, especially among elderly people.

Three possible futures are proposed as further stages of the health transition. Each country will follow its own route to the various 'ages', and this might involve stagnation or reversal of a country's status, depending on economic, political, social or environmental events and trends.

Three possible futures
• **The age of emerging infectious diseases or the re-emergence of 'old' diseases:** Changes in social, political and economic factors globally will bring about changes in trade, travel, microbiological

resistance, human behaviour, health systems and the environment that will be unfavourable to population health. Responses to increasing disease threats will be made difficult by resistance to antibiotics and insecticides, and inadequate or deteriorating public health infrastructures. These dynamics will lead to a drastic increase in infectious diseases and decrease in life expectancy (as is the case in many developing countries because of AIDS). Such patterns of ill-health will lead to lower levels of economic activity, which in turn will drive a downward spiral of environmental degradation, depressed incomes and poor health. Political and financial obstacles, and an inability to use existing technologies, will hamper infectious diseases control.

- **The age of medical technology:** While risks to health might arise from changes in lifestyle and environments, increased economic growth and technological improvements will offer new opportunities for health gain. If long-term, sustainable economic development does not become a reality,

increased environmental pressure and social imbalance might propel poor societies into the age of emerging infectious diseases. On the other hand, if a balance can be achieved between environmental and social resources and economic growth, sustained health might be achieved.

- **The age of sustained health:** Investments in social services will lead to significant and rapid reductions in lifestyle-related diseases and the eradication of most environmentally related infectious diseases. Health policies will be framed so that the health of future generations is not compromised by, for example, the depletion of resources needed by future generations. Although infections might emerge, improved worldwide surveillance and monitoring systems will lead to an effective and timely handling of any outbreak. Health systems will be well adjusted to an older population and disparities in health between rich and poor countries will eventually disappear.

Source: Martens & Huynen (2003: 899).

explicitly be harnessed so that developing countries 'leapfrog' to an age in which chronic diseases are less prevalent and sustained health is more possible.

Others have adopted a range of approaches to envision the future, often through more qualitative means, such as nominal group process or Delphi studies.

Gazing into public health futures: Preparing for tsunamis of change

Drawing together themes from the various projections, this section will briefly explore the signs of change to which Australian public health practitioners need to pay attention because of their implications for public health over the next several decades. In the tradition of George Rosen, these issues might not be regarded as mainstream public health issues at present (or public health issues at

all), but they are likely to become the issues of the future, and certainly will demand a public health approach to their resolution.

New issue: New forms of health care

The first issue concerns the new forms of health care that are emerging in various societies as a result of multiple drivers of change. Future-gazing about health care identifies many intriguing possibilities that could play a role in an organised approach to improving the health of current and future populations and preventing and managing specific diseases and conditions.

Central to the new forms of health care are innovations in diagnostic and communications technologies. People living in modern societies are already able to experience many forms of health care that were once only imagined, such as diagnostic services that can be delivered in the home, from distant locations, even from different countries, using communications and health-care technologies. The future of emergency health care as well as chronic illness care will be strongly influenced in this way.

The boundaries of early intervention are being stretched, and prevention opportunities expanded, by epigenetics. This is the study of gene activity changes (not arising from changes in the underlying primary DNA sequence) that are heritable. The epigenome is cellular material located on top of the genome that governs the expression of genes. Environmental factors like diet, stress and the nutrition of women prior to pregnancy can impact on genes through epigenetic marks, and these are then passed to the next generation. In 2004, the US Food and Drug Administration first approved an epigenetic drug that treats people with a group of rare and life-threatening malignancies by quelling the activity of genes in blood precursor cells. Other diseases with a genetic component (such as cancer, diabetes, autism and Alzheimer's disease) could in future be prevented by 'turning off' the relevant epigenetic markers.

Brain research and precision medicine are other domains where the outcomes of multi-year research investments are potentially game-changing. Where once it was thought that the brain was 'hard-wired' and (unlike the mind) not able to change, the discovery of new neural tissue in the brain region responsible for memory led to new work exploring

---

Box 18.4 The new frontier in clinical care: Personalised medicine

Ms H is a 35-year-old woman from Japan who has had a cough for three weeks. Her physician sends her for an x-ray and CT scan that reveal an advanced lesion, which a biopsy confirms to be non-small-cell lung cancer. She has never smoked. Can anything be done for her?

Had Ms H's cancer been diagnosed before 2004, her oncologist might have offered her a treatment to which about 10 per cent of patients have a response, with the remainder gaining a negligible survival benefit and experiencing clinically significant side-effects. But her diagnosis was made in 2011, when her biopsy tissue could be analysed for a panel of genetic variants that can reliably predict whether the disease will respond to treatment. Her tumour was shown to be responsive to a specific targeted agent, the administration of which led to a remission lasting almost a year; her only side-effect was a rash.

This scenario illustrates the fundamental idea behind personalised medicine: coupling established clinical–pathological indexes with state-of-the-art molecular profiling to create diagnostic, prognostic and therapeutic strategies precisely tailored to each patient's requirements—hence the term 'precision medicine'. Recent biotechnological advances have led to an explosion of disease-relevant molecular information, with the potential for greatly advancing patient care. However, progress brings new challenges, and the success of precision medicine will depend on establishing frameworks for regulating, compiling and interpreting the influx of information that can keep pace with rapid scientific developments. In addition, we must make health-care stakeholders aware that precision medicine is no longer just a blip on the horizon—and ensure that it lives up to its promise.

Ultimately, precision medicine should ensure that patients get the right treatment at the right dose at the right time, with minimum negative consequences and maximum efficacy. But it will change how medicine is practised and taught, and how health care is delivered and financed. It will change the way in which research and development are financed and regulated. It will deeply affect public trust and the nature of the patient–clinician relationship, and it will require unprecedented collaboration among health-care stakeholders.

Source: Mirnezami, Nicholson & Darzi (2012).

the potential for psychosocial interventions to produce therapeutic effects. This heralds myriad possibilities for revising standard approaches to mental health care practice for conditions including anxiety and panic disorder, as well as for individuals and communities pursuing wellness through meditation and similar strategies. Precision medicine is coming to the fore, with prospects for changing the practice, delivery and financing of health care.

As well as technologies, prominent drivers of change of future health care are the values, expectations, characteristics and capacities of patients and the public. Health-care consumers of the future are predicted to be better informed, more educated, more time-pressured, more affluent, less deferential to authority and professionals, more aware of what they can compare their health system against, and more demanding of control and choice (Horey & Hill 2005). When one considers that in some countries there has been an exponential increase in the use of the internet for health-care matters by consumers and a huge growth in the number of health websites, it is clear that access to health information is on the rise. Whether this information is of high quality, relevant to specific consumers or able to be understood and acted upon are salient issues.

Health-care consumers in the future, with the benefit of greater access to information and experience and as consumers of many other goods and services, will expect the health-care system to be capable of providing:

- highly accessible, safe, high-quality treatment that rapidly takes up effective new technologies
- an integrated, connected approach that features more proactive primary care services
- services where there are effective links and good communications between the different parts of the service and beyond
- a patient-centred service that responds to people's individual needs and offers choice regarding accommodation, services, timing of treatment and range of treatment. (Owen 2002).

While these expectations might not differ in nature from those of the present day, a challenge for health systems is how to use the possibilities offered by new and emerging medical and communications technologies to continually adapt system designs and models of care to meet the expectations and needs of health service users. The use of social marketing and social media is coming to the fore in many areas of health, and is improving the effectiveness of prevention strategies. Vaccination reminders to teenagers and parents and reminders to women that they are due for a pap smear or mammogram are coming via SMS and other alert systems. Disaster preparedness at the community and household levels is also being set up to utilise the versatility of social media for increasing reach and responsiveness.

Key trends will continue to change what health-care services can be offered in modern societies in the next two decades and how, by whom and where they can be delivered (Dargie 2000; Owen 2002). The practice of integrative medicine (combining orthodox Western medicine with a range of complementary and alternative health-care practices) will increase and gain more policy attention. New technologies—and their more rapid diffusion—will enable more people to access remote diagnostic services, computer-mediated counselling and social support, and home-based health monitoring; track personal health histories; take charge of health-care decisions; and receive and give social support in cyberspace. The use of new technologies to provide services—such as radiology, other diagnostic services and counselling for consumers with psychiatric conditions—will benefit people living in rural and isolated locations in particular, as well as people who are housebound. Such trends will influence the continuity and timeliness of care, types of providers, consumers' choices among providers, and the size and composition of the health-care workforce.

A greater focus on prevention in the health-care system will be possible, with more tailored drugs available to treat the risk of disease and greater access to quality health information, accessible via personal computers and mobile technologies. As drug therapies and other technologies improve and more diseases are treated as chronic rather than acute conditions, there is likely to be an increasing prevalence of some diseases.

Technical availability of a variety of ways of creating human life, including cloning and genetically altered 'designer babies', will raise fundamental and complex ethical and moral issues for populations to confront.

Emerging international developments—such as free trade agreements, the harnessing of indigenous knowledge and traditional medical practices, and new directions in pharmaceutical research and development—will present complex challenges to public health systems in future decades, especially in terms of developing an organised approach to ensuring timely access to treatment regimes for all segments of the population.

Longer-range speculations, illustrating the merging of social and technological innovations—such as molecular nanotechnology, biotechnology, information technology and cognitive science—present an even greater scope in terms of opportunities for and challenges to the organisation of public health systems. While the difference these technologies could make to human lives is impressive, crucial privacy, ethical and moral questions will need to be framed and debated. For example, literacy (health literacy in particular) and disadvantaged living conditions are likely to act as 'social brakes' on enabling people to access and benefit from health-care technologies. These technologies might contribute to enhancing overall population health status, but they simultaneously increase inequities between population sub-groups.

Some of the questions implied by these developments for the organised public health effort are:

• Can these technologies be harnessed to ensure that equitable access to health care is improved?

• How might the health-care system be differently organised and financed at the global and national levels?
• Which technologies are most likely to bring greatest benefit, such that they should now receive accelerated support?
• How should workforce training be modified to take account of these developments?
• What information systems do we need to monitor the distributional impacts (in terms of health risks, health outcomes and health services) of these new developments?
• What processes need to be in place to enable debate about ethical and moral issues associated with technologies and to develop guidelines for practice?

Nanotechnology (see Table 18.3) is one specific area of scientific innovation that raises a set of critical questions, and not only for health-care systems. Nanotechnology refers to the emerging range of technologies, techniques and processes that allow new materials to be built by moving and combining individual atoms and molecules at the scale of 1 to 100 nanometres into tiny mechanical, electrical and biological machines. (One nanometre is one billionth of a metre.) These materials will have new optical, magnetic, thermal or electrical properties. As such, they will have potential applications in numerous fields—materials and manufacturing, computer technology, aeronautics and space exploration, education, environment and energy, and biotechnology and agriculture (Gordijn 2003). Global investments in nanotechnology now total billions of dollars annually.

As with the silicon revolution that brought us personal computers and genetic engineering, which in turn brought us innovations in medical diagnostics and treatment, advances in nanotechnology raise numerous complex ethical issues. Ways of dealing with these issues lag behind technological developments. Claims that nanotechnology is a benign or overwhelmingly positive force for change compete

Table 18.3 Nanotechnology: The stuff of dreams—or nightmares?

Field of application	Types of application	Potential positives	Potential negatives
Developing world applications	Techniques to decontaminate water, repair environmental damage, produce cheaper medicines	Healthier living and working conditions, clean water, reduction of diseases associated with unclean living and working conditions	A 'nanodivide' between rich and poor nations
Surveillance and data gathering	Techniques such as implanted tracking devices, nanocameras and nanomicrophones	Improved delivery of business functions and services	Compromised privacy of individuals and organisations; enhanced potential for espionage
Defence	Techniques for chemical, biological and nuclear sensing	Better early warning of threats; defence capabilities	Personal and national security threats, such as an unstable arms race
Biotechnology and technology health care	Techniques that enable chemicals or viruses to be detected in bloodstream, physical composition of tissues to be changed and drugs to be delivered	Improved (including more precise) detection of causes of disease, disease processes, drug delivery and disease treatment	Risks to health, too invasive, medicalisation of normal human functions

Source: adapted from Gordijn (2003).

with suggestions that we need to be cautious about going too far, too fast in developing and applying the technologies. Political leaders are weighing in on debates about nanotechnology futures: 'The current work in nanoscience—manipulating and building devices atom by atom—is startling in its potential ... This kind of disruptive technology may create whole new industries and products we can't begin to imagine.' (Blair 2002)

Ethical and social questions raised by nano-technology have crucial equity dimensions. Who benefits from, and who could be harmed by, nanotechnology applications in the future? While some developing countries might benefit from the way it could improve living conditions, could nanotechnology ultimately entrench unequal distribution of wealth—and health—within and between developed and developing countries? Aspects of opposing sides of the debate presented in

Table 18.3 indicate the complexity and scope of the ethical debates ahead.

New issue: Globalisation and security

Globalisation is a major emerging issue that poses difficulties for policy-makers because it relates to numerous fields and is simultaneously positive and negative: 'It's just like electricity. If you put your finger in a socket, it's bad. But if you use it to plug in things that improve your wellbeing, it's wonderful ... It's a challenge for us all to make sure it all moves in the right direction.' (Anon 2001)

Such contradictions can be seen in relation to cultural globalisation. On the one hand, we are witnessing cultural homogenisation through many parts of the world, brought about through mass media and a greater exposure of cultures. On the other hand, the rise of fundamentalism and increased importance of identity politics suggest the separation of individuals from their cultural homes.

The same contradictions can be seen in terms of globalisation of trade. Feachem (2001) points out that economic growth arising from globalisation of trade has had positive impacts on population health, and has allowed action on human rights matters (such as oppression, corruption and genocide) to be coordinated at an international level. At the same time, increasing globalisation of trade has been accompanied by increasing threats to personal and national security.

The effects of globalisation can be seen in relation to most aspects of life associated with health: values and attitudes, products and lifestyles, practitioners and practices, places in which we live and organisations in which we work. Consequently, globalisation in its many forms poses numerous public health policy challenges because of the impacts of new connections 'among people; across states, in production networks and financial markets; between greed and grievance; among failing states, terrorism, and criminal networks; between nature and society' (Ruggie 2003). Public health implications of globalisation stem from features such as its 'footloose' capitalism, which demands increased labour mobility and the increased movement of populations through travel. Impacts include economic integration as well as polarisation (poverty and mobility), and an accelerated pace of change in social order at the national and local levels. Impacts on the health of

Box 18.5 Globalisation

According to Lee (2003), modern globalisation started in the 1960s as a range of technological innovations interacted with other changes to initiate significant transformations in patterns of human activity and the relationship between people and social and physical environments. This period is described as a 'turning point in the historical unfolding of globalisation processes, marked by such diverse events as the landing on the moon, increased use of transoceanic cables, satellite communications and other information technologies, spread of transborder production and consumption patterns, and the expansion of global organisations'.

Globalisation is now evident in terms of three dimensions:
- spatial changes (the movement of people, other life forms, information, capital, goods and spaces leading to new 'social geographies' and interactions)
- temporal changes (interactions are sped up by communications technologies and slowed down by complexities)

- cognitive changes (merging of, and possible future backlash against, cultures, wants, needs, values, beliefs, knowledge and aspirations).

As such, it represents a complex and constantly changing set of forces, bringing about changes in ways of living and working—and in population health—that are not necessarily apparent in the short term.

Lee (2004) calls for greater clarity of the nature of globalisation and an objective appraisal of its positives and negatives:

The church of globalisation is a broad one, and its denominational factions full of perceived sinners and saints, but lacking clear revelation of the future to lead us all forward. The health community needs to find a way into this debate without feeling overwhelmed by it. This means moving into unfamiliar territory and engaging in debate on subjects that have traditionally been seen as outside the health field ... Engaging with the globalisation debate is only the starting point. Adding informed voices, backed by sound evidence, about the value of promoting and protecting human health will help move the debate forward at a time when it is much needed.

Sources: Feacham (2001); Lee (2004: 158).

individuals, families, communities and populations stem from changes to these structural determinants of health, although they might not be discernible or measurable in the short term.

Globalisation has important implications for governance. Increasing trade and communication are giving rise to the changing role of nations and civil society organisations (such as trade unions and non-government organisations) and exposure to different forms of governance. The internet in particular is providing a vehicle of expression for previously unheard and new voices and associations, and influencing how governance processes, such as agenda-setting and decision-making, are performed.

As well, the locus of governance is undergoing change as a result of impacts from globalisation (Gilbert et al. 1996). In some countries, the number of people moving into cities is so large that 'mega-cities' are forming, such as Tokyo, Shanghai, Mumbai and Mexico City. By virtue of their population size (some have more than 10 million residents), roles as producers and consumers, and influence on social and environmental conditions, many cities (and their governments) are no longer side players but operate alongside nations as key global actors. In responding to local needs and competing interests and tensions, local governments are responding to global forces at work, but with the common good of the local community in view. All things considered, the importance—for both health and security—of effective governance at this *glocal* interface cannot be under-estimated.

Box 18.6 Framework Convention on Global Health

The Framework Convention/Protocol approach has become an essential strategy of trans-national social movements to safeguard health and the environment. The Kyoto Protocol to the UN Framework Convention on Climate Change sets specific levels for greenhouse gas emissions. The WHO Framework Convention on Tobacco Control sets global standards for reducing the demand for and supply of tobacco. The Framework Convention/Protocol approach is flexible, allowing states to agree to politically feasible obligations, saving contentious issues for later protocols. It enables a 'bottom-up' process of social mobilisation for health and health justice.

A global coalition of civil society and academics—the Joint Action and Learning Initiative on National and Global Responsibilities for Health—has formed an international campaign to advocate for a Framework Convention on Global Health (FCGH). It has been endorsed by the UN Secretary-General. The FCGH would reimagine global governance for health, offering a new post-Millennium Development Goals vision.

An FCGH would be a binding treaty using an incremental process whereby states negotiate a framework with key normative standards. More stringent obligations can subsequently be created through protocols. The FCGH creates fair terms of international cooperation to solve the defining global health issues in a more systematic and integrated way.

The FCGH envisions linkages between existing institutional structures and newly created ones: the WHO Secretariat, the Conference of Parties (implementing FCGH duties and drafting protocols), an inter-governmental panel on global health (facilitating and evaluating scientific research on innovative solutions) and a high-level intersectorial consortium on global health (placing health on the agendas of multiple sectors). The modalities of the FCGH would include defining national responsibilities for the population's health; defining international responsibilities for reliable, sustainable funding; setting global health priorities; coordinating fragmented activities; reshaping global governance for health; and providing strong global health leadership through the World Health Organization.

Source: Gostin (2012).

The consequent challenges for public health are enormous, and more than ever demand that an organised response, finely tuned and well resourced, is developed within and between nations and significant supra-national and international organisations. From harnessing communications technologies to modernising and harmonising international public health law, public health systems need to determine ways to adapt, based on known and possible futures.

Some of the issues to be considered in relation to the organised public health effort are:

- How do public health systems infiltrate the processes that shape the workings of globalisation with multiple, representative voices and authority?
- How can influential partnerships be forged with consumer and other social movements to construct and implement agendas for change?
- How might international treaties be used to ensure protection from the harmful aspects of globalisation, and to harness the benefits?
- What information systems do we need to track the impacts of globalisation?

New issue: Science, technology and environment

The domains of science, technology and environment are the traditional focus of future-gazing. The last 100 years have seen an unprecedented escalation in the ways in which basic and applied sciences have led social and cultural change.

In the twenty-first century, the emergence of 'mega-risks' has accompanied globalisation, presenting major dilemmas for science, technology and adaptability systems. The preface to the book *Emerging Risks in the Twenty-first Century: An Agenda for Action* (OECD 2003) refers to the series of large-scale disasters throughout the world in recent years, such as windstorms and flooding in Europe; new diseases affecting both humans (such as HIV and the Ebola virus) and animals (BSE); and terrorist attacks in the United States and elsewhere. Based on research into these developments and their drivers, the OECD (2003) suggests that these trends are likely to continue.

Research (for example, Allen Consulting Group 2005; McMichael 2001) continues to expose how ecological disturbances at the local level are leading to diseases that, through the influence of globalisation, become regional and global concerns:

- Emerging diseases are being traced to bats, horses, birds, pigs, cows and poultry.
- Dengue is spreading with the presence of mosquitoes at higher altitudes.
- Deforestation is becoming recognised as an early warning signal for poverty, population mobility and disease.
- Inappropriate use of antibiotics in health care, and in animal feed, is leading to multiple problems with drug resistance, as seen with such 'super bugs' as Vancomycin-resistant *Enterococcus* (VRE) and Methicillin-resistant *Staphylococcus aureus* (MRSE).
- Drug resistance is also a concern in relation to malaria, tuberculosis and VRE.

One of the most significant research developments in human history—the mapping of the human genome—was completed in 2003 and will present future generations with unparalleled opportunities to gain more certainty about their potential personal destiny, and that of their children. Gene therapy and genetic engineering hold immense power to reshape the nature of human life and force the most complex ethical, legal, social and religious questions on (perhaps ill-prepared) communities and societies. This case of scientific innovation has at its core numerous moral dilemmas that are confronting us now (see Box 18.7). Other dilemmas will emerge to confront future populations, such as what rights we have to genetically change ourselves and future generations into new species. Should society create 'future elite' populations by applying artificial intelligence technologies and genetic engineering? Should we genetically interfere with newborns or

Box 18.7 Societal concerns arising from the new genetics

- **Fairness in the use of genetic information:** by insurers, employers, courts, schools, adoption agencies, and the military, among others. Who should have access to personal genetic information, and how will it be used?

- **Privacy and confidentiality:** of genetic information. Who owns and controls genetic information?

- **Psychological impact and stigmatisation:** due to an individual's genetic differences. How does personal genetic information affect an individual and society's perceptions of that individual? How does genomic information affect members of minority communities?

- **Reproductive issues:** including adequate informed consent for complex and potentially controversial procedures, use of genetic information in reproductive decision-making, and reproductive rights. Do health-care personnel properly counsel parents about the risks and limitations of genetic technology? How reliable and useful is foetal genetic testing? What are the larger societal issues raised by new reproductive technologies?

- **Clinical issues:** including the education of doctors and other health service providers, patients and the general public in genetic capabilities, scientific limitations and social risks; and implementation of standards and quality-control measures in testing procedures. How will genetic tests be evaluated and regulated for accuracy, reliability and utility? How do we prepare health-care professionals for the new genetics? How do we prepare the public to make informed choices? How do we, as a society, balance current scientific limitations and social risk with long-term benefits?

- **Uncertainties:** associated with gene tests for susceptibilities and complex conditions (for example, heart disease) linked to multiple genes and gene–environment interactions. Should testing be performed when no treatment is available? Should parents have the right to have their children tested for adult-onset diseases? Are genetic tests reliable and interpretable by the medical community?

- **Conceptual and philosophical implications:** regarding human responsibility, free will vs genetic determinism, and concepts of health and disease. Do people's genes make them behave in particular ways? Can people always control their behaviour? What is considered acceptable diversity? Where is the line between medical treatment and enhancement?

- **Health and environmental issues:** concerning genetically modified (GM) foods and microbes. Are GM foods and other products safe to humans and the environment? How will these technologies affect developing nations' dependence on the West?

- **Commercialisation of products:** including property rights (patents, copyrights and trade secrets) and accessibility of data and materials. Who owns genes and other pieces of DNA? Will patenting DNA sequences limit their accessibility and development into useful products?

Source: Human Genome Project (2005).

---

embryos because their genetic code shows a high probability of anti-social behaviours? Should intelligent technological 'beings' be created that can compete for an ecological niche with humans or other forms of life (Glenn & Gordon 2005)?

In the midst of enormous commercial interest in exploiting the potential of genetic sciences, the need for regulation of gene technology requires public health systems to demonstrate vigorous leadership and to act in the interests of the common good. The ways forward to protect the public interest are not clear, however, and differing Australian policy responses can be seen in relation to food labelling and gene technology, for instance.

Technological innovations that until recently have developed largely in parallel are being used in combination with myriad applications by scientists. The merging of nanotechnology, biotechnology, information technology and cognitive science is of particular importance because their potential applications are so wide-ranging: from biometrics to counter-terrorism systems; from restoring brain functioning and eyesight to increasing longevity (Glenn & Gordon 2003). With the potential for their applications to benefit people in their daily lives as well as in health care, such innovations are being pursued with vigour by government and entrepreneurial private-sector bodies.

Some of the issues for the organised public health effort are:

• What forms of global governance should exist to ensure the applications of science and technology are used for the benefit of humanity?
• How can citizens be empowered to understand the risks and benefits, and to engage effectively in policy discussions and action?
• What information systems are needed to track possible causes of health problems and health consequences in the short and long term?
• In the light of the need for research that is integrative and interdisciplinary, what new research priorities and approaches should be pursued?

Becoming future aware: A first step in preparedness

New thinking for a new public health era

It is doubtful whether current paradigms for thinking about public health threats, risks, opportunities and action are adequate. This is demonstrated by the difficulties encountered in implementing integrated action on the risks described by the WHO as accounting for over one-third of premature deaths worldwide: underweight, unsafe sex, high blood pressure, consumption of tobacco and alcohol, unsafe water, sanitation and hygiene, iron deficiency, indoor smoke from solid fuels, high cholesterol and obesity (WHO 2002). Obstacles such as the separate working habits of disciplines and sectors and inadequate scaling up of proven small-scale interventions (Bammer 2005) have combined with resistance to target more fundamental social, economic and political factors to inhibit coordinated action.

The need for 'new thinking', as described by James Gleik (2012), as well as 'new thinkers', has never been more significant or pressing. Current tools for detecting, investigating, measuring and responding to present public health problems and possible futures take inadequate account of the cross-sectoral nature of health development. New thinking in public health is required to frame—and answer—fresh questions, such as: What precipitates change? How can we understand and apply our understanding of self-organising and emergent systems? How can we engage with complexity and work from the top down and bottom up, and with non-linear dynamics? Attempts to reduce complex questions to simple ones avoid the central dilemma that public health issues are constantly changing, but an organised approach to responding to them remains a priority goal.

Bammer (2005) suggests that a new specialisation of 'integration and implementation sciences' could help to tackle some of the enduring and new complex issues of the twenty-first century. It could support an organised approach to public health by scoping problems and issues in new ways, applying tools such as systems-based modelling and participatory approaches, and identifying the disciplines and sectors that need to be involved in bringing about change. Re-aggregating existing knowledge and understanding developed in various disciplines and practice arenas would be needed for framing both problems and solutions.

As well as new thinking, new tools and resources are required for an organised approach that is 'future aware'. The further development of public health systems could tailor the training of public health workers to equip them to consider and operate in conditions of uncertainty. Public health workers in the future will likely operate in an environment where international treaties and conventions increasingly will be used, so they will need skills and methods to influence governments around priorities and approaches, and to form trusted partnerships with novel constituencies to influence change. Information systems and knowledge management will need to be improved and democratised to empower partnerships and collaborations. Skills in using futures methods—particularly those that are useful to support integrated thinking, such as scenario planning and causal layered analysis—could be foundation skills for public health workers at all levels (Hunter 2009).

An organised approach to studying futures in public health

If a society's public health response is most effective when it is organised, a key question is how to bring futures work into the organised response and evaluate its impact. Systematic approaches to exploring the future and linking this work into the dynamic processes of public health policy development and planning are yet to be designed and implemented, though there are signs that structured futures studies approaches are attracting more serious attention and investment, sometimes in the guise of tools for strategic decision-making and policy support.

While the rationale for their establishment differs, research entities have been initiated by numerous governments and institutions around the world to assess challenges to humanity and ecological systems, and to inform strategy development (Fawkes 2009). These have included government-housed groups or statutory agencies (for example, in Singapore, Sweden, Canada, the United Kingdom and the United States), specialised government-affiliated bodies (such as NASA), inter-governmental and international organisations (for example, the WHO and the OECD), independent/private bodies (resource, pharmaceutical and technology companies) and research groups

(for example, the American Council for the United Nations University, RAND and the James Martin 21st Century School at Oxford University). Projects and programs undertaken by these bodies produce information and perspectives about futures that can contribute to specific policy processes in public health as well as the 'stock or reservoir of knowledge' (Hanney et al. 2003) generally available to inform policy-making.

For a systematic approach to examining the future, there must be in place the 'ability to continuously monitor and analyse emerging and persisting trends and to draw out the policy and societal implications' (Marsh & Yencken 2004). International models of a systematic approach at the national level could be analysed for their relevance to the Australian context and used to support public health strategy. For instance, the Finnish parliament's permanent seventeen-member Committee for the Future (2005) has representation from all political parties and conducts dialogue with the government on major future issues—such as health-care provision—and how these might be addressed. In the United Kingdom, pre-existing departments combined to form the Strategy Unit, which operated from 2002 until 2010. Reporting to the Prime Minister through the Cabinet Secretary, the unit provided the Prime Minister and government departments with policy analysis and research on how policy would develop over time, emerging social challenges and new perspectives on addressing them. This work aided strategy development in key areas of government, including public health. One of the important fundamental issues for public health is that improving population health requires cross-sectoral collaboration; thus, any systematic approach to analysing futures needs to consider the ramifications of policy across a range of portfolios, even if it is led or instigated by the Health ministry. A systematic approach will need to include mechanisms for perspectives on drivers of change and futures among the public and other interests (such as the private sector) to be considered.

427

In Australia, thinking about futures in relation to public health—especially at the national level—has generally been unsystematic. Activities such as professional workshops, simulation exercises, research projects, high-level think-tanks and community visioning exercises have been undertaken on an occasional basis in the public health sector. Professional and sector conferences have studied projections and trends on specific issues (such as food supply) and cross-cutting issues (such as workforce), and debated their implications for policy and planning. Building capacity for futures thinking among those who have responsibilities for health policy and planning will be a first step towards better preparedness for whatever public health futures confront us.

Conclusion: A societal effort for healthy futures

In an increasingly interconnected and interdependent world, where widening health inequalities characterise the type of 'Gordian knot' problems we are facing, is it possible for public health systems to make a difference to the health and well-being of populations? The central thesis of this book is that only weak, uncoordinated and short-term effects will be possible if an organised approach is not pursued and elevated as one of society's most critical investments.

The alternative futures we are facing will be characterised by more uncertainty, a greater range of interrelated risks and less certainty about which decisions and interventions will benefit public health. Threats to population health—such as an avian influenza pandemic or extreme weather events—alert us to the need for an organised approach to continuously assessing and interpreting emerging and longer-term health risks and

implementing the systematic responses that will be needed. This will require a new policy approach to risk management, stronger international cooperation in all elements of the risk-management cycle, better use of technological potential and enhanced research efforts (OECD 2003).

It will also require changes in leadership and participation in the public health effort. An organised approach cannot be static or rely on 'top-down' methods to effect change. The concept of the state is itself changing, as is the relationship between the state and civil society. 'Thinking globally and acting locally', facilitated by international community and networks, is not only more necessary than ever but more possible. Cooperation will be needed between the public and private sectors in the interests of the common good, and the engagement of stakeholders and the general public in assessing and responding to issues (OECD 2003: 259). New thinking is required, however, to sort through the short- and long-term ramifications of distributing responsibilities, resources and accountability in new ways.

While public health issues change over time, some constants endure, such as the '3 Ps' of public health practice: in the public interest, organised by the public, and using public processes and governance arrangements. This book has provided evidence that organised approaches that integrate and implement a basic, holistic framework for analysing complex public health issues and designing multi-level, multi-sector strategies to improve health are most likely to be successful.

Into the future, and ideally with an era of *sustained* health in view, further consolidation of an organised effort based on an integrated approach will best position public health systems to anticipate and respond to emerging and existing threats and opportunities.

19

A final note on ethical practice

Introduction

Just as there are frequent debates about ethics in medicine—about who should have the last available hospital bed, or whether life should be extended or allowed to end—public health practitioners are engaged in a range of ethical debates. Over the course of the twentieth century, there were debates about whether water should be fluoridated, whether the use of seatbelts should be mandatory, whether smoking should be banned, whether people with infectious diseases should be quarantined, whether all population groups (despite marital status, sexual orientation or ethnic background) should be able to access services equally, whether employees or employers should bear responsibility for workplace accidents, whether marijuana should be decriminalised and so on.

Public health practitioners are called upon on a daily basis to make judgements about how to act now in the interests of groups and populations in the immediate and longer-term future. In one study, researchers interviewed public health practitioners to identify the ethical challenges they encountered in their practice (see Box 19.1). A central dilemma in public health practice is to sort through questions of right and wrong, and find a workable and acceptable balance between societal interests and individual rights, and between state regulation and individual choice.

Many ethical issues in society are debated over a number of years before they are finally resolved. These debates occur in the political arena, in social and institutional settings, within professional and industry associations, across community networks, in the courts and in the media. They are often informed by international agreements, such as the UN Declaration of Human Rights, which sets out essential principles. The Commonwealth government has established the Australian Health Ethics

Box 19.1 Ethical challenges identified by public health practitioners

- **Determining the appropriate use of public health authority.** Population health benefits need to be balanced with business and economic benefits, with individual financial viability or with respect for individuals' autonomy.
- **Making decisions related to resource allocation.** There is a lack of clarity or a perception of inappropriateness about priorities for allocating funds or focusing practitioners' time; practitioners have little control over allocation decisions.
- **Negotiating political interference in public health practice.** Political issues interfere with best practices; political pressure exists to bend rules or to focus on politically expedient issues.
- **Ensuring standards of quality of care.** Quality of care may vary inappropriately from one population group to another; clinicians have difficulty ensuing that services are done 'right' in the face of constraints.
- **Questioning the role or scope of public health.** Individual concepts of appropriate public health services and activities are challenged; clinicians question whether public health actions are consistent with the over-arching mission of public health.

Source: adapted from Baum et al. (2009).

Committee, under the aegis of the NHMRC, as a focal point for the development of advice about ethical issues in medicine. Public health ethics, in contrast, is still an evolving field.

Public health practitioners need to have an understanding of the global picture and, at the same time, an appreciation of how these larger societal forces shape the lives, health and well-being of individuals and groups of people. In a special issue of its *Bulletin* devoted to public health ethics, key global issues identified by the World Health Organization include disparities in access to the benefits of medical research; collective action and the use of quarantine to combat infectious disease; exploitation of low-income countries and the commodification of the human body; balancing personal choice in combating the growing threat of preventable non-communicable diseases; and the continuing development of participatory, transparent and accountable practice in medical research (WHO 2008b).

Values and principles: Guidance for public health practice

Because of the uncertain ethical territory in which public health practitioners operate, it is particularly important that they are reflective about their practice and incorporate ethical principles in their activities. Most professions have codes of ethics to which they expect their members to adhere. Traditionally, ethics has been concerned with enunciating the nature of the common good, and how professionals can work to maintain this commitment to the common good. To support practitioners in exercising judgement, the American Public Health Association has proposed a code of ethics for the public health profession (see Box 19.2). As yet, no such code exists in Australia, but the field of public health ethics is gaining recognition and public health practitioners are being called upon to routinely include ethical deliberations when making decisions, and when explaining and justifying their practice. Public discussions about health frequently invoke ethical concepts. Recent examples in Australia include the critique of the Northern Territory Intervention that focuses on its potential to undermine the human rights of Indigenous Australians (NSW Health 2012a) and the concern about lack of consultation and potential health risks to participants in the Retractable Needle and Syringe Technology Initiative (Fry et al. 2006).

A range of values and assumptions underlie this code, and they reflect the principles discussed

---

Box 19.2 Principles of ethical practice in public health

1 Public health should address principally the fundamental causes of disease and requirements for health, aiming to prevent adverse health outcomes.

2 Public health should achieve community health in ways that respect the rights of individuals in the community.

3 Public health policies, programs and priorities should be developed and evaluated through processes that ensure an opportunity for input from community members.

4 Public health should advocate and work for the empowerment of disenfranchised community members, aiming to ensure that the basic resources and conditions necessary for health are accessible to all.

5 Public health should seek information needed to implement effective policies and programs that protect and promote health.

6 Public health institutions should provide communities with the information they have that is needed for decisions on policies or programs and should obtain the community's consent for their implementation.

7 Public health institutions should act in a timely manner on the information they have within the resources and the mandate given to them by the public.

8 Public health programs and policies should incorporate a variety of approaches that anticipate and respect diverse values, beliefs and cultures in the community.

9 Public health programs and policies should be implemented in a manner that most enhances the physical and social environment.

10 Public health institutions should protect the confidentiality of information that can bring harm to an individual or community if made public. Exceptions must be justified on the basis of the high likelihood of significant harm to the individual or others.

11 Public health institutions should ensure the professional competence of their employees.

12 Public health institutions and their employees should engage in collaboration and affiliations in ways that build the public's trust and the institutions' effectiveness.

Source: extract from American Public Health Association (2006).

---

throughout this book. In a nutshell, these include (American Public Health Association 2006):

- Health is a right.
- Human beings are interdependent.
- Collaboration—across professions, government, industry and communities—is integral to effective public health practice.
- Trust between communities and public health institutions is a basic requisite for public health institutions to be effective.
- Opportunities for all to participate in public health debates are a core feature of community empowerment.

- Knowledge derived from systematic investigation provides a foundation for public health action.
- Action may be required to protect health and dignity before full information is available.

These underlying values and the principles embodied in the code of practice inform how public health practitioners go about collecting data, analysing health trends, investigating outbreaks, providing health education, mandating screening and treatment services, conducting research, exercising regulatory powers and all other aspects of public health practice.

Kass (2001) offers a six-step framework for ethical practice in public health. These are questions that help public health practitioners to consider the ethical implications of any proposed policies and programs. In brief, she suggests that the key questions in ethical analysis are:

- What are the public health goals of a proposed program (or policy)—what health improvements will occur as a result of the proposed intervention?
- How effective is the program (or policy) in achieving its stated goals—what are the basic assumptions in the program, and what data exist to substantiate them? Are the assumptions valid and does the analytical or logical basis stand up to scrutiny?
- What are the known or potential burdens of the program—could harm arise from the public health program (or policy)?
- Can burdens be minimised, and are there alternative approaches—what modifications to the program (or policy) are required to pose fewer risks to other moral claims (such as liberty, opportunity and justice)?
- Is the program (or policy) implemented fairly—are the benefits and the burdens fairly distributed?
- How can the benefits and burdens of a program be fairly balanced—is it possible to ensure the public benefits outweigh the burdens (or costs or other problems)?

Being clear about the values and principles, and applying these steps in an ethical analysis, ultimately helps to build the trust the community then vests in public health action, and to assure the integrity of public health practitioners.

Role of ethical theory: Debates and reference points

The practice of public health adopts a pragmatic approach to solving health problems in communities and societies. As such, it draws from an eclectic range of theories, models and tools— ethical theories among them. Such theories help practitioners to make decisions by offering frameworks for examining the wrongs and rights of specific decisions.

The ethical theory that has historically underpinned decision-making in public health is utilitarianism, notably espoused by eighteenth-century legal scholar, social philosopher and political activist Jeremy Bentham (1982). Utilitarian theory—sometimes referred to as the 'greatest happiness principle'—broadly asserts the moral primacy of actions that achieve the 'greatest good for the greatest number' and value the optimisation of benefits over harms. However, a weakness of utilitarianism is that it offers little guidance about which goods should be maximised or on their distribution.

That public health actions might restrict or disadvantage some people, or constrain individual choice, has been seen as problematic by those with a different philosophical disposition. Immanuel Kant's duty-based theory of ethics (see Kant 1780) dictates that our *actions* should be judged in terms of our *intention* to act in ways that are consistent with our duties. Our main duty or obligation is to uphold respect for the moral worth and dignity of all persons, whom we should always treat as ends not as means. From a public health perspective, making laws or regulations that impact on privacy (such as communicable disease reporting and contact tracing) or personal choices (such as having one's child immunised, or wearing a helmet while riding a motorcycle) carry the risk of compromising autonomy and self-determination despite the common goods that are associated with such activities.

Jürgen Habermas (1990) argues that no single philosophical theory can be valid for everyone in a pluralist society. For a norm to be considered legitimate, therefore, its consequences must be acceptable to all those affected. This can only be determined if those affected are enabled to participate in a process of communication directed towards shared understanding, in conditions of freedom, equality and fair play. In other words, those likely to be affected by decisions must be able to participate in shaping them.

Many of the current debates in public health reflect the tensions between the orientation towards individual autonomy that is found in bioethics, and the utilitarian, paternalistic and communitarian orientations that have marked the field of public health throughout its history. An alternative ethical framework for public health, based on international human rights and reflected in the Universal Declaration on Bioethics and Human Rights (UNESCO 2005), was proposed by Jonathan Mann. He advocated that values associated with 'modern human rights' link directly with societal structure and function and thus are more appropriate to guide public health practice than the more individually oriented ethical framework of bioethics.

Contemporary public health decision-making considers not only technical analyses of benefits and harms, but also respect for autonomy and concepts of justice. John Rawls (1973) argues that while inequalities of various kinds may inevitably exist in a society—for example, as a result of different skills, talents, motivations and capacities—liberal democracies should nevertheless aim to ensure that certain fundamental conditions are met which provide, at the very least, 'fair equality of opportunity' for all citizens.

Ethical theories such as those introduced above provide a range of principles that help determine which public health decisions might be right or wrong. They also offer reference points for consideration, rather than a strict list of principles for application. Public health practice takes place within contexts defined by history, culture, social norms, economic resources and political structures. Despite these differences, public health ultimately is concerned with how to achieve the best health outcomes for the population and, as such, is concerned with the central ethical principle of social justice.

Conclusion: Being a reflective practitioner

Different societies at different points in their history will resolve ethical debates in public health in different ways. The varied stances adopted across countries and communities may be explained in part by broader drivers of change and of ethical debates—that is, the intersection of technology, resources and values. Ultimately, some of the key ethical issues confronting public health practice are:

- Whose choice is it—that of the individual or the community (or government on behalf of the community)?
- Who imposes the societal frame—who defines what is in the public interest? Whose ethical principles will dominate?
- Can the actions pursued by public health practitioners go too far—in imposing their own set of values and principles on society? Where does the mandate of public health stop?
- Are core ideas of public health—such as rights and participation—culture-bound concepts? If so, what are the ethical implications for international cooperation in relation to global health issues?
- Is there a tradeoff between health and livelihood, and other social and economic goals (such as jobs and economic development)?
- Is there a tradeoff between the principles of public health (such as utilitarianism and the precautionary principle) and other social values (such as civil liberties and human rights)?

Theories about ethics assist in resolving these and other questions that arise for public health practitioners on a regular basis. A code of ethics for public health professionals provides some operational principles that can be applied in what is ultimately a moral and ethical enterprise, and one that can be expected to become more complex and demanding in the future.

433

Appendices

Appendix A

Australian core public health functions

Assess, analyse and communicate population health needs and community expectations

Established practice

- Monitor physical, mental and social morbidity and the causes of mortality.
- Research and monitor the determinants of health.
- Assess population health needs and risks.
- Undertake research to identify the causes of and solutions to health problems in populations.

Evolving practice

- Conduct public health program evaluation and outcome research.
- Evaluate health services and conduct research on the outcomes of health services.
- Conduct cross-disciplinary and multi-method research.

Prevent and control communicable and non-communicable diseases and injuries through risk factor reduction, education, screening, immunisation and other interventions

Established practice

- Conduct disease, injury and risk factor surveillance.
- Conduct disease outbreak investigation and control.
- Screen for selected communicable and non-communicable diseases.
- Implement comprehensive communicable disease control programs, including the provision of immunisation.
- Treat cases of infectious disease.
- Provide public health laboratory services.
- Provide veterinary public health services.
- Enable and encourage communities and individuals to adopt and maintain healthy practices, such as appropriate diet, moderate alcohol intake, physical activity, no smoking and improved oral health (including fluoride supplementation).
- Provide individual and community education to promote behaviours that reduce the risk of injury.
- Advocate, legislate for, develop and promote safer products and environments.

Evolving practice

- Monitor, research and respond to newly emerging disease threats (e.g. nosocomial infections, including antibiotic resistance).
- Address the social and economic determinants of non-communicable diseases.
- Address risk factors for intentional injuries.

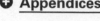

Promote and support healthy lifestyles and behaviours through action with individuals, families, communities and the wider society

Established practice

- Undertake personal and mass media education and advocacy in the areas of tobacco, nutrition, drugs, alcohol, physical activity and healthy sexuality.
- Provide health information and education that is sensitive to language and culture, to develop individual health knowledge, attitudes and behaviours.
- Use social marketing to complement education and community development strategies to promote health.

Evolving practice

- Shift focus from action at the level of the individual to broader societal and structural issues—for example, food supply.

Promote, develop and support healthy public policy, including legislation, regulation and fiscal measures

Established practice

- Contribute to the development of and promote the implementation of healthy public policy.
- Evaluate the impact of health and other public policy on population health, with a particular emphasis on identifying inequalities.
- Provide evidence-based advice for policy and program initiatives for health protection and promotion.
- Advocate for and work in partnership with all sectors to develop legislation and regulations that protect and promote health.
- Review, formulate, enact and enforce health legislation and regulations.
- Ensure sustainable financing for health protection and promotion.

Evolving practice

- Conduct health impact assessments of other sectors' policies and actions.
- Develop fiscal strategies that support health improvement.
- Develop financial incentives to encourage preventive health care.
- Promote public policy measures to reduce inequalities in health.
- Promote access to health services according to need.

Plan, fund, manage and evaluate health gain and capacity-building programs designed to achieve measurable improvements in health status and to strengthen skills, competencies, systems and infrastructure

Established practice

- Undertake strategic and operational planning.
- Directly manage and contract for service provision.
- Develop resource-allocation and priority-setting systems.
- Improve the quality and scope of public health information.
- Ensure adequate public health knowledge and skills in the health workforce.
- Ensure that the public health workforce participates in continuing professional development.
- Build organisational structures and processes for public health within agencies.
- Build links between the health sector and other sectors.
- Build organisational links between health agencies.

Evolving practice

- Develop and implement quality assurance processes for public health.
- Develop strategic alliances and partnership agreements.
- Develop performance management systems.

Strengthen communities and build social capital through consultation, participation and empowerment

Established practice

- Promote community and consumer participation in decisions affecting people's health.
- Develop community capacity to identify and act on public health problems.
- Fund community programs.
- Consult on planning and priorities of services.

Evolving practice

- Work with communities and other sectors to enhance social networks and contribute to building social support in communities.

Promote, develop, support and initiate actions that ensure safe and healthy environments

Established practice

- Protect and ensure water quality.
- Practise vector control.
- Promote food access and quality and ensure safety.
- Control hazardous environmental substances and wastes.
- Control radiation.
- Ensure drainage, sewerage and solid waste disposal.
- Control atmospheric pollution.

- Control drugs and poisons and the quality of therapeutic goods and appliances.

Evolving practice

- Promote safe and healthy working conditions.
- Promote environments that support physical, mental and social health.
- Promote ecologically sustainable development.

Promote, develop and support healthy growth and development throughout all life stages

Established practice

- Provide public health services for mothers and children.
- Provide services for early childhood development and care.
- Provide school health services, including dental health.
- Provide school health education, including drug and sex education.

- Provide prenatal and neonatal screening.
- Provide women's health and family-planning services.

Evolving practice

- Provide mental health-promotion programs.
- Provide public health services for older people.
- Provide genetic screening and counselling services.

Promote, develop and support actions to improve the health status of Aboriginal and Torres Strait Islander people and other vulnerable groups

Established practice

- Provide public health services and advocate for health care for Indigenous peoples.
- Provide emergency and natural disaster services to protect health.
- Provide public health services and advocate for health care for refugees, the homeless and people with a disability.

Evolving practice

- Provide public health services and advocate for health care for victims of violence and other crises.
- Provide public health services and advocate for health care of multiculturally diverse communities.
- Advocate for occupational health service.
- Advocate for mental health care services.

Source: NPHP (2000c).

Appendix B

Millennium Development Goals (MDGs)

MDG target	Illustrative indicators
Halve the proportion of people whose income is less than $1.00 a day	• Share of poorest quintile in national consumption • Proportion of population whose income below $1.00 per day
Halve the proportion of people who suffer from hunger	• Prevalence of under-weight children under five years of age • Proportion of population below minimum level of dietary energy consumption
Ensure that children everywhere will be able to complete a full course of primary schooling	• Primary completion • Literacy rate of fifteen- to 24-year-olds
Eliminate gender disparity in primary and secondary education	• Ratios of girls to boys in primary, secondary and tertiary education • Ratio of literate women to men aged fifteen to 24 years
Reduce the under-five mortality rate	• Under-five mortality rate • Infant mortality rate • Proportion of one-year-old children immunised against measles
Reduce the maternal mortality rate	• Maternal mortality ratio • Proportion of births attended by skilled health personnel

MDG target	Illustrative indicators
Halt and reverse the spread of HIV/AIDS	• HIV prevalence among fifteen- to 24-year-old pregnant women • Condom use rate at last high-risk sex incident • Contraceptive prevalence rate • Condom use rate of the contraceptive prevalence rate • Percentage of population aged fifteen to 24 with comprehensive, correct knowledge of HIV/AIDS
Halt and reverse the incidence of malaria and other major diseases and tuberculosis	• Prevalence and death rates associated with malaria • Proportion of population in malaria-risk areas using effective malaria-prevention and treatment measures • Proportion of tuberculosis cases detected and cured under directly observed treatment short course (DOTS)
Integrate the principles of sustainable development into country policies and programs	• Proportion of land area covered by forest • Proportion of population using solid fuels • Carbon dioxide emissions per capita and consumption of ozone-depleting CFCs
Halve the proportion of people without sustainable access to safe drinking water and basic sanitation	• Proportion of population with sustainable access to an improved water source • Proportion of urban and rural population with access to improved sanitation
Significantly improve the lives of slum-dwellers	• Proportion of households with access to secure tenure

Source: adapted from United Nations (2003).

Appendix C

Commonwealth Department of Health structure, 1921–2012

Year	Name	Divisions
2012	Department of Health and Ageing	Acute Care Division (ACD) Ageing and Aged Care Division (AACD) Audit and Fraud Control Health Workforce Division ICT and Corporate Support Division (ICT&CSD) Medical Benefits Division (MBD) Mental Health and Drug Treatment Division Pharmaceutical Benefits Division (PBD) Office for Aboriginal and Torres Strait Islander Health Office of Health Protection (OHP) Population Health Division (PHD) Portfolio Strategies Division (PSD) Primary and Ambulatory Care Division (PACD) Regulatory Policy & Governance Division (RPGD) State and territory offices Therapeutic Goods Administration (TGA)
2004	Department of Health and Ageing	Acute Care Ageing and Aged Care Business Group Health Services Improvement Information and Communications Medical and Pharmaceutical Services Office for Aboriginal & Torres Strait Islander Health Population Health Portfolio Strategies Primary Care

Year	Name	Divisions
1997	Department of Health and Family Services	Aged and Community Care Commonwealth Rehabilitation Service Corporate Services Family and Children's Services Health Benefits Health Services Development Information Services Information Technology Group Office for Aboriginal & Torres Strait Islander Health Services Office of NHMRC Portfolio Strategies Public Health Therapeutic Goods Administration
1985	Department of Community Services and Health	Australian Institute of Health Corporate Resources Executive & International Health Advancement Health Services Financing Internal Audit NHMRC Therapeutics
1971	Department of Health	Health Insurance and Benefits Laboratory Services and Quarantine Management Services National Health NHMRC Tuberculosis
1961	Department of Health	Medical and Hospital Benefits Nursing Pharmaceutical Plant Quarantine Public Health Tuberculosis Veterinary Hygiene

Year	Name	Divisions
1921	Department of Health	Chief Medical Officer
		Laboratories (including CSL)
		Marine Hygiene
		Public Health and Population Policy
		Quarantine Services
		Tropical Hygiene

Sources: Beddie (2001: 18–23); Duckett (2000: 93); DoHA (2004b; 2013b).

Appendix D

Commonwealth population health divisions, 1961–2012

Year	Division	Sections/branches
2012	Population Health	Cancer and Palliative Care Chronic Disease Drug Strategy Health in Social Policy Healthy Living Tobacco Control Taskforce
2004	Population Health	Biosecurity and Disease Control Drug Strategy Food and Healthy Living Strategic Planning Targeted Prevention Programs
1997	Population Health	National Centre for Disease Control National Health Promotion and Protection National Public Health Planning
1985	Health Advancement	Better Health Commission Secretariat Communicable Diseases Drug Dependence Health Strategies Nursing and Health Services Workforce Social and Community Health
1971	Public Health Branch (part of National Health Division)	Environmental Health Food Administration Nursing Nutrition Social and Preventive Medicine Toxicology

Year	Division	Sections/branches
1961	Public Health	Epidemiology
		Immigration Medical Service
		Institute of Anatomy
		National Fitness Movement
		Nursing
		Nutrition
		Therapeutic Substances

Sources: Department of Health (1961, 1971, 1985, 1997); DoHA (2005f, 2012j).

Appendix E

Approaches and theories for health promotion

Domain for intervention	Names of theories, frameworks or models	Main focus/concept	Key concepts	Major proponent	Instances where model has been useful
Individual behaviour	Health belief model	People's perceptions of the threat to health and their appraisal of recommended behaviour(s) for preventing and managing the problem are central.	• Perceived susceptibility • Perceived severity • Perceived benefits of action • Perceived barriers to action • Cues to action • Self-efficacy		Importance of beliefs among those at risk of HIV infection
	Theory of reasoned action	People's intentions to act to promote their health are the key and are influenced by social pressures.		Ajzen & Fishbein (1991)	Importance of short-term consequences in intentions of youth who smoke
	Trans-theoretical model or Stages of change model	Individuals' readiness to change or attempt to change towards healthy behaviours are important.	• Precontemplation • Contemplation • Decision/ determination • Action • Maintenance	Prochaska & DiClemente (1984)	Recognition that relapsing is a common problem in a change process

Domain for intervention	Names of theories, frameworks or models	Main focus/concept	Key concepts	Major proponent	Instances where model has been useful
	Consumer information processing model	Process by which consumers acquire and use information in their decision-making.	• Information process • Information search • Decision rules/ heuristics • Consumption and learning • Information environment		Consumer food choices at point of sale in supermarkets
	Social learning theory	Behaviour is explained via a three-way, dynamic reciprocal theory in which personal factors, environmental influences and behaviour continually interact.	• Behavioural capability • Reciprocal determinism • Expectations • Self-efficacy • Observational learning • Reinforcement	Bandura (1997)	Quitting smoking is easier in smoke-free environments but harder among heavy-smoking friends
Community behaviour	Community mobilisation/ organisation	Emphasises active participation and development of communities so they can better evaluate and solve health and social problems.	• Empowerment • Community competence • Participation and relevance • Issue selection • Critical consciousness		The focus of 'Safe Communities Project' on specific locations
	Social planning	A rational-empirical approach will be task-oriented and expert-driven.		Rothman & Tropman (1987)	
	Social action	Disadvantaged groups benefit from community-driven advocacy.		Minkler & Cox (1980)	Use of the sense of community among gay groups to minimise spread of HIV

Domain for intervention	Names of theories, frameworks or models	Main focus/concept	Key concepts	Major proponent	Instances where model has been useful
	Community development	Communities that reflect jointly can mobilise effectively.			
	Diffusion of innovation	Addresses how new ideas, products, and social practices spread within a society or from one society to another.	• Relative advantage • Compatibility • Complexity • Trialability • Observability	Rogers (1983)	Useful in maximising uptake of new programs
Public perception and knowledge strategies	Communication for behavioural change	A successful message needs to be well-crafted for its audience.		Egger, Donovan & Spark (1993)	Effect of men's health information depends on perceptions of authority of information source
	Social marketing	Market analysis and right product, placement, price and promotion to groups can increase the sale of health products—for example, immunisation.		Andreasen (1995)	Defining consumer based on their consumption patterns rather than age, sex, etc.
Organisational change and practices	Theories of organisational change	Concerns processes and strategies for increasing the chances that healthy policies and programs will be adopted and maintained in formal organisations.	• Problem definition (awareness stage) • Initiation of action (adoption stage) • Implementation of change	Goodman, Steckler & Kegler (1997)	Work through the layers of an organisation in successful implementation of, say, smoke-free policy

Domain for intervention	Names of theories, frameworks or models	Main focus/concept	Key concepts	Major proponent	Instances where model has been useful
	Models of intersectoral action	Organisations can work in partnerships for health goals if they share goals and plan actions.	• Institutionalisation of change	Harris et al. (1995)	Action following an outbreak of measles in 1991 effectively used child-care and health sectors
Healthy public policy	Ecological framework	The social climate of a policy includes policy stakeholders, such as politicians; policy influencers, such as pressure groups or other key stakeholders; and the public as taxpayers or voters.		Milio (1987)	Social climate after tragic mass shootings can aid gun control
	Determinants of policy-making	Key determinants are the assumptions of policy-makers, the vested interests in the policy, and the power of major stakeholders.		de Leeuw (1993)	Understand how no effective action is taken despite clear epidemiological evidence
	Indicators of health promotion policy	Health promotion ranges from rational-deductive to incremental 'muddle-through' approaches to policy, but a 'mixed scanning' model in which rationality is combined with frequent referral back to the community is probably the best.		Ziglio (1993)	Balance political realities with evidence-based planning

Source: based on Nutbeam & Harris (2004), which was in its turn adapted from Glanz et al. (1997) and <www.cancer.org>.

Appendix F

Ottawa Charter for Health Promotion, 1986 (extract)

Health promotion

Health promotion is the process of enabling people to increase control over, and to improve, their health. To reach a state of complete physical, mental and social well-being, an individual or group must be able to identify and to realize aspirations, to satisfy needs, and to change or cope with the environment. Health is, therefore, seen as a resource for everyday life, not the objective of living. Health is a positive concept emphasizing social and personal resources, as well as physical capacities. Therefore, health promotion is not just the responsibility of the health sector, but goes beyond healthy life-styles to well-being.

Prerequisites for health

The fundamental conditions and resources for health are:
* peace,
* shelter,
* education,
* food,
* income,
* a stable eco-system,
* sustainable resources,
* social justice, and equity.

Improvement in health requires a secure foundation in these basic prerequisites.

Advocate

Good health is a major resource for social, economic and personal development and an important dimension of quality of life. Political, economic, social, cultural, environmental, behavioural and biological factors can all favour health or be harmful to it. Health promotion action aims at making these conditions favourable through advocacy for health.

Enable

Health promotion focuses on achieving equity in health. Health promotion action aims at reducing differences in current health status and ensuring equal opportunities and resources to enable all people to achieve their fullest health potential. This includes a secure foundation in a supportive environment, access to information, life skills and opportunities for making healthy choices. People cannot achieve their fullest health potential unless they are able to take control of those things which determine their health. This must apply equally to women and men.

Mediate

The prerequisites and prospects for health cannot be ensured by the health sector alone. More importantly, health promotion demands coordinated action by all concerned: by governments, by health and other social and economic sectors, by nongovernmental and voluntary organizations, by local authorities, by industry and by the media. People in all walks of life are involved as individuals, families and communities. Professional and social groups and health personnel have a major responsibility to mediate between differing interests in society for the pursuit of health.

Health promotion strategies and programmes should be adapted to the local needs and possibilities of individual countries and regions to take into account differing social, cultural and economic systems.

Health promotion action means:

Build healthy public policy

Health promotion goes beyond health care. It puts health on the agenda of policy makers in all sectors and at all levels, directing them to be aware of the health consequences of their decisions and to accept their responsibilities for health.

Health promotion policy combines diverse but complementary approaches including legislation, fiscal measures, taxation and organizational change. It is coordinated action that leads to health, income and social policies that foster greater equity. Joint action contributes to ensuring safer and healthier goods and services, healthier public services, and cleaner, more enjoyable environments.

Health promotion policy requires the identification of obstacles to the adoption of healthy public policies in non-health sectors, and ways of removing them. The aim must be to make the healthier choice the easier choice for policy makers as well.

Create supportive environments

Our societies are complex and interrelated. Health cannot be separated from other goals. The inextricable links between people and their environment constitutes the basis for a socioecological approach to health. The overall guiding principle for the world, nations, regions and communities alike, is the need to encourage reciprocal maintenance—to take care of each other, our communities and our natural environment. The conservation of natural resources throughout the world should be emphasized as a global responsibility.

Changing patterns of life, work and leisure have a significant impact on health. Work and leisure should be a source of health for people. The way society organizes work should help create a healthy society. Health promotion generates living and working conditions that are safe, stimulating, satisfying and enjoyable.

Systematic assessment of the health impact of a rapidly changing environment—particularly in areas of technology, work, energy production and urbanization—is essential and must be followed by action to ensure positive benefit to the health of the public. The protection of the natural and built environments and the conservation of natural resources must be addressed in any health promotion strategy.

Strengthen community actions

Health promotion works through concrete and effective community action in setting priorities, making decisions, planning strategies and implementing them to achieve better health. At the heart of this process is the empowerment of communities—their ownership and control of their own endeavours and destinies.

Community development draws on existing human and material resources in the community to enhance self-help and social support, and to develop flexible systems for strengthening public participation in and direction of health matters. This requires full and continuous access to information, learning opportunities for health, as well as funding support.

Develop personal skills

Health promotion supports personal and social development through providing information, education for health, and enhancing life skills. By so doing, it increases the options available to people to exercise more control over their own health and over their environments, and to make choices conducive to health.

Enabling people to learn, throughout life, to prepare themselves for all of its stages and to cope with chronic illness and injuries is essential. This has to be facilitated in school, home, work and community settings. Action is required through educational, professional, commercial and voluntary bodies, and within the institutions themselves.

Reorient health services

The responsibility for health promotion in health services is shared among individuals, community groups, health professionals, health service institutions and governments.

They must work together towards a health care system which contributes to the pursuit of health. The role of the health sector must move increasingly in a health promotion direction, beyond its responsibility for providing clinical and curative services. Health services need to embrace an expanded mandate which is sensitive and respects cultural needs. This mandate should support the needs of individuals and communities for a healthier life, and open channels between the health sector and broader social, political, economic and physical environmental components.

Reorienting health services also requires stronger attention to health research as well as changes in professional education and training. This must lead to a change of attitude and organization of health services which refocuses on the total needs of the individual as a whole person.

Moving into the future

Health is created and lived by people within the settings of their everyday life; where they learn, work, play and love. Health is created by caring for oneself and others, by being able to take decisions and have control over one's life circumstances, and by ensuring that the society one lives in creates conditions that allow the attainment of health by all its members.

Caring, holism and ecology are essential issues in developing strategies for health promotion. Therefore, those involved should take as a guiding principle that, in each phase of planning, implementation and evaluation of health promotion activities, women and men should become equal partners.

Source: <www.who.int/healthpromotion/conferences/previous/ottawa/en/index.html>

Appendix G

Evidence-based public health: Recommendations from Taskforce on Community Preventive Services

Health issue	Intervention objective or approach	Evidence base		
		Strong	**Good**	**Insufficient**
Tobacco use	• Reduce exposure to environmental tobacco smoke	• Smoking bans and restrictions	• Provider reminder systems • Mobile phone based interventions	• Community education to reduce home exposures
	• Increase cessation	• Increase unit price of tobacco products • Provider reminders and education (+/−) patient education • 'Quit' lines (telephone support) • Mass media campaign		• Provider feedback • Provider education • Mass media contests • Internet-based interventions
	• Reduce initiation	• Reduce patient out-of-pocket costs for effective therapies • Mass media campaigns		
Physical activity	• Informational strategies	• Community-wide campaigns	• Point-of-decision prompts	• Classroom-based health education • Mass media campaigns
	• Behavioural and social strategies	• School-based physical education • Individually adapted behaviour-change programs • Social support in community settings		
	• Environmental and policy strategies			• Access to facilities + information outreach

Health issue	Intervention objective or approach	Evidence base		
		Strong	**Good**	**Insufficient**
Motor vehicle injury	• Reduction of alcohol-impaired driving	• Blood alcohol laws and testing • Legal drinking age at 21 • Ignition interlocks	• Training for servers of alcoholic drinks • Blood alcohol laws for young/new drivers	
	• Increase child safety seat use	• Child safety seat laws • Distribution and education programs		
	• Increase seatbelt use	• Seatbelt laws and enforcement		
Vaccine-preventable diseases	• Increase access to vaccination services	• Reduce out-of-pocket costs • Expand access to clinical services • Vaccination in schools and child-care centres • Home visits	• Vaccination in low-income maternal and child health settings client or family incentives	
	• Increase community demand for vaccines	• Client reminder/recall systems • Vaccination requirement for school and college attendance		• Clinic-based education • Client-held records • Community-wide education • Provider education
	• Provider-based strategies	• Standing orders for adults and children • Provider reminder/recall system • Assessment and feedback for providers		
Oral health	• Prevent caries	• Community water fluoridation • School-based dental sealant delivery programs		• Community-wide dental sealant promotion program
	• Prevent and control pharyngeal cancers			• Community-based early detection programs
	• Prevent craniofacial injury in contact sports			• Education on use of helmets, mouthguards and face masks

Health issue	Intervention objective or approach	Evidence base		
		Strong	**Good**	**Insufficient**
Diabetes	• Health-care policies	• Case management • Disease management		
	• Self-management education		• Education in community setting • Education in the home for adolescents (type 1)	• Education in the home (type 2) • Education for adolescents at camps • Education of school personnel • Worksite education
Social environment	• Improved cognitive development for children	• Early childhood development programs		
	• Reduce neighbourhood concentration of poverty	• Tenant-based rental vouchers		• Mixed-income housing developments

Source: adapted from Taskforce on Community Preventive Services (2011).

Appendix H

Examples of public health laws in Australia

Commonwealth

- Quarantine of goods, vessels and people (*Quarantine Act 1908*)
- Control of the quality and safety of therapeutic goods (*Therapeutic Goods Act 1989*)
- Protection of public health and environment (*Gene Technology Act 2000*)
- Health funding (e.g. *Health Insurance Act 1973*)
- *Food Standards Australia New Zealand Act 1991*
- *Tobacco Advertising Prohibition Act 1992*

New South Wales

- Public health and environmental sanitation (e.g. *Public Health Act 2010*)
- Control of tobacco or smoking (e.g. *Smoke-Free Environment Act 2000*)
- Control of drugs, poisons and dangerous goods (e.g. *Poisons and Therapeutic Goods Act 1966*; *Drugs (Misuse and Trafficking) Act 1985*)
- Food safety (e.g. *Food Act 2003*)
- Radiation safety (e.g. *Radiation Control Act 1990*)

Victoria

- Public health and environmental sanitation (*Public Health and Wellbeing Act 2008*; *Gene Technology Act 2001*)
- Control of tobacco or smoking (*Tobacco Act 1987*)

- Control of drugs, poisons and dangerous goods (*Drugs, Poisons and Controlled Substances Act 1981*; *Dangerous Goods Act 1985*)
- Radiation safety (*Public Health & Wellbeing Act 2008*)
- Food safety (*Dairy Act 2000*; *Meat Industry Act 1993*; *Food Act 1984*)

Australian Capital Territory

- Public health and environmental sanitation (*Public Health Act 1997*)
- Control of tobacco or smoking (*Tobacco Act 1927*; *Smoke-Free Public Places Act 2003*; *Smoking in Cars with Children (Prohibition) Act 2011*)
- Control of drugs, poisons and dangerous goods (*Drugs of Dependence Act 1989*)
- Radiation safety (*Radiation Act 1983*)
- Food safety (*Food Act 2001*)

Northern Territory

- Public health and environmental sanitation (*Public and Environmental Health Act 2011*)
- Control of tobacco or smoking (*Tobacco Control Act 2005*)
- Control of drugs, poisons and dangerous goods (*Dangerous Goods Act 2004*)
- Radiation safety (*Radiation Protection Act 2009*)
- Food safety (*Food Act 2004*)

South Australia
- Public health protection and environmental sanitation (e.g. *Public and Environmental Health Act 1987*)
- Control of tobacco or smoking (e.g. *Tobacco Products Regulation Act 1997*)
- Control of drugs, poisons and dangerous goods (e.g. *Controlled Substances Act 1984*)
- Food safety (e.g. *Food Act 2001; Primary Produce (Food Safety Schemes) Act 2004*)
- Radiation safety (e.g. *Radiation Protection and Control Act 1982*)

Queensland
- Public health and environmental sanitation (e.g. *Public Health Act 2005; Environment Protection Act 1994; Housing Act 2003*)
- Control of tobacco or smoking (*Tobacco and Other Smoking Products Act 1998*)
- Control of drugs, poisons and dangerous goods (*Dangerous Goods Safety Management Act 2001*)
- Radiation safety (*Radiation Safety Act 1999*)
- Food safety (*Food Act 2006*)

Tasmania
- Public health and environmental sanitation (*Public Health Act 1997*)
- Control of tobacco or smoking (*Public Health Act 1997*)
- Control of drugs, poisons and dangerous goods (*Dangerous Goods Act 1998; Poisons Act 1971*)
- Radiation safety (*Radiation Protection Act 2005*)
- Food safety (*Food Act 2003*)

Western Australia
- Public health and environmental sanitation (*Health Act 1911*)
- Control of tobacco and smoking (*Tobacco Products Control Act 2006*)
- Control of drugs, poisons and dangerous goods (*Poisons Act 1964*)
- Radiation safety (*Radiation Safety Act 1975*)
- Food safety (*Food Act 2008*)

Appendix I

Examples of new diseases identified in humans since 1975

Year of first cases	Disease	Incubation period Main signs and symptoms Case fatality rate (CFR)	Mode of transmission Reproducibility rate where known	Epidemiology
1976	**Ebola virus**, a severe acute viral illness caused by *Filoviridae* viruses	• Incubation: 2–21 days. • Sudden onset of fever, headaches, feeling very unwell, followed by diarrhoea and vomiting, sore throat and a rash and bleeding. • CFR is about 70 per cent.	• Intra-epidemic viral survival mechanism is unknown. • All body secretions are highly infectious, easily transmitted from person to person by close contact or handling of infected body fluids. • Reproducibility rate is unknown but very high.	• Originally identified in equatorial Africa, in Zaire and the Sudan, immunologically different from Marburg (Green Monkey) diseases. • Occurs in sporadic outbreaks of a few dozen to a few hundred people, mainly in villages.
1976	**Legionnaire's disease**, an acute bacterial infection	• Incubation period: 2–10 days. • Fever and chills, headaches, extreme tiredness and aching and painful muscles. • Dry cough and abnormal chest x-rays complete the picture. • CFR varies between 4 and 10 per cent; lower during outbreaks, presumably because of enhanced case detection.	• Not particularly infectious, and has never been documented to have been transmitted from person to person, therefore reproducibility rate is zero. • Occurs most often in late summer and autumn. • Several strains, found in damp human-made and natural environments, often associated with sprayed water, such as shower heads, fountains and water cooling towers. • Known to occur all over the world.	• First identified in the United States following the identification of an outbreak of atypical pneumonia in a group of Legionnaires who attended the same convention—the outbreak was eventually shown to be caused by the hotel's cooling tower system. • This disease is more common in the warmer months, and is associated with the use of cooling tower systems, spa pools and fountains as well as potting mixes. It is said to be more common in older men who smoke and have coexisting diseases. Although this reflects the cases routinely notified to Health Departments,

Year of first cases	Disease	Incubation period Main signs and symptoms Case fatality rate (CFR)	Mode of transmission Reproducibility rate where known	Epidemiology
				during outbreaks this pattern changes. The epidemiology of this disease has not yet been studied in detail.
1982	**Lyme disease** (Lyme borreliosis), a non-acute disease caused by a spirochete; also called tick-borne meningopoly-neuritis	• Incubation: 3–32 days. • Early symptoms are vague and changing. Significant symptoms (months to years later) include distinctive red skin lesions and fever, headache, stiff neck, tiredness, and muscle and joint aches.	• Spirochete are transmitted during biting of ticks, probably several hours after initial attachment; vertical (mother to foetal) transmission also occurs rarely; not transmitted from person to person. • Majority of cases occur mainly in summer, not transmitted person to person, therefore reproducibility rate is zero.	• Named after Old Lyme, Connecticut, United States, where it was first described. • Occurs all year but mainly in summer, in most parts of the United States and Canada, and in Europe and East Asia.
1982	***E. coli* O157:H7**, the most common pathogen to cause enterohaemorrhagic *Escherichia coli*	• Incubation: 2–8 days (a long time for ingested pathogens), usually 3–4 days. • Haemorrhagic colitis (bloody diarrhoea). • About 2 per cent of diagnosed people develop haemolitic uraemic syndrome (especially children); it is the most common cause of kidney failure in children under five, with a high CFR.	• Cattle are the most important reservoir of this disease; transmitted by eating infected food, most commonly undercooked or raw beef and milk products, and fruit and vegetables contaminated with the faeces of cows. • Infected water supplies. • Can be transmitted by infected persons for up to three weeks. • Only a low dose needed for infection; a high reproducibility rate.	• First identified in the United States, now an important problem in European countries, the North American continent and southern South America, Australia, South Africa and Japan.
1983	Human immunodeficiency virus (**HIV-1** and **HIV-2**) with acquired immune deficiency syndrome (**AIDS**)	• Incubation period: up to three months for detectable antibodies; up to fifteen years for HIV infection to progress to AIDS (tending to be shorter without preventive and palliative treatments). • HIV infection presents as a self-limiting infection with general symptoms, such as sore throat, tiredness, fever, and enlarged spleen and glands.	• HIV is transmitted from person to person by contact with blood and body fluids of an infected person (most commonly through sexual intercourse or sharing of needles); vertical transmission occurs particularly in women who are not on treatment; unscreened blood and blood products.	• The case series of Californian homosexual men who developed particular cancers and immune deficiency problems who were subsequently shown to have what became labelled HIV-1 infection is well known. The story of HIV-2 and its devastating effect on less developed countries, particularly in

Year of first cases	Disease	Incubation period Main signs and symptoms Case fatality rate (CFR)	Mode of transmission Reproducibility rate where known	Epidemiology
		• AIDS presents in various ways, from presentation with cancers typically seen in people living with AIDS, such as Kaposi's sarcoma, and the onset of unusual and opportunistic infections, particularly unusual pneumonias. • Over 90 per cent of people who are HIV positive will go on to develop AIDS. The CFR for AIDS is 80–90 per cent with treatment, and almost 100 per cent without.	• In developed countries most cases occur in men who have sex with men and in people who inject drugs and share injecting equipment, and therefore most cases are male. Countries in transition show a different pattern: most transmission occurs through heterosexual intercourse; and most cases are female, with about 10 per cent of infants born to HIV-positive mothers contracting HIV before or during birth. • The case definitions for HIV/AIDS include important laboratory diagnosis components.	women, is much less well known, although in most ways it is by far the greater public health problem. • Worldwide, the pattern of heterosexual transmission is most common, and the majority of cases are female.
1988	**Hepatitis E** (HEV)	• Incubation period: 2–9 weeks. • The main features of all forms of hepatitis are fever and feeling sick, abdominal discomfort, nausea and anorexia with jaundice appearing after a few days. • Fatalities occur in 0.1–0.3 per cent of cases overall, but is much more likely to occur in older people; pregnant women are reported to have an extremely high CFR of 20 per cent.	• HEV is an enteric disease, mainly transmitted through contaminated water, and is possibly a zoonotic infection that coincidentally infects humans. • This virus has been detected in the faeces of infected humans for about two weeks after jaundice begins.	• HEV is endemic in Asia and North Africa, and has been identified in travellers returning form these areas.
1989	**Hepatitis C** (HCV)	• Incubation period: 2–26 weeks; most commonly 6–9 weeks. • Signs and symptoms are very similar to other forms of hepatitis, although perhaps a little more vague.	• HCV is transmitted mainly by injection, and occurs mainly through reusing or sharing needles with infected people, or through the use of contaminated equipment during surgery; sexual transmission is thought to be rare.	• HCV has been identified all over the world, about 60 million people have this disease, and it is the second most common form of hepatitis (after hepatitis B). In developed countries, it is associated mainly with intravenous

Year of first cases	Disease	Incubation period Main signs and symptoms Case fatality rate (CFR)	Mode of transmission Reproducibility rate where known	Epidemiology
		• The fatality rate from secondary complications, such as hepatic (liver) cancers, is variable, but high		drug use, while in transitional countries poor health-care practices are more commonly implicated.
1992	*Vibrio cholerae* O139 Bengal	• Incubation period: a few hours to five days; usually 2–3 days. • Specific strain of cholera bacteria (causing acute enteric disease); typical signs and symptoms including sudden onset of painless, very watery diarrhoea, nausea and vomiting, which can lead to very severe dehydration. • Healthy Westerners who acquire cholera during their travels rarely die; however, the fatality rate in dislocated and starving peoples, such as refugees, can reach 15 per cent—overall, the CFR is probably 1–5 per cent.	• Direct transmission through contact with infected faeces or vomitus; contaminated zooplankton populations are found in stagnant water leading to indirect transmission occurring through contaminated water supplies. • Infected stools are highly infectious during illness and for the next few days; carriers are rare.	• Outbreak of several thousand cases in India and Bangladesh.
1994	**Sabia virus** (Sabia, or Brazilian haemorrhagic fever)	• Incubation: 1–2 weeks. • One of a group of diseases of gradual onset that cause fever and sweats, headache, red conjunctivae and pain behind the eyes, jaundice, inability to get out of bed, and rash of redness and blotches—disease causes bleeding so small blood spots in the mouth usually occur. Some cases develop severe nosebleeds, blood in the stool and urine, vomiting blood, and so on. • CFR is about 25 per cent.	• The mode of transmission is not known, although the related Arenaviruses have rodent hosts—transmission is thought to occur through inhaling dusts containing aerosolised virus from rodent faeces. • Transmission only very rarely occurs from person to person.	• Sporadic cases and outbreaks in villages in South American continent.

Year of first cases	Disease	Incubation period Main signs and symptoms Case fatality rate (CFR)	Mode of transmission Reproducibility rate where known	Epidemiology
1994 1999	**Hendra virus** **Nipah virus**	• Incubation period for this group of paramyxoviridae (which also includes Menangle virus): from a few days to three months. • All of these cause an influenza-like illness with fever, headaches, dizziness, drowsiness, lung inflammation, sore throat and sometimes itchy and runny eyes. • The CFR is high.	• Normally zoontic diseases, Hendra virus usually affects horses; however, it has caused disease in seven humans and death in four humans (Commonwealth of Australia 2013). • Nipah virus affects pigs.	• Hendra virus is not known outside Queensland, and Nipah viruses occur mainly in Malaysia. In Bangladesh 70 per cent of infected people died in the 2001 outbreak. (CSIRO 2013)
1995	**HHV8** (Kaposi's sarcoma virus, a herpes virus)	• Incubation period: unknown. • Produces dark red or dusky brown plaques and nodules on the skin and elsewhere.	• Mode of transmission is unknown, although there is some evidence that sexual activity may be implicated for some groups of people.	• Historically, eastern European males were particularly at risk of this sarcoma; nowadays, it is often associated with HIV infection.
1996	**Australian bat lyssavirus (ABL)**	• Incubation period: unknown, but probably several weeks. • Causes a viral encephalomyelitis (infection of the brain) with headache, fever, muscle spasms, and a number of associated fears and behaviour changes. • Two deaths are known to have occurred from this disease.	• A zoonotic disease known to be common in some Australian species of flying foxes and bats; it is widespread and can cause disease in humans. • Although it is related to rabies, dogs and cats do not seem to be susceptible to ABL, and therefore cannot pass it on to humans. • Transmission is from exposure to faeces or urine of, or bites and scratches from, infected animals.	• People who are exposed to bats—in particular, veterinarians, are most at risk.
1996	**nvCJD**	• Incubation: very long, from 15 months to 30 years. • A degenerative brain disease leading to dementia; the new variant CJD (nvCJD) is a more prolonged disease than the CJD it clinically resembles.	• Thought to be ingested by eating meat infected with 'prions'; it is hypothesised that it is caused by a protein ('prion') replicating in a specific, as yet unknown way. • There is no evidence that this disease is spread from person to person.	• 'Ordinary' and long-described CJD is known all over the world, but nvCJD (the cause of bovine spongiform encephalopathy or BSE, also known as 'mad cow disease', has been restricted almost entirely to the United Kingdom and is associated with the consumption of meat products containing offal and other meat scraps.

Year of first cases	Disease	Incubation period Main signs and symptoms Case fatality rate (CFR)	Mode of transmission Reproducibility rate where known	Epidemiology
1997	**H5N1 avian influenza**	• Influenza virus causes an acute, severe disease, with fever, severe headache and muscle and body aches, sore throat, runny and itchy eyes, and a dry cough. • Strains that normally affect only animals carry a high fatality rate if they escape into the human population.	• Normally highly contagious; however, the strains that escape from the bird population are not normally transmitted from person to person.	• Live birds, especially chickens, heavily affected—particularly in Hong Kong.
1999	**West Nile virus** (New York City)	• The flavivirus group, of which West Nile is a recently identified member, has a short incubation period of 3–12 days. • This group of viral diseases includes fevers, headaches, muscle aches and pains, sometimes with nausea and vomiting, confusion and dislike of light.	• An arthropod-borne disease, carried from infected birds to humans by mosquitoes. • It is not transmitted from person to person.	• Most commonly found in Africa, India, Israel, Pakistan, the former Soviet Union, Cyprus and France. • People are susceptible throughout life. • More recently it has been found in New York state, in the United States.
2003	**SARS CoV**	• Incubation period: up to 12 days. • Main signs include indications of gastroenteritis, fever and sometimes shortness of breath. • Lung changes on x-ray.	• Has affected about 8500 people worldwide, mainly in China (including Taiwan), Hong Kong, Vietnam, Singapore and Canada between November 2002 and June 2003—one fifth were health-care workers. • Transmitted person to person only in symptomatic people, not highly infectious. • CFR 11 per cent, reproducibility rate of about 3; however, some cases were thought to be 'super-spreaders'.	• Identified as an outbreak of atypical pneumonia in Hong Kong, subsequently traced back to China. • Chinese doctors had been aware of the outbreak but had not undertaken extensive epidemiological studies nor instituted rigorous outbreak control measures. • The WHO mounted a global investigation and control program, a global first and considered to be highly successful.

Year of first cases	Disease	Incubation period Main signs and symptoms Case fatality rate (CFR)	Mode of transmission Reproducibility rate where known	Epidemiology
2004	**Avian influenza (bird 'flu)**	• Fever, sore throat, cough and severe malaise. • In severe cases, viral pneumonia continuing to severe respiratory distress. • Case fatality rate 72 per cent.	• Secondary person-to-person transmission thought to be very rare. • Emerged in poultry in late 2003; by the end of 2004, 47 human cases had been identified, with 34 deaths.	• First cases in chickens identified in November 2003, and first human cases notified in January 2004 in South-East Asia. • Influenza virus A strain known as H5N1; potential for human strain acquiring some characteristics of H5N1 and triggering a serious pandemic led to enhanced surveillance.
2009	**Human swine 'flu**	• Fever (over 38°C), cough, sore throat, aches and tiredness, headache and chills. • In severe cases, viral pneumonia and lung failure. High-risk groups identified to be those with chronic respiratory conditions; pregnant women; those who are obese (BMI>30); Indigenous people; and those with chronic cardiac, neurological and immune conditions. Children and younger people are at increased risk of complications and are also rapid spreaders of the virus.	• Person-to-person droplet transmission. • In 2009, there were 37 636 cases in Australia, including 191 associated deaths (case fatality rate %), median age of those dying was 53 years compared with 83 years for seasonal influenza; 30 per cent of deaths occurred in previously healthy people.	• Derived mainly from strains that affect pigs, new H1N1 virus derived from human, swine and avian strains reported in Mexico April 2009 then spread to most other countries. • Influenza virus A strain known as H1N1 or influenza 09.

Sources: Benenson (1995); Acha & Szyfres (2003); Victorian Department of Human Services (2005a); DoHA (2012m).

Appendix J

Core environmental health services provided by departments of health and environment protection agencies

Jurisdiction	Departments of health	Environment protection agencies/departments
Australian Capital Territory	• Food safety • Tobacco control • Radiation safety • Drinking water quality • Air quality	• Air quality control and management • Regulation of hazardous chemicals, including pest chemicals • Noise pollution, including motor sports and outdoor concerts • Ozone depletion • Waterways pollution • Landfill and sewerage treatment • Remediation of contaminated sites
New South Wales	• The safe and adequate provision of drinking water • The recreational use of water • Sewage and waste water • Toxicology—chemical hazards and contaminated sites • State of the environment reporting • Regulation of a number of funeral and skin-penetration industries • Arbovirus control • Waste management	• Investigation and remediation of contaminated sites • Control of hazardous chemicals and dangerous goods • Regulation of air emissions, water quality • Noise control

Jurisdiction	Departments of health	Environment protection agencies/ departments
Northern Territory	• Aboriginal and general community environmental health • Environmental health-risk assessment • Solid waste and wastewater management • Water quality • Food safety • Radiation protection • Poisons control	• Review and assessment of the effectiveness of agency responses in dealing with environmental incidents and the coordination of the responses • Monitoring and assessment of the cumulative effects of development—public release of reports on environmental quality • Advice on best-practice environmental policy and management • Advice on setting objectives, targets and standards for public and private sectors • Advice on emerging environmental issues—advice on issues affecting capacity to achieve ecologically sustainable development
South Australia	• Wastewater management and septic tanks • Inspections, audits and investigations to ensure compliance with licence • Drinking water quality, rainwater tanks, fluoridation • Food safety • Drugs and poisons licences • Environmental monitoring—Port Pirie Lead Project • Tobacco control • Public health pest control • Public events • Public pools and spas water standards • Wastewater management, including recycled water	• Assessment of environmental impacts of major projects and developments, conditions, laws and regulations • Work with local government to protect local environments • Emergency response to incidents (chemical spills, sewer overflows) • Monitoring and research of environmental conditions and issues • Provision to businesses, industries and communities of solutions for environmental sustainability and improved environmental performance • Advice to government on environmental matters, issues and trends

Jurisdiction	Departments of health	Environment protection agencies/ departments
Queensland	<ul><li>Drugs, poisons and therapeutic goods regulation</li><li>Water and waste regulation</li><li>Health impact assessments</li><li>Environmental toxicology and health-risk assessments of environmental hazards</li><li>Food safety</li><li>Radiation health</li></ul>	<ul><li>Climate change</li><li>Protection of biodiversity, natural environment and resources</li><li>Management of parks, forestry and wildlife</li><li>Land management, including improvement of Indigeous land ownership and conservation of cultural heritage</li><li>Management of waste and waste reduction</li><li>Water security, including protection of water resources</li><li>Promotion of sustainable industry</li><li>Compliance inspections and audits of regulated industries</li></ul>
Tasmania	<ul><li>Communicable disease prevention and control</li><li>Environmental health</li><li>Food safety</li><li>Immunisation programs</li><li>Nutrition regulation</li><li>Radiation regulation</li><li>Tobacco control</li></ul>	<ul><li>Regulation of developments and activities that impact on environmental quality</li><li>Remediation of historical environmental damage</li><li>Sustainable environmental management</li><li>Monitor and reduce air pollution</li><li>Management of contaminated land</li><li>Noise control policy and management</li><li>Protection and enhancement of water quality</li></ul>

Jurisdiction	Departments of health	Environment protection agencies/ departments
Victoria	• Identification, assessment and response to public health threats • Emergency management and planning • Monitoring of drinking water quality • Assessment of industry developments • Food safety • Radiation safety • Regulation of pesticides and cooling towers • Development of recreational water standards • Climate change, including heatwave planning • Communicable disease prevention and control	• Climate change and greenhouse gas reduction • Regulation and licensing of industries and emissions • Pollution investigation • Protection and sustainability of water environments • Development of regulatory framework for waste • Coordination of activities to prevent and control noise • Prevention of land and groundwater contamination
Western Australia	• Food safety • Meat safety • Radiation safety • Water safety • Control of hazardous chemicals and pesticides • Control of mosquito-borne diseases • Regulation of tattooing and personal health services • Management of wastewater • Drinking and recreational water quality	• Conduct of environmental impact assessments • Preparation of statutory policies for environmental protection • Preparation of guidelines for the management of environmental impacts • Prevention, control and abatement of pollution and environmental harm • State of the environment reporting • Monitoring of compliance with ministerial approvals • Implementation of environmental offsets

Sources: compiled from the following web pages (accessed March 2012):
ACT Health Directorate <www.environment.act.gov.au/about_us>; ACT Environment and Sustainable Development Directorate <www.environment.act.gov.au/environment2/environment_protection_authority_legislation_and_policies>; NSW Health <www.health.nsw.gov.au/publichealth/environment/index.asp>; NSW EPA <www.environment.nsw.gov. au/epa/index.htm>; Northern Territory Department of Health & Families <www.health.nt.gov.au/Environmental_Health/ index.aspx>; South Australian Department of Health & Ageing <www.dh.sa.gov.au/pehs/environ-health-index.htm>; South Australia EPA <www.epa.sa.gov.au/what_we_do>; Queensland Health <www.health.qld.gov.au/ph/ehu/default. asp>; Tasmanian Department of Health and Human Services <www.dhhs.tas.gov.au/peh>; EPA Tasmania <epa.tas.gov. au/epa/about-us>; Victorian Department of Health <www.health.vic.gov.au/divisions/wica/cho.htm>; EPA Victoria <www. epa.vic.gov.au/about_us/default.asp>; Western Australia Department of Health <www.public.health.wa.gov.au/1/1060/2/ environmental_health_food_water_and_hazards.pm>; EPA Western Australia <www.epa.wa.gov.au/AbouttheEPA/ aboutetheEPA/Pages/default.aspx?cat=About%20the%>; and the following reports: Queensland Department of Environment and Resource Management, *Annual Report 2010–11*; DERM Brisbane (2011); Australian Capital Territory Chief Health Officer's Report 2010, Population Health Division, ACT Health, Canberra; Environment Protection Authority, *Annual Report 2010–11*, EPA Northern Territory, Darwin.

Appendix K

Vaccine start dates in Australia

1804	Smallpox from England
1917	Smallpox produced in Australia
1917	Tetanus antitoxin for armed forces
1924	Diphtheria toxin–antitoxin Melbourne City Council
1925	Tetanus toxoid
1925	Pertussis toxoid used in case contacts and epidemics
1927	Diphtheria toxoid
1932	Community immunisation for the public
1945 June	Tetanus toxoid available for civilians after World War II
1953	Diphtheria/Tetanus/Pertussis (DTP)
1956 May	SALK (polio)
1966 September	Polio sabin (OPV)
1969	Measles
1971 February	Rubella
1980	Smallpox vaccination ceased
1981 July	Mumps
1982	Pneumovax 14
1983 February	Measles/Mumps
1983 March	Hepatitis B Vax (Plasma)
1984–85	End of BCG school program
1986	CDT-DTP 4th dose (1st Pertussis booster)
1987	Infants 'at risk' birth dose hepatitis B
1987	Pneumovax 23
1987 November	Hepatitis B Vax II (Recombinant)
1989 June	Measles/Mumps/Rubella (MMR)
1992 May	Haemophilus influenzae (Hib) (18/12—5)
1993 July	Hib (2/12—18/12)
1993 July	Hepatitis A (Havrix)
1994	MMR males/females Grade 6
1995	CDT-DTP fifth dose (second Pertussis booster)
1997	Influenza program for over 65s

1997 October	Infanrix replaces fourth and fifth dose Triple Antigen
	HibTITER multidose expired (contained thiomersal)
1998	Pneumococcal Pneumonia (over 65s)
1998	MMR primary school program
1998	Four-year-old booster DTP, MMR, OPV program prior to school
1998	Hepatitis B paediatric vaccine (three doses) Year 7 secondary school program introduced
1999	MMR eighteen to 30-year-old campaign
1999	Infanrix—2½ to four years of age inclusive
2000	Comvax (hib-hepatitis B)
2000	OPV ceased in Year 9/10 school program
2000	Hepatitis B boosters ceased
2000	ADT boosters 10 yearly ceased
2000 May	Hepatitis B birth dose introduced
2001	Hepatitis B Adult vaccine (2 doses) Year 7 school program
2001	Hepatitis B vaccine for injecting drug users
2001	Varicella (chickenpox) (unfunded)
2001	Childhood pneumococcal pneumonia—Aboriginal and Torres Strait Islander children only
2001	Hib TITER vaccine ceased (only Pedvax available)
2001 December	Meningitec—Meningococcal C conjugate vaccine (unfunded)
2002 August	NeisVac C—Meningococcal C conjugate vaccine (unfunded)
2002 October	Menjugate—Meningococcal C conjugate vaccine (unfunded)
2003 January	Meningococcal C conjugate vaccine at twelve months of age
2003 January	One to nineteen years meningococcal C conjugate vaccination program (until 2006)
2003 September	Eighteenth-month dose DTPa ceased
	Expanded medical risk group for childhood pneumococcal under five years of age
2004 January	dTpa (Boostrix) for fifteen to seventeen years (Year 10 school program) in place of ADT
2004 September	4, 5 and 6 antigen combination vaccines
2005 January	Pneumococcal vaccine—Prevenar scheduled at two, four and six months of age—catch-up in 2005 for children born between 1 January 2003 and 31 December 2004
2005 January	Pneumococcal vaccine—Pneumovax 23 now funded by federal government for adults over 65 years of age
2005 November	Inactivated polio vaccine in combination with diphtheria, tetanus and pertussis scheduled at two, four and six months and four years of age
2005 November	Oral polio (sabin) ceased at two, four and six months and four years of age
2005 November	Chickenpox (varicella) vaccine scheduled at eighteen months of age and for children in Year 7 of secondary school who have not had chickenpox vaccine or the disease
2007	Hepatitis B vaccine for household contacts of a person living with hepatitis B
2007	Hepatitis B vaccine for prisoners
2007 April	Human papillomavirus vaccine (HPV) for girls aged between twelve and thirteen in Year 7 of secondary school. A two-year catch-up period to the end of June 2009 for girls aged fourteen to eighteen

2007 July	HPV for young women aged between eighteen and 26 for a two-year period to the end of June 2009
2007 July	Rotavirus (RotaTeq) vaccine scheduled at two, four and six months of age
2008 March	Diphtheria, tetanus, acellular pertussis, hepatitis B, poliomyelitis and haemophilus influenzae type b (Infanrix hexa) combination vaccine for babies at two, four and six months of age
2008 September	Hiberix vaccine (haemophilus influenzae type b) given at twelve months of age for an infant who has at minimum received Infanrix hexa vaccine at six months of age and is up to date with all vaccines
2008 September	Pedvax HIB ceased
2009 June	Diphtheria, tetanus, pertussis (Boostrix®) free vaccine for parents with an infant born from 15 June 2009; program ended 30 June 2012
2009 September	Pandemic influenza Panvax® H1N1 vaccine for people aged ten years and over
2009 December	Panvax® H1N1 approved for children aged six months to under ten years of age
2009 December	HPV vaccine (Gardasil®) catch-up program for females between thirteen and 26 years of age (ended 31 December 2009)
2010	Hepatitis B vaccine for HIV positive persons
2010 January	Human papillomavirus (HPV) vaccine (Gardasil®) Year 7 secondary schoolgirl program or age equivalent
2010 January	Influenza. Expanded eligibility for free seasonal influenza vaccine to include pregnant women, Indigenous people from fifteen years of age and over, residents of nursing homes and other long term care facilities, all people from six months of age and over with conditions predisposing to severe influenza
2010 December	Panvax® H1N1 vaccine program ended on 31 December 2010
2011 July	Prevenar® vaccine ceased for use at two, four and six months of age
2011 July	Prevenar 13® introduced for the primary schedule at two, four and six months of age
2011 October	A supplementary catch-up dose of Prevenar 13® for all children aged twelve months to 35 months; program ended 30 September 2012

Source: Victorian Department of Health (2012b).

Appendix L

Common food- or water-borne pathogens

Causative agent	Incubation period	Main symptoms	Foods commonly implicated
Campylobacter jejuni	1–10 days	Sudden onset of diarrhoea, abdominal pain, nausea, vomiting	Raw or undercooked poultry, raw milk, raw or undercooked meat, untreated water
Escherichia coli enterohaemorrhagic	2–10 days	Severe colic, mild to profuse bloody diarrhoea, which can lead to haemolytic uraemic syndrome	Many raw foods (especially minced beef), unpasteurised milk, contaminated water
E. coli entero-pathogenic enterotoxigenic enteroinvasive	12–72 hours (enterotoxigenic)	Severe colic, profuse diarrhoea	Many raw foods, food contaminated by faecal matter, contaminated water
Salmonella serovars (non-typhoid)	6–72 hours	Abdominal pain, diarrhoea, chills, fever, malaise	Raw or undercooked meat and chicken, raw or undercooked eggs and egg products
Salmonella typhi/ paratyphi	Typhoid 8–14 days Paratyphoid 1–10 days	Fever, headache and constipation	Raw shellfish, salads, contaminated water
Shigella species	12–96 hours	Malaise, fever, vomiting, diarrhoea	Foods contaminated by infected food handlers, untreated water contaminated by human faeces
Yersinia enterocolitica	3–7 days	Acute diarrhoea (sometimes bloody), fever, vomiting	Raw meat (especially pork), raw or undercooked poultry, milk and milk products
Vibrio cholerae	A few hours to 5 days	Asymptomatic to profuse painless watery diarrhoea, dehydration	Raw seafood, contaminated water

Causative agent	Incubation period	Main symptoms	Foods commonly implicated
Vibrio parahaemolyticus	4–30 hours	Abdominal pain, diarrhoea, vomiting and sometimes fever	Raw and lightly cooked fish, shellfish, other seafoods
Listeria monocytogenes	3–70 days	Flu-like symptoms to meningitis/septicaemia; infection in pregnancy can result in abortions, neonatal infection	Unpasteurised milk, soft cheese, paté, coleslaw, salads, ready-to-eat seafood, cold meats, fresh fruit drinks
Norovirus (and other viral gastroenteritis)	24–48 hours	Severe vomiting, diarrhoea	Oysters, clams, foods contaminated by infected food handlers, untreated water contaminated by human faeces
Rotaviruses	24–72 hours	Malaise, headache, fever, vomiting, diarrhoea	Foods contaminated by infected food handlers, untreated water contaminated by human faeces
Hepatitis A	15–50 days	Fever, nausea, abdominal discomfort, possibly jaundice	Shellfish, foods contaminated by infected food handlers, untreated water contaminated by human faeces
Cryptosporidium	1–12 days	Profuse watery diarrhoea, abdominal pain	Foods contaminated by infected food handlers, untreated water contaminated by human faeces
Giardia lamblia	1–3 weeks	Loose, pale, greasy stools, abdominal pain	Foods contaminated by infected food handlers, untreated water contaminated by human faeces
Entamoeba histolytica	2–4 weeks	Colic, mucous or bloody diarrhoea	Foods contaminated by infected food handlers, untreated water contaminated by human faeces
Bacillus cereus (toxin in food)	1–6 hours	Two known toxins causing nausea and vomiting or diarrhoea and cramps	Cereals, rice, meat products, soups, vegetables
Clostridium botulinum	12–36 hours	Blurred or double vision, difficulty swallowing, respiratory paralysis, muscle weakness and lethargy	Canned food (often home-canned, i.e. low acid)

Causative agent	Incubation period	Main symptoms	Foods commonly implicated
Clostridium perfringens (toxin in gut)	6–24 hours	Sudden-onset colic, diarrhoea	Meats, poultry, stews, gravies (often inadequately reheated or held warm)
Staphylococcus aureus (toxin in food)	30 min–8 hours	Acute vomiting, cramps, may lead to collapse	Cold foods, milk products, salted meats
Scombroid fish poisoning (histamine poisoning)	Few hours	Tingling and burning around mouth, sweating, diarrhoea, vomiting, headache, dizziness	Fish such as tuna, mackerel, skipjack, bonito, herring and sardines
Ciguatera poisoning	Less than 24 hours	Numbness and tingling around mouth, diarrhoea, vomiting and nausea, followed by neurological symptoms such as dizziness, blurred vision and temperature reversal	Large tropical reef fish
Paralytic shellfish poisoning	Minutes to several hours	Burning and tingling around the mouth and extremities, nausea dizziness, potentially muscle and respiratory paralysis	Bivalve molluscs
Diarrhetic shellfish poisoning	30 minutes–2 hours	Diarrhoea, nausea, vomiting	Mussels, scallops, clams

Source: Victorian Department of Human Services (2005a: 60–1).

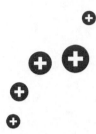

Useful resources

Websites

Australia

ACT Department of Health: <www.health.act.gov.au/c/health>
Australian Bureau of Statistics: <www.abs.gov.au>
Australian Consumers Association: <www.choice.com.au>
Australian Council of Social Service: <www.acoss.org.au>
Australian Healthcare and Hospitals Association: <www.ahha.asn.au>
Australian Indigenous Health Infonet : <www.healthinfonet.ecu.edu.au>
Australian Institute of Health and Welfare: <www.aihw.gov.au>
Australian National Preventive Health Agency: <www.anpha.gov.au>
Australian Research Alliance for Children and Youth: <www.aracy.org.au/about.htm>
Better Health Channel: <www.betterhealth.vic.gov.au>
Centre of Excellence in Intervention and Prevention Science: <www.ceips.org.au>
Consumer Health Forum: <www.chf.org.au>
Council of Academic Public Health Institutions Australia: <www.caphia.com.au>
Commonwealth Department of Health and Ageing: <www.health.gov.au>
Commonwealth of Australia National Occupational Health & Safety Commission: <www.nohsc.gov.au>
Food Standards Australia: <www.foodstandards.gov.au>
Health Insite: <www.healthinsite.gov.au>
Health Issues Centre: <www.healthissuescentre.org.au>
The Lowitja Institute: <www.lowitja.org.au>
National Aboriginal Community Controlled Health Organisation: <www.naccho.org.au>

National Health and Medical Research Council: <www.nhmrc.gov.au>
National Public Health Partnership: <www.nphp.gov.au>
NSW Health Department: <www.health.nsw.gov.au>
Northern Territory Department of Health and Community Services: <www.health.nt.gov.au>
Parliament of Australia: <www.aph.gov.au>
Public Health Association of Australia: <www.phaa.net.au>
Queensland Health: <www.health.qld.gov.au>
Sax Institute: <www.saxinstitute.org.au>
South Australian Department of Health: <www.health.sa.gov.au>
Tasmanian Department of Health & Human Services: <www.dhhs.tas.gov.au>
Victorian Department of Health: <www.health.vic.gov.au>
Victorian Department of Human Services: <www.dhs.vic.gov.au>
Western Australia Health Department: <www.public.health.wa.gov.au>
Women's Health Victoria: <www.whv.org.au>
Women's Portal: <www.women.gov.au>

International

Agency for Healthcare Research and Quality: <www.ahrq.gov/consumer>
American Public Health Association: <www.apha.org>
Asian Development Bank: <www.adb.org>
Centers for Disease Control and Prevention (USA): <www.cdc.gov>
Centre for Reviews and Dissemination (UK): <www.york.ac.uk/inst/crd>
Cochrane Library: <www.cochrane.org>
European Observatory on Health Systems and Policies: <www.euro.who.int/en>
Food and Agriculture Organization of the United Nations: <www.fao.org>
Global Fund (to fight against AIDS, tuberculosis and malaria): <www.theglobalfund.org/en>
Habitat for Humanity: <www.habitat.org.au>
Health Canada: <www.hc-sc.gc.ca/english/index.html>
Healthfinders: <www.healthfinder.gov>
International Labor Organization: <www.ilo.org>
International Network of Health Promoting Hospitals and Health Services: <www.hphnet.org>
International Organization for Migration: <www.iom.int>
International Union of Health Promotion and Education: <www.iuhpe.org>
National Institute for Health and Clinical Excellence (UK): <www.nice.org.uk>
National Institutes of Health (USA): <www.nih.gov>
National Public Health Institute: <www.ianphi.org>
New Zealand Ministry of Health: <www.moh.govt.nz/moh.nsf>
People's Health Movement: <www.phmovement.org>
Public Health Agency of Canada: <www.phac-aspc.gc.ca/index-eng.php>
Public Health Foundation (USA): <www.phf.org/index.htm>
Public Health Institute: <www.phi.org>
Society for Public Health Education: <www.sophe.org>
United Kingdom Department of Health: <www.dh.gov.uk>

UNAIDS: <www.unaids.org>
United Nations: <www.un.org>
United Nations Children's Fund: <www.unicef.org.au>
United Nations Development Program: <www.undp.org>
United Nations Refugee Agency: <www.unhcr.org>
United States Department of Health and Human Services: <www.hhs.gov>
World Bank: <www.worldbank.org>
World Economic Forum: <www.weforum.org>
World Federation of Public Health Associations: <www.wfpha.org>
World Health Organization: <www.who.int/en>
World Health Organization Bulletin: <www.who.int/bulletin>

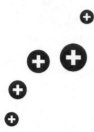

Sources for definitions

Public health terminology can be confusing. For generally authoritative definitions, please consult the following references. Public health agencies often develop their own glossaries, and these can be found on their websites.

Aulich, C., Halligan, J. and Nutley, S. 2001 *Australian Handbook of Public Sector Management*, Allen & Unwin, Sydney.

Breslow, L. (ed.-in-chief) 2002 *The Encyclopedia of Public Health*, Macmillan, New York.

Culyer, A.J. 2005 *The Dictionary of Health Economics*, Edward Elgar, Cheltenham.

Detels, R., Beaglehole, R., Lansang, M.A. and Guillford, M. 2011 *Oxford Textbook of Public Health*, Oxford University Press, Oxford.

European Commission 2001 *Glossary of Public Health: Technical Terms*, EC, Brussels.

Glasziou, P., Irwig, L., Bain, C. and Colditz, G. 2001 *Systematic Reviews in Health Care: A Practical Guide*, Cambridge University Press, Cambridge.

Heggenhougen, K. (ed.) 2008 *International Encyclopedia of Public Health*, Elsevier <www.sciencedirect.com/science/referenceworks/9780123739605> [20 February 2013].

Kirch, W. 2008 (ed) *Encyclopedia of Public Health: Volume 1: A–H, Volume 2: I–Z*, Springer, New York.

Last, J. 2006 *Dictionary of Public Health*, Oxford University Press, New York.

Modeste, N., Tamayose, T. and Marshak, H.H. 2004 *Dictionary of Public Health Promotion and Education: Terms and Concepts*, 2nd edn, Wiley Higher Education, Hoboken, NJ.

Nutbeam, D. 1998 *Health Promotion Glossary*, World Health Organization, Geneva, <www.who.int/hpr/NPH/docs/hp_glossary_en.pdf> [20 February 2013].

Oxford Bibliographies, Public Health, Oxford University Press: <www.oxfordbibliographies.com/obo/page/public-health>.

Pancheon, D., Guset, C., Melzer, D. and Gray, J.A. (eds) 2001 *Oxford Handbook of Public Health Practice*, Oxford University Press, Oxford.

Porta, M. (ed) 2008 *A Dictionary of Epidemiology*, 5th edn, International Epidemiological Association, Oxford University Press, Oxford.

Wallace, R.B. (ed.) 2007 *Maxcy-Rosenau-Last: Public Health and Preventive Medicine*, 15th edn, McGraw-Hill, New York.

White, K. 2005 *The Sage Dictionary of Health and Society*, Sage, London.

World Health Organization 2010 *International Statistical Classification of Diseases and Related Health Problems*, 10th rev. edn, <http://apps.who.int/classifications/icd10/browse/2010/en> [20 February 2013].

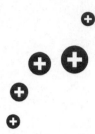

Bibliography

Abbott, T. 2004a 'Commonwealth Government to provide pneumococcal vaccine for both young and old', media release, 11 June, <www.health.gov.au/internet/wcms/publishing.nsf/Content/health-mediarel-yr2004-ta-abb078.htm> [13 October 2004].

——— 2004b 'MedicarePlus: Protecting and strengthening Medicare', media release, Minister for Health and Ageing, 18 November.

——— 2004c '$115 million boost to health and medical research programs', media release, Minister for Health and Ageing, 5 July, <www.health.gov.au/nhmrc/media/rel2004/boost.htm> [15 June 2005].

ABC Radio 2004 'Pneumococcal vaccination for Australian children', ABC Gold and Tweed Coasts, 12 August, <www.abc.net.au/cgi-bin/common/printfriendly>.

Abelson, P. (ed.) 2003a *Returns on Investment in Public Health*, Commonwealth Department of Health and Ageing, Canberra.

——— 2003b 'Road safety programs and road trauma', in P. Abelson (ed.), *Returns on Investment in Public Health*, Commonwealth Department of Health and Ageing, Canberra.

Abelson, P. and Taylor, R. 2003 'Public health programs to reduce tobacco consumption', in P. Abelson (ed.), *Returns on Investment in Public Health*, Commonwealth Department of Health and Ageing, Canberra.

ABS: *see* Australian Bureau of Statistics.

Acha, P.N. and Szyfres, B. 2003 *Zoonoses and Communicable Diseases Common to Man and Animals*, Pan American Health Organization, Washington, DC.

ACT Government 2010 *Issues and Options for Regulating Boarding Style Accommodation in the Australian Capital Territory: A Joint Initiative of the ACT Chief Minister's Department, ACT Health, Department of Justice and Community Safety, ACT Planning and Land Authority and Department of Disability, Housing and Community Services*, Chief Minister's Department, Canberra.

ACT Health 2010 *Citizens' Jury on Health Priorities 2010*, report by ACT Health Council, <http://health.act.gov.au/publications-reports/reports/citizens-jury-onhealth-priorities-2010> [20 February 2013].

Aday, L.A. 1994 'Health-status of vulnerable populations', *Annual Review of Public Health*, 15, pp. 487–509.

Adhikari, R., Gertler, P. and Lagman, A. 1999 *Economic Analysis of Health Sector Projects: A Review of Issues, Methods and Approaches*, Economic Staff Papers 58, Asian Development Bank, Manila.

Adler, N.E., Epel, E., Castellazzo, G. and Ickovics, J.R. 2000 'Relationships of subjective and objective social status with psychological and physiological functioning: Preliminary data in healthy white women', *Health Psychology*, 19, pp. 586–92.

AHMAC: *see* Australian Health Ministers' Advisory Council.

AHRC: *see* Australian Human Rights Commission.

AIEH: *see* Australian Institute of Environmental Health.

AIHPS: *see* Australian Institute of Health Policy Studies.

AIHW: *see* Australian Institute of Health and Welfare.

Aitken, C.K., Kerger, M. and Crofts, N. 2002 'Peer-delivered hepatitis C testing and counselling: A means of improving the health of injecting drug users', *Drug and Alcohol Review*, 21(1), pp. 33–7.

Ajzen, I. and Fishbein, M. 1980 *Understanding Attitudes and Predicting Social Behaviour*, Prentice-Hall, Englewood Cliffs, NJ.

Alford, R. 1975 *Health Care Politics*, University of Chicago Press, Chicago.

Allen Consulting Group 2005 *Climate Change Risk and Vulnerability: Promoting an Efficient Response in Australia*, Department of the Environment and Heritage, Canberra, <www.agric.wa.gov.au/objtwr/imported_assets/content/lwe/cli/climatechangeframework_no%20cover_web.pdf> [1 December 2012].

Allin, S., Mossialos, E., McKee, M. and Holland, W. 2004 *Making Decisions on Public Health: A Review of Eight Countries*, European Observatory on Health Systems and Policies, WHO, Geneva.

Allwell, L., Spink, J. and Robinson, S. 2004 'Consumer participation in the Sharing Health Care Initiative demonstration projects', *Health Issues*, 78, pp. 28–32.

Alonzo, A. and Reynolds, N.R. 1995 'Stigma, HIV and AIDS: An exploration and elaboration of a stigma trajectory', *Social Science and Medicine*, 41(3), pp. 303–15.

AMA: *see* Australian Medical Association.

American Public Health Association 2000 'Drinking water quality and public health' (Position Paper), *American Journal of Public Health*, 91(3), pp. 499–500.

——— 2006 Public Health Code of Ethics, <www.apha.org/codeofethics/ethics.htm> [6 April 2006].

AMSANT 2011 *Framework for the Development of the Primary Health Care Workforce in Aboriginal Health in the Northern Territory* <www.humancapitalalliance.com.au/documents/HR14-Aboriginal%20PHC%20Workforce%20Framework.pdf>.

ANAPHI: *see* Australian Network of Academic Public Health Institutions.

ANCARD: *see* Australian National Council on AIDS and Related Diseases.

Anderson, J., Petrosyan, V. and Hussey, P. 2002 *Multinational Comparisons of Health System Data, 2002*, The Commonwealth Fund, New York.

Andreasen, A.R. 1995 *Marketing Social Change: Changing Behavior to Promote Health, Social Development and the Environment*, Jossey-Bass, San Francisco.

Anon 2001 'Globalization—how healthy?' (editorial), *Bulletin of the World Health Organization*, 79(9), pp. 902–3.

——— 2003 'Fear factor', *Sydney Morning Herald*, 28 March.

——— 2004a 'Fifth framework programme', *CDR Weekly*, 14 (6), 16 April.

——— 2004b 'Immunisation Report', *Communicable Diseases Report*, 14 (20), pp. 1–25.

——— 2005 'Lung bus to visit Baryulgil', *SBS World News online*, <http://news.sbs.com/livingblack/index.php?action=news&id=105355> [16 March 2005].

ANPHA: *see* Australian National Preventive Health Agency.

Ansari, Z. 2002 *The Victorian Ambulatory Care Sensitive Conditions Study: Opportunities for Targeting Public Health and Health Services Interventions*, Rural and Regional Health and Aged Care Services Division, Victorian Government Department of Human Services, Melbourne.

—— 2005 Ambulatory Care Sensitive Conditions 2004–2005, update, Department of Health, Victoria.

Ansari, Z., Carson, N., Serraglio, A., Barbetti, T. and Cicuttini, F. 2002 'The Victorian ambulatory care sensitive conditions study: Reducing demand on hospital services in Victoria', *Australian Health Review*, 25(2), pp. 71–7.

Anti-Discrimination Board of New South Wales 2001 *Report of the Enquiry into Hepatitis C Related Discrimination*, Anti-Discrimination Board of New South Wales, Sydney.

Antonovsky, A. 1996 'The salutogenic model as a theory to guide health promotion', *Health Promotion International*, 11(1), pp. 11–18.

ANZFA: *see* Australia New Zealand Food Authority.

Appleby, J. and Brambleby, P. 2001 'Economic evaluation—the science of making choices', in D. Pencheon, C. Guest, D. Melzer and J.A.M. Gray (eds), *Oxford Handbook of Public Health Practice*, Oxford University Press, Oxford.

ARC: *see* Australian Research Council.

Armstrong, B. 2003 'Interim report of the expert medical panel to evaluate the *Kimberley Chemical Use Review* recommendations', <www.health.wa.gov.au/publications/documents/Interim%20report%20final%20report.pdf> [14 March 2005].

Arnold, D. 1993 *Colonizing the Body: State Medicine and Epidemic Disease in Nineteenth-Century India*, Oxford University Press, Bombay.

Aroni, R., de Boer, R. and Harvey, K. 2003 'The Viagra affair: Evidence as the terrain for competing "partners"', in V. Lin and B. Gibson (eds), *Evidence-based Health Policy*, Oxford University Press, Melbourne.

ARPANSA: *see* Australian Radiation Protection and Nuclear Safety Agency.

Arrow, K.J. 1963 'Uncertainty and the welfare economics of medical care', *American Economic Review*, 53, pp. 941–73.

Asbestos Diseases Society of Australia 2004 'Asbestos related information', <www.asbestosdiseases.org.au/asbestosinfo> [14 March 2005].

Aschengrau, A. and Seage, G.R. 2003 *Essentials of Epidemiology in Public Health*, Jones and Bartlett, Sudbury, MA.

Ashton, J. (ed.) 1992 *Healthy Cities*, Open University Press, Milton Keynes.

Attorney-General's Department 2004 *Australian Institute of Health and Welfare Act 1987*, Government of Australia, Canberra, <http://scaleplus.law.gov.au/html/pasteact0/291/0/PA000110.htm> [14 December 2004].

Australia New Zealand Food Authority (ANZFA) 1998 *Development of Uniform Food Acts for Australia and New Zealand, Part 1: Discussion and Recommendations*, AGPS, Canberra.

—— 2002 *Food Standards News*, 34, February, ANZFA, Canberra.

Australian and New Zealand Environment and Conservation Council 2000 *Core Environmental Indicators for Reporting on the State of the Environment*, State of the Environment Reporting Task Force, Environment Australia, Canberra.

Australian Bureau of Statistics (ABS) 2003 *Health Risk Factors*, ABS, Canberra.

—— 2005 *Year Book Australia*, ABS, Canberra.

—— 2006 National Aboriginal and Torres Strait Islander Health Survey, 2004–05, 4715.0, <www.abs.gov.au/ausstats/abs@.nsf/mf/4715> [4 October 2013].

—— 2010 *Measures of Australia's Progress, Data Cubes, Health*, <www.abs.gov.au/ausstats/abs@.nsf/Lookup/by%20Subject/1370.0~2010~Chapter~MAP%20downloads%20(8)> [1 November 2012].

—— 2011 *Labor Force Survey*, <www.abs.gov.au/ausstats/abs@.nsf/detailspage/6287.02011>.

—— 2012a *Leading Causes of Death by Gender*, <www.abs.gov.au/ausstats/abs@.nsf/Products/BBC4B00DFF0E942ACA2579C6000F6B15?opendocument#> [25 August 2012].

—— 2012b *National Health Survey First Results*, <www.abs.gov.au/ausstats/abs> [28 November 2012].

—— 2012c *State and Territory Statistical Indicators: Infant Mortality*, <www.abs.gov.au/ausstats/abs@.nsf/Lookup/by+Subject/1367.0~2012~Main+Features~Infant+Mortality~3.17> [1 November].

Australian Cochrane Centre 2006 'Cochrane Consumers and Communication Review Group: About the Group', <www.latrobe.edu.au/cochrane/about.html> [4 April 2006].

Australian Football League (AFL) 2012 *Respect and Responsibility Program*, <www.afl.com.au/respect%20%20responsibility/tabid/16781/default.aspx>.

Australian Government Chemicals and Plastic Regulation Productivity Commission Research Report July 2008, <www.apvma.gov.au/about/work/better_regulation> [13 June 2013].

Australian Health Ministers' Advisory Council 2005 'Health Ministers fund second round of priority driven research', press release, 25 February, <www.health.gov.au/nhmrc/media/rel2005/ahmac.htm> [15 June 2005].

—— 2008 *Population based screening framework*, Australian Population Health Development Principal Committee, Screening Subcommittee, Commonwealth of Australia, Canberra.

Australian Human Rights Commission (AHRC) 1997 *Bringing Them Home: Report of the National Inquiry into the Separation of Aboriginal and Torres Strait Islander Children from Their Families*, AHRC, Canberra, <http://humanrights.gov.au/social_justice/bth_report/report/index.html> [20 March 2013].

Australian Indigenous HealthInfoNet 2010 *Major Developments in National Indigenous Health Policy Since 1967*, <www.healthinfonet.ecu.edu.au/health-systems/policies/reviews/health-policytimelines> [28 November 2012].

Australian Institute of Health and Welfare (AIHW) 1999 *National Public Health Information Development Plan*, NPHP, Melbourne.

—— 2000 *BreastScreen Australia Achievement Report 1997–1998*, Cancer Series no. 13, AIHW, Canberra.

—— 2001 *National Public Health Expenditure 1998–99*, AIHW, Canberra.

—— 2002 *Australia's Health 2002*, AIHW, Canberra.

—— 2003 'Are all Australians gaining weight?' *Bulletin*, 11, AIHW, Canberra.

—— 2004a *Australia's Health 2004*, AIHW, Canberra.

—— 2004b *Health System Expenditure on Disease and Injury in Australia, 2000–01*, Health & Welfare Expenditure Series no. 19, AIHW, Canberra.

—— 2005a *A Picture of Australia's Children*, AIHW, Canberra.

—— 2005b *National Public Health Information Plan 2005*, National Public Health Information Working Group, AIHW, Canberra.

—— 2009 *A Picture of Australia's Children 2009*, AIHW, Canberra.

—— 2010a *Australia's Health 2010*, AIHW, Canberra.

—— 2010b *Health System Expenditure on Disease and Injury in Australia, 2004–05*, Health and Welfare Expenditure series no. 36, AIHW, Canberra, <www.aihw.gov.au/publication-detail/?id=6442468349> [11 December 2012].

—— 2011a *Cervical Screening in Australia 2008–2009*, Cancer series no. 61, AIHW, Canberra.

—— 2011b *Diabetes Prevalence in Australia: Detailed Estimates for 2007–08*, Diabetes series no. 17, AIHW, Canberra, <www.aihw.gov.au/publication-detail/?id=10737419311> [6 December 2012].

—— 2011c *Key Indicators of Progress for Chronic Disease and Associated Determinants: Data Report*, AIHW, Canberra.

—— 2011d *Life Expectancy and Mortality of Aboriginal and Torres Strait Islander People*, AIHW, Canberra.

—— 2011e *Public Health Expenditure in Australia 2008–09*, AIHW, Canberra, <www.aihw.gov.au/WorkArea/DownloadAsset.aspx?id=10737418246&libID=10737418246> [15 December 2012].

—— 2012 *Australia's Health 2012*, Australia's Health series no. 13, AIHW, Canberra.

Australian Institute of Health Policy Studies (AIHPS) 2009 *How Can We Prevent Illness and Promote Good Health? Deliberative Community Forums: Summary of Outcomes for Participants*, Australian Institute of Health Policy Studies, Canberra.

Australian Institute of Primary Care 2004 'Community participation in action: An evaluation of community participation methods', trialled at a forum conducted by Southern Health, La Trobe University, <www.latrobe.edu.au/aip> [12 January 2012].

Australian Medical Association (AMA) 2002 *No More Excuses: Aboriginal and Torres Strait Islander Health*, Public Report Card 2002, AMA, Canberra.

—— 2003 *Time for Action: Aboriginal and Torres Strait Islander Health*, Public Report Card 2002, AMA, Canberra.

Australian National Council on AIDS and Related Diseases (ANCARD) 1999a *Proving Partnership: Review of the Third National HIV/AIDS Strategy*, Commonwealth of Australia, Canberra.

—— 1999b *Status Report on Implementation of the Final Report Recommendations of the Legal Working Party*, Commonwealth of Australia, Canberra.

Australian National Preventative Health Agency 2009 Foundation competencies for master of public health graduates in Australia, <www.phaa.net.au/documents/ANAPHI_MPH%20competencies.pdf> [6 October 2012].

—— 2011 'Strategic Plan 2011–2015', <www.anpha.gov.au/internet/anpha/publishing.nsf/Content/strategic-plan> [2 October 2013].

—— 2012, *Attachment 2: National Agreements and Corresponding Indicators*, <www.anpha.gov.au/internet/anpha/publishing.nsf/Content/surveillance-forumtoc~attachment2>.

Australian Pesticides and Veterinary Medicines Authority 2013 'The APVMA is changing', <www.apvma.gov.au/about/work/better_regulation> [6 October 2013].

Australian Network of Academic Public Health Institutions 2002 *National Public Health Education Framework: Final Report*, July, Australian Government Department of Health and Ageing, Canberra.

Australian Radiation Protection and Nuclear Safety Agency (ARPANSA) 2001 *National Competition Policy Review of Radiation Protection Legislation: Final Report*, ARPANSA, Canberra.

Australian Research Council (ARC) 2012 *The National Research Priorities and their Associated Priority Goals*, <www.arc.gov.au/pdf/nrps_and_goals.pdf> [6 November 2012].

Awofeso, N. 2004 'What's new about the "New Public Health"?', *American Journal of Public Health*, 94(5), pp. 705–9.

Ayres, I. and Braithwaite, J. 1992 *Responsive Regulation: Transcending the Deregulation Debate*, Oxford University Press, New York.

Bailie R., Si D., Dowden M. and Lonergan M. 2007 *ABCD: Audit and Best Practice for Chronic Disease: Final Project Report*, Menzies School of Health Research, <http://menzies.edu.au/sites/menzies.edu.au/files/file/abcd/ABCD%20Project%20Report.pdf> [20 November 2012].

Bammer, G. 2005 'Integration and implementation sciences: Building a new specialization', *Ecology and Society*, 10(2), <www.ecologyandsociety.org/vol10/iss2/art6> [27 September 2005].

Bandura, A. 1977 'Self-efficacy: Towards a unifying theory of behavior change', *Psychological Review*, 84, pp. 191–215.

—— 1986 *Social Foundations of Thought and Action: A Social Cognitive Theory*, Prentice-Hall, Englewood Cliffs, NJ.

Barker, D.J.P. (ed.) 1992 *Fetal and Infant Origins of Adult Disease*, BMJ Publishing Group, London.

Barrand, P. 1997 'Mental health reform and human rights', in H. Gardner (ed.), *Health Policy in Australia*, Oxford University Press, Melbourne.

Barry, C., Konstantinos, A. and the National Tuberculosis Advisory Committee 2009 'Tuberculosis Notifications in Australia, 2007', *Communicable Disease Intelligence*, 33(3), pp. 304–15.

Bastian, H. 1998 'Speaking up for ourselves: The evolution of consumer advocacy', *Health Care: International Journal of Technology Assessment in Health Care*, 14(1), pp. 3–23.

Baum, F. 1998 *The New Public Health: An Australian Perspective*, Oxford University Press, Melbourne.

Baum, N., Gollust, S., Goold, S. and Jacobson, P. 2009 'Ethical Issues in Public Health Practice in Michigan', *American Journal of Public Health*, 99(2), pp. 369–74.

BBC News 1986 'On this day 30 December: Coal mine canaries made redundant', <http://news.bbc.co.uk/onthisday/hi/dates/stories/december/30/newsid_2547000/2547587.stm> [22 March 2006].

—— 2005 'McLibel: Longest case in English history', *World Edition Online*, 25 February, <http://news.bbc.co.uk/go/pr/fr/-/2/hi/uk_news/4266741.stm> [10 October 2005].

Beaglehole, R. and Bonita, R. 1997 *Public Health at the Crossroads: Achievements and Prospects*, Cambridge University Press, Cambridge.

Beauchamp, D. and Steinbock, B. (eds) 1999 *New Ethics for the Public's Health*, Oxford University Press, New York.

Beaver, C. and Zhao, Y. 2004 *Investment Analysis of the Aboriginal and Torres Strait Islander Primary Health Care Program in the Northern Territory*, Consultant report no. 2, Commonwealth of Australia, Canberra.

Beddie, F. 2001 *Putting Life into Years: The Commonwealth's Role in Australia's Health Since 1901*, Commonwealth of Australia, Canberra.

Beder, S. 1989 'From pipe dreams to tunnel vision: Engineering decision-making and Sydney's sewerage system', unpublished PhD thesis, University of New South Wales, Sydney.

—— 1990 'Early environmentalists and the battle against sewers in Sydney', *Royal Australian Historical Society Journal*, 76(1), pp. 27–44.

Begg, S., Vos, T., Barker, B., Stevenson, C., Stanley, L. and Lopez A.D. 2007 *The Burden of Disease and Injury in Australia 2003*, AIHW, Canberra.

Bell, C. and Lewis, M. 2005 *The Economic Implications of Epidemics Old and New*, Working Paper no. 54, Center for Global Development, Washington, DC.

Bell, M. and Khodeli, I. 2004 *Public Health Worker Shortages*, Trends Alert, Council of State Governments, Lexington, KT.

Bell, W. 1996 'An overview of futures studies', in R.A. Slaughter (ed.), *The Knowledge Base of Futures Studies, Volume 1: Foundations*, DDM Media Group, Melbourne.

Benenson, A.S. (ed.) 1995 *Control of Communicable Diseases Manual*, 16th edn, American Public Health Association, Washington, DC.

Bennett, C., Mein, J., Beers, M., Harvey, B., Vemulpad, S., Chant, K. and Dalton, C. 2000 'Operation Safe Haven: An evaluation of health surveillance and monitoring in an acute setting', *Communicable Diseases Intelligence*, 24(2), pp. 21–6.

Bennett, S., Bostock, L., Gatrell, A., Thomas, C., Popay, J. and Williams, G. 1999 'The place is all right it's just the people that I can't stand: (Dis)associating with people and with place', paper presented at the British Sociological Association Medical Sociology Conference, York, September.

Bentham, J. 1982 *An Introduction to the Principles of Morals and Legislation*, J.H. Burns and H.L.A. Hart (eds), Methuen, London.

Berkman, L. and Glass, T. 2000 'Social integration, social networks, social support, and health' in L.F. Berkman, and I. Kawachi (eds), *Social Epidemiology*, Oxford University Press, New York.

Berkman, L. and Kawachi, I. (eds) 2000 *Social Epidemiology*, Oxford University Press, New York.

Bettcher, D., Sapirie, S. and Goon, E. 1998 'Essential public health functions: Results of an international Delphi study', *World Health Statistics Quarterly*, 51, pp. 44–54.

Better Heath Channel 2012 *Men's Health*, <www.betterhealth.vic.gov.au/bhcv2/bhcarticles.nsf/pages/Men%27s_health> [6 October 2012].

Better Health Commission 1986 *Looking Forward to Better Health, Volume 1: Final Report*, AGPS, Canberra.

Bidmeade, I. and Reynolds, C. 1997 *Public Health Law in Australia: Its Current State and Future Directions*, AGPS, Canberra.

Birch, S. 1997 'As a matter of fact: Evidence-based decision-making unplugged', *Health Economics*, 6, pp. 547–59.

Birch, S., Stoddart, G. and Beland, F. 1998 'Modelling the community as a determinant of health', *Canadian Journal of Public Health*, 89(6), pp. 402–5.

Blair, T. 2002 'Prime Minister's speech to Royal Society: Science matters, 10 April, <www.pm.gov.uk/output/Page1715.asp> [20 March 2006].

Bloom, A. 2000 *Health Reform in Australia and New Zealand*, Oxford University Press, Melbourne.

Bollen, M. 1996 'Recent changes in Australian general practice', *Medical Journal of Australia*, 164, pp. 212–15.

Bonita, R., de Courten, M., Dwyer, T., Jamrozik, K. and Winkelmann, R. 2001 *Surveillance of Risk Factors for Noncommunicable Diseases: The WHO STEPwise Approach Summary*, WHO, Geneva.

Bowers, E. J. and Cheng, I. 2010 'Meeting the primary health care needs of refugees and asylum seekers', Research Roundup Issue, 16 December 2010, Primary Health Care Research and Information Service, Adelaide.

Bracht, N. (ed.) 1990 *Health Promotion at the Community Level*, Sage, Newbury Park, CA.

Braithwaite, J. 2003 '"Spotlight on Spring Street", seminar 3: Contemporary issues for the Victorian public sector', Institute of Public Administration Australia, Sydney.

BreastScreen Victoria 2001 *Annual Statistical Report*, BreastScreen Victoria, Melbourne.

Breslow, L. 2004 *A Life in Public Health: An Insider's Retrospective*, Springer, New York.

Bridgeman, P. and Davis, G. 1998 *Australian Policy Handbook*, Allen & Unwin, Sydney.

Briggs, B. and Skull, S. 2003 'Refugee health: Clinical issues', in P. Allotey (ed.), *The Health of Refugees: Public Health Perspectives from Crisis to Settlement*, Oxford University Press, Melbourne.

Brill, D. 2012 'Faulty breast implants trigger class action', *Australian Doctor*, 20 February 2012.

Brockington, F. 1958 *World Health*, Penguin, Ringwood.

Brown, V. 1992 'Health care policies, health policies, or policies for health?' in H. Gardner (ed.), *Health Policy: Development, Implementation and Evaluation in Australia*, Churchill Livingston, Melbourne.

Brown, V.A., Nicholson, R., Stephenson, P., Bennett, K. and Smith, J. 2001 *Grass Roots and Common Ground, Guidelines for Community-based Environmental Health Action: A Discussion Paper*, University of Western Sydney, Sydney.

Brownson, R.C., Baker, E.A., Leet, T.L. and Gillespie, K.N. 2003 *Evidence-based Public Health*, Oxford University Press, New York.

Brownson, R.C., Baker, E. and Novick, L. 1999 *Community-based Prevention: Programs that Work*, Aspen, Gaithersburg, MD.

Brownson, R.C. and Petitti, D.B. (eds) 1998 *Applied Epidemiology: Theory to Practice*, Oxford University Press, Oxford.

Brundtland, G. 1999, *World Meteorological Day, Weather, Climate and Health*, WHO, Geneva, <www.who.int/ directorgeneral/speeches/1999/English/19990323_wmo.html> [20 August 2004].

Buchanan, J. and Tullock, G. 1962 *Calculus of Consent: Logical Foundations of Constitutional Democracy*, University of Michigan Press, Ann Arbor, MI.

Burdekin, B. 1993 *Report of the National Inquiry into the Human Rights of People with Mental Illness*, AGPS, Canberra.

Bureau of Infrastructure, Transport and Regional Economics 2012 *Road Deaths Australia, 2011 Statistical Summary*, BITRE, Canberra.

Burgess, M. 2003 'Immunisation: A public health success', *NSW Public Health Bulletin*, 14(1–2), pp. 1–5.

Burke, H., Balding, B. and Lyle, D. 2003 'Reducing lead exposure in children in Broken Hill', *Public Health Bulletin*, 14(3), pp. 52–4.

Burnett, S.L., Gehm, E.R., Weissinger, W.R. and Beuchat, L.R. 2000 'Survival of *Salmonella* in peanut butter and peanut butter spread', *Journal of Applied Microbiology*, 89(3), pp. 472–7.

Burris, S. 2004 'Governance, microgovernance and health', *Temple Law Review*, 77, pp. 335–58.

Butler, J. 2003 'Public health programs to reduce HIV/AIDS', in P. Abelson (ed.), *Returns on Investment in Public Health*, Commonwealth Department of Health and Ageing, Canberra.

Butler, T. and Milner, L. 2003 *The 2001 New South Wales Inmate Health Survey*, Corrections Health Service, Sydney.

Caldwell, T., Jorm, A. and Dear, K. 2004 'Suicide and mental health in rural, remote and metropolitan areas in Australia', *Medical Journal of Australia*, 181(7), pp. S10–14.

Calman, K. 1998 *The Potential for Health*, Oxford University Press, Oxford.

Cameron, W. 2003 *Guiding Principles of Good Governance in the Public Sector*, Institute of Public Administration Australia (Victoria), Melbourne, <www.audit.vic.gov.au/speeches/agspeech_06.html> [20 September 2005].

Cancer Council Australia 2004 *National Cancer Prevention Policy 2004–06*, Cancer Council Australia, Sydney.

—— 2005 'Position statement on screening and early detection of skin cancer', <www.cancer.org.au/documents/screening_skin_cancer.pdf> [3 November 2005].

—— 2008 *Best Practice in Cervical Cancer Immunisation*, report of a roundtable discussion about the impact of the human papillomavirus vaccine in Australia, Cancer Council Australia, Sydney.

—— 2012a *National Cancer Prevention Policy Bowel Cancer*, <http://wiki.cancer.org.au/prevention/Bowel_cancer/Impact> (5 August 2012).

—— 2012b *Screening Programs*, <www.cancer.org.au//aboutcancer/Earlydetection/Screeningprograms.htm> [30 July 2012].

Cancer Council Australia and Australian Health Ministers' Advisory Committee, 2010 *Position Statement: Prostate Cancer Screening in Australia—Joint Key Messages*, Cancer Council Australia, Sydney.

Cancer Council Australia and Federation of Ethnic Communities' Councils of Australia 2010 *Cancer and Culturally and Linguistically Diverse Communities*, Cancer Council Australia, Sydney.

Carey, J. 1990 *John Donne*, Oxford University Press, Oxford.

Carson, R. 1965 *Silent Spring*, Penguin, Harmondsworth.

Cassel, J. 1976 'The contribution of the social environment to host resistance', *American Journal of Epidemiology*, 104, pp. 107–23.

Cassin, R. 2003 'Howard's plan to stealth-bomb health', *The Age*, 9 March.

Catford, J. 1995 'Health promotion in the market place: Constraints and opportunities', *Health Promotion International*, 10(1), pp. 41–50.

CDC: *see* Centers for Disease Control and Prevention.

CEIPS: *see* Centre of Excellence in Intervention and Prevention Science.

Centers for Disease Control and Prevention (CDC) 1977 *Ten Leading Causes of Death in the United States*, CDC, Atlanta.

—— 1999 'Ten great public health achievements: US, 1900–1999', *Morbidity and Mortality Weekly Report*, 48 (2), pp. 241–3.

—— 2001a *Public Health's Infrastructure: A Status Report*, CDC, Atlanta, GA.

—— 2001b 'Updated guidelines for evaluating public health surveillance systems: Recommendations from the Guidelines Working Group', *Morbidity and Mortality Weekly Report*, 50 (No. RR-13), <www.cdc.gov/mmwr/preview/mmwrhtml/rr5013a1.htm> [23 September 2004].

—— 2004 *PATCH: Planned Approach to Community Health*, <www.cdc.gov/nccdphp/patch> [10 November 2004].

Central Sydney Area Health Service and New South Wales Health 1994 *Program Management Guidelines*, NSW Health, Sydney.

Centre for Comparative Constitutional Studies 1999 *Implementation Options for National Legislative Schemes in Public Health*, revised final paper, Centre for Comparative Constitutional Studies, University of Melbourne, Melbourne.

Centre for Health Communication and Participation 2012, Cochrane Collaboration, <www.latrobe.edu.au/chcp/cochrane/index.html> [8 October 2012].

Centre for Health, Economics Research and Evaluation (CHERE) 2007 *Funding Public Health in Australia*, University of Technology, Sydney <http://hpm.org/en/Surveys/CHERE_Australia/09/Funding_Public_Health_in_Australia.html> [3 November 2012].

Centre for Health Equity Training, Research and Evaluation (CHETRE), University of New South Wales 2008 *Evaluation of Phase Three of the New South Wales Health Impact Assessment Project*, <www.hiaconnect.edu.au/files/NSW_HIA_Project_Evaluation_Summary.pdf> [20 November 2012].

Centre for Health Research in Criminal Justice 2004 *Research Plan 2004–2006*, Justice Health, Sydney.

Centre for Refugee Research 2001 *The Refugee Convention: Where to from Here Conference Report*, University of New South Wales, Sydney.

Centre for Research on Ageing n.d. *The Concord Health and Ageing in Men Project (CHAMP)*, <www.cera.usyd.edu.au/research_epid_CHAMP.html> [1 November 2012].

Centre of Excellence in Intervention and Prevention Science, 2012 *Projects*, <www.ceips.org.au> [1 November 2012].

Challis, L., Fuller, S., Henwood, M., Klein, R., Plowden, W., Webb, A., Whittingham, P. and Wistow, G. 1988 *Joint Approaches to Social Policy: Rationality and Practice*, Cambridge University Press, Cambridge.

Champion, R. and Gray, J. 2003 'May 1999 NSW Drug Summit', *Public Health Bulletin*, 14(3), pp. 59–61.

Chapman, S. 2003a 'Reducing tobacco consumption', *NSW Public Health Bulletin*, 14(3), pp. 46–8.

—— 2003b 'The decline in gun deaths', *NSW Public Health Bulletin*, 14(3), pp. 48–50.

Chapman, S., Barratt, A. and Stockler, M. 2010 *Let Sleeping Dogs Lie?* Sydney University Press, Sydney.

Cheadle, A., Psaty, B.M., Diehr, P., Koepsell, T., Wagner, E., Wickizer, T. and Curry, S. 1993 'An empirical exploration of a conceptual model for community-based health promotion', *International Quarterly of Community Health Education*, 13(4), pp. 329–63.

CHETRE: *see* Centre for Health Equity Training, Research and Evaluation, University of New South Wales.

Chin, J. 1986 'The status and challenge of communicable disease control', in J. Last (ed.), *Maxy-Rosenau Public Health and Preventive Medicine*, 12th edn, Appleton-Century-Crofts, Norwalk, CT.

Chong, A., Cruse, S. and Duffy, M. 2002 'Dissemination matters … thinking beyond the project', workshop summary, Primary Health Care Research and Information Service, Flinders University, Adelaide.

Claeson, M., Elmendorf, A.E., Miller, D. and Musgrove, P. 2002 *Public Health and World Bank Operations*, World Bank, Washington, DC.

Clayton, S. 2010 'Public health law, human rights and HIV: a work in progress', *NSW Public Health Bulletin*, 21(3–4), pp. 97–100.

Closing the Gap 2012 *Prime Minister's Report*, February, <www.fahcsia.gov.au/ourresponsibilities/indigenous-australians/publications-articles/closing-the-gap/closing-the-gapprime-ministers-report-2012> [20 November 2012].

Council of Australian Governments (COAG) Reform Council 2008 *COAG Reform Agenda*, <www.coagreformcouncil.gov.au/agenda/index.cfm> [26 August 2011].

—— 2012a *Indigenous Reform 2010–11: Comparing Performance Across Australia*, COAG Reform Council, Sydney.

—— 2012b *Seamless National Economy: Report on Performance*, COAG Reform Council, Sydney.

—— 2012c *COAG Reform Agenda: Report on Progress 2011*, COAG Reform Council, Sydney.

Coast, J. 1996 'Core services: Pluralistic bargaining in New Zealand', in J. Coast, J. Donovan and S. Frankel (eds), *Priority Setting: The Health Care Debate*, John Wiley, Chichester.

Cochrane, A. 1972 *Effectiveness and Efficiency: Random Reflections on Health Services*, Nuffield Trust, London.

Cochrane Consumer Network 2012 'About the Cochrane Consumer Network (CCNet)', <http://consumers.cochrane.org/healthcare-users-cochrane> [8 October 2012].

Cohen, M., March, J. and Olsen, J. 1972 'A garbage can model of organizational choice', *Administrative Science Quarterly*, 17, pp. 1–25.

Committee for the Future 2005 'List of members', <www.parliament.fi/FutureCommittee> [12 October 2005].

Committee on Future Directions for Behavioral and Social Sciences Research at the National Institutes of Health 2001 *New Horizons in Health: An Integrative Approach*, CFDBSSR, National Institutes of Health, National Academy Press, Washington, DC.

Commonwealth of Australia 1992a *National Strategy for Ecologically Sustainable Development*, AGPS, Canberra.

—— 1992b *Mutual Recognition Act*, <www.austlii.edu.au/au/legis/cth/consol_act/mra1992221/s3.html>
[14 February 2005].

—— 1998 *The Virtuous Cycle Working Together for Health and Medical Research* (Wills Report), Health and Medical
Research Strategic Review-Summary, December, <www.health.gov.au/internet/main/publishing.nsf/
Content/hmrsr.htm> [20 August 2012].

—— 1999 *The National Environmental Health Strategy: enHealth*, AGPS, Canberra.

—— 2003 *The Future Role of the Divisions Network: Report of the Review of the Role of Divisions of General Practice*, Canberra.

—— 2009 Fourth National Mental Health Plan: An Agenda for Collaborative Government Action in Mental
Health 2009–2014 <www.health.gov.au/internet/main/publishing/nsf/Content/360EB322114EC906CA
2576700014A817/$File/plan09v2.pdf>

—— 2010 *National Health and Hospitals Network for Australia's Future: Delivering the Reforms*, Commonwealth of Australia,
Canberra.

—— 2012 'The role of the Therapeutic Goods Administration regarding medical devices, particularly Poly
Implant Prothese (PIP) breast implants', submission to Senate—Community Affairs References Committee,
Canberra.

—— 2013 National Pests and Disease Outbreaks <www.outbreak.gov.au/pests_diseases_animals/hendra>
[24 June 2013].

Community Services and Health Training Australia 2004 *Qualifications Framework—Health Training Package: Population
Health*, interim document prepared for stakeholders' information, Australian National Training Authority,
Canberra.

Consumers' Health Forum of Australia 2001 *Guidelines for Consumer Representatives*, 4th edn, Consumers' Health
Forum of Australia, Canberra.

Cooperative Research Centre for Aboriginal Health (CRCAH) 2006 'The research agenda', <www.crcah.org.au>
[21 March 2006].

Copeland, J. 2001 *Substance Abuse and Comorbidity: The Big Picture—Diversity in Health. Sharing Global Perspectives*,
Commonwealth Department of Family and Community Services, Sydney.

Cornish, E. 2004 *Futuring: The Exploration of the Future*, World Future Society, Bethesda, MD.

Council of Australian Governments 2005 *Mutual Recognition Agreement*, <www.coag.gov.au/recognition.htm>
[20 July 2005].

Coye, M.J. 1994. 'Our own worst enemy: Obstacles to improving the health of the public', in M.J. Coye,
W.H. Foege and W.L. Roper (eds), *Leadership in Public Health*, Milbank Memorial Fund, New York.

Craun, G.F., Nwachuku, N., Calderon, R.L. and Craun, M.F. 2002 'Outbreaks in drinking water systems,
1991–1998', *Journal of Environmental Health*, 65(1), pp. 16–23.

Crofts, N., Dore, G. and Locarnini, S. (eds) 2001 *Hepatitis C: An Australian Perspective*, IP Communications,
Melbourne.

CSDH 2008 *Closing the Gap in a Generation: Health Equity Through Action on the Social Determinants of Health—Final Report of
the Commission on Social Determinants of Health*, WHO, Geneva.

CSIRO 1999 *A Guidebook to Environmental Indicators*, CSIRO, Melbourne.

—— 2013 Fighting Nipah Virus <www.csiro.au/en/Outcomes/Food-and-Agriculture/Fighting-Nipah-virus/
Fighting-Nipah> [14 June 2013].

Cumpston, J.H.L. 1978 *The Health of the People: A Study in Federalism*, Roebuck, Canberra.

—— 1989 *Health and Disease in Australia: A History*, AGPS, Canberra.

Cunha, B.A. 2004 'Influenza: Historical aspects of epidemics and pandemics', *Infectious Disease Clinics of North
America*, 18(1), pp. 141–55.

Curtin Indigenous Research Centre 2000 *Training Re-Visions: A National Review of Aboriginal and Torres Strait Islander Health Worker Training*, report submitted to the Office for Aboriginal and Torres Strait Islander Health, Commonwealth of Australia, Canberra.

Dahl, R. 1982 *Dilemmas of Pluralist Democracy: Autonomy vs Control*, Yale University Press, New Haven, CT.

Daniels, N. and Sabin, J. 2002 *Setting Limits Fairly: Can We Learn to Share Medical Resources?*, Oxford University Press, Oxford.

Dargie, C. (in association with Dawson, S. and Garside, P.) 2000 *Policy Futures for UK Health: 2000 Report*, Nuffield Trust, London.

Davis, A. and George, J. 1998 *States of Health: Health and Illness in Australia*, 3rd edn, Longman, Sydney.

Davis, G. and Rhodes, R. 2000 'From hierarchy to contracts and back again: Reforming the Australian Public Service', in M. Keating, J. Wanna and P. Weller (eds), *Institutions on the Edge: Capacity for Governance*, Allen & Unwin, Sydney.

Davis, S.R. and Brands, J. 2008 *Research Priorities in Aboriginal Prisoner Health: Recommendations and Outcomes from the CRCAH Aboriginal Prisoner Health Industry Roundtable, November 2007*, Discussion Paper No. 6, Cooperative Research Centre for Aboriginal Health, Darwin.

Davison, G. 1979 *The Rise and Fall of Marvellous Melbourne*, Melbourne University Press, Melbourne.

Dawson, D. 1998 'Tuberculosis in Australia: Bacteriologically confirmed cases and drug resistance, 1996', *Communicable Disease Intelligence*, 22(9), pp. 183–8.

De Buyser, M.L., Dufour, B., Maire, M. and Lafarge, V. 2001 'Implication of milk and milk products in food-borne diseases in France and in different industrialised countries', *International Journal of Food Microbiology*, 67(1–2), pp. 1–17.

Deeble, J. 1999a *Resource Allocation in Public Health: An Economic Approach*, National Public Health Partnership, Melbourne.

—— 1999b *The Financing of Public Health Laboratory Services: Issues Paper*, National Public Health Partnership, Melbourne.

—— 2000 *Resource Allocation in Public Health: An Economic Approach*, 2nd edn, National Public Health Partnership, Melbourne.

—— 2003 'John Deeble exposes the false crisis in Medicare', special address to launch the Whitlam Institute Health Forum series, 15 July, <www.whitlam.org/its_time/14/deeble.html> [10 October 2004].

Deeble, J. and Goss, J. 1998 *Expenditures on Health Services for Aboriginal and Torres Strait Islander People*, AIHW, Canberra.

De Leeuw, E. 1993 'Health policy, epidemiology and power: The interest web', *Health Promotion International*, 8(1), pp. 49–53.

Department of Agriculture, Fisheries and Forestry 2011 *Issues Paper to Inform Development of a National Food Plan*, Department of Agriculture, Fisheries and Forestry, Canberra.

Department of Environment and Heritage 2004 *Environmental Indicators for National State of the Environment Reporting*, Commonwealth of Australia, Canberra.

Department of Finance and Administration 2006 *Public Private Partnerships: Business Case Development, Financial Management Guidance No. 17*, Australian Government, Canberra.

Department of Health 1961 *Annual Report 1960–61*, Commonwealth of Australia, Canberra.

—— 1971 *Annual Report 1970–71*, Commonwealth of Australia, Canberra.

—— 1985 *Annual Report 1984–85*, Canberra Publishing and Printing, Canberra.

—— 1997 *Annual Report 1996–97*, AGPS, Canberra.

Department of Health and Ageing (DoHA) 2002a *The National Strategy for Quality Use of Medicines*, Commonwealth of Australia, Canberra.

—— 2002b *Quality Use of Medicines, Statement of Priorities and Strategic Action Plan 2001–2003*, Commonwealth of Australia, Canberra.

—— 2003a *Annual Report 2002–03*, Commonwealth of Australia, Canberra.

—— 2003b *Research Report: Evaluation Report for the 2000/2001 Phase of the BreastScreen Australia Campaign*, Screening Monograph No. 1/2004, Commonwealth of Australia, Canberra.

—— 2004a *BreastScreen Australia Program*, Primary Care Division, <www.health.gov.au/pcd/campaigns/breastsc/index.htm> [3 November 2004].

—— 2004b 'Organisational Chart September 2004', <www.health.gov.au/internet/wcms/Publishing.nsf/Content/health-struct.htm> [10 November 2004].

—— 2004c *Immunise Australia Program and Seven Point Plan*, <www.health.gov.au/internet/wcms/publishing.nsf/Content/health-pubhlth-strategimmunis> [16 July 2004].

—— 2004d *General Practice Immunisation Incentives Scheme*, <www.health.gov.au/internet/wcms/publishing.nsf/Content/health-pubhlth-strateg-immunis-gp.htm> [16 July 2004].

—— 2004e *Cervical Screening, Cervical Cancer: The Facts*, <www.cervicalscreen.health.gov.au/facts> [22 July 2004].

—— 2004f *Cervical Screening Marketing Strategy*, <www.health.gov.au/pubhlth/cervical/marketing/strategy.html> [26 July 2004].

—— 2005a *BreastScreen Australia: Why Should I Have a Mammogram?*, <www.breastscreen.info.au/why/index.htm> [23 April 2005].

—— 2005b 'History of the Department: Fact Sheets and Poster', <www.health.gov.au/internet/wcms/publishing.nsf/Content/health-history.htm#facts> [2 November 2005].

—— 2005c *Australian Management Plan for Pandemic Influenza*, Section 3: Building Blocks for Pandemic Planning, Commonwealth of Australia, Canberra, <www.health.gov.au/internet/wcms/publishing.nsf/Content/phd-pandemic-plan-3-d> [24 March 2006].

—— 2005d *Australia's Bowel Cancer Screening Pilot and Beyond*, final evaluation paper, Bowel Cancer Screening Pilot Monitoring and Evaluation Steering Committee, <www.cancerscreening.gov.au/bowel/pdfs/eval_oct05.pdf> [10 February 2006].

—— 2005e 'Lifestyle Prescriptions', <www.health.gov.au/internet/wcms/Publishing.nsf/Content/health-pubhlth-strateglifescripts-index-htm> [24 April 2006].

—— 2005f Annual Report 2004–05, <www.health.gov.au/internet/annrpt/publishing.nsf/Content/40A2AE5C8A370019CA257052000B1FFE/$Filc/part1.pdf> [31 July 2006].

—— 2006 *Better Health for All Australians* <www.health.gov.au/internet/ministers/publishing.nsf/content/health-mediarel-yr2006-ta-abb011.htm?OpenDocument&yr=2006&mth=2> [23 October 2012].

—— 2009 *BreastScreen Australia Evaluation—Evaluation Final Report*, Screening Monograph No. 1/2009, Commonwealth Government, Canberra.

—— 2010a *Health Reform Update*, <www.health.gov.au/internet/yourhealth/publishing.nsf/Content/UpdateDecember2010> [23 October 2012].

—— 2010b *Third National Hepatitis C Strategy 2010–2013*, Commonwealth Government, Canberra.

—— 2010c Second National Sexually Transmissable Infections Strategy, 2010–2013 <www.health.gov.au/internet/main/publishing.nsf/Content/ohp-national-strategies-2010-sti/$File/sti.pdf>

—— 2011a *Sixth National HIV Strategy 2010–2013*, <www.health.gov.au/internet/main/publishing.nsf/Content/ohp-national-strategies-2010-hiv/$File/hiv.pdf> [29 August 2012].

—— 2011b 'Immunisation coverage annual report, 2009', *Communicable Diseases Intelligence*, 35 (2) pp. 132–48.

—— 2012a *Australian Longitudinal Study on Male Health*, <www.health.gov.au/internet/main/publishing.nsf/Content/male-health-research> [9 December 2012].

—— 2012b *BreastScreen*, <www.cancerscreening.gov.au/internet/screening/publishing.nsf/Content/breastscreen-about> [9 December 2012].

—— 2012c *How the TGA Regulates*, <www.tga.gov.au/about/tga-regulates-how.htm> [9 December 2012].

—— 2012d *Immunise*: <www.health.gov.au/internet/immunise/publishing.nsf/Content/immunise-hpv> [9 December 2012].

—— 2012e *National Bowel Cancer Screening Program*, <www.cancerscreening.gov.au/internet/screening/publishing.nsf/Content/bowelabout> [5 August 2012].

—— 2012f *National Cervical Screening Program*, <www.cancerscreening.gov.au/internet/screening/publishing.nsf/Content/cervical-about> [9 December 2012].

—— 2012g *National Male Health Policy*, <www.health.gov.au/internet/main/publishing.nsf/Content/male-policy> [9 December 2012].

—— 2012h *National Male Health Policy Supporting Document: Healthy Minds* <www.betterhealth.vic.gov.au/bhcv2/bhcarticles.nsf/pages/Men's_health> [9 December 2012].

—— 2012i *National Immunisation Program Schedule*, Department of Health and Ageing, <www.immunise.health.gov.au/internet/immunise/publishing.nsf/Content/nips2> [5 November 2012].

—— 2012j 'Population Health Division (PHD)', <www.health.gov.au/internet/main/publishing.nsf/Content/phd-structure> [9 December 2012].

—— 2102k *Poly Implant Prothese (PIP) Breast Implants: The Australian Perspective*, <www.tga.gov.au/safety/alerts-device-breast-implants-120104.htm> [9 December 2012].

—— 2012l *Sharing Health Care Initiative*, <www.health.gov.au/internet/main/publishing.nsf/Content/chronicdisease-sharing.htm> [2 November 2012].

—— 2012m *Types of Influenza*, <www.flupandemic.gov.au/internet/panflu/publishing.nsf/Content/types-1> [10 October 2012].

—— 2012n *Vaccination for Boys*, <www.health.gov.au/nsf//HPV-vaccination-for-boysfactsheet.pdf> [9 December 2012].

—— 2012o '2010–13 Department of Health and Ageing Corporate Plan', <www.health.gov.au/internet/main/publishing.nsf/Content/corporate-plan-2010-13> [5 October 2013].

—— 2013a <www.yourhealth.gov.au/internet/publishing.nsf/Content/nhra-agreement-fs> [14 June 2013].

—— 2013b 'Management Structure Chart', <http://www.health.gov.au/internet/main/publishing.nsf/Content/health-struct.htm> [6 October 2013].

Department of Health and Ageing and enHealth Council 2002 *Environmental Health Risk Assessment: Guidelines for Assessing Human Health Risks from Environmental Hazards*, Commonwealth of Australia, Canberra.

—— 2012 *Skin Penetration*, <www.public.health.wa.gov.au/3/1085/2/skin_penetration.pm> [4 November 2012].

Department of Human Services 2012a, *Australian Childhood Immunisation Register,* <www.medicareaustralia.gov.au/provider/patients/acir/statistics.jsp> [4 November 2012].

—— 2012b *Maternity Immunization Allowance*, <www.humanservices.gov.au/customer/services/centrelink/maternity-immunisationallowance?> [5 June 2012>.

—— 2012c *General Practice Immunization Incentive*, <www.medicareaustralia.gov.au/provider/incentives/gpii/index.jsp#N10009> [9 December 2012].

—— 2013 'Australian Childhood Immunisation Register (ACIR) statistics', <www.medicareaustralia.gov.au/provider/patients/acir/statistics.jsp> [6 October 2013].

Department of Immigration and Citizenship (DIAC) 2012 *Australia's Humanitarian Program 2013–14 and Beyond* <www.immi.gov.au/media/publications/pdf/humanitarian-program-information-paper-2013-14.pdf>.

Department of Immigration, Multicultural and Indigenous Affairs (DIMIA) 2002 *Fact Sheet 22*, DIMIA, Canberra.

—— 2005 Refugee and Humanitarian Issues, Australia's Response June 2005 <www.immi.gov.au/media/publications/pdf/refhumiss-fullv2.pdf>.

—— 2006 *Resettlement Data Base*, <www.immi.gov.au/department/pid/bccd3.htm> [20 April 2006].

Department of Primary Industries 2012 *Victorian Committee of Food Regulators*, <http://health.vic.gov.au/phwa> [21 August 2012].

Department of the Prime Minister and Cabinet 2011 *Reform of Australian Government Administration, Staying Ahead of the Game* <www.dpmc.gov.au/reformgovernment/index.cfm> [2 November 2012].

Department of Sustainability, Environment, Water, Population and Communities (DSEWPaC) 2012 Ecologically Sustainable Development, <www.environment.gov.au/about/esd/index.html> [4 November 2012].

De Swaan, A. 1988 *In Care of the State: Health Care, Education and Welfare in Europe and the USA in the Modern Era*, Polity Press, Oxford.

Detels, R., Holland, W., McEwen, J. and Omenn, G.S. (eds) 1997 *Oxford Textbook of Public Health*, 3rd edn, Oxford University Press, New York.

DHS: *see* Department of Human Services.

DIAC: *see* Department of Immigration and Citizenship.

Diamond, J. 1997 *Guns, Germs and Steel: A Short History of Everybody for the Last 13 000 Years*, Random House, London.

DIMIA: *see* Department of Immigration, Multicultural and Indigenous Affairs.

Dixon, J. 2001 'Learning from international models of funding and delivering health care', in D. Pencheon, C. Guest, D. Melzer and J.A.M. Gray (eds), *Oxford Handbook of Public Health Practice*, Oxford University Press, Oxford.

DoHA: *see* Department of Health and Ageing.

Domoto, A. 2003 'Welcoming remarks', *Proceedings of International Symposium on Gender-Sensitive Medicine*, Chiba Prefecture, Japan, 1 March, WHO Kobe Centre, Kobe.

Donovan, B., Harcourt, C., Egger, S., Watchirs Smith, L., Schneider, K., Kaldor, J.M., Chen, M.Y., Fairley, C.K. and Tabrizi, S. 2012 *The Sex Industry in New South Wales: A Report to the NSW Ministry of Health*, Kirby Institute, University of New South Wales, Sydney.

Dooris, M. 2004 'Joining up settings for health: A valuable investment for strategic partnerships?' *Critical Public Health*, 14(1), pp. 49–61.

Dore, G., Law, M., MacDonald, M. and Kaldor, J.M. 2003 'Epidemiology of hepatitis C virus infection in Australia', *Journal of Clinical Virology*, 26(2), pp. 171–84.

Doyle, J.W.E, Yach, D., McQueen, D., De Francisco, A., Stewart, T., Reddy, P., Gulmezoglu, A.M., Galea, G. and Portela, A. 2005 'Global priority setting for Cochrane systematic reviews of health promotion and public health research', *Journal of Epidemiology and Community Health*, 59, pp. 193–7.

Draper, G., Turrell, G. and Oldenburg, B. 2004 *Health Inequalities in Australia: Mortality*, Health Inequalities Monitoring Series No. 1, QUT and AIHW, Canberra.

Drummond, M.F., O'Brien, B.J., Stoddard, G.L. and Torrance, G.W. 1997 *Methods for the Economic Evaluation of Health Care Programmes*, 2nd edn, Oxford University Press, Oxford.

Duckett, S.J. 1990 'Methods to establish priorities for health care', *Australian Health Review*, 13(40), pp. 255–62.

—— 2000 *The Australian Health Care System*, Oxford University Press, Melbourne.

—— 2007 *The Australian Health Care System*, Oxford University Press, Melbourne.

Duckett, S. and Sharon Willcox, S. 2011 *The Australian Health Care System*, revised 4th edition, Oxford University Press, South Melbourne.

Dunstan, D. 1984 *Governing the Metropolis: Politics, Technology and Social Change in a Victorian City—Melbourne 1850–1891*, Melbourne University Press, Melbourne.

Durkheim, E. 1970 *Suicide: A Study in Sociology*, translated (from the French) by J. A. Spaulding and G. Simpson (eds), with an introduction by G. Simpson, Routledge and Kegan Paul, London.

Dwyer, J. 1989 'The politics of participation', *Community Health Studies*, 13(1), pp. 59–65.

Eager, K., Garrett, P. and Lin, V. 2001 *Health Planning: An Australian Perspective*, Allen & Unwin, Sydney.

Edmonds, S. 1989 'Health Impact Statements: Challenges Ahead?', *Community Health Studies* 23(4), pp. 448–55.

Edwards, M. 2001 *Social Policy, Public Policy: From Problem to Practice*, Allen & Unwin, Sydney.

Egger, G., Donovan, R. and Spark, R. 1993 *Health and the Media: Principles and Practices for Health Promotion*, McGraw-Hill, Sydney.

Engel, G.L. 1977 'The need for a new medical model: A challenge for biomedicine', *Science*, 196, pp. 129–36.

Engels, F. 1987 [1844] *The Condition of the Working Class in England*, Penguin, Harmondsworth.

EngenderHealth 2004 *Guiding Principles for a Comprehensive Approach to HIV/AIDS Prevention, Care, and Treatment*, <www.engenderhealth.org/ia/swh/guiding_principles.html> [12 April 2006].

EnHealth 2001 *Health Impact Assessment Guidelines*, September, Commonwealth of Australia, Canberra.

—— 2004 *National Review of Indigenous Environmental Health Workers*, discussion paper, March, <www.health.gov.au/pubhlth/strateg/envhlth/discussion_indgen.pdf> [19 April 2005].

—— 2007 National Environmental Health Strategy 2007–2012, Canberra.

—— 2009 *enHealth Environmental Health Officer Skills and Knowledge Matrix*, Department of Health and Ageing, <www.health.gov.au/internet/main/publishing.nsf/Content/ohp-enhealth-skill> [3 November 2012].

Enthoven, A. 1997 'Markets and collective action in regulating managed care', *Health Affairs*, 16, pp. 26–32.

Environment Protection Authority (Victoria) and Australian Institute of Environmental Health 2001 *A Survey of Local Government Management of Domestic On-site Wastewater Systems*, EPA, Melbourne.

Eriksson, J.G. 2005 'The fetal origins hypothesis—10 years on', editorial, *British Medical Journal*, 330, pp. 1066–7.

Ervin, L., Robinson, P. and Carter, B. 'Curriculum mapping: not as straightforward as it sounds', *Journal of Vocational Education & Training*, in press.

European Centre for Health Policy 1999 'Health Impact Assessment: Main concepts and suggested approach', Gothenburg consensus paper, December, WHO Regional Office for Europe, Brussels.

Evans, R.G. and Stoddart, G.L. 1994 'Producing health, consuming health care', in R.G. Evans, M.L. Barer and T.R. Marmor (eds), *Why are Some People Healthy and Others Not? The Determinants of Health of Populations*, Aldine de Gruyter, New York.

Ewan, C., Young, A., Bryant, E. and Calvert, D. 1992 *National Framework for Health Impact Assessment in Environmental Impact Assessment*, vol. 1, Executive Summary and Recommendations, National Better Health Program, University of Wollongong, Wollongong, NSW.

Ewles, L. and Simnett, I. 1985 *Promoting Health: A Practical Guide to Health Education*, John Wiley & Sons, Chichester.

External Advisory Committee on Smart Regulation 2004 *Smart Regulation: A Regulatory Strategy for Canada*, report to the Government of Canada, September, <www.smartregulation.gc.ca> [11 April 2006].

Eylenbosch, W.J. and Noah, N.D. 1988 *Surveillance in Health and Disease*, Oxford University Press, Oxford.

FaHCSIA, AIFS and ABS 2012, *Growing Up in Australia,* <www.growingupinaustralia.gov.au/index.html> [9 December 2012].

Farmer, P. 1996 'On suffering and structural violence: A view from below', *Daedalus*, 125(1), pp. 261–84.

Fawkes, S. 1997 'Aren't health services promoting health?' *Australian and New Zealand Journal of Public Health*, 27, pp. 391–7.

—— 2009 'Taking the long view in health policy making: The use of futures studies', unpublished PhD thesis, School of Public Health, La Trobe University.

Fawkes, S., Palmer, J., Inayatullah, S., Burke, R., Miller, M., Worland, P. and Ellis, N. 2011 *The Futures of Safety, Compensation and Recovery: Final Report on the Futures Research Initiative*, Research Report no. 0811-017-R2, ISCRR, Melbourne, <www.iscrr.com.au/reports-pubs/research-reports/iscrr-futuresinitiative-brief-report.pdf> [1 December 2012].

Feacham, R. 1995 *Valuing the Past, Investing in the Future: Evaluation of the National HIV/AIDS Strategy 1993–94 to 1995–96*, Commonwealth Department of Human Services and Health, Canberra.

Feacham, R.G. 2001 'Globalisation is good for your health, mostly', *British Medical Journal*, 323(1), pp. 504–6.

Filipov, D. 2003 'Lives lost', *Boston Globe Online*, 29 May, <www.boston.com/news/specials/lives_lost/russia> [13 April 2005].

Fisher, E.B., Brownson, C.A., O'Toole, M.L., Shetty, G., Anwuri, V. and Glasgow, R.E. 2005 'Ecological approaches to self-management: The case of diabetes', *American Journal of Public Health*, 95(9), pp. 1523–35.

Fitzgerald, J.L. and Sewards, T. 2003 'Evidence-based practice in the Australian Drug Policy Community', in Lin, V. & Gibson, B. (eds), *Competing Rationalities: Evidence-Based Practice Health Policy*, Oxford University Press, Melbourne.

Flinn, M.W. (ed.) 1965 [1842] *Report on the Sanitary Condition of the Labouring Population of Great Britain by Edwin Chadwick*, Edinburgh University Press, Edinburgh.

Foster, Peter 2005 *Queensland Health Systems Review: Final Report*, Queensland Health, Brisbane, <www.qld.gov.au/health_sys_review/final> [19 October 2005].

Fraser, N. 1989 *Unruly Practices: Power, Discourse and Gender in Contemporary Social Theory*, Polity Press, Cambridge.

Frazer, W.M. 1950 *A History of English Public Health 1834–1939*, Bailliere, Tindall and Cox, London.

Friere, P. 1973 *Education for Critical Consciousness*, Sheed and Ward, London.

Frommer, M. and Rychetnik, L. 2002 *A Schema for Evaluating Evidence on Public Health Interventions*, National Public Health Partnership, Melbourne.

Fry, C.L., Madden, A., Brogan, D. and Loff, B. 2006 'Australian resources for ethical participatory processes in public health research', *Journal of Medical Ethics*, 32 (3), p. 186.

FSANZ 2012 Food allergies, <www.foodstandards.gov.au/consumerinformation/foodallergies/> [6 October 2013].

Fuller, J., Edwards, J., Proctor, N. and Moss, J. 2002 'Mental health in rural and remote Australia', in D. Wilkinson and I. Blue (eds), *The New Rural Health*, Oxford University Press, Melbourne.

Galbally, R. 2000 'Placing prevention at the centre of health sector reform', in A. Bloom (ed.), *Health Reform in Australia and New Zealand*, Oxford University Press, Melbourne.

Garrett, L. 1994 *The Coming Plague*, Penguin, New York.

—— 2001 *Betrayal of Trust: The Collapse of Global Public Health*, Oxford University Press, New York.

Gatherer, A., Moller, L. and Hayton, P. 2005 'The World Health Organization European Health in Prisons Project after 10 years: Persistent barriers and achievements', *American Journal of Public Health*, October, 95(10), pp. 1696–1700.

Gatrell, A., Thomas, C., Bennet, S., Bostock, L., Popay, J., Williams, G. and Shahtahmasebi, S. 2001 'Understanding health inequalities: Locating people in geographical and social spaces', in H. Graham (ed.), *Understanding Health Inequalities*, Open University Press, Buckingham, pp. 156–69.

Geary, P.M. 1988 'Domestic wastewater management alternatives for the Mt Lofty Ranges watershed: Alternative waste treatment systems', *Proceedings of the International Conference Held at Massey University, Palmerston North, NZ*, 26–27 May, Elsevier, New York.

Geiger, H.J. 1984 'Community health centres: Health care as an instrument of social change', in V. Sidel and S. Sidel (eds), *Reforming Medicine*, Pantheon, New York.

General Practice Consultative Committee 1992 *The Future of General Practice: A Strategy for the Nineties and Beyond*, Department of Human Services and Health, Canberra.

General Practice Partnership Advisory Council 2002 'The role of general practice in the Australian primary health care system', work in progress document, paper from the Primary Health Care Standing Committee, Melbourne.

General Practice Victoria 2011 *Introducing Medicare Locals: Objectives of Medicare Locals*, November, handout, General Practice Victoria, Melbourne.

Germov, J. 1998 'Imagining health problems as social issues', in J. Germov (ed.), *Second Opinion*, Oxford University Press, Melbourne.

Gibson, B. 2003 'Beyond "Two Communities"', in V. Lin and B. Gibson (eds), *Evidence-based Health Policy*, Oxford University Press, Melbourne.

Gifford, S.M., O'Brien, M., Bammer, G. and Banwell, C. 2003 'Australian women's experiences of living with hepatitis C: Results from a cross-sectional survey', *Journal of Gastroenterology and Hepatology*, 18(7), pp. 841–50.

Gilbert, R., Stevenson, D., Girardet, H. and Stren, R. 1996 *Making Cities Work: The Role of Local Authorities in the Urban Environment*, Earthscan, London.

Gillings School of Global Public Health n.d. 'Public health leadership program, University of North Carolina at Chapel Hill', <http://sph.unc.edu/department-pages/public-health-leadership-program> [6 October 2013].

Glanz, K., Lewis, F.M. and Rimer, B.K. (eds) 1990 *Health Behaviour and Health Education: Theory, Research and Practice*, Jossey-Bass, San Francisco.

—— 1997 *Theory at a Glance: A Guide for Health Promotion Practice*, National Institute of Health, Bethesda, MD.

Glasgow, R., Lichtenstein, E. and Marcus, A. 2003 'Why don't we see more translation of health promotion research to practice? Re-thinking the efficacy-to-effectiveness transition', *American Journal of Public Health*, 93(8), pp. 1261–7.

Glasgow, R.E., Vogt, T.M. and Boles, S.M. 1999 'Evaluating the public health impact of health promotion interventions: The RE-AIM framework', *American Journal of Public Health*, 89, pp. 1323–7.

Glasson, B. 2003 'Medicare Plus: a positive "second best" option', AMA media release, 18 November, <www.ama.com.au/web.nsf/doc?WEEN-5STE8CG> [4 October 2004].

Gleik, J. 2012 *The Information: A History, A Theory, A Flood*, Vintage, New York.

Glenn, J.C. and Gordon, T.J. 2003 *State of the Future*, American Council for the United Nations University, Washington, DC.

—— 2004 *State of the Future*, American Council for the United Nations University, Washington, DC.

—— 2005 *State of the Future*, American Council for the United Nations University, Washington, DC.

Glenn, J.C., Gordon, T.J. and Florescu, E. 2012 *State of the Future: The Millennium Project, Global Futures Studies and Research* <www.millennium-project.org/millennium/2012SOF.html>.

Goldsmid, J. 1988 *The Deadly Legacy: Australian History and Transmissible Disease*, UNSW Press, Sydney in association with the Australian Institute of Biology.

Goldstein, G. and von Schirnding, Y.E. 1997 'Environmental health indicators in evaluation of healthy cities programmes', working paper for 4th International Conference on Health Promotion, Jakarta.

Goodman, R. 1999 'Principles and tools for evaluating community-based prevention and health promotion programs', in R. Brownson, E. Baker and L. Novic (eds), *Community-based Prevention: Programs That Work*, Aspen, Gaithersburg, MD.

Goodman, R.A., Rothstein, M.A., Hoffman, R.E., Lopez, W. and Matthews, G.W. (eds) 2003 *Law in Public Health Practice*, Oxford University Press, New York.

Goodman, R.M., Steckler, A. and Kegler, M.C. 1997 'Mobilising organizations for health enhancement: Theories of organisational change', in K. Glanz, F.M. Lewis and B.K. Rimer (eds), *Health Behavior and Health Education: Theory, Research and Practice*, 2nd edn, Jossey-Bass, San Francisco.

Gordijn, B. 2003 'Nanoethics: From utopian dreams to apocalyptic nightmares—towards a more balanced view', paper presented at 3rd session of the UNESCO World Commission on the Ethics of Scientific Knowledge and Technology (COMEST), Rio de Janeiro, Brazil, 1–4 December, <http://portal.unesco.org/shs/en/file_download.php/19013ff6599f7bfd12e38868a1fbcaNanoethic.pdf> [18 February 2006].

Gordon, D. 1976 *Health, Sickness and Society: Theoretical Concepts in Social and Preventive Medicine*, University of Queensland Press, Brisbane.

Gostin, L. 2000a *Public Health Law: Power, Duty, Restraint*, University of California Press, Berkeley, CA.

—— 2000b 'Public health law in a new century, part III', *Journal of the American Medical Association*, 283(23), pp. 3118–22.

—— 2004 'Law and ethics in population health', *Australian and New Zealand Journal of Public Health*, 28(1), pp. 7–12.

—— 2012 'A Framework Convention on Global Health: Health for all, justice for all', *Journal of the American Medical Association*, 307(19): 2087–92.

Gostin, L.O. and Hodge, J.G. 2002 *Collaborating for a New Century in Public Health: State Public Health Law Assessment Report*, Turning Point National Program Office, University of Washington, Seattle, WA.

Gostin, L.O., Koplan, J.P. and Grad, F.P. 2003 'The law and the public's health: The foundation', in R.A. Goodman, M.A. Rothstein, R.E. Hoffman, W. Lopez and G.W. Matthews (eds), *Law in Public Health Practice*, Oxford University Press, New York.

Government of New South Wales (NSW) 1991 *Public Health Act 1991*, <www.austlii.edu.au/au/legis/nsw/consol_act/pha1991126> [11 February 2005].

Government of Tasmania 1997 *Public Health Act*, <www.austlii.edu.au/au/legis/tas/consol_act/pha1997126> [14 February 2005].

—— 2003 *Food Act 2003*, Section 3, <www.austlii.edu.au/au/legis/tas/consol_act/fa200357/s3.html> [14 February 2005].

—— 2005 *A Review of the* Health Complaints Act 1995: *Call for Public Comment*, <www.justice.tas.gov.au/health_complaints/publications.html> [11 February 2005].

Government of Victoria 1988 *Health (General Amendment) Act 1988*, VGPO, Melbourne.

—— 2001 Health (Infectious Diseases) Regulations 2001, 41/2000.

—— 2005a *Health Act 1958*, Government Printer, Melbourne.

—— 2005b *Australian Health Care Agreement Between the Commonwealth of Australia and the State of Victoria 1998–2003*, <www.health.vic.gov.au/agreement> [22 June 2005].

Gray, B. 1989 *Collaborating: Finding Common Ground for Multiparty Problems*, Jossey-Bass, San Francisco.

Gray, G. 1984 'The termination of Medibank', *Politics* 19(2), pp. 1–17.

—— 2004 *The Politics of Medicare: Who Gets What, When and How*, UNSW Press, Sydney.

Gray, N. 1997 'Forty years of plotting for public health', *Medical Journal of Australia*, 167, pp. 587–9.

Green, L. and Kreuter, M. 1991 *Health Promotion Planning: An Educational and Environmental Approach*, 2nd edn, Mayfield, CA.

—— 2005 *Health Program Planning: An Educational and Ecological Approach*, 4th edn, McGraw-Hill, New York.

Green, L.W., Kreuter, M.W., Partridge, K. and Deeds, S. 1980 *Health Education Planning: A Diagnostic Approach*, Mayfield, Mountain View, CA.

Green Dragon Consultants 2003 *Summary of the First Report from the Bellevue Health Surveillance Register*, report prepared for the Department of Health, Perth.

Gregg, M. (ed.) 2002 *Field Epidemiology*, 2nd edn, Oxford University Press, Oxford.

Greig, J.E., Carnie, J.A., Tallis, G.F., Ryan, N.J., Tan, A.G., Gordon, I.R., Zwolak, B., Leydon, J.A., Guest, C.S. and Hart, W.G. 2004 'An outbreak of Legionnaires' disease at the Melbourne Aquarium, April 2000: Investigation and case-control studies', *Medical Journal of Australia*, 180(11), pp. 566–72.

Griffiths, W. 1972 'Health education definitions, problems, and philosophies', *Health Education Monographs*, 31, pp. 12–14.

Gross, P.F., Leeder, S.R. and Lewis, M.J. 2003 'Australia confronts the challenge of chronic disease', editorial, *Medical Journal of Australia*, 179(5), pp. 233–4.

Grundy, F. 1964 *Preventative Medicine and Public Health, An Introduction for Students and Practitioners*, H.K. Lewis and Co., London.

Gruszin, S., Hetzel, D. and Glover, J. 2009 *Advocacy and Action in Public Health: Lessons from Australia, 1901–2006*, Public Health Information Development Unit, University of Adelaide, Adelaide.

Gruszin, S. and Szuster F. 2010 Audit of Australian Chronic Disease Associated Risk Factor Data Collections Final Report, Public Health Information Unit, University of Adelaide, Adelaide.

Guba, E.G. and Lincoln, Y.S. 1989 *Fourth Generation Evaluation*, Sage, Thousand Oaks, CA.

Haase, C.E. 2003 'The use of research in policy and program formation and implementation: HIV/AIDS education in Australia—a case study in the diffusion of innovation', PhD thesis submitted to the School of Social Work, University of Melbourne, Melbourne.

Habermas, J. 1990 *Moral Consciousness and Communicative Action*, MIT Press, Cambridge.

Hadden, F. and O'Brien, S. 2003 'Assessing acute health trends', in D. Pencheon, C. Guest, D. Melzer and J.A.M. Grey (eds), *Oxford Handbook of Public Health Practice*, Oxford University Press, Oxford.

Hamblin, A. 1998 *Environmental Indicators for National State of the Environment Reporting: The Land, Australia—State of the Environment* (Environmental Indicator Report), Department of the Environment, Canberra.

Hamlin, C. and Sheard, S. 1998 'Revolutions in public health: 1848, and 1998?', *British Medical Journal*, 317, pp. 587–91.

Hammond, T. 2004 'Discovery obligations and document retention', Australian Insurance Law Association breakfast seminar, 26 May, <www.aila.com.au/research/2004_papers/AILApaperMay04.doc> [10 November 2005].

Hancock, T. and Perkins, F. 1985 'The Mandala of health: A conceptual model and teaching tool', *Health Promotion*, 24, pp. 8–10.

Hanney, S.R., Gonzalez-Block, M.A., Buxton, M.J. and Kogan, M. 2003 'The utilisation of health research in policy-making: Concepts, examples and methods of assessment', *Health Research Policy and Systems*, 1(2), pp. 1–28.

Harper, A. 2002 *The Kimberley Chemical Use Review*, a report for and presented to the Hon. Kim Chance, Minister for Agriculture, Forestry and Fisheries, Government of Western Australia, Perth.

—— 2004 'Agent Orange in the Kimberley', *Perspective*, ABC Radio National, 23 September, <www.abc.net.au/rn/talks/perspective/stories/s1205759.htm> [10 March 2005].

Harris, E., Wise, M., Hawe, P., Finlay, P. and Nutbeam, D. 1995 *Working Together: Intersectoral Action for Health*, AGPS, Canberra.

Harris, M.F. and Mercer, P.J.T. 2001 'Reactive or preventive: The role of general practice in achieving a healthier Australia', *Medical Journal of Australia*, 175, pp. 92–3.

—— 2011 *Financing Global Health 2011: Continued Growth as MDG Deadline Approaches*, Chapter 2, <www.healthmetricsandevaluation.org/sites/default/files/policy_report/2011/FGH_2011_chapter_2_IHME.pdf> [24 November 2012].

Harrison, D. 2002 'Health promotion and the politics of integration', in R. Brunton and G. Macdonald (eds), *Health Promotion Disciplines, Diversity and Development*, 2nd edn, Routledge, London.

Harvey, D. 1974 'Ideology and population theory', *International Journal of Health Services*, 4(3), pp. 515–37.

Hassan, T. 2005 'Govt to investigate asbestos illness claims ABC', ABC Online, 4 March <www.abc.net.au/pm/content/2005/s1316497.htm> [11 April 2006].

Hawe, P., Degeling, D. and Hall, J. 1990 *Evaluating Health Promotion: A Health Worker's Guide*, MacLennan & Petty, Sydney.

Hawe, P., Noort, M., King, L. and Jordens, C. 1997 'Multiplying health gains: The critical role of capacity-building within health promotion programs', *Health Policy*, 39, pp. 29–42.

Hayden, D. 2003 *Pox: Genius, Madness and the Mysteries of Syphilis*, Basic Books, New York.

Hazelton, M. and Clinton, M. 2002 'Mental health consumers or citizens with mental health problems?' in S. Henderson and A. Petersen (eds), *Consuming Health: The Commodification of Health Care*, Routledge, London.

Health Commission of New South Wales 1977 *Community Health: Book 1—General Concepts*, Health Commission of NSW, Sydney.

Health Development Agency 2002 *Introducing Health Impact Assessment (HIA): Informing the decision-making process*, HDA, London.

HealthInfoNet *Overview of Australian Indigenous Health Status 2011. Mortality*, <www.healthinfonet.ecu.edu.au/ health-facts/overviews/mortality>.

Health Innovations International 2000 'Australian public health initiative: scoping paper', draft, March, Health Innovations International, Sydney.

Health Insurance Commission (HIC) 2000 *Australian Childhood Immunisation Register, Information Kit*, HIC, Canberra.

Health Issues Centre 2008 *Primary Care Partnerships: New Directions in Victorian Primary Health Care* <www. healthissuescentre.org.au/documents/items/2008/05/206773-upload-00001.pdf> [13 October 2012].

Health Targets and Implementation (Health for All) Committee 1988, *Health for All Australians*, AGPS, Canberra.

Heider F. 1958 *The Psychology of Interpersonal Relations*, John Wiley & Sons, New York.

Hendy, S. 1998 'Partnerships in public health: a Northern Territory perspective', *NPHP News*, 3, pp. 1, 12–16.

Hepatitis Australia 2012a *Hepatitis C*, <www.hepatitisaustralia.com/abouthepatitis/hepatitis-c> [25 November 2012].

—— 2012b *A Guide to Current and Emerging Hepatitis C Treatments*, February, Hepatitis Australia, Canberra.

Hermans, H. and den Exter, A. 1998 'Priorities and priority setting in health care in the Netherlands', *CMJ Online*, 39(3), <www.cmj.hr/1998/3903/390316.htm> [22 February 2005].

Hess, M. and Adams, D. 2002 'Knowing and skilling in contemporary public administration', *Australian Journal of Public Administration*, 61(4), pp. 68–79.

Hetzel, B. 2004 'Bridging the knowledge application gap: The global elimination of brain damage due to iodine deficiency', keynote address to the Asia Pacific Academic Consortium in Public Health, Brisbane, 2 December, <www.apacph.org/downloads/HetzelKeynote.pdf> [20 August 2007].

Heymann, D.L. 2004 *Control of Communicable Diseases Manual*, 18th edn, American Public Health Association, Washington, DC.

Higginbotham, N., Albrecht, G. and Conner, L. 2001 *Health Social Science: A Transdisciplinary and Complexity Perspective*, Oxford University Press, Melbourne.

Himmelman, A.T. 1996 'On the theory and practice of transformational collaboration', in C. Huxham (ed.), *Creating Collaborative Advantage*, Sage, London.

Holman C.D, Bass, A.J., Rosman, D.L., Smith, M.B., Semmens, J.B., Glasson, E.J., Brook, E.L., Trutwein, B., Rouse, I.L., Watson, C.R., de Klerk, N.H. and Stanley, F.J. 2008 'A decade of data linkage in Western Australia: Strategic design, applications and benefits of the WA data linkage system', *Australian Health Review*, 32(4), pp. 766–77.

Hopwood, M. and Southgate, E. 2001 *Living with Hepatitis C: A Sociological Review*, National Centre in HIV Research, University of New South Wales, Sydney.

Horey, D. and Hill, S. 2005 'Engaging consumers in health policy', paper prepared for 3rd Health Policy Roundtable, Canberra, 8 November.

Houghton, S., Braunack-Mayer A. and Hiller, J.E. 2002 'Undergraduate public health education: A workforce perspective', *Australian and New Zealand Journal of Public Health*, 26(2), pp. 174–9.

Hudson, P. 2004 'GP fee rise would wipe out Medicare package: ALP', *The Age*, 17 October.

Hughes, L. and McMichael, T. 2011 *The Critical Decade: Climate Change and Health*, Climate Commission Secretariat (Department of Climate Change and Energy Efficiency), Canberra.

Hull, B., Dey, A., Campbell-Lloyd, S., Menzies, R.I. and McIntyre, P.B. 2011 'NSW Annual Immunisation Coverage Report, 2010', *NSW Health Public Health Bulletin*, 22(9–10), pp. 179–95.

Hull, B., Dey, A., Mahajan, D., Menzies, R., and McIntyre, P.B. 2009, 'Immunisation Coverage Annual Report', *Communicable Disease Intelligence*, 35(2), pp. 132–48.

Human Genome Project 2005 'Information', <www.ornl.gov/sci/techresources/Human_Genome/elsi/elsi. shtml> [1 June 2005].

Hunt, J.M. and Lumley, J. 2002 'Are recommendations about routine antenatal care in Australia consistent and evidence based?' *Medical Journal of Australia*, 176, pp. 255–9.

Hunt, S. and Bolton, G. 1978 'Cleansing the dunghill: Water supply and sanitation in Perth 1878–1912', *Studies in West Australian History*, 2, pp. 1–17.

Hunter, D.J. 2009 'Leading for health and wellbeing: The need for a new paradigm', *Journal of Public Health*, 31(2), pp. 202–4.

Hunter Institute of Mental Health 2005 *Evaluation of MindMatters: Ninth Interim Report 1/2/2005 to 31/7/200*, report to the Australian Principals Association's Professional Development Council and the Evaluation Reference Group, <http://cms.curriculum.edu.au/mindmatters/resources/pdf/evaluation/9th_interim_report.pdf> [16 November 2005].

IHP+: *see* International Health Partnerships and Related Initiatives.

Iles, V. and Sutherland, K. 2001 *Organisational Change: A Review for Health Care Managers, Professionals and Researchers*, NHS, London.

Inayatullah, S. 2002 *Questioning the Future: Futures Studies, Action Learning and Organisational Transformation*, Tamkang University, Taipei.

—— 2003 'Aging: Alternative futures and policy choices', *Foresight*, 5(6), pp. 8–17.

—— 2005 *Questioning the Future: Methods and Tools for Organisational and Social Transformation*, Tamkang University, Taipei.

Indig, D., McEntyre, E., Page, J. and Ross, B. 2010a *2009 NSW Inmate Health Survey: Aboriginal Health Report*, Justice Health, Sydney.

Indig, D., Topp, L., Ross, B., Mamoon, H., Border, B., Kumar, S. and McNamara, M. 2010b *2009 NSW Inmate Health Survey: Key Findings Report*, Justice Health, Sydney.

Ingram, A. 2003 *UK Pathfinder for Global Health*, working paper for Nuffield Trust, London.

INHPF: *see* International Network of Health Promotion Foundations.

Institute of Medicine 1988 *The Future of Public Health*, National Academy Press, Washington, DC.

—— 2002 *Future of the Public's Health in the 21st Century*, National Academy of Sciences, Washington, DC.

—— 2003a *Unequal Treatment*, National Academy Press, Washington, DC.

—— 2003b *Fostering Rapid Advances in Health Care: Learning from System Demonstrations*, National Academy Press, Washington, DC.

Interdepartmental Group on Health Risks from Chemicals 2003 *Uncertainty Factors: Their Use in Human Health Risk Assessment by UK Government*, Institute for Environment and Health, University of Leicester, Leicester.

Intergovernmental Committee on HIV/AIDS 1992 *Final Report of the Legal Working Party*, Commonwealth of Australia, Canberra.

International Health Partnerships and Related Initiatives (IHP+) 2012, *IPH Results: Progress in the International Health Partnerships and Related Initiatives (IHP+)*, <www.internationalhealthpartnership.net/fileadmin/uploads/ihp/Documents/Results___Evidence/IHP__Results/IHP_Results_2012_Rpt.Eng.pdf> [25 October 2012].

International Network of Health Promotion Foundations (INHPF) 2012 'FAQ', <www.hpfoundations.net/faq> [23 October 2012].

International Union for Health Promotion and Education (IUHPE) 2000 *The Evidence of Health Promotion Effectiveness: Shaping Public Health in the New Europe*, 2nd edn, European Commission, Brussels.

—— 2009, *Toward Domains of Core Competency for Building Global Capacity in Health Promotion: The Galway Consensus Conference Statement*, draft, April.

—— 2011 'Draft of the White Paper on surveillance and health promotion', <www.iuhpe.org/?page=497#White%20Paper%20on%20Surveillance%20and%20Health%20Promotion> [6 October 2013].

Investment Review of Health and Medical Research Committee 2004 *Sustaining the Virtuous Cycle: For a Healthy, Competitive Australia*, final report, Commonwealth of Australia, Canberra.

IUHPE: *see* International Union for Health Promotion and Education.

Jackson, D. 2004 *Report of the Special Commission of Inquiry into the Medical Research and Compensation Foundation*, Appendix J: Asbestos and James Hardie, Cabinet Office, New South Wales Government, Sydney.

Jackson, T., Duckett, S., Shepheard, J. and Baxter, K. 2006 'Measurement of adverse events using "incidence flagged" diagnosis codes', *Journal of Health Services Research Policy*, 11(1), pp. 21–6.

Jackson Bowers, E. and Cheng, I. 2010 'Meeting the primary health care needs of refugees and asylum seekers, *Research Round Up*, 16, December, Primary Health Care Research and Information Service, Melbourne.

Jacobs, L., Marmor, T. and Oberlander, J. 1999 'The Oregon Health Plan and the political paradox of rationing: What advocates and critics have claimed and what Oregon did', *Journal of Health, Politics, Policy and Law*, 24(1), pp. 161–80.

Jaensch, D. and Teichmann, M. 1979 *The Macmillan Dictionary of Australian Politics*, Macmillan, Melbourne.

Janes, C.R., Stall, R. and Gifford, S.M. (eds) 1986 *Anthropology and Epidemiology: Interdisciplinary Approaches to the Study of Health and Disease*, D. Reidel, Amsterdam.

Jayasinghe, S. 2011 'Conceptualising population health: from mechanistic thinking to complexity science', *Emerging Themes in Epidemiology*, 8(2), <www.eteonlne.com/content/8/1/2> [24 November 2012].

Joanna Briggs Institute 2004 'Evidence-based health care movement: Overview and development', <www.joannabriggs.edu.au/about/history_ebhc_overview> [10 February 2005].

Johnston, J. 2000 'The New Public Management in Australia', *Administrative Theory & Praxis*, 22(2), pp. 345–68.

Jorm, L. and Visotina, M. 2003 'The Sydney Olympics: A win for public health', *NSW Public Health Bulletin*, 14(3), pp. 43–5.

Kalucy, E., Hann, K. and Guy, S. 2005 *Divisions: The Network Evolves: Report of the 2003–2004 Annual Survey of Divisions of General Practice*, Primary Health Care Research and Information Service, Flinders University, Adelaide.

Kant, I. 1780 *The Metaphysical Elements of Ethics* available at <www.gutenberg.org/etext/5684> [6 April 2006].

Kaplan, D.W. 2009 'Barriers and potential solutions to increasing immunization rates in adolescents', *Journal of Adolescent Health*, 46, pp. S24–S33.

Kaplan, G., Pamuk, E., Lynch, J.W., Cohen, R.D. and Balfour, J.L. 1996 'Inequality in income and mortality in the US: Analysis of mortality and potential pathways', *British Medical Journal*, 312, pp. 999–1003.

Karasek, R., Baker, D., Marxer, F., Ahlbom, A. and Theorell, T. 1981 'Job decision latitude, job demands, and cardiovascular disease: A prospective study of Swedish men', *American Journal of Public Health*, 71, pp. 694–705.

Kasl, S.V. and Cobb, S. 1966 'Health behaviour, illness behaviour, and sick-role behaviour I: health and illness behaviour', *Archives of Environmental Health*, 12, pp. 246–66.

Kass, N. 2001 'An ethics framework for public health', *American Journal of Public Health*, 91(11), pp. 1776–82.

Kawachi, I. and Berkman, L. 2000 'Social cohesion, social capital and health' in L. Berkman and I. Kawachi (eds), *Social Epidemiology*, Oxford University Press, New York.

Kawachi, I. and Kennedy, B.P. 1997 'Socioeconomic determinants of health: Health and social cohesion—why care about income inequality?', *British Medical Journal*, 314, pp. 1037–40.

Kawachi, I., Kennedy, B.P., Lochner, K. and Prothrow-Stith, D. 1997 'Social capital, income inequality and mortality', *American Journal of Public Health*, 87, pp. 1491–8.

Keating, M. 1996 'Past and future directions of the APS: Some personal reflections', *Australian Journal of Public Administration*, 55(4), pp. 3–9.

Kellehear, A. 1999 *Health Promoting Palliative Care*, Oxford University Press, Melbourne.

—— 2003 'Public health challenges in the care of the dying', in P. Liamputtong and H. Gardner (eds), *Health, Social Change and Communities*, Oxford University Press, Melbourne.

—— 2005 *Compassionate Cities: Public Health Approaches to End-of-Life Care*, Routledge, London.

Kerr, C., Taylor, R. and Heard, G. (eds) 1998 *Handbook of Public Health Methods*, McGraw-Hill, Sydney.

Kickbusch, I. 1996 'Tribute to Aaron Antonovsky: "what creates health?"', *Health Promotion International*, 11(1), pp. 5–6.

—— 1997 'Think health: what makes a difference?', *Health Promotion International*, 12(4), pp. 265–72.

—— 2004 'Constructing global public health in the 21st century', paper presented to meeting on global health governance and accountability, Harvard University, June.

King, K. and Vodicka, P. 2001 'Screening for conditions of public health importance in people arriving in Australia by boat without authority', *Medical Journal of Australia*, 175, pp. 600–2.

The Kirby Institute 2011 *HIV, Viral Hepatitis and Sexually Transmissible Infections in Australia Annual Surveillance Report 2011*, The Kirby Institute, University of New South Wales, Sydney.

Klaucke, D.N., Buehler, J.W.,Thacker, S.B., Parrish,R.G., Trowbridge, F.L., Berkelman, R.L. and the Surveillance Coordination Group 1988, 'Guidelines for Evaluating Surveillance Systems', <http://www.cdc.gov/mmwr/preview/mmwrhtml/00001769.htm> [6 October 2013].

Koh, T., Plant, A. and Lee, E.H. (eds) 2003 *The New Global Threat: Severe Acute Respiratory Syndrome and Its Impacts*, World Scientific Publishing Co., Singapore.

Kohatsu, N.D., Robinson, J.G. and Torner, J.C. 2004 'Evidence-based public health: An evolving concept', *American Journal of Preventive Medicine*, 27(5), pp. 417–21.

Koplan, J. and McPheeters, M. 2004 'Plagues, public health and politics', *Emerging Infectious Diseases*, 10(11), pp. 2039–43.

Krieger, N. 2000 'Discrimination and health', in L. Berkman and I. Kawachi (eds), *Social Epidemiology*, Oxford University Press, New York.

Kuh, D. and Ben-Shlomo, Y. (eds) 1997 *A Life Course Approach to Chronic Disease Epidemiology*, Oxford University Press, Oxford.

Kuzmin, I.V., Bozick, B., Guagliard, S.A., Kunkel, R., Shak, J.R., Tong, S. and Rupprecht, C.E. 2011 'Bats, emerging infectious diseases, and the rabies paradigm revisited', *Emerging Health Threats Journal*, 4, p. 7159.

Labonte, R. 1990 'Empowerment: Notes on professional and community dimensions', *Canadian Review of Social Policy*, 26, pp. 64–75.

—— 1998 *A Community Development Approach to Health Promotion: A Background Paper on Practice, Tensions, Strategic Models and Accountability Requirements for Health Authority Work on the Broad Determinants of Health*, Health Education Board of Scotland, Research Unit on Health and Behaviour Change, University of Edinburgh, Edinburgh.

Lalonde, M. 1974 *A New Perspective on the Health of Canadians: A Working Document*, Government of Canada, Ottawa.

Lanciani, R. 1967 *Ancient Rome in the Light of Recent Discoveries*, Benjamin Blom, New York.

Langenberg, C., Shipley, M.J., Batty, G.D. and Marmot, M.G. 2005 'Adult socio-economic position and the association between height and coronary heart disease mortality: Findings from 33 years of follow-up in the Whitehall study', *American Journal of Public Health*, 95(4), pp. 628–32.

Lasker, R.D. and the Committee on Medicine and Public Health 1997 *Medicine and Public Health, the Power of Collaboration*, The New York Academy of Medicine, New York.

Last, J. (ed.) 1986 *Maxy-Rosenau Public Health and Preventive Medicine*, Appleton-Century-Crofts, Norwalk.

—— (ed.) 1995 *A Dictionary of Epidemiology*, 3rd edn, Oxford University Press, New York.

—— (ed.) 2001 *A Dictionary of Epidemiology*, 4th edn, International Epidemiological Association, Oxford University Press, Oxford.

La Trobe University 2012 Centre for Health Communication and Participation website, <www.latrobe.edu.au/chcp/about.html> [12 October 2012].

Laverack, G. 2009 'Community empowerment', in *Working document for 7th Global Conference on Health Promotion, 'Promoting Health and Development: Closing the Implementation Gap'*, Nairobi, Kenya, 26–30 October, <www.who.int/healthpromotion/conferences/7gchp/Track2_Inner.pdf> [20 October 2012].

Lawson, J.S. and Bauman, A.E. 2001 *Public Health Australia: An Introduction*, 2nd edn, McGraw-Hill, Sydney.

Lee, K. 2003 *Globalisation and Health: An Introduction*, Palgrave Macmillan, London.

—— 2004 'Globalisation: What is it and how does it affect health?', *Medical Journal of Australia*, 180(4), pp. 156–8.

Lee, K. and McInnes, C. 2003 *Health, Foreign Policy and Security*, UK Global Health Programme Working Paper No. 1, Nuffield Trust, London.

Levy, M. 2005 'Prisoner health care provision: Reflections from Australia', *International Journal of Prisoner Health*, 1(1), pp. 65–73.

Lewis, M.J. (ed.) 1989 *Health and Disease in Australia: A History*, AGPS, Canberra.

Lewis, R.A. 1952 *Edwin Chadwick and the Public Health Movement 1832–1854*, Longmans, Green and Co., London.

LGA: *see* Local Government Association.

Li, J., Hampson, A., Roche, P., Yohannes, K. and Spencer, J. 2005 'Annual report of the National Influenza Surveillance Scheme', *Communicable Diseases Intelligence*, 29(2), pp. 124–35.

Li, J., Roche, P., Spencer, J. and the National Tuberculosis Advisory Committee 2004 'Tuberculosis notifications in Australia, 2003', *Communicable Diseases Intelligence*, 28(4), pp. 464–73.

Liberman, J. 2002 'Rolah Ann McCabe v British American Tobacco Australia Services Limited: Judgement of Justice Eames, Supreme Court of Victoria', Summary and implications prepared for the VicHealth Centre for Tobacco Control, Melbourne, <www.vctc.org.au> [20 June 2005].

Lin, M., Spencer, J., Roche, P., McKinnon M. and the National Tuberculosis Advisory Committee 2002 'Tuberculosis notifications in Australia, 2000', *Communicable Diseases Intelligence*, 26(2), pp. 214–15.

Lin, V. 1999 'Health protection and health promotion: Harmonizing our responses to the challenges of the 21st century', in *Proceedings of Regional Meeting on Health Promotion and Protection*, World Health Organization, Manila.

——— 2000 'Maximising women's capacity and leadership in health: Vision and propositions for action', from a presentation prepared for WHO Kobe Centre's 2nd International Meeting on Women in Health, 4–6 April 2000, Canberra.

——— 2002 'Structural reform and cultural transition: Reflections on the National Public Health Partnership', in H. Gardner and S. Barraclough (eds), *Health Policy in Australia*, 2nd edn, Oxford University Press, Melbourne.

——— 2003a 'Agenda for research transfer and governance', in V. Lin and B. Gibson (eds), *Evidence-based Health Policy: Problems and Possibilities*, Oxford University Press, Melbourne.

——— 2003b 'Competing rationalities', in V. Lin and B. Gibson (eds), *Evidence-based Health Policy: Problems and Possibilities*, Oxford University Press, Melbourne.

Lin, V. and Duckett, S.J. 1996 'Health system reform in Victoria: Casemix and beyond', in H. Gardner (ed.), *Health Policy in Australia*, Oxford University Press, Melbourne.

Lin, V. and Fawkes, S. 2002 'Effectiveness of health promotion in changing environment and lifestyles in developing countries in the Western Pacific: A review and a proposed framework', presented at Regional Meeting on Capacity-building for Health Promotion, Manila.

——— 2003a 'Effectiveness of health promotion in changing environment and lifestyles in developing countries of the Western Pacific Region: A review and a proposed framework', prepared for WHO Regional Office for the Western Pacific, School of Public Health, La Trobe University, Melbourne.

——— 2003b *Strengthening Effectiveness: Health Promotion Effectiveness in the Western Pacific Region*, World Health Organization Western Pacific Regional Office, Manila.

——— 2005a 'Evidence and effectiveness in health promotion', in S. Thomas and C. Browning (eds), *Behavioural Change: Evidence-based Handbook for Social and Public Health*, Churchill Livingston, Edinburgh.

——— 2005b 'Prolead: Health promotion leadership development in the Western Pacific region', *Health Promotion Journal of Australia*, 16(3), pp. 176–8.

Lin, V. and Gibson, B. (eds) 2003 *Evidence-based Health Policy: Problems and Possibilities*, Oxford University Press, Melbourne.

Lin, V. and King, C. 2000 'Intergovernmental reforms in public health', in A. Bloom (ed.), *Health Reform in Australia and New Zealand*, Oxford University Press, Melbourne.

Lin, V., Gruszin, S., Ellickson, C., Glover, J., Silburn, K., Wilson, G. and Poljski, C. 2003 *Comparative Evaluation of Indicators for Gender Equity and Health*, Women and Health Programme, WHO Centre for Health Development, Kobe, Japan.

Lin, V. and Robinson, P. 2005 'Australian public health policy in 2003–2004', *Australia New Zealand Health Policy*, 2(7), <www.anzhealthpolicy.com/content/2/1/7> [2 November 2005].

Lin, V. Watson, R. and Oldenberg, B. 2009 'The future of public health: The importance of workforce', *Australia and New Zealand Journal of Public Health Policy*, <www.anzhealthpolicy.com/content/6/1/4>.

Lindblom, C.E. 1959 'The science of muddling through', *Public Administration Review*, 19(2), pp. 79–88.

Link, B.G. and Phelan, J. 2001 'Conceptualizing stigma,' *Annual Review of Sociology*, 27, pp. 363–85.

Lister, G., Lee, K. and Williams, O. 2003 'Global health and foreign policy', paper prepared for Nuffield Trust and RAND Corporation, London.

Local Government Association of South Australia n.d. *Common Illegal Dumping Problems, Asbestos Waste*, <www.lga. sa.gov.au/site/page.cfm?u=1900> [1 November 2012].

Lomas, J. 1997 *Beyond the Sound of One Hand Clapping: A Discussion Document on Improving Health Research Dissemination and Uptake*, NSW Health Department, Research and Development Centre, Sydney.

—— 2003 'Health services research' (editorial), *British Medical Journal*, 327, pp. 1301–2.

Lorig, K. and Holman, H. 2000 'Self-management education: Context, definition, and context and mechanisms', *Proceedings of the 1st Chronic Disease Self-Management Conference, Sydney, Australia*, August, Stanford University School of Medicine, Stanford, CA.

Louie, R., Krouskos, D., Gonzales, M. and Crofts, N. 1998 'Vietnamese-speaking injecting drug users in Melbourne: The need for harm reduction programs', *Australian and New Zealand Journal of Public Health*, 22(4), pp. 481–4.

Lowitja Insitute 2012 Australia's National Institute for Aboriginal and Torres Strait Islander Research <www.lowitja.org.au>

Lumb, R., Bastian, I., Carter, R., Jelfs, P., Keehner, T. and Sievers, A. 2011, 'Tuberculosis in Australia: Bacteriologically confirmed cases and drug resistance, 2008 and 2009. A report of the Australian Mycobacterium Reference Laboratory Network', *Communicable Disease Intelligence*, 35(2), pp. 154–61.

Lumley, J., Brown, S. and Gunn, J. 2003 'Getting research transfer into policy and practice in maternity care', in V. Lin and B. Gibson (eds), *Evidence-based Health Policy: Problems and Possibilities*, Oxford University Press, Melbourne.

Lurie, N., Valdez, R., Wasserman, M., Stoto, M., Myers, S., Molander, R., Asch, S., Mussington, D. and Solomon, V. 2004 *Public Health Preparedness in California: Lessons Learned from Seven Health Jurisdictions*, Rand Health, Santa Monica, CA.

Lutter, C. 2012 'The International Code of Marketing of Breast-milk Substitutes: Lessons learned and implications for the regulation of marketing of foods and beverages to children', *Public Health Nutrition*, 4, pp. 1–6. [epub ahead of print].

Lynch, J. and Kaplan, G. 2000 'Socioeconomic position', in L. Berkman and I. Kawachi (eds), *Social Epidemiology*, Oxford University Press, New York.

Lynch, J., Kaplan, G. and Salonen, J.T. 1997 'Why do poor people behave poorly? Variation in adult health behaviours and psychosocial characteristics by stage of the socioeconomic lifecourse', *Social Science and Medicine*, 44, pp. 809–19.

Macintyre, S. and Ellaway, A. 2003 'Neighborhoods and health: Overview' in I. Kawachi and L.F. Berkman (eds), *Neighborhoods and Health*, Oxford University Press, New York.

MacMahon, B. and Pugh, T.F. 1970 *Epidemiology: Principles and Methods*, Little, Brown, Boston.

Madden, L. and Salmon, A. 1999 'Public health workforce: Results of a NSW state-wide consultation on the development of national public health workforce', *NSW Public Health Bulletin*, 10(3), pp. 19–21.

Maddox, G. 2005, *Australian Democracy in Theory and Practice*, 5th edn, Pearson Education, Sydney.

Mahoney, M. and Durham, G. 2002 *Health Impact Assessment: A Tool for Policy Development in Australia*, report prepared on behalf of the HIA research team, Faculty of Health and Behavioural Sciences, Deakin University, Melbourne, <www.deakin.edu.au/hbs/hia/publications> [2 November 2004].

Mahoney, M., Simpson, S., Harris, E. and Williams, J. 2004 *Equity-Focused Health Impact Assessment Framework*, The Australian Collaboration for Health Equity Impact Assessment, Sydney, <http://chetre.med.unsw.edu.au/files/EFHIA_Framework.pdf> [9 December 2004].

Mann, J.M., Gruskin, S., Grodin, M.A. and Annas, G.J. 1999 'Health and human rights', in Mann et al. (eds), *Health and Human Rights: A Reader*, Routledge, New York.

March, J. and Olsen, J. 1989 *Rediscovering Institutions: The Organizational Basis of Politics*, The Free Press, New York.

Marks, C., Tideman, R. and Mindel, A. 1997 'Evaluation of sexual health services within Australia and New Zealand', (*eMJA*) *Medical Journal of Australia*, 166, pp. 348–52.

Marmor, T. and Christianson, J.B. 1982 *Health Care Policy: A Political Economy Approach*, Sage, Beverly Hills, CA.

Marmot, M. 2000 'Multilevel approaches to understanding social determinants' in L. Berkman and I. Kawachi (eds), *Social Epidemiology*, Oxford University Press, New York.

Marmot, M., Bosma, H., Brunner, E. and Stansfeld, S. 1997 'Contribution of job control and other risk factors to social variations in coronary heart disease incidence', *Lancet*, 26 July, 350(9073), pp. 235–9.

Marmot, M. and Wilkinson, R.G. (eds) 1999 *Social Determinants of Health*, Oxford University Press, New York.

Marsh, I. and Yencken, D. 2004 *Into the Future: The Neglect of the Long Term in Australian Politics*, The Australian Collaboration, Melbourne.

Martens, P. and Huynen, M. 2003 'A future without health? Health dimension in global scenario studied', *Bulletin of the World Health Organization*, 81(12), pp. 896–901.

Martin, J.A. and Mak, D.B. 2006 'Changing faces: A review of infectious disease screening of refugees by the Migrant Health Unit, Western Australia in 2003 and 2004', *Medical Journal of Australia*, 185(11/12), pp. 607–10.

McCall, B.J., Epstein, J.H., Neill, A.S., Heel, K., Field, H., Barrett, J., et al. 2000 'Potential human exposure to Australian bat lyssavirus, Queensland, 1996–1999', *Emerging Infectious Diseases*, 6(3), pp. 259–64.

McCormack, C. 1994 'The health promotion gap', *Healthlines*, 13, p. 10.

McCulloch, J. 1986 *Asbestos: Its Human Cost*, University of Queensland Press, Brisbane.

McDonald, A (ed.) 2011 *HIV, Viral Hepatitis and Sexually Transmissible Infections in Australia*, Annual Surveillance Report, <www.kirby.unsw.edu.au/sites/hiv.cms.med.unsw.edu.au/files/hiv/resources/2011Annual SurvReport_0.pdf> [29 August 2012].

McIntyre, P., Gidding, H., Gilmour, R., Lawrence, G., Hull, B., Hornby, P., Wang, H., Andrews, R. and Burgess, M. 2002 'Vaccine preventable diseases and vaccination coverage in Australia, 1999 to 2000', *Communicable Diseases Intelligence*, 26, Supplement, Commonwealth of Australia, Canberra.

McKeown, T. 1979 *The Role of Medicine: Dream, Mirage or Nemesis?*, Princeton University Press, Princeton, NJ.

MacMahon, B. and Pugh, T.F. 1970 *Epidemiology: Principles and Methods*, Little, Brown, Boston.

McMichael, A.J. 1993 *Planetary Overload: Global Environmental Change and the Health of the Human Species*, Cambridge University Press, Cambridge.

—— 2001 *Human Frontiers, Environments and Disease: Past Patterns, Uncertain Futures*, Cambridge University Press, Cambridge.

McMichael, C. and Lin, V. 2004 *Case Studies in Successful Public Health Interventions*, report prepared for the European Observatory on Health Systems, Brussels.

McQueen, D.V. 2001 'Strengthening the evidence base for health promotion', *Health Promotion International*, 16(3), pp. 261–8.

McSpotlight 2005 'The McLibel Trial', <www.mcspotlight.org/case/trial/story.html> [20 May 2012].

Medical Journal of Australia (2003) 'Editorial: Australia confronts the challenge of chronic disease', 179(5), pp. 233–4.

Merson, M., Black, R. and Mills, A. (eds) 2001 *International Public Health: Diseases Programs, Systems, and Policies*, Aspen, Gaithersburg, MD.

Milburn, K. 1996 'The importance of lay theorising for health promotion research and practice', *Health Promotion International*, 11(1), pp. 41–6.

Miliband, R. 1969 *The State in Capitalist Society*, Weidenfeld & Nicolson, London.

Milio, N. 1987 'Making healthy public policy: Developing the science by learning the art—an ecological framework for policy studies', *Health Promotion*, 2(3), pp. 263–74.

Miller, M., Lin, M., Spencer, J. and the National Tuberculosis Advisory Committee 2002 'Tuberculosis notifications in Australia, 2001', *Communicable Disease Intelligence*, 26(4), pp. 525–36.

Miller, M.T. and Strömland, K. 1999 'Thalidomide: A review, with a focus on ocular findings and new potential uses', *Teratology*, 60(3), pp. 306–21.

Miller, P. and Peters, B. 2004 'Overview of the public health implications of cockroaches and their management', *NSW Public Health Bulletin*, 15(11–12), pp. 208–11.

Mills, C.W. 1959 *The Power Elite*, Oxford University Press, New York.

Minkler, M. 1989 'Health education, health promotion and the open society: An historical perspective', *Health Education Quarterly*, 16, pp. 17–30.

Minkler, M. and Cox, K. 1980 'Creating critical consciousness in health: Applications of Friere's philosophy and methods to the health care setting', *International Journal of Health Services*, 10, pp. 311–22.

Mirnezami, R., Nicholson, J. and Darzi, A. 2012 'Preparing for precision medicine', *New England Journal of Medicine*, 366, pp. 489–91.

Moodie, R. 2004 'Here's a way to reduce those waiting lists', *The Age*, 10 November.

Moodie, R., Pisani, E. and de Castellarnau, M. 2000 'Infrastructures to promote health: The art of the possible', technical paper prepared for the Fifth Global Conference on Health Promotion, Mexico City, June.

Mooney, G. and Blackwell, S. 2004 'Whose health service is it anyway? Community values in health care', *Medical Journal of Australia*, 180, pp. 76–8.

Mooney, G., Gerard, K., Donaldson, C. and Farrar, S. 1992 *Priority Setting in Purchasing: Some Practical Guidelines*, Research Paper 6, National Association of Health Authorities and Trusts, Birmingham.

Morey, S. and Madden, L. 2003 'Building the infrastructure for public health', *Public Health Bulletin*, 14(3), pp. 50–1.

Mulgan, R. 1998 *Politicising the Australian Public Service*, Research Paper 3 1998–99, Parliamentary Library, Canberra.

Murnane, M. and Cooper, D. 2005 'Is the Australian hospital system adequately prepared for terrorism? The Australian Government's response', *Medical Journal of Australia*, 183(11/12), pp. 572–3.

Murphy, J. 2005 'Health promotion', *Economic Roundup*, Winter, Commonwealth of Australia, Canberra.

Murray, C.J. and Lopez, A.D. 1996 *The Global Burden of Disease: A Comprehensive Assessment of Mortality and Disability from Diseases, Injuries and Risk Factors in 1990 Projected to 2020*, Harvard University School of Public Health, Cambridge, MA.

Nabhan, G.P. 2004 *Why Some Like It Hot: Food, Genes, and Cultural Diversity*, Island Press/Shearwater Books, Washington DC.

Nader, C. 2004 'Needless care clogs beds', *The Age*, 9 December, p. 9.

Naidoo, J. and Wills, J. (eds) 2001 *Health Studies: An Introduction*, Palgrave, Basingstoke.

Nash, S. 1999 'Self help in Australia: The self help movement in Australia in the 1990s', *Community Quarterly*, Winter, <http://home.vicnet. net.au/~coshg/selfhelphistory.html> [10 March 2005].

National Aboriginal Health Strategy (NAHS) Working Party 1989 *A National Aboriginal Health Strategy*, NAHS Working Party, Canberra.

National Center for Environmental Health 2002 *Summary of Core Environmental Public Health Indicators*, <www.cdc.gov/nceh/indicators/summary.htm> [17 April 2004].

National Centre in HIV Epidemiology and Clinical Research (NCHECR) (ed.) 2000 *Annual Surveillance Report: HIV/AIDS, Hepatitis C and Sexually Transmissible Infections in Australia*, NCHECR, University of New South Wales, Sydney.

—— 2002 *HIV/AIDS, Viral Hepatitis and Sexually Transmissible Infections in Australia Annual Surveillance Report 2002*, National Centre in HIV Epidemiology and Clinical Research, University of New South Wales, Sydney.

National Environmental Health Forum (NEHF) 1999 *Indigenous Environmental Health*, NEHF Monographs, Indigenous Environmental Health Series No. 1, NEHF, Canberra.

—— 2000 *Indigenous Environmental Health, Report of the First National Workshop*, 20–22 May 1998, NEHF Monographs, Indigenous Environmental Health Series No. 1, NEHF, Canberra.

National Health Information Management Group 2003 *Health Information Development Priorities*, AIHW, Canberra.

National Health Information Standards and Statistics Committee (NHISSC) 2009 *The National Health Performance Framework*, 2nd edn, NHISSC, Canberra.

National Health and Medical Research Council (NHMRC) 1993 *Ethical Considerations Relating to Health Care Resource Allocation Decisions*, Commonwealth of Australia, Canberra.

—— 1994 *National Framework for Environmental and Health Impact Assessment*, AGPS, Canberra.

—— 1996 'New guidelines aim to eliminate tuberculosis in Australia', media release, 19 June.

—— 1997a *Health Australia Review*, Health Advancement Standing Committee, Canberra.

—— 1997b *Promoting the Health of Australians: A Review of Infrastructure Support for National Health Advancement*, AGPS, Canberra.

—— 1999 *A Guide to the Development, Implementation and Evaluation of Clinical Practice Guidelines*, Commonwealth of Australia, Canberra.

—— 2001 'State Commonwealth research issues forum', media release, <www.nhmrc.gov.au/media/2001rel/mediarel.htm> [8 June 2005].

—— 2005a 'WA leads the way on ageing research', ministerial media release, 17 January, <www.nhmrc.gov.au/media/re2005/ageresearchwa.htm> [8 June 2005].

—— 2005b 'Research projects focus on the health of Indigenous children', ministerial media release, 19 May, <www.nhmrc.gov.au/media/rel2005/focus.htm> [8 June 2005].

—— 2009a *Report of the Review of Public Health Research Funding in Australia* <www.phaa.net.au/documents/PublicHealthResearchFundingReport.pdf> [19 October 2012].

—— 2009b *Response to the Report of the Review of Public Health Research Funding in Australia (Nutbeam Committee Report) May 2009*, <www.nhmrc.gov.au/_files_nhmrc/file/research/phr/response-to-nutbeam.pdf> [19 October 2012].

—— 2009c 'NHMRC levels of evidence and grades for recommendations for developers of guidelines', <www.nhmrc.gov.au/_files_nhmrc/file/guidelines/developers/nhmrc_levels_grades_evidence_120423.pdf> [31 October 2012].

—— 2011 *Climate Change*, <www.nhmrc.gov.au/your-health/climate-change> [19 November 2012].

—— 2012a 'NHMRC grants: A–Z list of funding types', <www.nhmrc.gov.au/grants/typesfunding/-z-list-funding-types> [6 November 2012].

—— 2012b 'NHMRC Committees', <www.nhmrc.gov.au/about/committees-nhmrc> [19 October 2012].

National Health and Medical Research Council (NHMRC) and the Consumers' Health Forum of Australia 2002 *Statement on Consumer and Community Participation in Health and Medical Research*, Commonwealth of Australia, Canberra.

National Health Service 2012 'NHS alert: New "SARS-like" virus detected', *NHS Choices Bulletin*, 25 September, <www.nhs.uk/news/2012/09September/Pages/NewSARS-like-virus-detected.aspx> [31 October 2012].

National Occupational Health and Safety Commission 2004 *National Occupational Health and Safety Commission Annual Report 2003–2004*, National Capital Printing, Canberra.

National Prescribing Service 2005 'Who we are', <www.nps.org.au> [10 March 2005].

National Preventative Health Taskforce 2008 *Australia: The Healthiest Country by 2020—A Discussion Paper*, Commonwealth of Australia, <www.preventativehealth.org.au/internet/preventativehealth/publishing.nsf/Content/discussion-healthiest> [6 October 2013].

National Public Health Partnership (NPHP) 1998a, *Memorandum of Understanding Between the Commonwealth and States and Territories to Establish the National Public Health Partnership*, NPHP, Canberra.

—— 1998b *Issues for Consideration in Industry Partnerships for Public Health Initiatives*, NPHP, Melbourne.

—— 1998c 'National HIV/AIDS strategy and Australia's response to related disease', in *Key Achievements in Public Health*, National Public Health Partnership-Secretariat, Melbourne, <www.nphp.gov.au> [19 October 2013].

—— 1998d Summary Report of Workshop on Envisioning Public Health in the 21st Century, 20 October, <http://www.nphp.gov.au/publications/phpractice/envisioning_ph_1998.pdf> [6 October 2013].

—— 1998e 'Public health in Australia: The public health landscape', <www.nphp.gov.au/publications/broch/sectn002.htm> [2 November 2005].

—— 1999 *Guidelines for Improving National Public Health Strategies Development and Coordination*, NPHP, Melbourne.

—— 2000a *A Planning Framework for Public Health Practice*, NPHP, Melbourne.

—— 2000b *A Proposed Schema for Evaluating Evidence on Public Health Interventions*, discussion paper, NPHP, Melbourne.

—— 2000c *Public Health Practice in Australia Today: A Statement of Core Functions*, NPHP, Melbourne.

—— 2000d *Integrated Public Health Practice: Supporting and Strengthening Local Action*, background paper, June, NPHP, Melbourne.

—— 2001 *Preventing Chronic Disease: A Strategic Framework*, NPHP, Melbourne.

—— 2002a *A Schema for Evaluating Evidence on Public Health Interventions*, NPHP, Melbourne.

—— 2002b *The Role of Local Government in Public Health Regulation*, NPHP, Melbourne.

—— 2002c *Public Health Performance Project*, a discussion paper, NPHP, Melbourne.

—— 2004 The National Computer Assisted Telephone Interviewing Technical Reference Group, <www.nphp.gov.au/catitrg> [13 February 2005].

National Public Health Partnership and SIGNAL 2000 *An Intervention Portfolio to Promote Fruit and Vegetable Consumption: Part 1—The Process and Portfolio*, NPHP, Melbourne.

NCHECR: *see* National Centre in HIV Epidemiology and Clinical Research.

Nettleford, J. 2004 'Aerial spraying renews health concerns', *7.30 Report*, ABC TV, <www.abc.net.au/7.30/content/2004> [4 April 2005].

Ng, S., Rouch, G. and Dedman, R. 1996 'Human salmonellosis and peanut butter', *Communicable Diseases Intelligence*, 20(14), p. 326.

NHISSC: *see* National Health Information Standards and Statistics Committee.

NHMRC: *see* National Health and Medical Research Council.

NHS: *see* National Health Service.

Noack, R.H. 1997 *Research for Health Promotion*, working paper prepared for the 4th International Health Promotion Conference, Jakarta.

NOHSC: *see* National Occupational Health and Safety Commission.

NPHP: *see* National Public Health Partnership.

NSW Corrections Service 1997 *1996 Inmate Health Survey*, <www.justicehealth.nsw.gov.au/pubs/Inmate_Health_Survey_1997.pdf> [20 April 2006].

NSW Health 2000 'Report of the NSW Chief Health Officer: Blood lead levels in children', <www.health.nsw.gov/public-health/chorep00/env_bhelc.htm> [27 February 2006].

—— 2001 *NSW Public Health Bulletin*, Special issue: Health Inequalities: Something Old, Something New, NSW Health, Sydney.

—— 2010, *Public Health Classifications Project: Determinants of Health Phase Two—Final Report*, NSW Health, Sydney, <www0.health.nsw.gov.au/pubs/2010/pdf/public_health_classifications_project.pdf> [19 October 2013].

—— 2012a *NSW Public Health Bulletin*, Public health ethics: informing better public health practice, 23(5-6).

—— 2012b 'Year in review: Health protection in NSW, 2011', *NSW Public Health Bulletin* 23(7–8), n.p.

—— n.d., 'About us', <www.health.nsw.gov.au/aboutus/chart.asp> [31 July 2012].

NSW WorkCover 2005 'Facts and figures', <www.workcover.nsw.gov.au/AboutUs/FactsandFigures/default. htm> [22 April 2005].

—— 2012a 'About Us', <www.workcover.nsw.gov.au/aboutus/Pages/default.aspx> [6 October 2012].

—— 2012b 'Prosecutions', <www.workcover.nsw.gov.au/LAWPOLICY/PROSECUTIONS/Pages/default.aspx> [6 October 2013].

Nutbeam, D. 1986 'Health promotion glossary', *Health Promotion International*, 1(1), pp. 113–27.

—— 1996 'Health outcomes and health promotion: defining success in health promotion', *Health Promotion Journal of Australia*, 6(2), pp. 58–60.

Nutbeam, D. and Harris. E. 1999 *Theory in a Nutshell: A Guide to Health Promotion Theory*, McGraw-Hill, Sydney.

—— 2004 *Theory in a Nutshell: A Practitioner's Guide to Commonly Used Theories and Models in Health Promotion*, 2nd edn, McGraw-Hill, Sydney.

Nutbeam, D., Wise, M., Bauman, A., Harris, E. and Leeder, S. 1993 *Goals and Targets for Australia's Health in the Year 2000 and Beyond*, AGPS, Canberra.

O'Brien, K. and Webbie, K. 2003 'Are all Australians gaining weight? Differentials in overweight and obesity among adults, 1989–90 to 2001', *AIHW Bulletin* no. 11. Cat. no. AUS 39, Canberra, AIHW, <http://www.aihw.gov.au/publication-detail/?id=6442467542> [2 October 2013].

O'Connor, J. 1974 *The Corporations and the State: Essays in the Theory of Capitalism and Imperialism*, Harper and Row, New York.

OECD: *see* Organisation for Economic Cooperation and Development.

Ogden, J. 2001 'Health psychology', in J. Naidoo and J. Wills (eds), *Health Studies: An Introduction*, Palgrave, Basingstoke.

O'Grady, K., Counahan, M., Birbilis, E. and Tallis, G. 2003 *Surveillance of Notifiable Infectious Diseases in Victoria 2002*, Public Health Group, Victorian Department of Human Services, Melbourne.

Oldenburg, B., O'Connor, M., French, M. and Parker, E. 1997 *The Dissemination Effort in Australia: Strengthening the Links Between Health Promotion Research and Practice*, AGPS, Canberra.

O'Leary, P., Breheny, N., Reid, G., Charles, T. and Emery, J. 2006 'Regional variations in prenatal screening across Australia: Stepping toward a national policy framework', *Australian and New Zealand Journal of Obstetrics and Gynaecology* 46, pp. 427–32.

Olsen, N.J., Franklin, P.J., Reid, A., de Klerk, N.H., Threlfall, T.J., Shilkin, K. and Musk, B. 2011 'Increasing incidence of malignant mesothelioma after exposure to asbestos during home maintenance and renovation', *Medical Journal of Australia*, 195(5), pp. 271–4.

Orent, W. 2004 *The Plague*, The Free Press, New York.

Organisation for Economic Cooperation and Development (OECD) 1994 *The Reform of Health Care Systems: A Review of Seventeen OECD Countries*, OECD, Paris.

—— 2003 *Emerging Risks in the Twenty-first Century: An Agenda for Action*, OECD, Paris.

—— 2012 *Health Data*, <www.oecd.org/els/healthpoliciesanddata/oecdhealthdata2012-frequentlyrequesteddata. htm> [20 December 2012].

Otok, R. Levin, I. Sitko and S. Flahault, A. 2011, <www.publichealthreviews.eu/upload/pdf_files/9/03_Otok. pdf> [20 November 2012].

Owen, J.W. 2002 *The National Health Service and the New Health Economy: Securing Our Future*, Nuffield Trust, London, <www.nuffieldtrust.org.uk/policy_themes/docs/state24.doc> [2 May 2004].

Owen, N., Bauman, A., Booth, M., Oldenburg, B. and Magnus, P. 1995 'Serial mass-media campaigns to promote physical activity: Reinforcing or redundant?', *American Journal of Public Health*, 85, pp. 244–8.

Oxfam 2007 *Close the Gap: Solutions to the Indigenous Health Crisis Facing Australia—a Policy Briefing Paper from the National Aboriginal Community Controlled Health Organisation and Oxfam Australia*, Oxfam, Sydney.

OzFoodNet Working Group 2003 'Foodborne disease in Australia: Incidence, notifications and outbreaks. Annual Report of the OzFoodNet Network 2002', *Communicable Diseases Intelligence*, 27(2), pp. 209–43.

—— 2004 'Enhancing foodborne disease surveillance across Australia: Quarterly report, July to September 2004' *Communicable Diseases Intelligence*, 28(4), pp. 485–8.

—— 2010 'Monitoring the incidence and causes of diseases potentially transmitted by food in Australia: Annual Report of the OZFOODNET Network, 2009', *Communicable Disease Intelligence*, 34 (4), pp. 396–426.

PAHO: *see* Pan American Health Organization.

Paine, N. and Cassell, E. 2003 'Local government enforcement of private swimming pool safety regulations: Survey of council building surveyors/inspectors', *Hazard*, 55, pp. 3–13.

Palmer, B. 2005 'The rule of law', *Palmer's Oz Politics*, <www.ozpolitics.info/rules/rol.htm> [14 June 2005].

Palmer, G. and Short, S. 2000 *Health Care and Public Policy: An Australian Analysis*, 3rd edn, Macmillan, Melbourne.

Pan American Health Organization (PAHO) 1982 *Operational Aspects of Disease Surveillance After Disaster*, PAHO, Washington, DC, Chapter 4.

—— 1999 The Driving Forces, Pressure, State, Exposure, Effect, Action (DPSEEA) model of WHO, <www.fep.paho.org/english/env/indicators.htm> [10 May 2006].

Parliamentary Library 2004 'In the shadow of the corporate veil: James Hardie and asbestos compensation', Research Note no. 12, 12 August, Commonwealth of Australia, Canberra.

Parsons, T. 1978 *Action Theory and the Human Condition*, Macmillan, London.

Patrias, K., Gordner, R.L. and Groft, S.C. 1997 'Thalidomide: Potential benefits and risks', *Current Bibliographies in Medicine*, 97(4), National Library of Medicine, Bethesda, <www.nlm.nih.gov/pubs/resources.html> [17 April 2004].

Patton, G.C., Goldfeld, S.R., Pieris-Caldwell, I., Bryant, M. and Vimpani, G.V. 2005 'A picture of Australia's children', *Medical Journal of Australia*, 182(9), pp. 437–8.

Peacock, S., Richardson, J. and Carter, R. 1997 *Setting Priorities in South Australian Community Health II: Marginal Analysis of Mental Health Services*, Research Report 14, Centre for Health Program Evaluation, Monash University, Melbourne.

Pedersen, D. 2002 'Political violence, ethnic conflict, and contemporary wars: Broad implications for health and social well-being', *Social Science & Medicine*, 55, pp. 175–90.

Periman, F. and Gray, S. 2004 *The Specialist Public Health Workforce in the UK: A Report for the Board of the Faculty of Public Health*, Royal College of Physicians of the United Kingdom, London.

Peterson, A. and Lupton, D. 1996 *The New Public Health: Health and Self in the Age of Risk*, Allen & Unwin, Sydney.

PHAA: *see* Public Health Association of Australia.

Phelps, K. 2003 'Government admits it cannot afford to pay for Medicare', AMA press release, 28 April <www.ama.com.au/web.nsf/doc/WEEN-5M2AJJ> [6 October 2004].

PHF: *see* Public Health Foundation.

PHIDU: *see* Public Health Information Development Unit.

Physicians for Human Rights and the Bellevue 2003 *From Persecution to Prison: The Health Consequences of Detention for Asylum Seekers*, Physicians for Human Rights and the Bellevue/NYU Program for Survivors of Torture, Boston.

Pierce, J.P., Macaskill, P. and Hill, D. 1990 'Long-term effectiveness of mass media led antismoking campaigns in Australia', *American Journal of Public Health*, 80, pp. 565–9.

Platt, M. and Gifford, S.M. 2003 'Promoting health through promoting work: The dilemmas of disclosure in the workplace for Australian women living with hepatitis C', *Health Promotion Journal of Australia*, 14, pp. 180–6.

Plowman, D.A., Solansky, S., Beck, T.E., Baker, L., Kulkarni, M. and Travis, D.V. 2007 'The role of leadership in emergent, self organization', *Leadership Quarterly*, 18(4), pp. 341–56.

Plummer, D. 2003 'Designing effective STI strategies', discussion paper prepared for the Australian National Council on AIDS, Hepatitis C and Related Diseases.

PMSEIC: *see* Prime Minister's Science, Engineering and Innovation Council.

Pollard, R. 2004 'Hepatitis C epidemic sweeps NSW prisons', *Sydney Morning Herald Online*, 12 January, <www.smh.com.au/articles/2004/01/1073769455690.html> [21 April 2006].

Popay, J.B.S., Thomas, C., Williams, G., Gattrell, A. and Bostock, L. 2003 'Beyond "beer, fags, eggs and chips"? Exploring lay understandings of social inequalities in health', *Social Health and Illness*, 25(1), pp. 1–23.

Pope, J. 2003 *Social Capital and Social Capital Indicators: A Reading List*, Working Paper Series No. 1, Public Health Information Development Unit, Adelaide.

Pope, J. and Gruszin, S. 2002 'Chronic disease and associated risk factors information monitoring systems: The results of an audit of Australian data collections and policies and a review of the international experience', paper prepared for the audit phase of the Feasibility Study for Developing a Nation-wide Chronic Disease and Associated Risk Factors Information and Monitoring System for the Commonwealth Department of Health and Ageing, Canberra.

Population Heath Queensland 2008 *Health Impact Assessment, Flinders Street Redevelopment Project*, <www.hiaconnect.edu.au/reports/Flinders_Street_Redevelopment_HIA.pdf> [20 October 2012].

Porter, D. 1999 *Health, Civilization and the State: A History of Public Health from Ancient to Modern Times*, Routledge, London.

Porter, M. and Haslam, N. 2005 'Predisplacement and postdisplacement factors associated with mental health of refugees and internally displaced persons', *Journal of the American Medical Association*, 294(5), pp. 602–12.

Potter, I. 1997 'Looking back … looking ahead', plenary presentation, 4th International Conference on Health Promotion, Jakarta, 21–25 July, <http://whqlibdoc.who.int/hq/1998/WHO_HPR_HEP_41_CHP_SP_98.1.pdf> [18 April 2006].

Potter, J., Mahoney, M., Sangster, K. and McCormick, J. 2003 'Potential health impacts of the proposed family violence strategy', report of the Rapid Health Impact Assessment, School of Health Sciences, Deakin University, Melbourne.

Potvin, L. and McQueen, D. (eds) 2008 *Health Promotion Evaluation Practices in the Americas: Values and Research*, Springer, New York.

Prime Minister's Science, Engineering and Innovation Council (PMSEIC) 2010a *Australia and Food Security in a Changing World*, Prime Minister's Science, Engineering and Innovation Council, Canberra, Australia, <www.innovation.gov.au/Science/PMSEIC/Documents/AustraliaandFoodSecurityinaChangingWorld.pdf> [1 December 2012].

—— 2010b *Challenges at Energy-Water-Carbon Intersections*, Prime Minister's Science, Engineering and Innovation Council, Canberra, Australia, <www.innovation.gov.au/Science/PMSEIC/Documents/ChallengesatEnergyWaterCarbonIntersections.pdf> [1 December 2012].

Prochaska, J.O. and DiClemente, C. 1984 *The Transtheoretical Approach: Crossing Traditional Foundations of Change*, Don Jones/Irwin, Hanrewood.

Productivity Commission 2003 *Social Capital: Reviewing the Concept and Its Policy Implications*, research paper, AusInfo, Canberra.

—— 2008 *Chemicals and Plastics Regulation*, Research Report, Melbourne.

—— 2012 *Performance Benchmarking of Australian Business Regulation: The Role of Local Government as Regulator*, Commonwealth of Australia, Canberra.

Public Broadcasting Service 2005 'Hippocratic oath: classical version', *Nova online*, <www.pbs.org/wgbh/nova/doctors/oath_classical.html> [20 January 2005].

Public Health Agency of Canada 2005 'Revising the International Health Regulations', <www.phac-aspc.gc.ca/cepr-cmiu/ihr_e.html> [2 July 2005].

Public Health Association of Australia (PHAA) 2004 *Policy on Periconceptional Folate and the Prevention of Neural Tube Defects*, <www.phaa.net.au/policy/folate.htm> [22 October 2012].

—— 2008 'About us', <www.phaa.net.au/aboutUs.php> [22 October 2012].

—— 2010, *Policy-at-a-glance: Indigenous Health Policy*, PHAA, Canberra.

Public Health Foundation (PHF) n.d. 'About the core competencies for public health professionals', <www.phf.org/programs/corecompetencies/Pages/About_the_Core_Competencies_for_Public_Health_Professionals.aspx> [20 December 2012].

Public Health Information Development Unit (PHIDU) 2008 *Audit of Australian Chronic Disease and Associated Risk Factor Data Collections*, University of Adelaide, <www.publichealth.gov.au/pdf/reports_papers/Audit_of_Australian_Chronic_Disease_&_Associated_Risk_Factor_Data_Collections_2008_2010.pdf> [24 December 2012].

Public Interest Advocacy Centre 1996 *Working the System: A Guide for Citizens, Consumers and Committees*, Pluto Press, Sydney.

Puplick, C. 2001 'Hepatitis C: Developing a policy response' in N. Crofts, N.G. Dore and S. Locarnini (eds), *Hepatitis C: An Australian Perspective*, IP Communications, Melbourne.

Putnam, R. 1995 'Bowling alone: America's declining social capital', *Journal of Democracy*, 6(1), pp. 65–78.

Queensland Health 2002 *Smart State: Health 2020, a Vision for the Future*, Directions Statement 2002, <www.health.qld.gov.au/Health2020/2020_directions.pdf> [30 March 2006].

—— 2007 'About us', <www.health.nsw.gov.au/aboutus/chart.asp> [31 July 2012].

—— 2011 'Public Health Units', <www.health.qld.gov.au/cho> [31 July 2012].

QUIT 2003 *QUIT Victoria Research and Evaluation Studies No. 11, 2000–2001*, <www.quit.org.au> [23 May 2005].

Ralph, A. and Kelly, P. 2009 'What's new in TB?' *Australian Family Physician*, 38(8), pp. 578–85.

Ramsey, A. 2003 'A "fairer" Medicare? Truth is Howard would rather have it put down', *Sydney Morning Herald*, 30 April.

Raviglione, M.C. and Pio, A. 2002 'Evolution of WHO policies for tuberculosis control, 1948–2001', *Lancet*, 2 March, 359(9308), pp. 775–80.

Rawls, J. 1973 *A Theory of Justice*, Oxford University Press, London.

Recreation Australia Limited 2001 'A brief history of Life. Be In It', <www.lifebeinit.com.au> [5 April 2006].

Reich, M. (ed.) 2002 *Public–Private Partnerships for Public Health*, Harvard Center for Population and Development Studies, Cambridge, MA.

Reichenbach, L. 2001 *Priority Setting in International Health: Beyond DALYs and Cost-effectiveness Analysis*, Working Paper Series 11(9), Harvard Center for Population and Development Studies, Cambridge, MA.

Reid, J. and Trompf, P. (eds) 1990 *The Health of Immigrant Australia: A Social Perspective*, Harcourt Brace Jovanovich, Sydney.

Reid, J.C., Goldstein, G.B. and Keo, L. 1986 'Refugee medical screening in NSW: Refugee welfare versus public risk?', *Community Health Studies*, 10(3), pp. 265–74.

—— 1991 *The Health of Aboriginal Australia*, Harcourt Brace Jovanovich, Sydney.

Reiger, K. and Keleher, H. 2002 *Surviving the Contract State: A Report on the Victorian Maternal and Child Health Service in a Decade of Change*, School of Social Sciences, La Trobe University, Melbourne.

Ren, X.S., Amick, B.C. and Williams, D.R. 1999 'Racial/ethnic disparities in health: The interplay between discrimination and socio-economic status', *Ethnicity and Disease*, 9, pp. 151–65.

Reneau, R.B. Jr, Hayedorn, C. and Degen, M.J. 1989 'Reviews and analysis: Fate and transport of biological and inorganic contaminants from on-site disposal of domestic wastewater', *Journal of Environmental Quality*, 18(1), pp. 135–44.

Restum, Z.G. 2005 'Public health implications of substandard correctional health care', *American Journal of Public Health*, 95(10), pp. 1689–91.

Reynolds, C. 1998 'Ideas and arguments about public health law', in C. Reynolds (ed.), *Public Health Law in Australia: New Perspectives*, Australian Institute of Health Law and Ethics, Commonwealth of Australia, <www.health.gov.au/pubhlth/publicat/document/law2.pdf> [22 June 2005].

—— 2003 'Law and public health: Addressing obesity', paper presented at Law in Population Health: Forum for Thought and Discussion, 22 July, Royce Hotel, presented by Centre for Public Health Law, La Trobe University.

—— 2004 *Public Health Law and Regulation*, Federation Press, Sydney.

—— 2011 *Public and Environmental Health Law*, Federation Press, Sydney.

Richardson, J., Segal, L., Carter, R., Catford, J., Gallbally, R. and Johnson, S. 1995 *Prioritising and Financing Health Promotion in Australia*, Centre for Health Program Evaluation, Melbourne.

Ridoutt, L., Gadiel, D., Cook, K. and Wise, M. 2002 *Planning Framework for the Public Health Workforce*, a discussion paper, June, NPHP, Melbourne.

—— 2004 *Calculating Demand for an Effective Public Health Workforce*, final report for the NPHP, Human Capital Alliance, Melbourne.

Robotin, M. 2002 'Evaluation of the Australian CJD Surveillance System', *Communicable Diseases Intelligence*, 26, pp. 265–72.

Roche, P., Merianos, A. and the National Tuberculosis Advisory Committee 2001 'Tuberculosis notifications in Australia, 1999', *Communicable Diseases Intelligence*, 25(4), pp. 254–60.

Roemer, M.I. 1991 *National Health Systems of the World, Vol. 1: The Countries*, Oxford University Press, Oxford.

Roemer, R., Taylor, J.D.A. and Lariviere, J. 2005 'Origins of the WHO Framework Convention on Tobacco Control', *American Journal of Public Health*, 95(6), pp. 936–8.

Rogers, E.M. 1983 *Diffusion of Innovations*, 3rd edn, Free Press, New York.

Rogers, R.J., Douglas, I.C., Baldock, F.C., Glanville, R.J., Seppanen, K.T., Gleeson, L.J., et al. 1996 'Investigation of a second focus of equine morbillivirus infection in coastal Queensland', *Australian Veterinary Journal*, 74, pp. 243–4.

Rootman, I., Goodstadt, M., Hyndman, B., McQueen, D.V., Potvin, L., Springett, J. and Ziglio, E. (eds) 2001 *Evaluation in Health Promotion: Principles and Perspectives*, European Series, no. 92, WHO Regional Publications, Copenhagen.

Rose, G. 1992 *The Strategy for Preventive Medicine*, Oxford University Press, Oxford.

Rosen, G. 1958 *A History of Public Health*, MD Publications, New York.

Ross, H.S. and Mico, P.R. 1980 *Theory and Practice in Health Education*, Mayfield, Palo Alto, CA.

Rotem, A. 1995 *The Public Health Workforce Education and Training Study*, a research report commissioned by the Department of Human Services and Health, AGPS, Canberra.

Rotem, A., Dewdney, J., Jochelson, T., Mallock, N. and Chan, K. 2004 'Public health job vacancies: who wants what, where?', draft report for the National Public Health Partnership Steering Group, Melbourne.

Rothman, J. and Tropman, J.E. 1987 'Models of community organization and macro practice: Their mixing and phasing', in F.M. Cox, J.L. Ehrlich, J. Rothman and J.E. Tropman (eds), *Strategies of Community Organization*, 4th edn, Peacock, Itasca, IL.

Rousseau, C., Rufagari, M.C., Bagilishya, D. and Measham, T. 2004 'Remaking family life: Strategies for re-establishing continuity among Congolese refugees during the family reunification process', *Social Science & Medicine*, 59, pp. 1095–1108.

Routley, V., Staines, C., Brennan, C., Haworth, N. and Ozanne-Smith, J. 2003 *Suicide and Natural Deaths in Road Traffic: Review*, Report no. 216, Monash University Accident Research Centre, Melbourne, <www.monash.edu.au/miri/research/reports/muarc216.pdf> [20 September 2012].

Rowling, L. 2005 'Dissonance and debates encircling health promoting schools', *Health Promotion Journal of Australia*, 16(1), pp. 55–7.

Royal Australian College of General Practitioners 2004 *SNAP: A Population Health Guide to Behavioural Risk Factors in General Practice*, Royal Australian College of General Practitioners, Sydney.

Royal Australian and New Zealand College of Obstetricians and Gynaecologists 2009 *College Statement (C-Obs 3) Pre-pregnancy Counselling and Routine Antenatal Assessment in the Absence of Pregnancy Complications*, Royal Australian and New Zealand College of Obstetricians and Gynaecologists, Sydney.

Ruggie, J.G. 2003 'The United Nations and globalization: Patterns and limits of institutional adaptation', *Global Governance*, 9, pp. 301–21.

Russell, M. 2004 'The condition of the working class in England', *Journal of Health Services Research Policy*, 9(3), pp. 184–5.

Russell, S. 2004 *Public Health/Health Promotion Research Workforce: Development, Progression and Retention*, final report, VPHREC, Melbourne.

Rychetnik, L. and Frommer, M.A. 2002 *A Schema for Evaluating Evidence on Public Health Interventions, Version 4*, National Public Health Partnership, Melbourne.

Sabatier, P.A. 1988 'An advocacy coalition framework of policy change and the role of policy-oriented learning therein', *Policy Sciences*, 21, pp. 129–68.

Sackett, D.L., Rosenberg, W.M.C., Gray, J.A.M., Haynes, R.B. and Richardson, W.S. 1996 'Evidence-based medicine: What it is and what it is not', *British Medical Journal*, 312, pp. 71–2.

Safe Work Australia 2011 *Australian Work Health and Safety Strategy 2012–2022*, draft, Safe Work Australia, Canberra.

Sainsbury, P. 1999 'Divisions of population health: Quantum leap forward or rearranging the deckchairs?', *Australian and New Zealand Journal of Public Health*, 23(2), pp. 119–25.

Samaan, G., Roche, P., Spencer, J. and the National Tuberculosis Advisory Committee 2003 'Tuberculosis notifications in Australia, 2002', *Communicable Diseases Intelligence*, 27(4), pp. 449–58.

Sarawak 2002 'Kuching Health City Project', <www.healthycity.sarawak.gov.my> [10 April 2006].

Sax, S. 1984 *A Strife of Interests: Politics and Policies in Australian Health Services*, Allen & Unwin, Sydney.

Sax Institute 2012 'Research Partnerships', <www.saxinstitute.org.au> [20 December 2012].

Scambler, G. and Higgs, P. 2001 '"The dog that didn't bark": Taking class seriously in the health inequalities debate', *Social Science and Medicine*, 52, pp. 157–9.

Scammell, M. 2004 *Environmental Problems Georges Bay, Tasmania*, a report prepared for the Tasmanian Fishing Industry Council, <www.tfic.com.au/scammell_report_07.04> [4 April 2005].

Schoen, C. and Osborn, R. 2011 *International Health Policy Survey of Sicker Adults in Eleven Countries*, Commonwealth Fund, <www.commonwealthfund.org/Surveys/2011/Nov/2011-International-Survey.aspx> [20 December 2012].

Schoen, C., Osborn, R., Huynh, P.T., Doty, M., Davis, K., Zapert, K. and Peugh, J. 2004 'Primary care and health system: Adults' experiences in five countries', *Health Affairs*, 28 October, pp. W4-487–503, <http://content.healthaffairs.org/cgi/reprint/hlthaff.w4.487v1> [31 January 2005].

Scollo, M.M. and Winstanley, M.H. 2012 *Tobacco in Australia: Facts and Issues*, 4th edn, Cancer Council Victoria, Melbourne <www.TobaccoInAustralia.org.au> [6 October 2013].

Schoen, C., Osborn, R., Squires, D., Doty, M.M., Pierson, R. and Applebaum, S. 2011 'New 2011 survey of patients with complex care needs in eleven countries finds that care is often poorly coordinated', *Health Affairs*, 30(12), pp. 2437–48.

Scotton, R.B. 2000 'Medibank: From conception to delivery and beyond', *Medical Journal of Australia*, 173, pp. 9–11.

Scotton, R.B. and Macdonald, C.R. 1993 *The Making of Medibank*, School of Health Services Management, University of New South Wales, Sydney.

Scott-Samuel, A. 1998 'Health impact assessment: theory into practice', *Journal of Epidemiology and Community Health*, 52(11), pp. 704–5.

Segal, L. and Chen, Y. 2001 *Priority Setting for Health: A Critique of Alternative Models*, report to the Population Health Division, Department of Health and Aged Care, Research Report 22, Centre for Health Program Evaluation, Melbourne.

Segal, L. and Robertson, I. 2001 *Diabetes Integrated Care Trial Mid-North Coast, New South Wales: Economic Evaluation*, Research Report 21, Centre for Health Program Evaluation, Melbourne.

Sen, A. 1997 'Editorial: Human capital and human capability', *World Development* 25(12), pp. 1959–61.

—— 2001 'Health equity: Perspectives, measurability and criteria' in T. Evans, M. Whitehead, A. Bhuiya and M. Wirth (eds), *Challenging Inequities in Health: From Ethics to Action*, Oxford University Press, Oxford.

Senanayake, S.N. and Ferson, M. 2004 'Detention for tuberculosis: Public health and the law', *Medical Journal of Australia*, 180(11), pp. 573–6.

Senate Community Affairs References Committee 1999 *Rocking the Cradle: A Report into Childbirth Procedures*, Commonwealth of Australia, Canberra.

Sepulveda, S., Bustreo, F., Tapia, R., Rivera, J. et al. 2006 'Health system reform in Mexico 6: Improvement of child survival in Mexico—the diagonal approach', *The Lancet*, 368(9551), pp. 2017–27, <http://0-search. proquest.com.alpha2.latrobe.edu.au/docview/199071042> [30 October 2012].

Short, K. 1994 *Quick Poison Slow Poison: Pesticide Risk in the Lucky Country*, Kate Short, St Albans, NSW.

Short, S. 1997 'Elective affinities: Research and health policy development' in H. Gardner (ed.), *Health Policy in Australia*, Oxford University Press, Melbourne.

Siegrist, J.M.M. 2004 'Health inequalities and the psychosocial environment: Two scientific challenges', *Social Science Medicine*, 58(8), pp. 1463–73.

Simon, H. 1955 'A behavioural model of rational choice', *Quarterly Journal of Economics*, 69, pp. 99–118.

Skinner, S. 2001 'Toxic timebombs', *Background Briefing*, ABC Radio National, 9 December, <www.abc.net.au/rn/ talks/bbing/stories/s436839> [22 March 2005].

Slaughter, R.A. (ed.) 1996 *The Knowledge Base of Futures Studies, Volume 1: Foundations*, DDM Media Group, Victoria, Australia, 1996.

Small, R., Rice, P., Yelland, J. and Lumley, J. 1999 'Mothers in a new country: The role of culture and communication in Vietnamese, Turkish and Filipino women's experiences of giving birth in Australia', *Women and Health*, 28, pp. 77–101.

Smith, J.C. 1991 'A change in the role of the environmental health officer: An unexpected outcome of the Municipal Public Health Plan?', unpublished Master of Health Sciences thesis, La Trobe University, Melbourne.

—— 2001 'The intergovernmental context in reforming public health policy: The introduction of a new food safety policy in Victoria', *Environmental Health*, 1(1) pp. 115–22.

—— 2002 'The journey toward a national food safety policy' in H. Gardner and S. Barraclough (eds), *Health Policy in Australia*, 2nd edn, Oxford University Press, Melbourne.

Social Exclusion Unit 2004 *Tackling Social Exclusion: Taking Stock and Looking to the Future*, Office of the Deputy Prime Minister, UK Government, London.

South Australian Department of Health 2012 *Fact sheet: South Australian Public Health Act 2011*, <www.sahealth. sa.gov.au/wps/wcm/connect/e3faa98044762ca5970c9fad53c49818/PublicHealthAct2011FactSheet-PHCC-110608. pdf?MOD=AJPERES&CACHEID=e3faa98044762ca5970c9fad53c49818&CACHE=NONE> [20 December 2012].

Spencer, J., Azoulas, J., Broom, A., Buick, T., Daniels, P. et al. 2001 'Murray Valley encephalitis virus surveillance and control initiatives in Australia: A report on behalf of the National Arbovirus Advisory Committee of the Communicable Diseases Network Australia', *Communicable Diseases Intelligence*, 25(2), pp. 33–47.

Standing Committee on Aboriginal Affairs 1984 *The Effects of Asbestos Mining on the Baryulgil Community*, report to the House of Representatives, Commonwealth of Australia, Canberra.

Starfield, B. 1996 'Public health and primary care: A framework for proposed linkages', *American Journal of Public Health*, 86(10), pp. 365–9.

—— 1998 *Primary Care: Balancing Health Needs, Services, and Technology*, Oxford University Press, New York.

State of the Environment 2011 *Committee: Australia state of the environment 2011: in brief. Independent report to the Australian Government Minister for Sustainability, Environment, Water, Population and Communities*, Canberra: State Planning Unit.

State of the Environment Advisory Council 1996 *Australia: State of the Environment 1996*, independent report presented to the Commonwealth Minister for the Environment, CSIRO Publishing, Melbourne.

Stead, M., MacAskill, S., MacKintosh, A., Reece, J. and Eadie, D. 2001 '"It's as if you're locked in": Qualitative explanations for area effects on smoking in disadvantaged communities', *Health and Place*, 4, pp. 333–43.

Steering Committee of the Victorian Consortium for Public Health 2004 'Student survey: A report for VCPH', October, Melbourne.

Stewart, K. and Penny, R. 2003 'Containing HIV in NSW: A world class success', *Public Health Bulletin*, 14(3), pp. 57–9.

Susser, M. 1973 *Causal Thinking in the Health Sciences: Concepts and Strategies of Epidemiology*, Oxford University Press, New York.

Sweet, M. 2002 'Australian media raises alarm over meningitis', *British Medical Journal*, 325(604), <http://bmj.bmjjournals.com/cgi/content/full/325/7364/604> [18 October 2004].

Swerissen, H., Butler, A. and Macmillan, J. 2003 *Feasibility Study for Developing a Nationwide Chronic Disease and Associated Risk Factors Information and Monitoring System*, Australian Institute for Primary Care, La Trobe University, Melbourne.

Swerissen, H., Duckett, S.J., Daly, J., Bergen, K., Marshall, S., Borthwick, C. and Crisp, B.R. 2001 'Health promotion and evaluation: A programmatic approach', *Health Promotion Journal of Australia*, 11(1), special supplement, April, pp. 1–28.

Syme, L. 1986 'Strategies for prevention', *Preventive Medicine*, 15, pp. 492–507.

Syme, S.L. and Berkman, L. 1976 'Social class, susceptibility, and sickness', *American Journal of Epidemiology*, 104, pp. 1–8.

Szreter, S. 1997 'Economic growth, disruption, deprivation, disease and death: On the importance of the politics of public health for development', *Population and Development Review*, 23(4), pp. 702–28.

Tan, N., Wakefield, M. and Freeman, J. 2000 'Changes associated with the National Tobacco Campaign: Results of the second follow-up survey', in K. Hassard (ed.), *Australia's National Tobacco Campaign Evaluation Report*, vol. 2, Commonwealth Department of Health and Aged Care, Canberra.

Tannahill, A. 2002 'Epidemiology and health promotion: A common understanding', in R. Bunton and G. Macdonald (eds), *Health Promotion: Disciplines, Diversity and Developments*, 2nd edn, Routledge, London.

Taskforce on Community Preventive Services 2011 *The Guide to Community Preventive Services: What Works to Promote Health*, eds S. Zaza, P. Briss and K. Harris, Oxford University Press, New York, <www.thecommunityguide.org> [10 October 2012].

Taskforce on Migrant-Friendly and Culturally Competent Health Care 2005 'Migrant-friendly hospitals', WHO Network on Health Promoting Hospitals, <www.mfheu.net> [18 July 2005].

Taylor, R. 2003 'Halving deaths from cervical cancer', *Public Health Bulletin*, 14(3), pp. 55–6.

Taylor, R., Page, A., Morrella, S., Harrison, J. and Carter, G. 2005 'Mental health and socioeconomic variations in Australian suicide', *Social Science and Medicine*, 61(7), pp. 1551–9.

Tehan, M. 2002 lecture given to postgraduate students at La Trobe University, October.

Tesh, S. 1988 *Hidden Arguments: Political Ideology and Disease Prevention Policy*, Rutgers University Press, New Brunswick.

Teutsch, S.M. and Churchill, E. (eds) 2000 *Principles and Practice of Public Health Surveillance*, Oxford University Press, New York.

Thompson, S.J. and Gifford, S.M. 2000 'Trying to keep a balance: The meaning of health and diabetes in an urban Aboriginal community', *Social Science Medicine*, 51(10), pp. 1457–72.

Tollman, S. 1991 'Community oriented primary care: Origins, evolution, applications', *Social Science and Medicine*, 32, pp. 633–42.

Trewin, D. and Madden, R. 2005 *The Health and Welfare of Australia's Aboriginal and Torres Strait Islander Peoples*, ABS and AIHW, Canberra.

Tröhler, U. 2005 'Lind and scurvy: 1747 to 1795', *Journal of the Royal Society of Medicine*, 98(11), pp. 519–22.

Trostle, J. 1986 'Early work in anthropology and epidemiology: From social medicine to the germ theory, 1840 to 1920', in C.R. Janes, R. Stall and S.M. Gifford (eds), *Anthropology and Epidemiology: Interdisciplinary Approaches to the Study of Health Disease*, D. Reidel, Amsterdam.

Tsouros, A. 1994 *The WHO Healthy Cities Project: State of the art and future plans*, WHO/EURO/HCPO, Copenhagen.

Tulchinsky, T.H. and Varavikova, E. 2000 *The New Public Health: An Introduction for the 21st Century*, Academic Press, San Diego.

Turnock, B.J. 2012 *Public Health: What It Is and How It Works*, 5th edition, Jones & Bartlett Learning, Burlington, MA.

Turrell, G., Stanley, L., de Looper, M. and Oldenburg, B. 2006 *Health Inequalities in Australia: Morbidity, Health Behaviours, Risk Factors and Health Service Use*, Health Inequalities Monitoring Series No. 2, AIHW and Queensland University of Technology, Canberra.

Turshen, M. 1989 *The Politics of Public Health*, Rutgers University Press, New Brunswick, NJ.

Tyler, T.R. 2001 'Why do people rely on others: Social identity and the social aspects of trust', in K.S. Cook (ed.), *Trust in Society*, Russell Sage Foundation, New York.

UK Foresight 2007 *Obesity*, <http://webarchive.nationalarchives.gov.uk/+/www.dh.gov.uk/en/Publichealth/Healthimprovement/Obesity/DH_07971>.

UNAIDS 1998 *The Public Health Approach to STD Control*, UNAIDS Technical Update, UNAIDS Best Practice Collection, Geneva.

UNESCO 2005 *Universal Declaration on Bioethics and Human Rights*, <http://portal.unesco.org/hs/en/file_download.php/46133elf4691e4c6e57566763d474a4dBioethicsDeclaration_EN.pdf> [6 April 2006].

United Kingdom National Screening Committee 2005, <www.nsc.nhs.uk/index.htm> [22 April 2005].

United Kingdom Public Record Office n.d. Snapshot, 'The 1833 Factory Act', <www.learningcurve.pro.gov.uk/snapshots/snapshot13/snapshot13.htm> [19 August 2004].

United Nations 2003 *Indicators for Monitoring the Millennium Development Goals: Definitions, Rationale, Concepts and Sources*, United Nations, New York.

—— 2006 *Report of the Meeting on Indigenous Peoples and Indicators of Wellbeing*, Permanent Forum on Indigenous Issues, Fifth session, <www.un.org/esa/socdev/unpfii/documents/5session_crp3_indicators.doc> [20 November 2012].

United Nations Development Program 2011, *Human Development Index and its components, Table 1* <http://hdr.undp.org/en/media/HDR_2011_EN_Table1.pdf> [25 November 2012].

United Nations High Commission for Refugees (UNHCR) 2002 *Resettlement Handbook*, Department of International Protection, UNHCR, Geneva.

—— 2005 'The basic facts', <www.unhcr.org/cgibin/texis/vtx/basics/opendoc.htm?tbl=BASICS&id=3b028097c#Resettlement> [10 April 2006].

United Nations Permanent Forum on Indigenous Issues 2006 *Report of the Meeting on Indigenous Peoples and Indicators of Well-being*, Fifth session, <www.un.org/esa/socdev/unpfii/documents/5session_crp3_indicators.doc> [18 December 2012].

United Nations Secretary-General's High-level Panel on Global Sustainability 2012, *Resilient People, Resilient Planet: A Future Worth Choosing*, New York.

United States Department of Health and Human Services 2000 *Healthy People 2010: Understanding and Improving Health*, US Public Health Service, Washington, DC.

—— 2001 *The Public Health Workforce: An Agenda for the 21st Century*, a report of the Public Health Functions project, <www.health.gov/phfunctions/pubhlth.pdf> [2 November 2005].

—— 2002 *Physical Activity Evaluation Handbook*, CDC, Atlanta, GA.

United States Department of Labor Occupational Safety and Health Administration 2012 'Medical surveillance', <www.osha.gov/SLTC/medicalsurveillance/index.html> [30 July 2012].

United States Environmental Protection Agency 2004 'Love Canal' Public Information Office, <www.epa.gov/superfund/sites/npl/nar180.htm> [27 February 2006].

United States Government 2012 *Track the Money*, <www.recovery.gov/Transparency/RecoveryData/Pages/RecipientReportedDataMap.aspx> [20 December 2012].

United States National Institute of Occupational Safety and Health 2004 'NIOSH topic area: Surveillance', <www.cdc.gov/niosh/topics/surveillance> [22 July 2004].

University of Melbourne Key Centre for Women's Health in Society and Royal Women's Hospital 2001 *Responding to Cultural Diversity in Women's Health: A Resource for Health Professionals*, Key Centre for Women's Health in Society, University of Melbourne, Melbourne.

US News and World Report 2012 'Best graduate schools, top health schools, public health rankings', <http://grad-schools.usnews.rankingsandreviews.com/bestgraduate-schools/top-health-schools/public-health-rankings> [18 September 2012].

Vertio, H. and Catford, J. 1995 *Resourcing Health Promotion: Suggestions on Ways to Win More Resources For Health Promotion*, European Health Promotion Series, WHO/Europe, Helsinki.

VFSF: *see* Victorian Foundation for Survivors of Torture.

VicHealth 2006 *Measuring Wellbeing: Engaging Communities*, <www.communityindicators.net.au/files/civ/20060817_VCIP_Final_Report.pdf [7 August 2012].

—— 2011 'The partnerships analysis tool', <www.vichealth.vic.gov.au/partnerships> [9 October 2012].

Victorian Department of Education and Early Childhood Development 2012, Website, <www.education.vic.gov.au> [31 July].

Victorian Department of Health 2010, *Public Health and Wellbeing Act 2008*, <http://health.vic.gov.au/phwa> [21 August 2012].

—— 2011 *Surveillance of Notifiable Infectious Diseases in Victoria, 2009*, Department of Health, Melbourne.

—— 2012a Website, <www.health.vic.gov.au. [31 July].

—— 2012b *Immunisation Newsletter*, 56, April.

—— 2012c *Immunisation History*, <www.health.vic.gov.au/immunisation/resources/history.htm> [3 June 2012].

Victorian Department of Human Services (DHS) 1999 *Guidelines for the Investigation of Gastrointestinal Illness*, DHS, Melbourne.

—— 2001 'Tuberculosis strategy—community information', <www.health.vic.gov.au/ideas/downloads/tb_community.pdf> [10 January 2006].

—— 2002a *Immunisation Program Newsletter*, 1, August, <www.health.vic.gov.au/immunisation/downloads/newsletters/immnews_aug02.pdf> [4 April 2006].

—— 2002b *Management, Control and Prevention of Tuberculosis: Guidelines for Health Care Providers (2002–2005)*, DHS, Melbourne.

—— 2003 *Integrated Health Promotion Resource Kit*, DHS, Melbourne.

—— 2004a *Planning for Healthy Communities: Reducing the Risk of Cardiovascular Disease and Type 2 Diabetes through Healthier Environments and Lifestyles*, DHS, Melbourne.

—— 2004b *Sentinel Event Program: Annual Report 2003–04*, Metropolitan Health and Aged Care Services Division, DHS, Melbourne.

—— 2005a *The Blue Book: Guidelines for the Control of Infectious Diseases 2005*, Communicable Diseases Section, DHS, Melbourne.

—— 2005b 'Health Act: MPHP', <www.health.vic.gov.au/localgov/mphp.htm> [21 March 2006].

—— 2006 *Cultural Diversity Plan for Victoria's Specialist Mental Health Services 2006–2010*, Melbourne, <www.health.vic.gov.au/mentalhealth/publications/cald-strategy.pdf> [23 December 2012].

—— 2009 *Municipal Public Health Plans: New Requirements*, <www.health.vic.gov.au/phwa/downloads/municipal_health_plan.pdf> [1 November 2012].

—— 2012, <www.dhs.vic.gov.au/home> [31 July 2012].

Victorian Environment Protection Authority and Australian Institute of Environmental Health 2001 *Survey of Local Government Management of Domestic On-site Wastewater Systems*, EPA, Melbourne.

Victorian Foundation for Survivors of Torture (VFST) 1998 *Refugee Health and General Practice*, Victorian Foundation for Survivors of Torture, Melbourne.

—— 2004a *Improving Health and Community Services for People from Refugee Backgrounds Settling in Victoria*, Victorian Foundation for Survivors of Torture, Melbourne.

—— 2004b *Towards a Health Strategy for Refugees and Asylum Seekers in Victoria*, Victorian Department of Human Services, Melbourne.

Victorian Health Promotion Foundation 2003 *Promoting the Mental Health and Wellbeing of New Arrival Communities: Learning and Promising Practices*, Victorian Health Promotion Foundation, Melbourne.

—— 2005 *A Plan for Action 2005–2007: Promoting Mental Health and Wellbeing*, Victorian Health Promotion Foundation, Melbourne.

Victorian Settlement Planning Committee 2005 *The Good Practice Principles Guide for Working with Refugee Young People*, Victorian Settlement Planning Committee, Melbourne.

Vidal, J. 1997 *McLibel*, Macmillan, London.

Visotina, M. and Hills, M. 2000 *NSW Health Services for the Sydney Olympic and Paralympic Games*, NSW Health Department, Sydney.

Vitruvius 1960 *The Ten Books on Architecture*, translated by M.H. Morgan, Dover, New York.

Vos, T. and Begg, S. 1999a *The Victorian Burden of Disease Study: Morbidity*, Victorian Department of Human Services, Melbourne.

—— 1999b *The Victorian Burden of Disease Study: Mortality*, Victorian Department of Human Services, Melbourne.

Waas, A. 2003 *Promoting Health: The Primary Health Care Approach*, 2nd edn, Elsevier, Sydney.

Wadsworth, Y. 1997 *Do It Yourself Research*, Allen & Unwin, Sydney.

Walker, A.E. and Colagiuri, S. 2011 'Cost-benefit model system of chronic diseases in Australia to assess and rank prevention and treatment options', *International Journal of Microsimulation*, 4(3), pp. 57–70.

Walker, R. 2000 *Collaboration and Alliances: A Review*, VicHealth, Melbourne.

Walker R., Lewis, B. and Mitchell, S. 1996 'Community health service agreements, 1992 to 1995: Changes in practice and purpose', *Australian Journal of Primary Health: Interchange*, 2, pp. 42–53.

Wallace, R. (ed.) 1998 *Maxcy–Rosenau–Last: Public Health and Preventive Medicine*, 14th edn, Appleton and Lange, Stanford, CT.

Wallerstein, N. 2006 'What is the evidence on effectiveness of empowerment to improve health?', *Health Evidence Network Report*, WHO Regional Office for Europe, Copenhagen, <www.euro.who.int/Document/E88086.pdf> [4 April 2006].

Wanless, D. 2002 *Securing Our Future Health: Taking a Long-term View*, final report, HM Treasury, London.

—— 2004 *Securing Good Health for the Whole Population*, final report, UK Department of Treasury, London.

Ward, K.F., Menzies, R.I., Quinn, H.E. and Campbell-Lloyd, S. 2010 'School based vaccination in NSW', *NSW Health Public Health Bulletin*, 21(9–10), pp. 237–42.

Watchirs, H. 1993 'Public health, criminal law and HIV/AIDS', conference paper presented at Law, Medicine and Criminal Justice, Surfers Paradise, 6–8 July.

—— 2002 *Reforming the Law to Ensure Appropriate Responses to the Risk of Disease Transmission*, Occasional Papers No. 2, May, Australian National Council on AIDS and Hepatitis C and Related Diseases, Canberra.

Watson, K.J.R. 2000 'Preventing hepatitis C virus transmission in Australians who inject drugs', *Medical Journal of Australia*, 172, pp. 55–6.

Watters, C. 2001 'Emerging paradigms in the mental health care of refugees', *Social Science & Medicine*, 52, pp. 1709–18.

Weatherall, D. 1994 'The relative roles of nature and nurture in common disease in health and environment', in Bryan Cartledge (ed.), *The Linacre Lectures 1992–93*, Oxford University Press, New York.

Wellcome Trust 2004 *Public Health Sciences: Challenges and Opportunities*, report of the Public Health Sciences Working Group Convened by the Wellcome Trust, March, London.

Western Australian Department of Health 2008 *Health Impacts of Climate Change: Adaptation Strategies for Western Australia*, Western Australian Government, Perth.

—— 2010 *Department of Health Policy Recommendations 2010–2015: Model of Best Practice for Prenatal Screening Choices*, Office of Population Health Genomics, Department of Health, Perth.

White, K. 1994 'Nineteenth century medicine, science and values', in C. Waddell and A.R. Petersen (eds), *Just Health, Inequality in Illness, Care and Prevention*, Churchill Livingstone, Melbourne.

White, K.L. 1986 *Australia's Bicentennial Health Initiative: Independent Review of Research and Educational Requirements for Public Health and Tropical Health*, report to the Hon. Neal Blewett, Minister for Health, Canberra.

Whitehead, J.H. and Geary, P.M. 2000 'Geotechnical aspects of domestic on-site effluent management systems', *Australian Journal of Earth Sciences*, 47, pp. 75–82.

Whitehead, M. and Dahlgren, G. 1997 *City Planning for Health and Sustainable Development*, European Sustainable Development and Health Series, 2, World Health Organization, WHO Regional Office Europe, Copenhagen.

WHO: *see* World Health Organization.

Wilkinson, W. and Sidel, V.W. 1991 'Social applications and interventions in public health', in W.W. Holland, R. Detels et al. (eds), *Oxford Textbook of Public Health*, Oxford University Press, Oxford.

Willis, E. 1983 *Medical Dominance*, Allen & Unwin, Sydney.

—— 1989 *Medical Dominance*, rev. edn, Allen & Unwin, Sydney.

Willis, K. 2003 'Challenging the evidence: Women's health policy in Australia' in V. Lin and B. Gibson (eds), *Evidence-based Health Policy: Problems and Possibilities*, Oxford University Press, Melbourne.

Willis, P. 2004 'Bed bugs', *Catalyst*, ABC TV, 19 August, <www.abc.net.au/catalyst/stories/s1180604.htm> [14 March 2005].

Wills, P. 1998 *The Virtuous Cycle: Working Together for Health and Medical Research*, Health and Medical Research Strategic Review discussion document, December, Commonwealth of Australia, Canberra.

Winslow, C.E.A. 1923 *The Evolution and Significance of the Modern Public Health Campaign*, Yale University Press, South Burlington, VT.

Winstanley, M., Woodward, S. and Walker, N. 1995 *Tobacco in Australia: Facts and Issues*, Victorian Smoking and Health Program, Melbourne.

Woltring, C., Constantine, W. and Schwarte, L. 2003 'Does leadership training make a difference? The CDC/UC Public Health Leadership Institute: 1991–1999', *Journal of Public Health Management and Practice*, 9(2), pp. 103–22.

Women's Health Australia 2012 *Australian Longitudinal Study on Women's Health*, <http://www.alswh.org.au> [1 November 2012].

Women's Health Queensland Wide 2003 'Women's health policy and program development in Australia', Health Information: Student Factsheets, <www.womhealth.org.au/studentfactsheets/womenhealthpolicy.htm> [3 November 2004].

Wooldridge, M. 1991 *Health Policy in the Fraser Years 1975–83*, Department of Administrative Studies, Monash University, Clayton.

—— 2001 'Launch of the Cervical Screening Incentives Program for GPs', speech by the Minister for Health and Aged Care, Canberra, 26 September, <www.health.gov.au/internet/wcms/publishing.nsf/Content/health-mediarel-yr2001-mw-mwsp010926.htm> [16 June 2005].

World Health Organization (WHO) 1968 *Report of the Technical Discussions at the Twenty-first World Health Assembly on 'National and Global Surveillance of Communicable Diseases'*, WHO, Geneva.

—— 1978 *Declaration of Alma Ata*, International Conference on Primary Health Care, Alma-Ata, Soviet Union, 6–12 September, <www.who.int/publications/almaata_declaration_en.pdf> [24 November 2012].

—— 1980 *European Regional Strategy for Health for All by the Year 2000*, WHO Regional Office for Europe, Copenhagen.

—— 1981 *Global Strategy for Health for All by the Year 2000*, WHO, Geneva.

—— 1986 *Ottawa Charter for Health Promotion: First International Conference on Health Promotion, Ottawa, Canada*, World Health Organization Regional Office for Europe, Copenhagen, <www.who.int/hpr/NPH/docs/ottawa_charter_hp.pdf> [16 March 2006].

—— 1995 *Global Strategy on Occupational Health for All: The Way to Health at Work*, WHO, Geneva, <www.who.int/occupational_health/en/oehstrategy.pdf> [3 July 2006].

—— 1996 'Creating healthy cities in the twenty-first century', paper presented to the UN Conference on Human Settlements, Istanbul, Turkey.

—— 1997 *Jakarta Declaration on Leading Health Promotion into the 21st Century*, Fourth International Conference on Health Promotion, Jakarta, Indonesia, July, WHO, Geneva, at <www.who.int/healthpromotion/conferences/previous/jakarta/declaration/en/print.html> [20 July 2006].

—— 1998 *Health Promotion Glossary*, <www.who.int/hpr/NPH/docs/hp_glossary_en.pdf> [8 September 2004].

—— 2000 *World Health Report 2000 Health Systems: Improving Performance*, WHO, Geneva.

—— 2001a *Global Prevalence and Incidence of Selected Curable Sexually Transmitted Infections: Overview and Estimates*, WHO, Geneva.

—— 2001b *Guidelines for the Management of Sexually Transmitted Infections*, WHO, Geneva.

—— 2001c *Macroeconomics and Health: Investing in Health for Economic Development*, report of the Commission on Macroeconomics and Health, WHO, Geneva.

—— 2002 *The World Health Report 2002: Reducing Risks, Promoting Healthy Life*, WHO, Geneva.

—— 2003a *Health Promotion Financing Opportunities in the Western Pacific Region*, WHO/WPRO, Manila.

—— 2003b *Surveillance of Noncommunicable Disease Risk Factors Fact Sheet 273*, WHO, Geneva.

—— 2005a DOTS, <www.who.int/tb/dots/whatisdots/en/print.html> [20 May 2005].

—— 2005b *Global Conferences on Health Promotion*, <www.who.int/healthpromotion/conferences/en> [5 April 2005].

—— 2005c 'International health regulations', <www.who.int/csr/ihr/current/en/index.html> [2 July 2005].

—— 2005d *Tuberculosis Fact Sheet*, <www.who.int/mediacentre/factsheets/fs104> [17 October 2005].

—— 2007a *Everybody's Business: Strengthening health systems to improve health outcomes—WHO's framework for action*, WHO, Geneva.

—— 2007b *Global Strategy for the Prevention and Control of Sexually Transmitted Infections*: 2006–2015, WHO, Geneva.

——— 2008a *Commission on Social Determinants of Health: Final Report. Closing the Gap in a Generation: Health Equity Through Action on the Social Determinants of Health,* <www.who.int/social_determinants/thecommission/finalreport/en/index.html> [7 August 2012].

——— 2008b *The Contribution of Ethics to Public Health,* special issue of the *Bulletin of the World Health Organisation,* 86(8).

——— 2008c *The World Health Report 2008: Primary Health Care (Now More Than Ever),* <www.who.int/whr/2008/en> [24 November 2012].

——— 2009 *Global Health Risks: Mortality and Burden of Disease Attributable to Selected Major Risks,* World Health Organization, Geneva.

——— 2011a *Sexually Transmitted Infections Fact Sheet No. 110,* August, <www.who.int/mediacentre/factsheets/fs110/en/index.html> [21 June 2012].

——— 2011b *Prevalence and Incidence of Selected Sexually Transmitted Infections: Methods and Results Used by WHO to Generate 2005 Estimates,* WHO, Geneva.

——— 2011c 'FAQs: Japan nuclear concerns', <www.who.int/hac/crises/jpn/faqs/en/index7.html> [31 October 2012].

——— 2011d *The Global Plan to Stop TB 2011–2015: Transforming the Fight Towards Elimination of Tuberculosis,* WHO, Geneva.

——— 2011e *Building Healthy and Equitable Workplaces for Women and Men: A Resource for Employers and Worker's Representatives,* Protecting Workers' Health Series No.11, p. 6.

——— 2012 'Occupational health', <www.euro.who.int/en/what-we-do/health-topics/environment-and-health/occupational-health/policy> [6 October 2012].

World Health Organization Collaborating Centres for Occupational Health 1995 *Global Strategy on Occupational Health for All: The Way to Health at Work—Recommendations of the Second Meeting of the WHO Collaborating Centres for Occupational Health,* WHO, Geneva.

World Health Organization Regional Office for the Western Pacific *Australia: Health Situation,* <www.wpo.who.int/countries/aus/health_situation.htm> [3 November 2005].

World Health Organization South East Asia Regional Office 1993 *HIV/AIDS Care at the Institutional, Community and Home Level,* report of a WHO Regional Workshop, Bangkok, 29 March–2 April, <http://w3.whosea.org/EN/Section10/Section18/Section356/Section427.htm> [3 July 2006].

WPRO: *see* World Health Organisation Western Pacific Regional Office.

Young, T.K. 1998 *Population Health: Concepts and Methods,* Oxford University Press, New York.

Ziglio, E. 1993 *European Macro Trends Affecting Health Promotion Strategies,* WHO/EURO Working Paper, World Health Organization, Regional Office for Europe, Health Promotion and Investment Programme, Copenhagen.

Zwi, A., Fustukian, S. and Sethi, D. 2002 'Globalisation, conflict and humanitarian response', in K. Lee, K. Buse and S. Fustukian (eds), *Health Policy in a Globalising World,* Cambridge University Press, Cambridge.

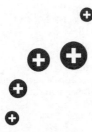

Index